Therapeutic Electrophysical Agents

Evidence Behind Practice

THIRD EDITION

Therapeutic Electrophysical Agents

Evidence Behind Practice

THIRD EDITION

Alain-Yvan Bélanger, PhD, PT

Retired Professor
Laval University
Canada

Owner and Consultant
Physiométrix Inc.

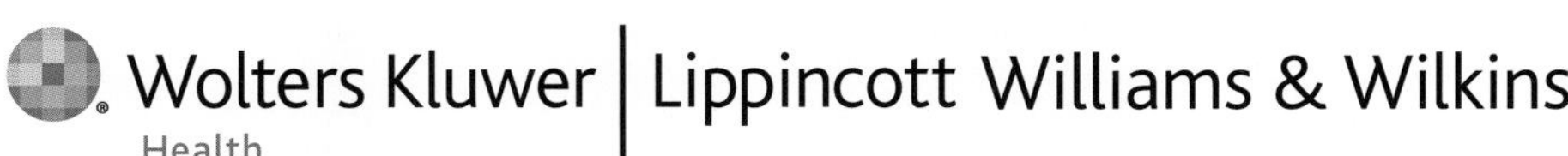
Wolters Kluwer | Lippincott Williams & Wilkins
Health

Philadelphia • Baltimore • New York • London
Buenos Aires • Hong Kong • Sydney • Tokyo

Acquisitions Editor: Emily Lupash
Product Manager: Matt Hauber
Marketing Manager: Leah Thomson
Production Project Manager: Marian Bellus
Design Coordinator: Terry Mallon
Illustration Coordinator: Jennifer Clements
Manufacturing Coordinator: Margie Orzech
Prepress Vendor: Aptara, Inc.

Third Edition

351 West Camden Street
Baltimore, MD 21201

Two Commerce Square
2001 Market Street
Philadelphia, PA 19103

Printed in China

9 8 7 6 5 4 3 2

Library of Congress Cataloging-in-Publication Data

Bélanger, Alain, author.
Therapeutic electrophysical agents : evidence behind practice / Alain-Yvan Bélanger.—Third edition.
p. ; cm.
Includes bibliographical references and index.
ISBN 978-1-4511-8274-3 (alk. paper)
I. Title.
[DNLM: 1. Therapeutics—Handbooks. 2. Therapeutics—Outlines. 3. Evidence-Based Medicine—Handbooks. 4. Evidence-Based Medicine—Outlines. 5. Physical and Rehabilitation Medicine—Handbooks. 6. Physical and Rehabilitation Medicine—Outlines. WB 39]
RM841.5
615.8′3—dc23

2013035769

To purchase additional copies of this book, call our customer service department at (800) 638-3030 or fax orders to (301) 223-2320. International customers should call (301) 223-2300.

Visit Lippincott Williams & Wilkins on the Internet: http://www.lww.com. Lippincott Williams & Wilkins customer service representatives are available from 8:30 am to 6:00 pm, EST.

DEDICATION

I dedicate this third edition to all educators, students, and clinicians in their journey to become the best evidence-based teachers, students, and practitioners of therapeutic electrophysical agents they can be.

QUOTES

Learning never exhausts the mind.

Leonardo da Vinci

Any fool can know. The point is to understand.

Albert Einstein

I never learn anything talking. I only learn things when I ask questions.

Lou Holtz

Great things are not accomplished by those who yield to trends and fads and popular opinion.

Jack Kerouac

Absence of evidence is not evidence of absence.

Carl Sagan

ABOUT THE AUTHOR

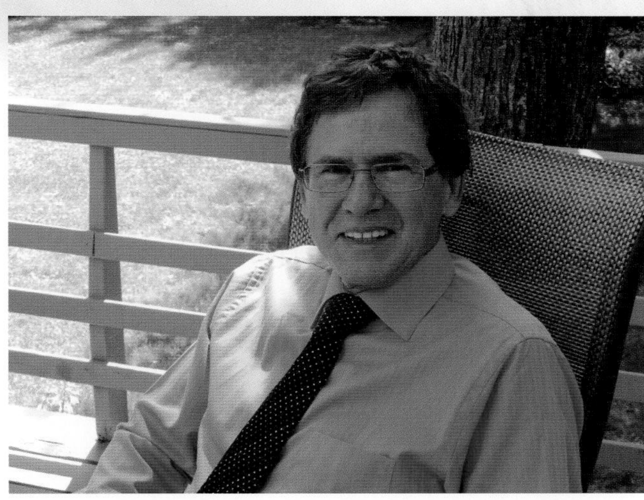

Alain-Yvan Bélanger, BSc, MSc, PhD, PT is a retired Professor from the Department of Rehabilitation, Physiotherapy program, Faculty of Medicine, Laval University, Quebec City, Canada. Dr. Bélanger holds a bachelor's degree in physiotherapy from the University of Montreal, a master's of science degree in kinesiology from Simon Fraser University, and a doctoral degree in neurosciences from McMaster University. He has extensive experience as a teacher, researcher, consultant, and author in the field of human neuromuscular physiology and therapeutic electrophysical agents. Dr. Bélanger has held the positions of Scientific Editor of the journal *Physiotherapy Canada* and President of the Canadian Physiotherapy Association. He has also served as Associate Editor of several journals. He is the sole author of the first and second editions of this book. An avid golf and poker player, Alain still dreams of playing a sub 80s round of golf and winning the next World Series of Poker Seniors Championship!

ACKNOWLEDGMENTS

I want to express my deepest gratitude to all of you who chose the previous two editions of this textbook to learn, teach, and practice therapeutic electrophysical agents.

Thank you to Julie Stegman, LWW Publisher, for her continued trust and support, and to Emily Lupash, Acquisition Editor, for her dedication to see a third edition.

Thanks to all of the reviewers for their thoughtful comments and suggestions related to the preparation of this third edition.

I want to express a very special thank you to my Product Development Editor, Matt Hauber, for his advice, direction, skillful work, and professionalism.

To everyone at LWW, thank you for giving me the opportunity to make my work a published reality.

Alain-Yvan Bélanger, BSc, MSc, PhD, PT

REVIEWERS

Misha Bradford, PT, DPT, OCS
Assistant Professor (Clinical)
University of Utah
Salt Lake City, Utah

Joseph Gallo, DSc, ATC, PT
Director, Athletic Training Program
Salem State University
Salem, Massachusetts

Leigh Ann Hewston, PT, Med
Instructor
Thomas Jefferson University
Philadelphia, Pennsylvania

Paul Higgins, DPT, MPT, ATC, CSCS
Assistant Professor of Physical Therapy
University of Hartford
West Hartford, Connecticut

Martha Hinman, PT, EdD
Professor
Hardin-Simmons University
Abilene, Texas

Teresa Hoppenrath, PT, DPT, GCS
Assistant Professor, Director of Clinical Education
Ithaca College
Ithaca, New York

Carrie Hoppes, PT, DPT, NCS, OCS, ATC
Adjunct Professor
Baylor University
Fort Sam Houston, Texas

Michael S. Krackow, PhD, ATC, PTA, CSCS
Associate Professor
Virginia Military Institute
Lexington, Virginia

Scott Livingston, PhD, PT, ATC, SCS, LAT
Assistant Professor
University of Kentucky
Lexington, Kentucky

Sara Maher, PT, DScPT, OMPT
Associate Professor
Oakland University
Rochester, Michigan

Byron Smith, PT, DPT, MPE, OCS
Instructor
University of Miami
Coral Gables, Florida

Andrew Priest, EdD
Dean of College of Health and Human Services
Touro University Nevada
Henderson, Nevada

Robert Rowell, DC, MS
Associate Professor
Palmer College of Chiropractic
Davenport, Iowa

PREFACE

There are several electrophysical agent (EPA) textbooks on the market, and I truly appreciate your continued interest in this one. I am particularly excited by this third edition because it brings us to another level in our journey to become the best evidence-based learners and practitioners of EPAs we can be. In the first edition, my goal was to introduce the concept of evidence-based practice into the field of EPAs using a pocket-style format. It is fair to say that the focus of textbooks published prior to the year 2000 was much more on how to safely and effectively apply EPAs rather than on the treatment effectiveness related to these agents. In other words, texts on this subject were much more oriented to application safety and efficacy, and less oriented to treatment effectiveness based on the evidence—that is, on results of published research-based human trials. In the second edition, the goal was to expand on the concept of evidence behind the practice of EPAs by adding more content on key related topics such as pain and soft tissue healing, as well as case studies and an illustrated glossary of terms related to EPAs. The purpose then was to create a textbook that faculty could use to teach undergraduate and graduate students. With this third edition, my goal is to offer the most comprehensive and practical textbook in the field of EPAs by providing updated and new materials, as well as unique and practical ancillary tools.

ENHANCED AND NEW CONTENT PRESENTATION

This edition now offers a full-color presentation designed to maximize text and image quality, clarity, and accuracy. The textbook has also been reorganized into five logical parts containing 21 chapters. Part I, *Foundations*, includes six chapters. A new Chapter 2, Toward a Practice Based on Evidence, explains how the adoption of evidence can optimize the clinical decision making process. In addition, a new Chapter 5, Purchase, Electrical Safety, and Maintenance, consolidates the content of two former chapters, Purchase of Therapeutic Electrophysical Agents and Electrical Shocks, Safety Measures, and Maintenance of Line-Powered Devices. Part II, *Thermal Agents*, includes three chapters: Thermotherapy, Cryotherapy, and Hydrotherapy. The chapter on thermotherapy now integrates four previous chapters, Hot Pack and Paraffin Baths, Fluidotherapy, Skin Sensory Heat and Cold Discrimination Testing, and Skin and Electrophysical Agents Temperature Measurement. Part III, *Electromagnetic Agents*, is also composed of three chapters: Shortwave Diathermy, Low-Level Laser Therapy, and Ultraviolet. Part IV, *Electrical Agents*, includes four chapters. A new Chapter 13, Neuromuscular Electrical Stimulation, now integrates two former chapters, Russian Current Therapy and Interferential Current Therapy. The former chapter on Diadynamic Current Therapy has been deleted because of lack of evidence to support its therapeutic effectiveness. A new Chapter 15, Electrical Stimulation for Tissue Healing and Repair, incorporates two former chapters, Microcurrent Therapy and High-Voltage Pulsed Current Therapy. Part V, *Mechanical Agents*, includes five chapters. A new Chapter 21, Extracorporeal Shockwave Therapy, is added to cover the latest mechanical source of energy used for the management of chronic soft tissue disorders.

Learning objectives are rewritten to reflect recent updates made to Bloom's Taxonomy. The illustrated glossary of electrophysical terminology, formerly Chapter 5, is now integrated into related chapters to enhance the learning experience, meaning that there is no longer a need for readers to go back and forth to this chapter when studying a particular agent. Each chapter now incorporates a new feature, *The Bottom Line*, which highlights key elements. New updated and revised *Application, Contraindications, and Risks* boxes, coupled with *Research-Based Indications* boxes, eliminate some of the redundancies in the previous edition while concisely providing all essential elements required to enhance treatment safety, efficacy, and effectiveness. Revised *Case Studies* are now based on the concepts of evidence-based practice; the International Classification of Functioning, Disability, and Health (ICF) model; and SOAP (*s*ubjective, *o*bjective, *a*ssessment, *p*lan) note format.

NEW AND UNIQUE ANCILLARY MATERIAL

This third edition offers new and unique tools designed to help you master the practice of EPAs. Readers can now access *Online Dosimetric Calculators*, a unique tool in the field, to simplify the often complex and confusing dosimetric aspect of EPA practice while maintaining an emphasis on scientific-based treatment. By entering dosimetric parameters, you can obtain the results and chart them into a patient's file without the need for memorizing formulas or doing hand calculations. Also available are links to *Online Videos* to help students better visualize EPA equipment and accessories, as well as application to patients. Finally, *Online Board-Style Questions* are included to help students with the all-important preparation for licensing.

Alain-Yvan Bélanger, BSc, MSc, PhD, PT

CONTENTS

PART I

Foundations

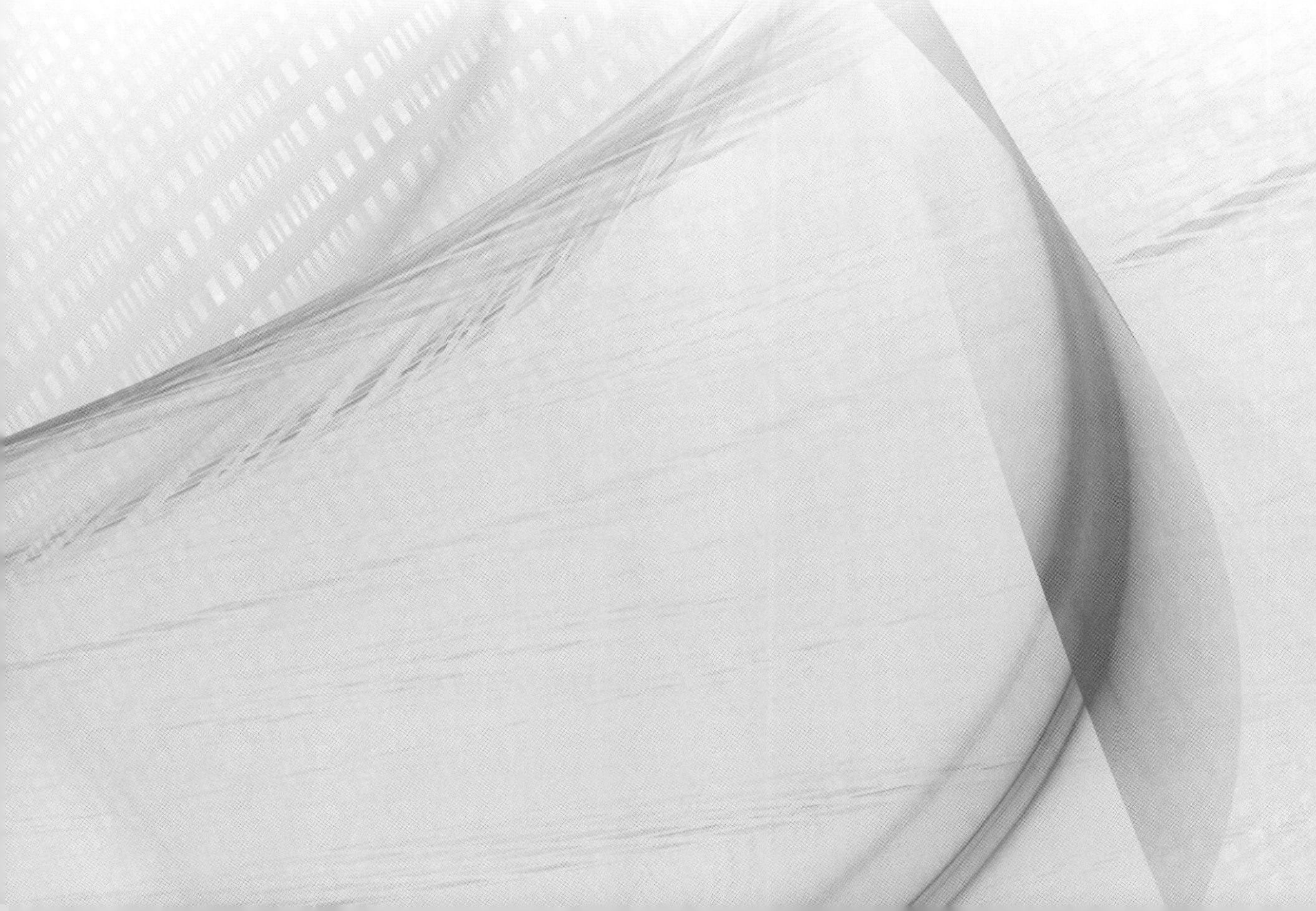

Chapter 1

Therapeutic Electrophysical Agents in Health Care

Chapter Outline

Learning Objectives

Remembering: List, by type and energy delivered, the electrophysical agents covered in this textbook.
Understanding: Define and distinguish between the six elements of the ICF model.
Applying: Illustrate and demonstrate the ICF model.
Analyzing: Differentiate between efficiency and effectiveness.
Evaluating: Appraise the value of using the ICF model in the delivery of therapeutic electrophysical agents.
Creating: Construct a model showing the place of electrophysical agents in the field of health care.

I. THE USE OF ELECTROPHYSICAL AGENTS

The use of electrophysical agents (EPAs) is widespread in the field of physical therapy, physical medicine, athletic training, chiropractic, and sports therapy (see Hayes, 2000; Kahn, 2000; Low et al., 2000; Nalty, 2001; Horodyski et al., 2004; Hecox et al., 2005; Behrens et al., 2006; Robertson et al., 2006; Fox et al., 2007; Robinson et al., 2008; Watson, 2008; Belanger, 2009; Prentice, 2011; Michlovitz et al., 2012; Cameron, 2013; Starkey, 2013; Knight et al., 2013). Their use is also well documented in numerous published surveys conducted in countries such as the United States, Canada, Australia, England, the Netherlands, and Ireland (Robinson et al., 1988; Ter Haar et al., 1988; Lindsay et al., 1990; Lindsay et al., 1995; Taylor et al., 1991; Pope et al., 1995; Robertson et al., 1998; Roebroeck et al., 1998; Shields et al., 2001; Shields et al., 2004; Nussbaum et al., 2007; Chipchase et al., 2009).

A. COMPLEMENTARY ROLE

The body of literature on EPAs indicates that their main use is for the treatment of human soft-tissue pathologies that have an impact on a patient's life and well-being. Because EPAs are used to manage a broad variety of pathologies or health conditions, their role in the global therapeutic spectrum is to *complement* other physical, medical, and surgical therapeutic interventions. As a result, EPAs seldom are the sole therapeutic intervention in any given clinical case. It is, therefore, the practitioner's responsibility to determine and implement an optimal combination of EPAs that would best match the set of other interventions and together lead to optimal therapeutic outcomes for patients. This textbook will show that the evidence-based use of EPAs to treat soft-tissue pathologies, applied as a complementary treatment to other physical, medical, and surgical therapeutic interventions, can benefit patients.

B. CONSERVATIVE APPROACH

The treatment of human soft-tissue pathology rests with three basic approaches: pharmacologic, surgical, and conservative. Contrary to the pharmacologic and surgical approaches, which are invasive in nature and often associated with major side effects, the conservative approach to treatment, as exemplified by the use of EPAs, is noninvasive and characterized by minimal side effects.

II. INTERNATIONAL SOCIETY FOR ELECTROPHYSICAL AGENTS IN PHYSICAL THERAPY

In 2011, the World Confederation for Physical Therapy (WCPT) admitted another subgroup in areas of interest to its organization—the International Society for Electrophysical Agents in Physical Therapy (ISEAPT). The purpose of this society is to promote the worldwide use of EPAs by providing education materials, as well as related information and news on this subject of interest, to its members.

A. DEFINITION

The ISEAPT defines the term *electrophysical agent* as the use of electrophysical and biophysical energies for the purposes of evaluation, treatment and prevention of impairments, activity limitations, and participation restrictions (www.wcpt.org/iseapt). Evaluative EPAs may include, but are not limited to, ultrasound imaging and electroneurophysiologic testing that can assist diagnosis, guide treatment procedures, and evaluate treatment outcomes. Treatment and prevention EPAs, on the other hand, may include cryotherapy, iontophoresis, and laser, to name only a few, whose main purposes are to promote soft-tissue healing and increase body function (www.wcpt.org/iseapt). This latest edition is dedicated to the treatment and prevention component of EPAs.

TABLE 1-1 CLASSIFICATION OF THERAPEUTIC ELECTROPHYSICAL AGENTS

Energy	Electrophysical Agent
Thermal	Thermotherapy Cryotherapy Hydrotherapy
Electromagnetic	Shortwave diathermy Low-level laser therapy Ultraviolet
Electrical	Neuromuscular electrical stimulation Transcutaneous electrical nerve stimulation Electrical stimulation for tissue healing and repair Iontophoresis
Mechanical	Spinal traction Limb compression Continuous passive motion Ultrasound Extracorporeal shock wave therapy

B. CLASSIFICATION

This text classifies EPAs based on the type or form of energy delivered to soft tissues. Thermal, electromagnetic, electrical, and mechanical energies are delivered through various applicators on most body areas. As shown in Table 1-1, this textbook focuses on the application of 15 EPAs, all of which commonly used worldwide for the purpose of soft-tissue treatment.

III. THE DISABLEMENT CONCEPT

The American Physical Therapy Association (APTA), in the second edition of its *Guide to Physical Therapist Practice,* refers to the concept of *disablement* as "various impact(s) of chronic and acute conditions . . . on the functioning of specific body systems, on basic human performance, and on people's functioning in necessary, usual, expected, and personally desired roles in society" (APTA, 2001). A number of disablement models, including the Nagi and the International Classification of Functioning, Disability, and Health (ICF), have emerged in the literature over the past 30 years. Essentially, these models are attempts to better delineate the interrelationship among pathologies, impairments, functional limitations, disabilities, and handicaps (Nagi, 1991; Lee Kirby, 1998; APTA, 2001; World Health Organization [WHO], 2001; Jette, 2006).

A. THE ICF MODEL

In 2001, the WHO published the ICF disablement model. Figure 1-1 illustrates its framework. This model portrays human function and decrease in function as the product of a dynamic interaction between various health conditions and contextual factors. Disability and functioning are viewed as outcomes of interactions between health conditions and contextual factors. The patient's impairment, functional, and disability levels are captured by the following three components: body functions and structures, activities, and participation. The ICF is endorsed worldwide in the field of health care. All case studies presented in this textbook comply with the ICF framework. The ICF disablement model rests on six components (Fig. 1-1). The first component, *health condition,* captures all forms of injury, disease, disorder, or conditions such as osteoarthritis, stroke, or tendinitis. The second component is *body functions and structures.* Body functions are physiologic or psychological functions of body systems. Body structures, on the other hand, are anatomic parts of the body. Decreased shoulder range of motion would exemplify this component. The third component, *activities,* reflects the execution of a task by the patient, such as difficulty walking. The fourth component, *participation,* captures the patient's involvement in life situations, such as the inability to work. The last two components are *environmental and personal factors.* These two components show how environmental factors, such as climate, social structures, and lifestyle, and personal factors, such as age, profession, and gender, may influence the disability experienced by the patient.

B. IMPACT OF ELECTROPHYSICAL AGENTS ON THE ICF MODEL

The therapeutic application of EPAs fits nicely in the ICF disablement model. This textbook will show that EPAs can significantly influence patients' health conditions by directly affecting the body functions and structures component of the model, which in turn will indirectly affect the activities and participation components. For example, the use of a given EPA, such as cryotherapy, may significantly decrease pain caused by inflammation, which in turn may increase the patient's ability to walk and engage in functional activities.

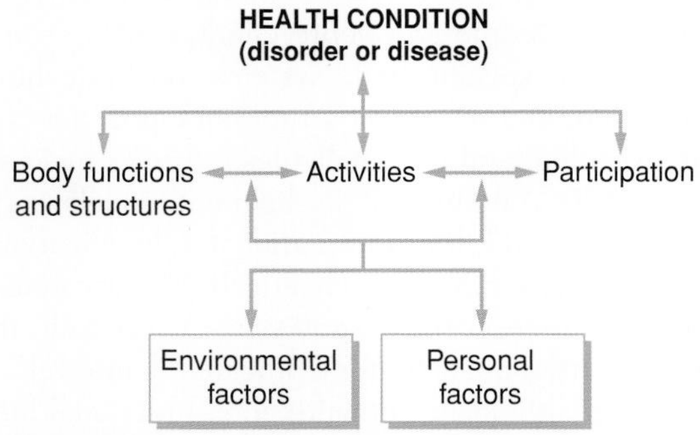

FIGURE 1-1 Model for the International Classification of Functioning, Disability, and Health (ICF). (From the World Health Organization: Towards a Common Language for Functioning, Disability and Health (IFC), Geneva, 2002, WHO.)

IV. TODAY'S DELIVERY OF ELECTROPHYSICAL AGENTS

For a multitude of reasons, the focus has shifted in the field of health care delivery as a whole from doing the *thing right* to doing the *right thing.* In other words, today's practitioners are becoming more and more preoccupied with the issue of therapeutic effectiveness while continuing to be concerned about the issue of therapeutic efficiency. A major impetus behind this shift is the ever-increasing cost of health care delivery. Another key impetus is the growing recognition and application of a new health care paradigm called *evidence-based practice* (EBP).

A. THERAPEUTIC EFFICIENCY

Doing the *thing right* is to show *efficiency.* Clinical efficiency is the degree to which things are done by the book, or according to recognized standards. It is the production of the desired effects or results with minimum waste of time, effort, or skill. Much has been written on the application and safety issues related to the use of EPAs in physical rehabilitation. For decades, educating students about how to apply EPAs safely was the focus—in other words, student demonstration of clinical efficiency was the primary goal.

B. THERAPEUTIC EFFECTIVENESS

Doing the *right thing* for the patient is to show *effectiveness.* Clinical effectiveness is the degree to which therapeutic objectives are achieved and the extent to which problems are solved. It is the quality of being successful in producing an intended result. How can practitioners who use EPAs improve their therapeutic effectiveness? Today, literature related to health care strongly suggests complementing the traditional experienced-based practice model with the newer EBP model. The aim of EBP is to apply the best available evidence gained from the scientific method to clinical decision making (see Chapter 2). The main objective of this textbook is to promote the evidence-based delivery of therapeutic EPAs. To conclude, higher levels of clinical efficiency and effectiveness must be demonstrated in the delivery of therapeutic EPAs to optimize patient care and to assure the survival of this therapeutic field in the future.

C. COST-BENEFIT AND RISK-BENEFIT RATIOS

Cost-benefit and risk-benefit ratios are two of the most relevant issues in ongoing health organization procedures.

The delivery of EPAs can be cost and labor intensive as well as taxing to patients. To determine cost-benefit ratios, practitioners must analyze the cost-effectiveness of different EPAs to see whether their benefits outweigh their costs—that is, to assess the overall value for the money. To determine risk-benefit ratios, practitioners must now determine whether the use of EPAs, particularly those presenting higher risks and precautions, are worth the risk to patients as compared with possible benefits if the EPA is successful—to put it simply, to determine if the treatment is worse than the disease. Unfortunately, no peer-reviewed literature could be found that would have addressed one, or both, of these important issues for a given or group of EPAs. In the absence of such literature, it is therefore the responsibility of each clinical setting to regularly monitor these two important ratios to optimize the delivery of therapeutic EPAs.

V. EMERGING THERAPIES

It seems that in the field of EPAs, no single year can pass without hearing on radio and television or reading on the web, magazines, or newspapers that at a new therapy has been discovered that shows the beneficial effects for a wide array of soft-tissue pathologies. Magnetic bracelets, abdominal electric stimulators, deep oscillation therapy, and zero gravity traction are examples of such therapies. No one will disagree that the emergence of new therapies is a necessary process and that we must all keep an open mind toward them. The major problem with many of these new therapies, however, is the therapeutic claims made by their proponents. To claim therapeutic effectiveness based on the opinions of gurus, patient testimonies, or sophisticated marketing schemes is no longer acceptable to health care stakeholders. As stated in this textbook, claims of therapeutic effectiveness must rest on scientific evidence. When confronted with a new or emerging therapy, the evidence-based practitioner is very likely to say something like "show me the evidence" as opposed to "show me how to use it." As discussed in Chapter 2, this textbook proposes to apply evidence and critical thinking to our decision-making process with regard to the application of EPAs.

VI. LIMITED THERAPEUTIC SCOPE

The scope of therapeutic EPAs, as with all therapeutics used in health care, is limited. For example, EPAs are not designed to replace therapeutic exercises, in the same way that surgical procedures are not designed to replace medications—*they complement each other.* This textbook will show that the evidence-based use of EPAs to treat soft-tissue pathologies, applied as a complementary treatment to other physical, medical, and surgical therapeutic interventions, can promote healing while minimizing the functional limitations and disabilities associated with such pathologies.

VII. THE BOTTOM LINE

- The practice of therapeutic EPAs has achieved international recognition in the field of physical therapy.
- EPAs are noninvasive therapies used to complement other therapeutic interventions.
- Application of EPAs can significantly affect the body function and structure, activity, and participation components of the ICF model.
- Adopting an evidence-based approach to practice can only benefit the demonstration of therapeutic effectiveness.
- Cost-benefit and risk-benefit issues related to the practice of EPAs must be addressed to optimize delivery.
- The appraisal of emerging therapies can only be done based on their related body of evidence.
- Higher levels of clinical efficiency and effectiveness in the delivery of therapeutic EPAs are needed to assure the survival of this therapeutic field in the future.

VIII. CRITICAL THINKING QUESTIONS

Clarification: What is meant by therapeutic EPAs?

Assumptions: You assume that the use of EPAs can significantly affect some elements of the ICF model. How do you justify that assumption?

Reasons and evidence: Therapeutic EPAs are classified according to the form of energy supplied to soft tissues. Why does it make sense to use such a classification?

Viewpoints or perspectives: You agree with the consensus that EPAs should be used in conjunction with, or as a complement to, other therapeutic interventions. What would say to a colleague who disagrees with you?

Implications and consequences: You state that therapeutic EPAs can affect the ICF disablement model. What are you implying?

About the question: Why are EPAs valuable complements to medical or surgical interventions in the treatment for soft-tissue pathology? Why do you think I ask this question?

IX. REFERENCES

Articles

American Physical Therapy Association (2001) Guide to Physical Therapy Practice, 2nd ed. Phys Ther, 81: 9–746

Chipchase LS, Williams MT, Robertson VJ (2009) A national study of the availability and use of electrophysical agents by Australian physiotherapists. Physioth Theory Practice, 25: 279–296

Jette AM (2006) Toward a common language for function, disability, and health. Phys Ther, 86, 726–734

Lindsay DM, Dearness J, McGinley CC (1995) Electrotherapy usage trends in private physiotherapy practice in Alberta. Physiother Can, 47: 30–34

Lindsay DM, Dearness J, Richardson C (1990) A survey of electromodality usage in private physiotherapy practices. Aust J Physiother, 36: 249–256

Nussbaum EL, Burke S, Johnstone L, Lahiffe G, Robitaille E, Yoshida K (2007) Use of electrophysical agents: Findings and implications of survey of practice in Metro Toronto. Physiother Can, 59: 118–131

Pope GD, Mockett SP, Wright JP (1995) A survey of electrotherapeutic modalities: Ownership and use in the NHS in England. Physiotherapy, 81: 82–91

Robertson VJ, Spurritt D (1998) Electrophysical agents: Implications of their availability and use in undergraduate clinical placements. Physiotherapy, 84: 335–334

Robinson AJ, Snyder-Mackler L (1988) Clinical application of electrotherapeutic modalities. Phys Ther, 68: 1235–1238

Roebroeck ME, Dekker J, Ostendorp RA (1998) The use of therapeutic ultrasound by physical therapists in Dutch primary health care. Phys Ther, 78: 470–478

Shields N, Gormley J, O'Hare N (2001) A survey into the availability of shortwave diathermy equipment in Irish hospitals and private practices. Br J Ther Rehab, 8: 331–339

Shields N, O'Hare N, Gormley (2004) Contra-indications to shortwave diathermy: Survey of Irish physiotherapists. Physiotherapy, 90: 42–53

Taylor E, Humphry R (1991) Survey of physical agent modality use. Am J Occup Ther, 45: 924–931

Ter Haar G, Dyson M, Oakley S (1988) Ultrasound in physiotherapy in the United Kingdom: Results of a questionnaire. Physiother Pract, 4: 69–72

Chapters of Textbooks

Lee Kirby R (1998) Impairment, disability and handicap. In: Rehabilitation Medicine: Principles and Practice, 3rd ed. Delisa JA, Gans BM (Eds). Lippincott-Raven Publishers, Philadelphia, pp 55–60

Nagi S (1991) Disability concepts revisited. Implications for prevention. In: Disability in America: Towards a National Agenda for Prevention. Pope AM, Tarlov AR (Eds). National Academy Press, Washington, pp 309–327

Textbooks

Behrens BJ, Michlovitz SL (2006) Physical Agents: Theory and Practice, 2nd ed. FA Davis, Philadelphia

Belanger AY (2009) Therapeutic Electrophysical Agents: Evidence Behind Practice. 2nd ed. Lippincott Williams & Wilkins, Philadelphia

Cameron MH (2013) Physical Agents in Rehabilitation: From Research to Practice, 4th ed. Saunders, St-Louis

Fox JE, Sharp TN (2007) Practical Electrotherapy: A Guide to Safe Application. Churchill Livingstone, London

Hayes KW (2000) Manual for Physical Agents, 5th ed. Prentice-Hall Health, Upper Saddle River, New York

Hecox B, Weisberg J, Mehreteab TA, Sanko J (2005) Integrating Physical Agents in Rehabilitation, 2nd ed. Prentice Hall, New York

Horodyski M, Starkey C (2004) Laboratory Activities for Therapeutic Modalities, 3rd ed. FA Davis, Philadelphia

Khan J (2000) Principles and Practice of Electrotherapy, 4th ed. Churchill Livingstone, New York

Knight KL, Draper DO (2013) Therapeutic Modalities: The Art and Science, 2nd ed. Lippincott Williams & Wilkins, Philadelphia

Low J, Reed A (2000) Electrotherapy Explained: Principles and Practice, 3rd ed. Butterworth Heinemann, Oxford

Michlovitz SL, Bellew JW, Noland TP (2012) Modalities for Therapeutic Intervention, 5th ed. F.A. Davis, Philadelphia

Nalty T (2001) Electrotherapy: Clinical Procedures Manual. McGraw-Hill, New York

Prentice WE (2011) Therapeutic Modalities in Rehabilitation. 4th Ed. McGraw-Hill Medical, New York

Robertson V, Ward A, Low J, Reed A (2006) Electrotherapy Explained: Principles and Practice, 3rd ed. Butterworth-Heinemann, Oxford

Robinson AJ, Snyder-Mackler L (2008) Electrophysiology: Electrotherapy and Electrophysiologic Testing, 3rd ed. Lippincott Williams & Wilkins, Philadelphia

Starkey C (2013) Therapeutic Modalities, 4th ed. FA Davis, Philadelphia

Watson T (2008) Electrotherapy: Evidence-Based Practice, 12th ed. Churchill Livingstone, London

Monograph

World Health Organization (2001) International Classification of Functioning, Disability and Health; ICF. Geneva, Switzerland

Internet Resource

www.wcpt.org/iseapt: World Confederation for Physical Therapy/International Society for Electrophysical Agents in Physical Therapy

Chapter 2

Toward a Practice Based on Evidence

Chapter Outline

Learning Objectives

Remembering: List and describe the seven elements found in the proposed evidence-based clinical decision making protocol.

Understanding: Discuss why it is preferable to focus on human versus animal studies when investigating the therapeutic effectiveness of a given electrophysical agent.

Applying: Illustrate how to apply the SOAP note format for a given clinical case.

Analyzing: Examine the value of adopting an evidence-based approach to the delivery of therapeutic electrophysical agents.

Evaluating: Appraise the assessment schemes presented in this chapter for assessing the strength of evidence and therapeutic effectiveness.

Creating: Construct an evidence-based clinical decision making protocol.

I. TODAY'S CLINICAL DECISION MAKING

The contemporary practice of electrophysical agents (EPAs) requires that clinicians be involved in complex decision making. Clinical decisions relate primarily to documenting cases, choosing and implementing EPAs, documenting their outcomes, and assessing their effectiveness. Practitioners make clinical decisions daily using the knowledge and skills they have gained through education and practice. What else should practitioners take into account to make their decision making as effective as possible? This edition recommends to document cases using the International Classification of Functioning, Disability, and Health (ICF) model to capture the whole dimension of the patient's problem while taking account of the available research-based evidence. In other words, this text proposes that practitioners engage in evidence-based clinical decision making when considering the delivery of therapeutic EPAs.

II. THE CONCEPT OF EVIDENCE

Dictionaries generally define *evidence* as anything that establishes a fact or gives reason to believe something. Historically, heath practitioners relied primarily on evidence based on their clinical experiences and expert opinions. Over the past two decades, however, the introduction, development, and growing use of evidence based on research findings have marked a significant shift in health care delivery worldwide. The phenomenal amount of money spent annually on health care research has resulted in an exponential growth of literature. Practitioners can no longer ignore this huge body of clinical literature. What is evidence-based practice and how useful is this research-based literature to the practice of EPAs?

III. EVIDENCE-BASED PRACTICE: WHAT IS IT?

Evidence-based practice (EBP) is now a reality in the field of health care. The first (Belanger, 2002) and second (Belanger, 2009) editions of this textbook have championed the use of this concept in the delivery of therapeutic EPAs. This third edition is committed to putting evidence into practice. So what is EBP? It is the product of integration of information from three sources: scientific research; clinical experience of the practitioner; and patient values, concerns, and expectations (Sackett et al., 1997). When do practitioners become evidence-based practitioners? It is when they realize that evidence does not mean answer, but instead informed decision making among options. It is when they accept that a lack of research evidence on a given therapeutic intervention does not constitute evidence for lack of therapeutic effectiveness. In other words, something that has yet to be proven does not mean that it is not proven. Finally, it is when practitioners accept to be guided by research findings however scarce and imperfect these may be.

IV. BARRIERS TO EVIDENCE-BASED CLINICAL DECISION MAKING

As practitioners become more involved in decision making, it is important for them to use the best evidence to make effective and justifiable decisions. It is fair to say that a very large majority of health practitioners view clinical decision making based on research evidence positively and consider it important to better patient care. How can one explain the rather slow pace of accepting and implanting EBP in clinical settings? Several personal and institutional barriers have been identified (Jette et al., 2003). For example, the lack of time to search for, to understand, and to interpret research findings are found to be major personal barriers. Moreover, inadequate access to research databases and lack of training on EBP at work are examples of institutional barriers frequently reported by practitioners.

V. EVIDENCE-BASED CLINICAL DECISION MAKING PROTOCOL

To help practitioners in their journey toward using more evidence based on research findings in their decision-making process, this edition proposes an evidence-based clinical decision making protocol made of seven components. A sample version of this protocol, titled *Evidence-Based Clinical Decision Making Protocol,* is illustrated below. This protocol is used to resolve all the case studies presented in this text. It always starts with the formulation of the case and ends with its documentation.

A. FORMULATE THE CASE HISTORY

Optimal decision making begins with a clear and succinct formulation of the case history, which lists key subjective and objective elements.

EVIDENCE-BASED CLINICAL DECISION MAKING PROTOCOL

1. **Formulate the Case History**
2. **Outline the Case Based on the ICF Framework**
3. **Outline Therapeutic Goals and Outcome Measurements**
4. **Justify the Use of Electrophysical Agents Based on the EBP Framework**
5. **Outline Key Intervention Parameters**
6. **Report Pre- and Post-Intervention Outcomes**
7. **Document Case Intervention Using the SOAP Note Format**

   S: Subjective
   O: Objective
   A: Assessment
   P: Plan

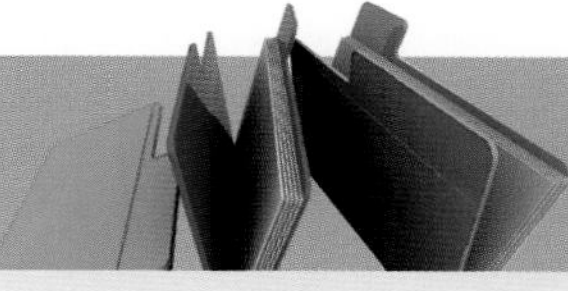

Research-Based Indications

Health Condition	Benefit—Yes		Benefit—No	
	Rating	Reference	Rating	Reference
Rheumatoid/osteoarthritic conditions	I	Dellhag et al., 1992 (pb)		
	I	Harris et al., 1955 (pb)		
	II	Hawkes et al., 1985 (pb)		
	II	Yung et al., 1986 (pb)		
	II	Bromley et al., 1994 (pb)		
	II	Williams et al., 1986 (hp)		
	II	Myrer et al., 2011 (pb)		
	II	Cetin et al., 2008 (hp)		
	II	Myrer et al., 2011 (pb)		

Strength of evidence: Moderate
Therapeutic effectiveness: Substantiated

Health Condition	Benefit—Yes		Benefit—No	
	Rating	Reference	Rating	Reference
Neck/back/shoulder pain	II	Landen, 1967 (hp)	II	Garra et al., 2010 (hp)
	II	Cordray et al., 1959 (hp)		
	II	Miller et al., 1996 (hp)		

B. OUTLINE THE CASE BASED ON THE ICF FRAMEWORK

To better capture the whole impact of the case on the patient's life, the case formulation is broken down using the ICF model (see Chapter 1). How the patient's health condition relates to body functions and structures, to activities, and to participation is revealed. How the contextual personal and environmental factors related to the case may influence its resolution is also reflected.

C. OUTLINE THERAPEUTIC GOALS AND OUTCOME MEASUREMENTS

No case study can be resolved without outlining clear therapeutic goals and related outcome measurements. Therapeutic goals should be realistic, achievable, timely, and cost-effective. They should be discussed with the patient and, depending of the case, the family, treating physician, or attending nurse. The outcome measurements used, on the other hand, should be valid and specific to each therapeutic goal.

D. JUSTIFY THE USE OF ELECTROPHYSICAL AGENTS BASED ON THE EBP FRAMEWORK

The justification to use a given EPA over another in the treatment for a given condition should rests on evidence. This means that all three elements of EBP—practitioner experience with the therapeutic agent, patient expectations with regard to the use of the agent, and research-based indications—must be taken into consideration. Throughout this text (see Chapters 7 through 21), *Research-Based Indications* boxes such as the sample one shown above, are used to display the body of human research based evidence available behind each EPA. To construct such indications boxes, the body of scientific literature was to be searched, collected, assessed, and then analyzed.

1. Searching and Collecting the Evidence

The first step was to search and collect the body of research evidence available behind each EPA. The method used was an exhaustive computerized search of English language, human-only, peer-reviewed clinical studies or articles using keywords such as *electrophysical agents, physical agents, physical modalities, therapeutic modalities,* and *electrotherapy,* to name only a few. In addition, keywords included the name of each therapeutic agent, such as *iontophoresis, spinal traction,* or *ultrasound.* Several research databases, including PubMed, CINAHL, and PED*ro,* were searched for evidence. Published abstracts and poster abstracts were excluded from the search. As shown in the Research-Based Indications box, the pathologic conditions studied with regard to the agent used are listed in the Health Condition column.

a. Focusing on Human Studies Only: Why?

In the pyramid of research evidence related to the field of therapy, human studies are seen as demonstrating a higher level of evidence than animal studies, with the latter studies being considered at higher evidence than animal in vivo and in vitro studies (Chiappelli et al., 2010). Maintaining the focus only on human studies to promote the use of EBP in the field of EPA is in keeping with this fact. This human-only approach to the literature search is also consistent with the American Physical Therapy Association's (APTA) Hooked on Evidence approach to EBP.

b. What Is "Hooked on Evidence," and What Articles Are Eligible for the Database?

As defined on the Hooked on Evidence Web site,

> Hooked on Evidence is APTA's "grassroots" effort to develop a database containing current research evidence on the effectiveness of physical therapy interventions. The Hooked on Evidence project was motivated by a concern that clinicians lacked access to the knowledge available from current research, thus hindering evidence-based practice.
>
> (www.hookedonevidence.com/faq.cfm)

What articles are eligible for the Hooked on Evidence database?

> All studies of the effectiveness of physical therapy that meet the following criteria are eligible for inclusion in the database: 1) includes human subjects with the target condition, 2) includes at least one physical therapy intervention, 3) includes an outcome of the intervention, and 4) published in English in a peer-reviewed journal that is indexed.
>
> (www.hookedonevidence.com/faq.cfm)

2. Rating of Articles

Each collected article was rated using one criteria only—the type of research design used by the authors. This led to an evidence rating scale made of three classes (I, II, and III), as shown in the Research-Based Indications box. A class I rating was evidence from *controlled studies,* regardless of randomization and blindness. A class II rating was evidence from *noncontrolled studies,* also regardless of randomization and blindness. A class III rating was evidence from *case reports* and *case series.* There is more than one definition associated with the term *control group* or *controlled study* in research. A control group can be defined as an experimental group of patients who receive no treatment, a sham, or a placebo treatment. The rating of articles listed in the Research-Based Indication box is based on this definition. A control group can also be defined as a group of patients who receive no treatment, a sham, a placebo, or *another* treatment that is different from the treatment under investigation. To simplify the rating scale, and as indicated earlier, no effort was made to subclassify each article based on respective levels of randomization and blindness. The *reference* attached to each article is presented in each box.

3. Assessing Clinical Benefit

Clinical, or therapeutic, benefit was assessed on the basis of a simple Yes and No scale, as illustrated in the Research-Based Indications box. A study reporting overall positive therapeutic benefit was assigned the label *Yes.* In contrast, a study reporting no or negative therapeutic benefit was labeled as *No.* Considering that all articles collected were from peer-reviewed journals, the determination of therapeutic benefit was made based on the authors' own overall interpretation and conclusion.

4. Analyzing the Strength of Evidence

The evidence was assessed for its strength based on the articles' rating scheme described previously. It is well established in research that the strength of a controlled study is greater than that of a noncontrolled study, regardless of randomization and blindness. It is also well recognized that the strength of a noncontrolled study is greater than that found in case reports or case series (Chiappelli et al., 2010). Thus, the higher the strength of evidence, the better the scientific evidence behind a given EPA for a given health condition. In this textbook, and as presented in Table 2-1, the strength of evidence was classified according to four levels—*strong, moderate, weak,* and *pending*—based on the number of studies found per rating or class (I, II, III) and expressed as a percentage. The criteria defining each level are presented in the table. For example, the strength of evidence was considered strong for a given EPA and related condition when the number of class I (controlled study) articles equaled or exceeded 50%. The strength of evidence was considered pending for any given health condition when fewer than five peer-reviewed studies were available for analysis.

5. Analyzing Therapeutic Effectiveness

Analysis of therapeutic effectiveness was based on the percentage of studies showing benefit (Yes), as shown in Table 2-2, regardless of their classes. Four levels of therapeutic effectiveness were identified—*substantiated, conflicting,*

TABLE 2-1 LEVEL OF STRENGTH OF EVIDENCE

Strength of Evidence	Percentage of Studies per Class
Strong	≥50% in class I
Moderate	≥50% in class I + class II
Weak	>50% in class III
Pending	Fewer than 5 studies available

TABLE 2-2	LEVEL OF THERAPEUTIC EFFECTIVENESS
Therapeutic Effectiveness	**Percentage of Studies Showing Benefit (Yes)**
Substantiated	≥60%
Conflicting	≥40% but <60%
Unsupported	<40%
Pending	Fewer than 5 studies available

unsupported, and *pending*. For example, a level of substantiated effectiveness for a given EPA and related health condition was granted when the percentage of studies showing benefit (Yes) was equal to or greater than 60%. It is important to distinguish between the strength of evidence and therapeutic effectiveness. For example, the strength of evidence behind a given EPA may be strong because the percentage of class I studies is equal to or greater than 50% (Table 2-1), but its level of therapeutic effectiveness may be conflicting if its percentage of studies showing benefit (Yes) is equal to or greater than 40% but less than 60%.

E. OUTLINE KEY INTERVENTION PARAMETERS

This fifth element of the protocol rests on the listing of key intervention parameters related to application and therapeutic intervention. Parameters such as methods of application, risks and precautions, device model used, applicator used, and dosage and treatment frequency are examples.

F. REPORT PRE- AND POST-INTERVENTION OUTCOMES

The assessment of therapeutic effectiveness begins with the use of recognized outcome measures. Comparison of results between pre- and post-intervention is done to formulate a statement on treatment effectiveness.

G. DOCUMENT CASE INTERVENTION USING THE SOAP NOTE FORMAT

There are several methods that health practitioners can use to document their notes on patient files. One method commonly used today is the SOAP (*s*ubjective, *o*bjective, *a*ssessment, *p*lan) note format. To document a patient's file or case intervention using the SOAP format implies writing short notes on these four components. The *subjective* (S) component refers to the practitioner's account of the patient history. It includes short notes on the patient's current condition, including, but limited to, issues such as diagnosis, onset, location, symptoms, previous treatments, and other elements. An example might be, "The patient presents knee pain and has difficulty walking." The *objective* (O) component relates to the measurable elements of the case and includes the essentials related to treatment. Short notes are written that outline key assessment results gathered in relation to the patient's problem as well as treatment type and key parameters. Treatment notes should be specific enough so that if the practitioner is not available, another practitioner can treat the patient. An objective note might be, "Knee strength decrease by 25%; extension ROM deficit of 10 degrees; pain at 7/10. CSWD to knee joint; rigid capacitive plates; dose of 60 kJ." The *assessment* (A) is concerned with the patient's response and tolerance to treatment. "Decrease knee pain by 30%; improve walking ability; treatment well tolerated" may be an example. Finally, the *plan* (P) component relates to the course of treatment. It includes notes on progress, end of treatment, and discharge planning. A plan note might be, "Continue with CSWD as above and strengthening exercises for the next 3 weeks; full recovery is expected."

VI. BENEFIT OF EVIDENCE-BASED CLINICAL DECISION MAKING

Evidence-based clinical decision making is becoming an important element of quality care. Its use is essential to optimize therapeutic efficacy and effectiveness, as well as to ensure accountability and transparency in decision making. As discussed in this chapter, to incorporate more research-based evidence does not eliminate the need for professional clinical judgment nor for the consideration of client preferences when the time comes to resolve a clinical case (see the Evidence-Based Clinical Decision Making Protocol box). In the field of therapeutic EPAs, the time has come to do more of the *right thing* for patients while continuing to do the *thing right.*

VII. CHALLENGE AND LIMITATION

To assess the body of literature associated with the practice of therapeutic EPAs is a major challenge. First, most agents, as exemplified in this textbook, present with a wide range of dosimetric parameters and are applied using different methods on a wide selection of patients suffering from a wide variety of pathologic conditions that affect various body areas. This means that determining research-based therapeutic effectiveness of all agents, for all dosimetric prescriptions and for all pathologic conditions, is simply an impossible task. Second, no single universally accepted method exists to rate the strength and assess the effectiveness of any given therapy. Various methods, using different qualifiers, scales, or ratings, are found in the scientific literature. For example, rarely will practitioners see similar methodologies used by authors writing meta-analysis and critical review articles. Readers, therefore, should not be surprised to see that the method proposed in this textbook may be significantly different from the one they are familiar with or relying on, because of its simplicity and practicality. Its goal is to provide practitioners with useful evidence-based statements on the strength of evidence and therapeutic effectiveness. Its purpose is to avoid deceptive statements such as "There is insufficient available evidence to determine the effectiveness" or "Further research is needed," which are too often found in today's meta-analysis and critical review papers on the use of EPAs. It may well be that the complex methodology, found in these last two types of review articles and used on the limited and often sparse body of evidence related to EPAs, can only lead the authors to such concluding remarks. The Research-Based Indication boxes presented in this text strongly indicate that it is perhaps premature, at this time, to venture in the conduct of meta-analysis or critical reviews in the field of EPA precisely because the body of literature is limited. For the time being, therefore, to assess therapeutic effectiveness as described in this chapter has the advantage of presenting the actual body of evidence, as illustrated in the Research-Based Indications box, for what it is—that is, unfiltered and trusting the authors' conclusions. This approach thus provides students, clinicians, and educators with a clear overview of the strength of evidence and therapeutic effectiveness associated with each EPA covered in this textbook.

VIII. THE BOTTOM LINE

- Today's health care delivery requires complex decision making.
- EPA practitioners can no longer ignore the growing body of clinical research-based evidence.
- More and more practitioners are shifting from experienced-based to evidence-based clinical decision making.
- Making use of the evidence, as shown in the Research-Based Indications boxes, implies searching, collecting, rating, and analyzing the body of human peer-reviewed literature.
- Rating the strength of evidence and assessing therapeutic effectiveness levels behind each EPA is the goal.
- Making use of scientific evidence can only improve therapeutic efficiency and effectiveness and ensure accountability and transparency in the decision-making process.
- Case study protocol based on evidence that is formulated using the IFC model, making use of Research-Based Evidence, and documented using the SOAP note format is strongly recommended.
- The limited, and sometime sparse, body of scientific literature available in the field of EPAs strongly suggests that it may be premature, today, to conduct meta-analysis and critical reviews for the purpose of assessing therapeutic effectiveness.

IX. CRITICAL THINKING QUESTIONS

Clarification: What is meant by the term *evidence-based practice*?

Assumptions: You assume that clinical decision making based on evidence can only benefit the delivery of health care. How do you justify that assumption?

Reasons and evidence: Peer-reviewed articles are rated according to the type of research design used by the authors. Why does it make sense to use such a rating?

Viewpoints or perspectives: You agree that doing the *right thing* for your patient is more important than doing the *thing right.* What would say to a colleague who disagrees with you?

Implications and consequences: You state that it is important to assess the strength of evidence behind EPAs. What are you implying?

About the question: Why can the use of an evidence-based clinical decision making model improves the quality of our case resolution process? Why do you think I ask this question?

X. REFERENCES

Articles

Jette DU, Bacon K, Batty C, Carlson M, Ferland A, Hemingway RD, Hill JC, Ogilvie L, Volk D (2003) Evidence-based practice: beliefs, attitudes, knowledge, and behaviors of physical therapists. Phys Ther, 83:786–805

Textbooks

Belanger AY (2002) Evidenced-Based Guide to Therapeutic Physical Agents. Lippincott Williams & Wilkins, Baltimore

Belanger AY (2009) Therapeutic Electrophysical Agents: Evidence Behind Practice. 2nd ed. Lippincott Williams & Wilkins, Philadelphia

Chiappelli F, Caldeira Brant XM, Neagos N, Oluwadara OO, Ramchandani M (2010) Evidence-Based Practice: Towards Optimizing Clinical Outcomes. Springer, Berlin

Sackett DL, Richardson WS, Rosenberg WM.C, Haynes RB (1997). Evidence-Based Medicine: How to Practice and Teach EBM. Churchill Livingstone, Edinburg

Internet Resources

www.hookedonevidence.com/faq.cfm: Hooked on Evidence

www.ncbi.nlm.nih.gov/pubmed: PubMed

www.ebscohost.com/cinahl: CINAHL

www.pedro.org.au: PEDro

Chapter 3

Soft-Tissue Healing Process

Chapter Outline

Learning Objectives

Remembering: List the main anatomic components related to skin, tendon, ligament, articular cartilage, bone, skeletal muscle, peripheral nerve, artery, and vein.

Understanding: Compare the healing process with regard to the quality of healing commonly obtained for each of the soft tissues discussed.

Applying: Demonstrate how electrophysical agents facilitate the healing of soft tissues.

Analyzing: Explain why skin, bone, and skeletal muscle have a better healing capacity than ligament, tendon, and articular cartilage.

Evaluating: Formulate the relationship between each of the four basic phases of soft-tissue healing.

Creating: Discuss the characteristics of the hemostatic, inflammatory, proliferative, and remodeling/maturation phases of soft-tissue healing.

I. FOUNDATION

In the course of one's lifetime, soft-tissue pathologies caused by disease and injury will bring their share of suffering (Chapter 4) and body dysfunctions, affecting personal as well as environmental activities and participation (Chapter 1). **Soft tissue** is a generic term used to designate various body tissues that connect and support other structures. In this chapter, soft tissues refer specifically to skin, tendon, ligament, articular cartilage, skeletal muscle, peripheral nerve, blood vessel, and bone. Although many soft-tissue pathologies will heal naturally, without therapeutic intervention by health practitioners, a fair number will require specialized therapeutic interventions such as medication, surgery, exercise, and electrophysical agents (EPAs). There is ample evidence in daily experiences and in health literature to demonstrate that our body tissues, after injury and disease, immediately and automatically respond by triggering their own healing processes with the aim of restoring their lost structural integrity and function (Leadbetter et al., 1990; Salter, 1999; Leadbetter, 2001; Norris, 2004; Woo et al., 2004; Hess, 2005; Hildebrand et al., 2005; O'Connor et al., 2013). This innate capacity of our body to heal itself is remarkable but, unfortunately, often limited and imperfect. When both the nature and severity of soft-tissue pathology are such that the person's own capacity to heal the wound fails, then therapeutic interventions are needed to promote healing (Denegar, 2000; Leadbetter, 2001; Delforge, 2002a–d; Hess, 2005; Belanger, 2009; Sussman et al., 2012; O'Connor et al., 2013). The goal of all therapeutic interventions, therefore, is to minimize the adverse effects of tissue pathology while promoting tissue repair, thereby expediting a more rapid and effective return to activity and performance. To accomplish this goal, health practitioners must be familiar with the soft-tissue healing process.

II. THE HEALING PROCESS

The healing process, schematized in Figure 3-1, rests on four successive key physiologic phases, all of which overlap one another over time (Denegar, 2000; Leadbetter, 2001; Delforge, 2002a–d; Hildebrand et al., 2005; Carrilero et al., 2013; Dhawan et al., 2013; LaRose et al., 2013).

A. HEMOSTASIS PHASE

The first phase of healing, called *hemostasis,* is characterized by the arrest of bleeding at the wound site. This phase usually lasts a few seconds or, in case of moderate to severe pathologies that involve multiple well-vascularized tissues, up to several minutes. It involves the process of blood clotting and subsequent dissolution of the clot (Delforge, 2002a). The hemostatic response to injury is a complex series of regulatory events that require the interaction of both cellular elements and blood plasma proteins. The initial hemostatic mechanisms that occur within seconds after the blood vessel trauma include vasoconstriction and the development of a temporary hemostatic plug in the damaged vessels. Coagulation, or blood clotting, is the secondary hemostatic mechanism through which the initial platelet plug in the damaged vessels is reinforced (Delforge, 2002a). The presence of a blood mass outside the blood vessels is called *hematoma.* Hemostasis is the body's emergency response to pathology, of which the aim is to prevent hemorrhaging.

B. INFLAMMATORY PHASE

The *inflammatory phase* relates to the process of inflammation, of which the aim is to clean the wound of its cellular debris, preparing it for the deposition of new, repaired, or regenerated tissues. Inflammation, from the Latin word *inflammare,* means "to set on fire." It is a localized tissue response initiated by pathology. There are six clinical cardinal signs and symptoms associated this phase. These are erythema (rubor), hyperthermia (calor), edema (tumor), pain, muscle spasm, and dysfunction. *Erythema* is skin redness resulting from capillary engorgement. *Hyperthermia* results from erythema. *Edema* is caused by fluid accumulation in the interstitial spaces resulting from cell injuries. *Pain,* which results from activation of nociceptors caused by damaged tissues, triggers reflex *muscle spasm.* Finally, these combined symptoms cause temporary partial to total *dysfunction.* This phase is a

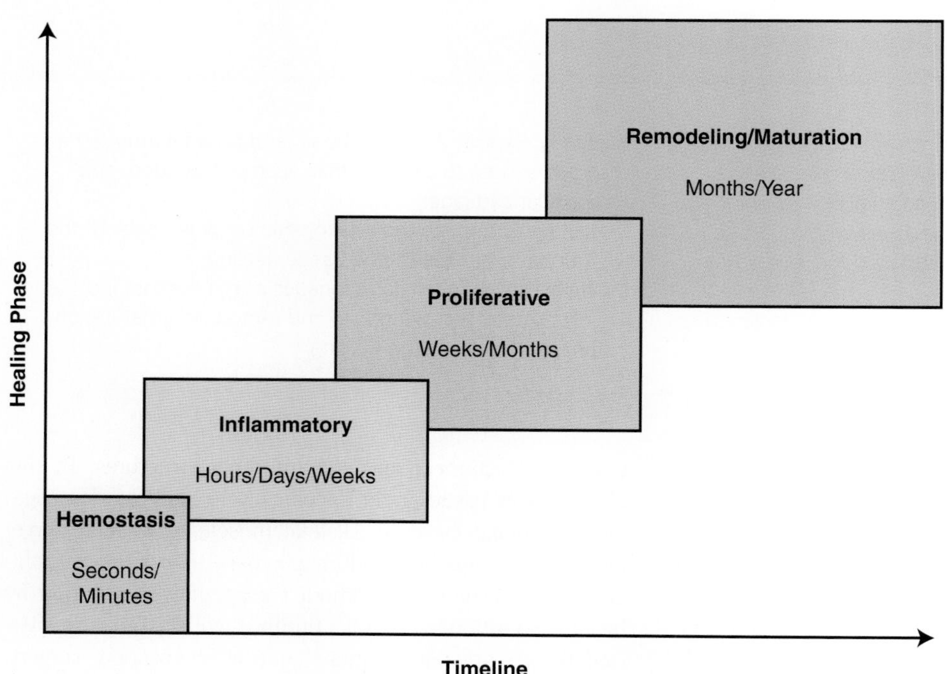

FIGURE 3-1 Soft-tissue healing process.

time-dependent evolving process, characterized by vascular, chemical, and cellular events that lead to the proliferative phase of healing. The inflammatory phase may last hours, days, or weeks depending on the severity of the pathology. *It is the crucial phase of healing—without it, no tissue healing is possible.*

C. PROLIFERATIVE PHASE

The inflammatory phase is followed by the *proliferative phase,* which deals with the formation and proliferation of new and immature repair tissues to replace the damaged tissues. Fibroplasia and angiogenesis are key processes during this phase. *Fibroplasia* is the formation of fibrous tissue. *Angiogenesis* is the process of growing new blood vessels. These processes are concomitant with all the other cellular responses during this phase of healing. The proliferative phase may last for weeks and sometimes months depending on the severity of pathology and the type of soft-tissue affected.

D. REMODELING/MATURATION PHASE

The fourth and final phase of healing is the *remodeling* (fiber alignment) and *maturation* (increase of mechanical strength) of immature tissue to form the most structurally functional tissue possible at the wound site. This phase usually lasts for months, sometimes more than a year, depending, again, on the severity of the pathology and the type of tissue affected.

E. TISSUE REGENERATION AND REPAIR

Tissue healing is defined as the natural response to pathology through which damaged and dead tissue is replaced by living tissue (Delforge, 2002a). The purpose of this healing process is to restore the structural and functional continuity of body tissues that has been disrupted by the pathologic processes (Martinez-Hernandez et al., 1990). Research has shown that injured soft-tissues heal through one of two primary mechanisms: regeneration and repair (Martinez-Hernandez, 1994). *Regeneration* refers to the restoration of tissue that is identical in structure and function to the tissue that has been damaged or destroyed. *Repair,* on the other hand, involves fibrous scar formation, which alters the normal structure and functional properties of the affected tissues. Soft-tissue healing occurs, in most cases, through a combination of regeneration and repair mechanisms.

F. HEALING QUALITY

Qualities of soft-tissue healing may be defined as ideal, acceptable, minimal, and failed (Leadbetter, 2001). *Ideal healing* is obtained when the wound is totally replaced by normal tissue structure, function, and appearance. This quality of healing implies regeneration, meaning that the repair tissue is identical to the original one. *Acceptable healing* is observed when the healed wound shows almost normal structure and appearance, and less than optimal function. *Minimal healing* is obtained when the healed wound shows minimal normal structure and appearance, and partial function. Finally, *failed healing* is present when the repair tissue shows abnormal structure, appearance, and function. Regardless of the therapeutic interventions used, ideal healing is rare. Minimal to acceptable healing, through the formation of scar tissue (repair mechanism) is, in the majority of cases, the best outcome that practitioners and patients can look for.

G. FACTORS INFLUENCING TISSUE HEALING

Research and practice have shown that factors other than therapeutic interventions can influence soft-tissue healing. Table 3-1 lists some of the factors that can either maximize or impede the healing process. Health practitioners must consider these factors when determining the potential healing outcome of any given soft-tissue injury. The timeline of the healing process described is characteristic of acute and subacute soft-tissue pathologies. Chronic pathology occurs when one or many of the phases (inflammatory, proliferative, remodeling, or maturation) of the healing process is incomplete, delayed, or absent. Therefore, management of chronic soft-tissue pathologies with EPAs aims at completing or enhancing the healing process by targeting the faulty phases of repair.

III. SKIN

The skin is the largest tissue in the body and has a number of important and interrelated functions, which are to provide protection from the outside environment; afford the sensation of mechanical, thermal, and painful

TABLE 3-1 FACTORS IMPEDING AND MAXIMIZING SOFT-TISSUE HEALING

Maximizing Factors	Impeding Factors
Good general health status	Poor general health status
No comorbidity	Comorbidities
Younger age	Older age
Proper nutrition	Malnutrition
Active lifestyles	Sedentary lifestyle
Good compliance with treatment	Poor compliance with treatment

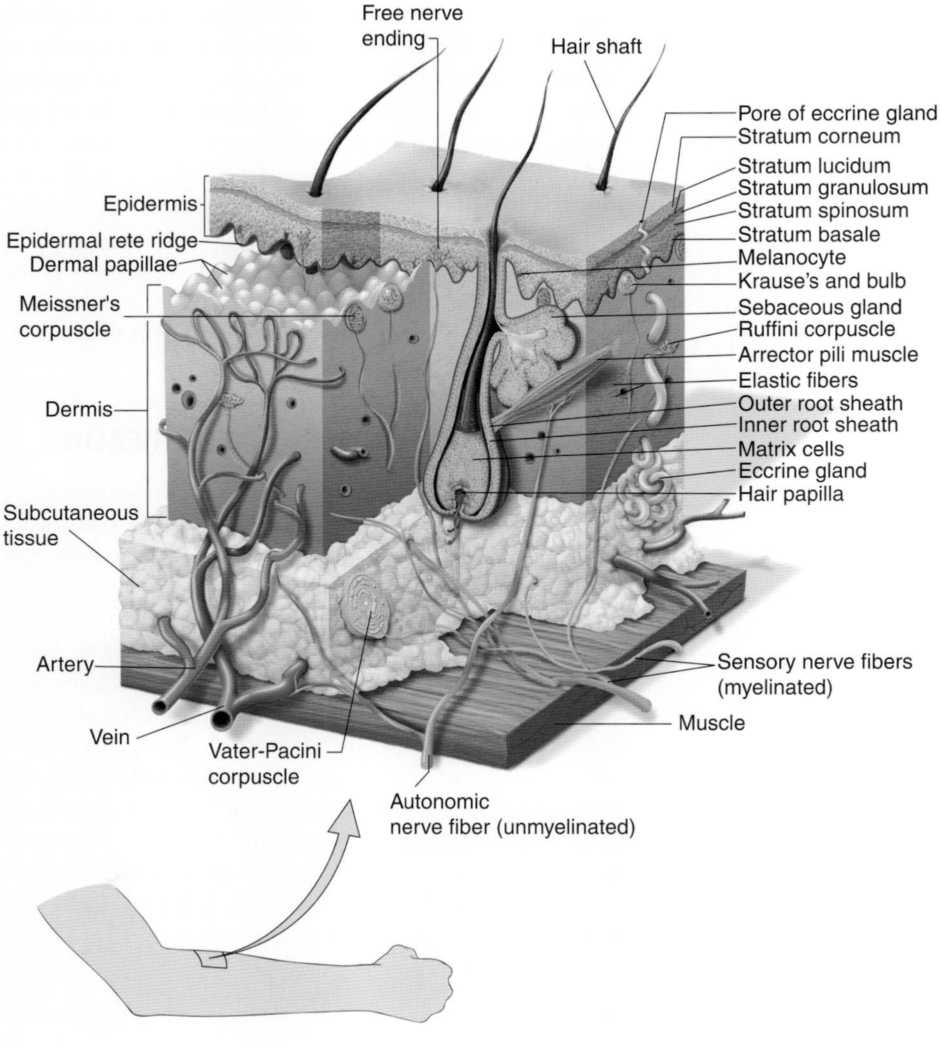

FIGURE 3-2 The structural hierarchy of the skin. (Used with permission from the Anatomical Chart Co.)

stimuli; and allow the secretion of fluids (sebum, sweat) for regulation of body temperature (Harvey, 2005; Johnstone et al., 2005; Whitney, 2005). Figure 3-2 illustrates a schematic anatomic cross-sectional view of the skin, revealing its layers and appendages. The *epidermis* has important protective functions against injury to subcutaneous tissues and excessive water loss. The *dermis,* on the other hand, provides nutrition through its vascular system and neural functions through its multiple neural receptors. The *subcutaneous layer,* made of adipose tissue, acts as a cushion for the skin while contributing to body heat regulation. The skin also contains numerous appendages, such as blood vessels, nerves, and glands, as well as thermal, mechanical, and nociceptive receptors. Table 3-2 lists common types of skin pathologies that may be classified based on four stages of severity (Harvey, 2005; Johnstone et al., 2005; Whitney, 2005). Table 3-3 presents an overview of the healing processes that take place following skin pathology (Harvey, 2005; Johnstone et al., 2005; Whitney, 2005). The final common outcome in most moderate to severe cases is the formation of weaker, less elastic but functional cutaneous repair tissue. Because the skin is a well-vascularized tissue, its quality of healing usually ranges from acceptable to ideal.

IV. TENDON AND LIGAMENT

Tendons and ligaments present striking structural and healing similarities. Figure 3-3 shows a schematic anatomic cross-sectional representation of both tendon and ligament. *Tendons* are fibrous, cordlike structure of collagenous tissue by which muscles attached to bones. Collagen fibers are fibrous proteins that have a great tensile strength, which give tendons the ability to withstand forces that stretch them. The major function of tendons is to transmit forces generated by muscles to bones, resulting in joint movements (Clancy, 1990; Herzog et al., 1994; Almekinders et al., 1998; Khan et al., 1999; Sevier et al., 2000; Woo et al., 2000; Sharma et al., 2005; Carrilero et al., 2013). The tendon splits into smaller entities called *fascicles.* Each fascicle then splits into fibers, which split further into fibrils, subfibrils, and microfibrils, and, ultimately,

TABLE 3-2 SKIN PATHOLOGY

Type	Description
Incision	Edges are regular, smooth
Laceration	Edges are irregular, ragged
Contusion	Skin is bruised, showing ecchymoses
Abrasion	Skin is lightly peeled away
Avulsion	Skin is severely peeled away
Ulcer	Skin hypoxia, leading to necrosis
Penetrating	Skin is punctured
Thermal	Skin is burned
Systemic	Skin is ulcerated
Severity	
Stage I	Wound shows no breaks in the skin
Stage II	Wound shows breaks in the epidermal and dermal layers of the skin
Stage III	Wound shows breaks in the epidermal, dermal, and subcutaneous tissues
Stage IV	Wound shows breaks in full-thickness, including surrounding tissues

TABLE 3-3 SKIN HEALING PROCESS

Hemostasis Phase

- Blood-clotting cascade leads to the arrest of bleeding by coagulation
- Blood clotting results in the release of proinflammatory molecules
- Fibrin clot establishes a provisional extracellular matrix, which will serve as a platform for the subsequent crucial inflammatory phase

Inflammatory Phase

- Inflammatory cells enter the site of injury
- Release of growth factors stimulates and regulates the functions of these migrating cells
- Wound is prepared for the subsequent proliferative phase of healing

Proliferative Phase

- Deposition of repair tissue in the wound
- Fibroblasts migrate to the wounded area and proliferate (fibroplasia)
- Granulation tissue, which will mature into scar tissue, forms
- Budding and growing of capillaries surrounding the repair zone (angiogenesis)
- The wound site fills up with new collagen fibers, which are weak and randomly oriented

Remodeling/Maturation Phase

- Maturation of new collagen from type III to type I
- Maturity and remodeling add strength to new collagen fibers and promote the normal orientation of collagen fibers

FINAL OUTCOME

✓ *Repair tissue:* Weaker and less elastic but functional. The structural, biomechanical, and functional properties of the healed skin often match those of intact skin.
✓ *Quality of healing:* Acceptable to ideal

into tropocollagen filaments. Tropocollagen is the fundamental unit of collagen (Herzog et al., 1994). Fibrils are the basic tensile load-bearing units of the tendon (Herzog et al., 1994). Every tendon is made up of three connective tissue sheaths holding the fascicules together (Sharma et al., 2005). The *paratenon* is a loose areolar connective tissue sheath, consisting of type I and type II collagen fibrils. Because it is the most superficial, it surrounds the tendon's epitenon sheath. The *epitenon* is a loose connective tissue sheath containing the vascular, lymphatic, and nerve supply to the tendon. This sheath surrounds all fascicles within the tendon. Finally, the *endotenon*, made of a thin reticular network of connective tissue, surrounds each fascicle.

Ligaments consist of collagen and elastin fibers. Their major function is to attach articulating bones together to provide joint stability and to guide joint movement (Frank et al., 1994; Woo et al., 2000; Frank, 2004). Their structures very much resemble those of a tendon, with fascicles, fibers, fibrils, subfibrils, microfibrils, and tropocollagen filaments (Fig. 3-3B). Each ligament is covered by a connective tissue sheath, called *epiligament,* that encloses neurovascular elements necessary for ligament survival and function. Just as for the tendon, fibrils are the tensile load-bearing units of ligaments. Table 3-4 lists the most common types of pathology affecting both tendons and ligaments. Tendon pathology falls under the generic name of *tendinopathy* or *strain injuries* (Clancy, 1990; Herzog et al., 1994; Almekinders et al., 1998; Khan et al., 1999; Sevier et al., 2000; Woo et al., 2000; Sharma et al., 2005; Carrilero et al., 2013). Pathologies caused to ligaments fall under the generic term *sprain* and range in severity from grade I to grade III (Frank et al., 1994; Woo et al., 2000; Frank, 2004; Carrilero et al., 2013). Table 3-5 presents an overview of the healing processes taking place in both tendon and ligament (Sevier et al., 2000; Woo et al., 2000; Sharma et al., 2005). These two tissues are relatively well vascularized via their respective epitenon and epiligament sheets, which bring blood vessels to them. As shown, their healing processes and final outcomes are very similar (Woo et al., 2000; Frank, 2004; Woo et al., 2004; Sharma et al., 2005).

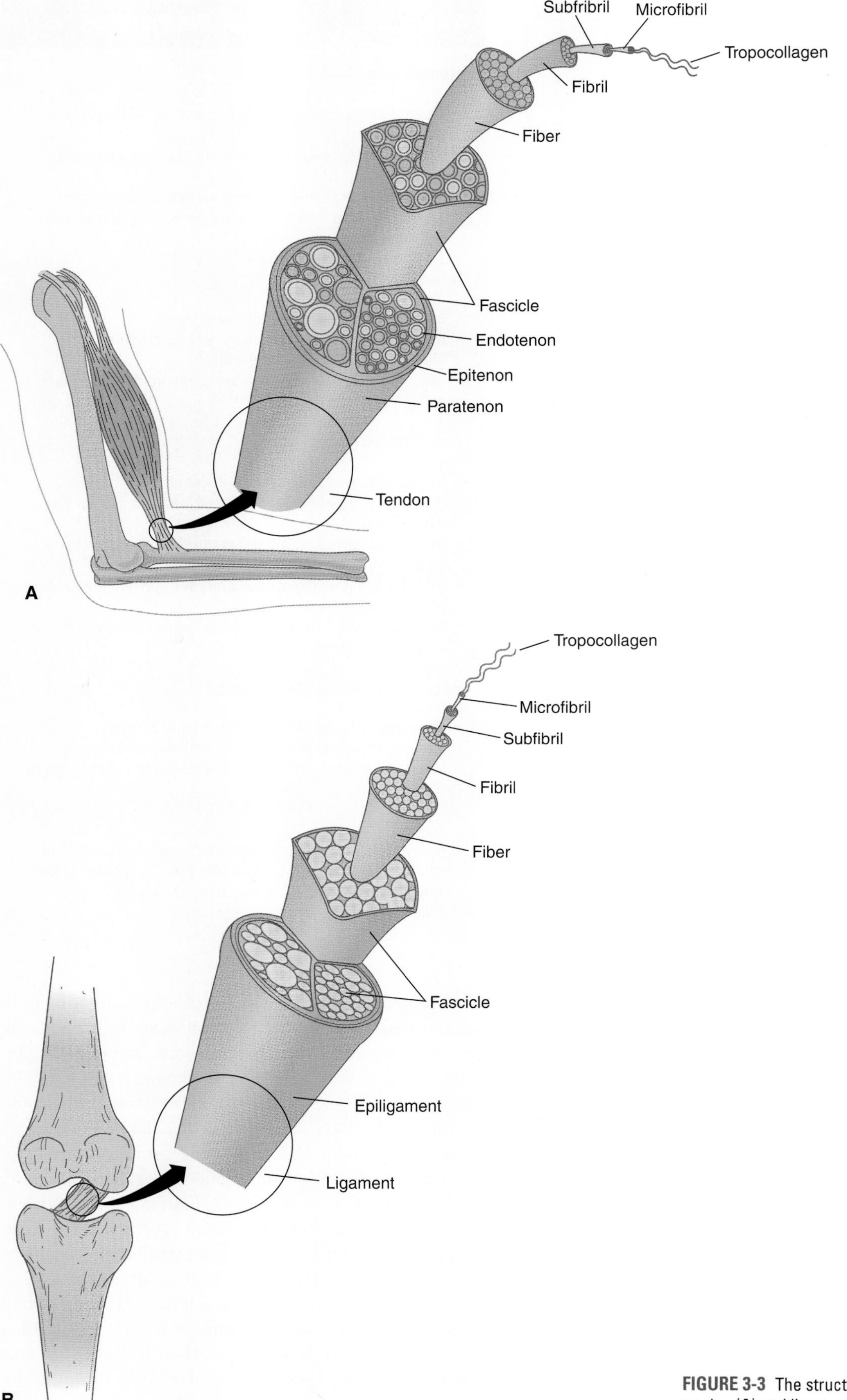

FIGURE 3-3 The structural hierarchy of a tendon (**A**) and ligament (**B**).

TABLE 3-4 TENDON AND LIGAMENT PATHOLOGY

Tendon		
Type	**Description**	**Severity**
Paratenonitis	Inflammation of the paratenon or tendon sheath. Peritendinitis and tenosynovitis are included in this category.	Grade I
Paratenonitis with tendinosis	Tendon degeneration with concomitant paratenon inflammation	Grade II
Tendinosis	Tendon degeneration without inflammation	Grade III
Tendinitis	Inflammation within the tendon	Grade IV
Tendon rupture	Complete rupture due to excessive tensile force	Grade V
Ligament		
Type	**Severity**	
Sprain	*Grade I:* Minor tearing without increase in translation of affected joint *Grade II:* Partial tearing with mild to moderate increased translation *Grade III:* Complete tear with marked increase in translation	

Following most pathologies, tendinous and ligamentous repair tissues form, whose structural, mechanical, and physiologic properties never match those of an intact tendon or ligament (Woo et al., 2000; Frank, 2004; Woo et al., 2004). Because tendons and ligaments are relatively well vascularized tissues, their quality of healing is usually minimal to acceptable.

V. ARTICULAR CARTILAGE

Articular cartilage is a complex structure lining the articular surfaces of diarthrodial joints. It is composed of water, collagen, proteoglycans, and chondrocytes. The articular or hyaline cartilage differs from the white and yellow fibrocartilages found in the intervertebral disks and the ears and larynx, respectively (Chen et al., 1999a,b; Farmer et al., 2001; Hayes et al., 2001; Buckwalter, 2002; Buckwalter et al., 2004; Mandelbaum et al., 2005). The major function of articular cartilage is to dampen the load imposed on the articular surfaces by distributing it within the subchondral bone and the cartilage itself. It also provides a smooth, low-friction surface while minimizing peak stress on the underlying subchondral bone (Dhawan et al., 2013). Figure 3-4 shows a cross-sectional view of a synovial articulation, revealing the articular or hyaline cartilage on the surface of the calcified cartilage layer on top of the subchondral bone. A very important anatomic consideration is the fact that articular cartilage, in comparison with all the other soft-tissues considered in this chapter, is *avascular* in nature. This aspect is crucial in relation to the capacity of the articular cartilage to repair itself or heal after injury or disease. Table 3-6 shows that pathology to articular cartilage, often resulting from impact or shearing force as well as overuse, causes damage to the cartilage matrix and chondral surfaces (Chen et al., 1999a,b; Hayes et al., 2001; Farmer et al., 2001; Buckwalter, 2002; Buckwalter et al., 2004; Mandelbaum et al., 2005; Dhawan et al., 2013). The Outerbridge classification is most widely used system for grading the severity of articular cartilage injuries. More recently, the International Cartilage Repair Society has modified this classification to a more comprehensive description and grading system

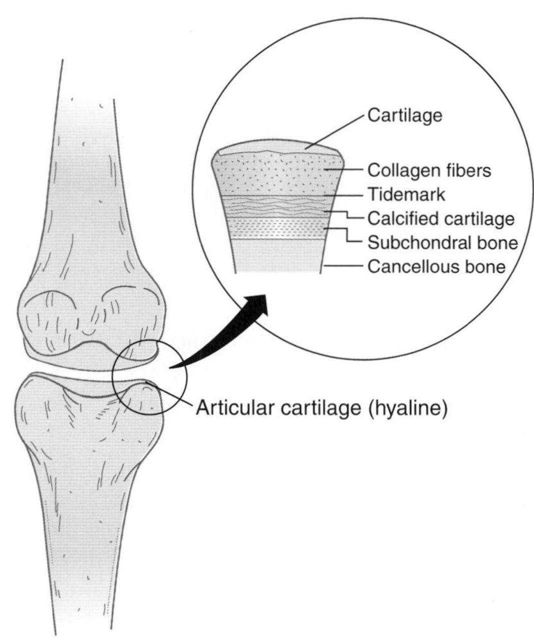

FIGURE 3-4 The structural hierarchy of articular cartilage.

TABLE 3-5	TENDON AND LIGAMENT HEALING PROCESS
Hemostasis/Inflammatory Phase	
Tendon	
• Blood-clotting cascade leads to the arrest of bleeding by coagulation • Fibrin clot establishes a provisional extracellular matrix • Inflammatory cells enter the site of injury • Phagocytosis of necrotic material • Tenocytes migrate to the injury site • Type III collagen synthesis is initiated	
Ligament	
• Blood clot formation • Retraction of disrupted ligament end	
Proliferative Phase	
Tendon	
• Deposition of repair tissue in the wound • Fibroblasts migrate to the wounded area and proliferate (fibroplasia) • Granulation tissue, which will mature into scar tissue, forms • Budding and growing of capillaries surrounding the repair zone (angiogenesis) • The wound site fills up with new collagen fibers, which are weak and randomly oriented	
Ligament	
• Granulation tissue, which will mature into scar tissue, forms • Budding and growing of capillaries surrounding the repair zone (angiogenesis) • Production of scar tissue by hypertrophic fibroblastic cells (fibroplasia) • Scar tissue becomes less disorganized as collagen fibers align with the long axis of the ligament • Collagen content abnormal (more type III in relation to type I, and more type V than normal)	
Remodeling/Maturation Phase	
Tendon/Ligament	
• *Consolidation stage:* Repair tissue changes from cellular to fibrous • Tenocytes and collagen fibers align in the direction of stress • Type I collagen synthesis occurs • *Maturation stage:* Fibrous tissue changes to scarlike tissue	
FINAL OUTCOME	
✓ *Repair tissue:* Weaker and less elastic but functional. The structural, biomechanical, and functional properties of the healed tendons and ligaments never match those of intact tendons or ligaments. ✓ *Quality of healing:* Minimal to acceptable	

(Dhawan et al., 2013). Because of the avascular nature of this tissue, the healing process of articular cartilage differs according to the type of pathology sustained (Chen et al., 1999a,b; Buckwalter, 2002; Buckwalter et al., 2004). Table 3-7 presents an overview of the healing process associated with articular cartilage damage. The full manifestation of the four classic healing phases will occur only if the pathology is severe enough to damage both the articular cartilage and the underlying deep full thickness of the osteochondral surfaces. The final common outcome in such severe cases is nonetheless disappointing because the repaired articular cartilage is made of a mixture of two cartilages (hyaline cartilage and fibrocartilage). This repaired cartilage, unfortunately, can only approximate the structural and mechanical properties of intact articular cartilage and, as a result, is very likely to be damaged again with normal activity.

VI. BONE

Bone is the hardest of all soft-tissues. Its connective tissue is made of organic, inorganic, and mineral elements (Childs, 2003; La Stayo et al., 2003; Phillips, 2005;

TABLE 3-6 ARTICULAR CARTILAGE PATHOLOGY

Type	Description
Microdamages to the cartilage matrix and cells	Microdamages to cartilage matrix; no damage to chondral surfaces
Microdamages to the superficial/partial-thickness chondral surfaces	Microdisruption of the articular surface without violation of the subchondral plates
Damages to the deep/full-thickness osteochondral surfaces	Damages to articulate surface, including the osteochondral bone surface
Severity	
Grade 0	Normal cartilage
Grade I	Superficial fissure
Grade II	Lesion to less than half cartilage depth
Grade III	Lesion to greater than half cartilage depth up to subchondral plate
Grade IV	Lesion through subchondral plate, exposing subchondral bone

TABLE 3-7 ARTICULAR CARTILAGE HEALING PROCESS

Hemostasis Phase

- Chondrocyte necrosis with minimal hemorrhagic response

Inflammatory Phase

- Minimal inflammation response
- Recruitment and proliferation of chondrocytelike cells begins

Proliferative Phase

- Minimal proliferative response
- Chondrocytelike cells progressively differentiate into chondroblasts, chondrocytes, and osteoblasts, which synthesize cartilage and bone matrices
- Limited angiogenesis

Remodeling/Maturation Phase

- Limited increase in metabolic and mitotic activities of surviving chondrocytes that border the defect or injury site
- Newly synthesized matrix remains on periphery and does not fill the lesion
- Osteochondral ossification occurs to heal the subchondral bone defect (several months)
- Unfortunately, subsequent degenerative changes occur within 6 months, including the fissuring of the articular surface

FINAL OUTCOME

✓ *Repair tissue:* Mixture of hyaline and fibrocartilage tissues at the wound site. Repair cartilage does not approximate the structure and function of intact articular cartilage.
✓ *Quality of healing:* Minimal to failed

LaRose et al., 2013). They have two important physiologic roles: to form blood cells (hematopoiesis) and store calcium (mineral homeostasis). They also provide protection for vital internal organs, support the body against the force of gravity, and act as a lever system for muscles during joint movements. Their major structural components are schematized in Figure 3-5. The proximal and distal epiphyses are made of spongy (cancellous) bone and the diaphysis of compact (cortical) bone. Fracture is the most common type of bone pathology (Table 3-8), and each fracture requires a particular conservative or surgical intervention (Childs, 2003; La Stayo et al., 2003; Phillips, 2005; LaRose et al., 2013). There is no standardized categorization with regard to the severity of bone fracture. The type, the location, and the damage caused by the fractured bone will dictate its severity. This textbook proposes a grading system from I to III, according to the complexity of the fracture. Bone tissue, because of its excellent vascularization, presents, with the skin, the best potential for healing. Table 3-9 shows an overview of the bone healing process. In most cases of fracture in relatively healthy individuals, the injured bone will repair itself with identical bone material, thus providing original structural, mechanical, and functional bone properties (Delforge, 2002d; Childs, 2003; La Stayo et al., 2003; Phillips, 2005). Its quality of healing is usually ideal.

VII. SKELETAL MUSCLE

Skeletal muscle is a type of tissue composed of contractile proteins (actin and myosin), regulatory proteins (tropomyosin and troponin), and a connective tissue matrix. Contraction of muscle fibers causes movement of the skeleton (Ehrhardt et al., 2005; Jarvinen et al., 2005; Carrilero et al., 2013). The basic function of skeletal muscles is to develop the force necessary to overcome gravity and to move the body through space. Figure 3-6 presents a cross-sectional view of a skeletal muscle. Each skeletal muscle splits into fascicles, which then split into muscle fibers, and into myofibrils. Each myofibril contains myosin (thick) and actin (thin) filaments that interact or slide with each other, causing the muscle to contract. Three connective tissue sheaths cover a skeletal muscle: epimysium, perimysium, and endomysium. The *epimysium* sheath

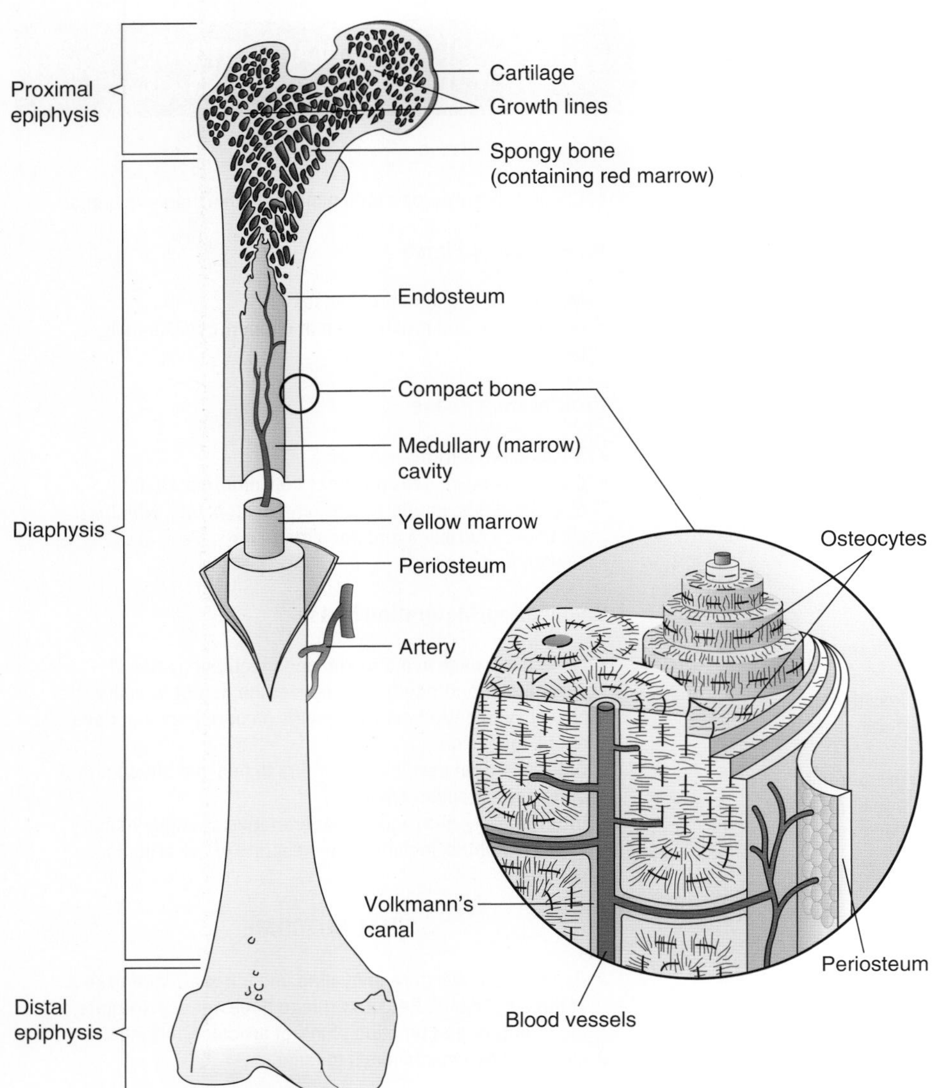

FIGURE 3-5 The structural hierarchy of a bone.

covers the outside of the muscle and plays a vital role in the transfer of muscular tension to the bone. The *perimysium* is a dense connective tissue sheath that provides a pathway for nerve fibers and blood vessels and surrounds each fascicle. The *endomysium* is a fine sheath covering each fiber. It carries the capillaries and the nerves that nourish and innervate each muscle fiber. The sarcolemma is a delicate plasma membrane, located directly underneath the endomysium, which covers or envelops every muscle fiber. It is through the sarcolemma that nerve impulses eventually reach each individual contractile unit. The sarcomere is the contractile unit of each skeletal muscle; it represents a band of thick (myosin) and thin (actin) filaments.

As shown in Table 3-10, two main types of pathologies affect skeletal muscles: strain and contusion (Leadbetter, 2001). Delayed-onset muscle soreness after vigorous exercise is more a transient, temporary syndrome than a disease. Myositis ossificans traumatica, on the other hand, is a pathologic condition resulting from inadequate healing of a previous injury, such as a contusion. Muscle strain injuries are graded as first, second, or third degree, depending on severity (Herzog et al., 1994; Ehrhardt et al., 2005; Jarvinen et al., 2005; Carrilero et al., 2013). In addition to skin and bone, skeletal muscle tissue, which is also well vascularized, presents the third-best potential for healing, as shown in Table 3-11. The final common outcome in most cases is a repaired muscle tissue that has structural, physiologic, and mechanical properties very similar to intact skeletal muscle. Its quality of healing is usually acceptable to ideal (Burnett et al., 2004; Wernig et al., 2005).

VIII. PERIPHERAL NERVE

Nerves arise from the spinal cord by rootlets and then converge to form a peripheral nerve (Burnett et al., 2004; Rummler et al., 2004; Wernig et al., 2005; Eby et al., 2013). Their role is to convey neural impulses from the central nervous system to tissues and organs (efferent nerves), and from organs and tissues back to the central

TABLE 3-8 BONE PATHOLOGY

Type	Description
Simple	Bone broken in one place, skin intact
Compound	Bone broken in one or more places, skin opened
Transverse	Fracture at angle to the long axis of bone
Greenstick	Fracture at only one side of bone
Comminuted	Part of the bone broken into many small pieces
Avulsion	Fracture resulting from tendon pull, following a powerful muscle contraction
Compression	Fracture resulting from two bones forced against each other (e.g., vertebrae)
Severity	
Grade I	Simple
Grade II	Compound
Grade III	Comminuted

TABLE 3-9 BONE HEALING PROCESS

Hemostasis/Inflammatory Phase

- Arrest of bleeding by the formation of a hematoma
- Hematoma provides an environment for the proliferation of osteogenic cells and granulation
- Formation necessary for collagen synthesis and new bone formation
- Proliferation of osteoblast at the fracture site

Proliferative Phase

- Angiogenesis leading to the formation of a soft callus around the repair site
- Development of fibrocartilaginous callus and formation of bone matrix at the fracture site
- Process of ossification (from soft to hard callus) is under way with the mineralization of the bone matrix

Remodeling/Maturation Phase

- Restoration of stability at the fracture site
- Resorption of existing bone by osteoclasts
- Deposition of new bone by osteoblasts (callus)
- The fractured bone resumes its normal structure, size, and shape

FINAL OUTCOME

✓ *Repair tissue:* Identical to intact bone
✓ *Quality of healing:* Ideal

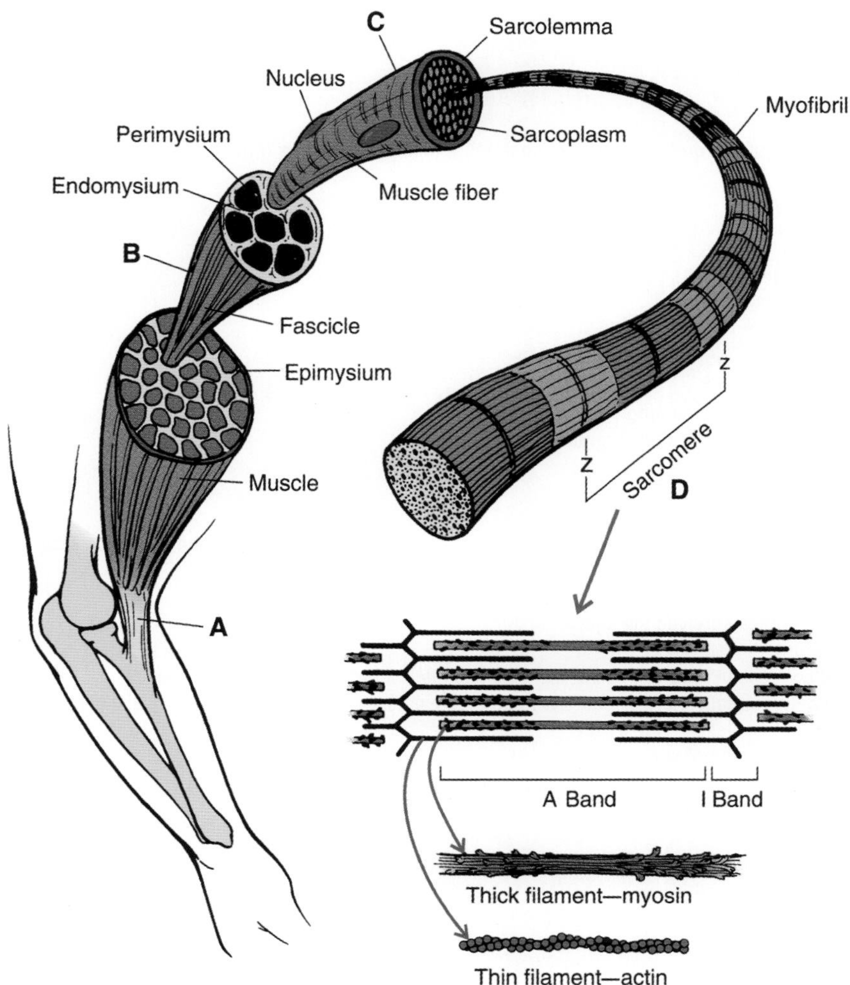

FIGURE 3-6 The structural hierarchy of a skeletal muscle. (Reprinted with permission from Hamill J (2008) Biomechanical Basis of Human Movement, 3rd ed. Lippincott Williams & Wilkins, Philadelphia.)

TABLE 3-10 SKELETAL MUSCLE PATHOLOGY

Type	Description
Strain	Muscle fiber tear
Contusion	Muscle is bruised, showing bleeding
Delayed muscle soreness	Muscle tenderness, stiffness, and soreness
Myositis ossificans traumatica	Muscle ossification
Severity of Strain	
First degree	Minimal tissue damage, minimal bleeding, rapid healing
Second degree	Moderate tissue damage, significant bleeding, partial tear most often at the myotendinous junction, some functional loss
Third degree	Severe tissue damage, massive bleeding, severe tear to rupture, severe functional loss

TABLE 3-11 SKELETAL MUSCLE HEALING PROCESS

Hemostasis Phase

- Blood clotting cascade leads the arrest of bleeding by coagulation
- Blood clotting results in the release of proinflammatory molecules
- Fibrin clot establishes a provisional extracellular matrix, which will serve as a platform for the subsequent crucial inflammatory phase

Inflammatory Phase

- Macrophages engage in proteolysis and phagocytosis of necrotic material
- Rupture and necrosis of myofibers
- Tear of sarcoplasmic membrane
- Contraction band seals off the membrane defect, forming a protective barrier so the torn membrane can be repaired
- Angiogenesis
- Bloodborne inflammatory cells access the site of injury
- Satellite cells begin the formation of new myofibers

Proliferative Phase

- Deposition of repair tissue in the wound
- Fibroblasts migrate to the wounded area and proliferate (fibroplasia)
- Granulation tissue, which will mature into scar tissue, forms
- Budding and growing of capillaries surrounding the repair zone (angiogenesis)
- The wound site fills up with new collagen fibers, which are weak and randomly oriented

Remodeling/Maturation Phase

- Concomitant activation of two supportive processes—regeneration of the disrupted myofiber and formation of connective tissue scar
- A balanced progression of both of these processes is necessary for optimal healing and recovery
- Satellite cells begin to proliferate, then differentiate into myoblasts to finally join together to form myotubes
- Myotubes then fuse with part of the myofibers that have survived the injury
- Regenerating parts of the myofibers grow to maturity
- Good vascularization of the injured muscle and successful regeneration of the intramuscular nerves are vital to this process
- Blood-derived fibrin and fibroblasts fill the gap between ruptured myofibers with connective tissue, forming a functionally disabling fibrous scar
- Large majority of muscle lesions heal without the formation of such a fibrous scar

FINAL OUTCOME

✓ *Repair tissue:* Mixture of regenerative and repair muscle fibers; partial to normal function
✓ *Quality of healing:* Acceptable to ideal

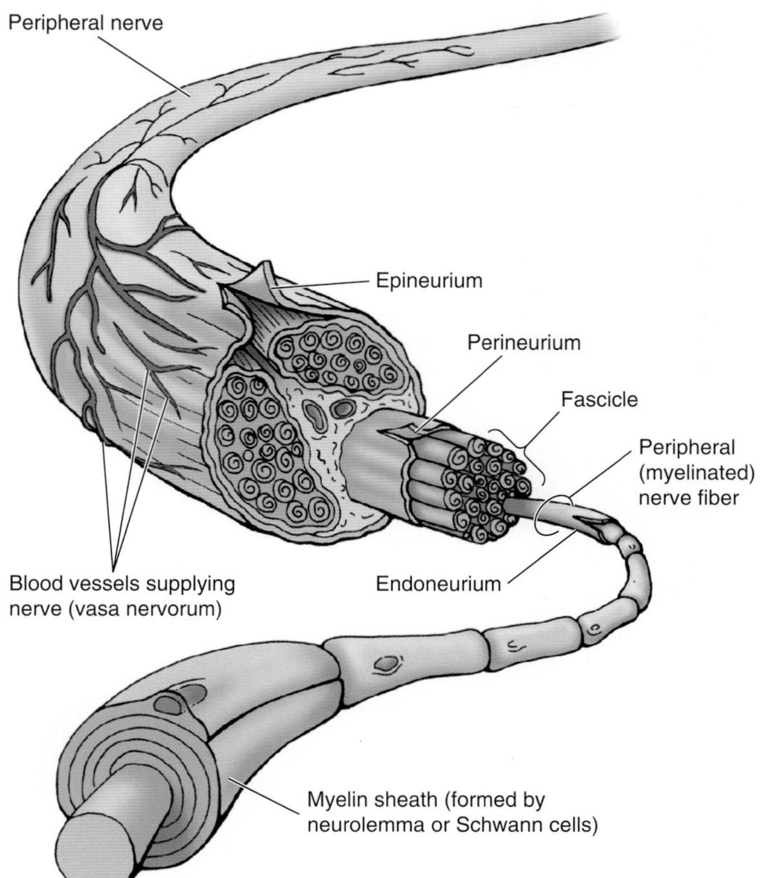

FIGURE 3-7 The structural hierarchy of a peripheral nerve.

nervous system (afferent nerves). Schematized in Figure 3-7 is a cross-sectional view of a peripheral nerve. Similar to skeletal muscle, tendon, and ligament, a peripheral nerve also splits into fascicles, which further split into nerve fibers. Each nerve fiber is made up of an axon and its covering, the myelin sheath (some nerve fibers are unmyelinated). Peripheral nerves are strong and resilient structures because of the support and protection they receive from their three connective tissue sheaths: epineurium, perineurium, and endoneurium. The *epineurium* is a thick sheath of loose connective tissue that surrounds all nerve fascicles forming the outermost covering of the peripheral nerve. It encloses blood and lymphatic vessels. The *perineurium* sheath encloses each nerve fascicle, providing an efficient barrier against penetration of the nerve fibers by foreign substances. The *endoneurium* is a delicate connective sheath that surrounds the axon and its myelin sheath. The axon is the fundamental unit of a peripheral nerve. Nerve impulses are generated because of axon depolarization. The *neurolemma* is formed by Schwann cells. It wraps isolated parts of the axon, playing a fundamental role in the process (speed) of nerve conduction velocity. Nerve injuries are categorized on the basis of two classification systems. In Seddon's classification (Table 3-12), peripheral nerve injuries are classified as neurapraxia, axonotmesis, and neurotmesis (Burnett et al., 2004; Eby et al., 2013). *Neurapraxia* is a functional injury, whereas axonotmesis and neurotmesis are anatomic and functional types of injuries. In Sunderland's classification, these are classified as first, second, third, fourth, and fifth degree injuries (Burnett et al., 2004; Rummler et al., 2004; Wernig et al., 2005; Eby et al., 2013). Severity ranges from neurapraxia (least severe) to neurotmesis (most severe). The healing process of peripheral nerves differs significantly from all the other soft-tissues, as illustrated in Table 3-13, in that none of the classic four phases of healing are present. In neurapraxia, the myelin sheath is damaged because of compression, and the axon remains intact. This type of nerve injury heals through a process of remyelination of the axon, which leads to full functional recovery. In axonotmesis and neurotmesis injuries, where the axon is damaged, healing occurs through the process of wallerian degeneration, followed by a combination of axonal and collateral regeneration. The final common outcome in axonotmesis is the formation of a repaired nerve, which may become functional if the nerve makes adequate connections with the target organ. In neurotmesis, the nerve may not heal unless expert neurosurgical intervention is available and adequate connection is established with its target tissue (Burnett et al., 2004; Wernig et al., 2005).

TABLE 3-12	PERIPHERAL NERVE PATHOLOGY
Type	**Description**
Neurapraxia	Axon and myelin intact; epineurium, perineurium, and endoneurium sheaths intact; damage to the myelin sheath only; full functional recovery expected
Axonotmesis	Axon and myelin disrupted, resulting in wallerian degeneration; epineurium, perineurium, and endoneurium sheaths intact; axon and myelin degeneration cause denervation; full to partial functional recovery expected
Neurotmesis	Axon and myelin completely disrupted; endoneurium sheath damaged; axon and myelin degeneration, causing denervation; partial functional recovery expected depending on the extent of damage to the endomysium; poor prognosis for recovery and usually requires urgent surgical intervention
Severity	
Grade I	Neurapraxia
Grade II	Axonotmesis
Grade III	Neurotmesis

TABLE 3-13	PERIPHERAL NERVE HEALING PROCESS

Grade I—Neurapraxia

- Focal demyelination caused by compression or stretch
- Transient disrupted focal nerve conduction
- Intact axons initiate remyelination through Schwann cell activity

FINAL OUTCOME

✓ *Repair tissue:* Identical to intact nerve
✓ *Quality of healing:* Ideal

Grades II and III—Axonotmesis and Neurotmesis

Wallerian Degeneration

- Degeneration process distal to the injured axon
- Removal of degenerated axonal/myelin debris within the endoneurial tubes
- Endoneurial tubes empty; ready to receive regenerating axons

Axonal Regeneration

- Regrowth of axons into empty endoneurial tubes

Collateral Regeneration

- Sprouting of empty endoneurial tubes into which new axons can grow
- All growing axons move toward their targets, attempting to reestablish neural contact and functional reinnervation
- Rate of axonal regeneration estimated to be 1 mm/day but may vary significantly according to the severity of the nerve injury
- Axonal and collateral regeneration is not synonymous with functional recovery

FINAL OUTCOME

✓ *Repair tissue:*
  - *Neurapraxia:* Focal remyelination leads to complete repair and full functional recovery
  - *Axonotmesis:* New tissue will be functional if adequate neural connection is made with target tissue
  - *Neurotmesis:* New tissue may be functional if there is proper neurosurgical intervention and adequate neural connection made by new axons with target tissue

✓ *Quality of healing:* Acceptable to minimal to failed

IX. VASCULATURE

The vascular system is made up of three basic tissues: artery, vein, and capillary. Blood, which carries nutrients, oxygen, and waste products to and from cells, circulates in our body through our arteries and veins. Adequate blood supply is critical to all living tissues. Figure 3-8 shows the structures of an artery and vein, which interact, one with the other, via the capillary bed. *Arteries* carry blood from the heart to the capillaries, where it is distributed to the target tissue. Each artery is made of three coats, or tunicae, named *adventitia, media,* and *intima*. A large part of the tunica media is made of smooth muscle that, under the influence of the autonomic nervous system, either constricts or dilates the arterial walls, thus narrowing or enlarging its lumen. The endothelium layer, within the tunica intima, plays a major role in the process of vascular repair. It is through the activation of endothelial cells that the growth or repair of blood vessels is initiated. *Veins,* on the other hand, return blood from the capillary beds to the heart. Like arteries, veins are also made of three coats, or tunicae, bearing identical names (see Fig. 3-8). Unlike arteries, veins are not wrapped with smooth muscle. Instead, they are filled with cuspid valves, which allow the blood to flow toward the heart. The *capillary bed* is the structure where the interchange of oxygen, nutrients, waste products, and other substances occurs. It is the junction between the arterioles and the venules. Following injury and disease to a soft-tissue, part of its vascular components (i.e., artery, veins, and capillaries) is damaged or destroyed, which leads to bleeding. For soft-tissue healing to occur, new blood vessels will need to grow back at the wound site and invade the newly formed repair tissue. Endothelial cells, which form the lining of the endothelium layer of both arteries and veins, play a key role as organizers and regulators of vascular healing. Damages to soft-tissues mentioned previously imply damages to their vascular system, because all of these tissues are well vascularized, with the exception of one—the articular cartilage. Table 3-14 shows common types of pathology affecting the peripheral vasculature.

TABLE 3-14 VASCULAR PATHOLOGY

Type	Description
Laceration	Tearing of vessels
Contusion	Bruising/crushing of vessels
Puncture	Hole in vessels
Transection	Cutting of vessels
Severity	
The severity of vascular injury is directly related to the amount of damaged tissues at the wound site. Transection of blood vessels is the most severe type of injury.	

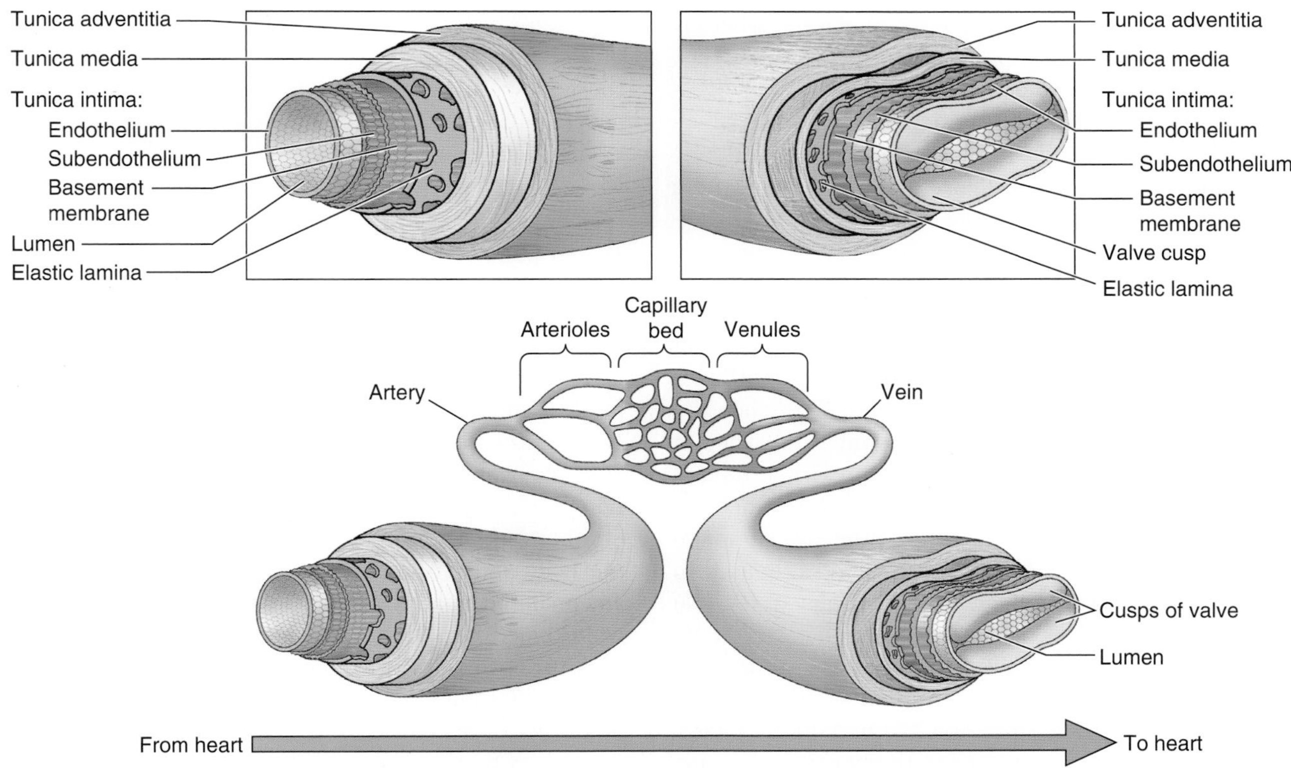

FIGURE 3-8 The structural hierarchy of the vasculature.

This textbook is concerned with vascular damages resulting primarily from injury or trauma to soft-tissues. The extent of vascular damages to arteries, veins, and capillary beds is proportional to the severity and size of the wound. Because some arterial, venous, and capillary damage occurs with soft-tissue pathology, new blood vessels (i.e., neovascularization) must grow into the wound space and eventually within the newly formed repair tissue to help it survive and function normally. The process of vascular repair or healing is concomitant with, and not independent of, the basic four healing phases described earlier. Research has shown that neovascularization occurs via two processes: angiogenesis and vasculogenesis (Tonnesen et al., 2000; Li et al., 2003; Bauer et al., 2005; Li et al., 2005; Walsh, 2007). *Angiogenesis* is defined as the growth of new blood vessels from preexisting ones (Walsh, 2007). Integral to successful wound repair, angiogenesis involves sprouting of wound-edge capillaries followed by their invasion into the site of damage. After a few days, a microvascular network is apparent throughout the wound that provides nutrients and oxygen to the growing tissues and aids in the formation of the provisional wound matrix, also known as granulation tissue. It occurs when endothelial cells sprout from preexisting blood vessels, then migrate and proliferate to form a cord-like structure (Bauer et al., 2005; Li et al., 2005). In other words, angiogenesis is the process by which resident endothelial cells of the wound's adjacent mature vascular network proliferate, migrate, and remodel into neovessels, which grow into the initially vascular wound. Angiogenesis also occurs by microvascular growth, also known as splitting angiogenesis, whereby a mature vessel divides, or splits, to form two vessels. *Vasculogenesis* refers to de novo formation of blood vessels as a result of the differentiation of bone marrow–derived precursor cells (Bauer et al., 2005). Initially believed to occur only during fetal development, there is recent but limited evidence to suggest that vasculogenesis may occur also in adults and contribute to the neovascularization process following soft-tissue injury and disease. Table 3-15 presents an overview of the different steps associated with the phenomenon of neovascularization following soft-tissue injury (Bauer et al., 2005; Li et al., 2005). These steps are related to the process of angiogenesis, which is well established in the literature. Until more evidence is presented to support the role of vasculogenesis in the process of neovascularization, this textbook recognizes the role of angiogenesis as the key process. Endothelial cells, housed in the endothelial sheath of endothelium, play a key role in the process of angiogenesis. Angiogenesis is at its peak during the proliferative phase of healing, bringing more than adequate oxygen and nutrients to the granulation tissue. With the remodeling and maturation phase, angiogenesis ceases, with most of the new vessels going through atrophy and becoming nonfunctional. A few of these new vessels will form into arterioles, venules, and capillaries within the newly formed repair tissue, ensuring adequate blood supply.

TABLE 3-15	VASCULAR HEALING PROCESS
Hemostasis/Inflammatory Phase	
STEP 1: Initiation of angiogenesis through the release of angiogenic cytokines and growth factors, such as vascular endothelial growth factor, from platelets, monocytes, fibroblasts, and ruptured cells **STEP 2:** Activation of endothelial cells and disruption of the extracellular matrix **STEP 3:** • Proliferation and budding of activated endothelial cells outward through the vascular basement membrane—full angiogenesis • Capillary sprouts orient and migrate directionally toward the source of growth stimuli—the wound bed • Vascular tubes and loops are formed, making immature arteriovenous tubules • Formation of granulation tissue at wound site	
Proliferative Phase/Maturation Phase	
• Maturation of new tubules with recruitment of smooth muscle cells to form a covering around the newly formed capillary • Formation of matured vascular network (capillary, arterioles, and venules at the wound site) • Blood flows to these newly formed vessels to irrigate the newly formed or repaired tissue • Large majority of newly formed vessels atrophy and eventually disappear	
FINAL OUTCOME	
✓ *Repair tissue:* Normal blood vessels ✓ *Quality of healing:* Ideal	

X. LYMPHATIC SYSTEM

Soft-tissue pathology often causes damage to the lymphatic system (Key, 2012). Fluid accumulation, or edema, is a common aspect of tissue damage and results from local vasodilation, increased vascular permeability, and/or damage to lymphatic vessels. Lymph is a clear fluid that contains lymphocytes (white blood cells) that fight infection and the growth of tumors. Lymph vessels are part of a network of thin tubes that help lymph flow through the body and return to the bloodstream. Lymph nodes are small, beanlike structures that filter lymph and store white blood cells that help fight infection and disease. There are two types of lymphedema. *Primary lymphedema* is caused by abnormal development of the lymph system. *Secondary lymphedema,* on the other hand, is caused by damage to the lymph system because of injury, trauma, or disease. *Lymphangiogenesis* is the formation of new lymphatic vessels from preexisting ones. Its process is under tight regulation by a plethora of events similar to angiogenesis.

XI. THE BOTTOM LINE

- The innate capacity of the body to heal itself is remarkable but, unfortunately, often limited and imperfect.
- The healing process of soft-tissues rest on four overlapping phases: hemostasis, inflammatory, proliferative, and remodeling/maturation.
- Hemostasis is the body's emergency response to pathology, of which the aim is to prevent hemorrhaging.
- The inflammatory phase is the crucial phase of healing—without it, no tissue healing is possible.
- The proliferative phase is concerned with the formation of new and immature repair tissues.
- Remodeling/maturation is concerned with the alignment and strength of the new repair tissues.
- Tissue healing occurs via regeneration and repair mechanisms.
- Qualities of soft-tissue healing may be defined as ideal, acceptable, minimal, and failed.
- Skin, bone, and skeletal muscle have the best healing capacity because they are very well vascularized.
- EPAs are used to enhance the soft-tissue healing process by targeting its specific phases.

XII. CRITICAL THINKING QUESTIONS

Clarification: What is meant by soft-tissue pathology and tissue healing?

Assumptions: You assume that soft-tissue healing occurs primarily through repair rather than by regeneration. How do you justify making that assumption?

Reasons and evidence: The consensus is that the natural process of soft-tissue healing involves four distinctive, successive, and overlapping phases. What leads you to believe this?

Viewpoints or perspectives: You believe that although the quality of healing of soft-tissue pathology is rarely ideal, it is nonetheless beneficial to patients. How can you answer an objection to this viewpoint?

Implications and consequences: The various connective tissue sheaths found in many soft-tissues, such as tendon, skeletal muscle, and peripheral nerves, play important roles in the healing process. What does this statement imply?

About the question: Is there a close relationship between the vascularity of a soft-tissue and its capacity for healing? Why do you think I ask this question?

XIII. REFERENCES

Review Articles

Almekinders LC, Temple JD (1998) Etiology, diagnosis, and treatment of tendonitis: An analysis of the literature. Med Sci Sports Exerc, 30: 1183–1190

Bauer SM, Bauer RJ, Valazquez OC (2005) Angiogenesis, vasculogenesis, and induction of healing in chronic wounds. Vasc Endovascular Surg, 39: 293–306

Buckwalter JA (2002) Articular cartilage injuries. Clin Orthop Rel Res, 402: 21–37

Buckwalter JA, Brown TD (2004) Joint injury, repair and remodeling: Roles in post-traumatic osteoarthritis. Clin Orthop Rel Res, 423: 7–16

Burnett MG, Zager EL (2004) Pathophysiology and peripheral nerve injury: A brief review. Neurosurg Focus, 16: 1–7

Chen FS, Frenkel SR, Di Cesare PE (1999a) Repair of articular cartilage defects: Part I. Basic science of cartilage healing. Am J Orthop, 28: 31–33

Chen FS, Frenkel SR, Di Cesare PE (1999b) Repair of articular cartilage defects: Pat II. Treatment options. Am J Orthop, 28: 88–96

Childs SG (2003) Stimulators of bone healing. Orthop Nurs, 22: 421–428

Ehrhardt J, Morgan J (2005) Regenerative capacity of skeletal muscle. Curr Opin Neurol, 548–553

Farmer JM, Martin DF, Boles CA, Curl WW (2001) Chondral endosteochondral injuries: Diagnosis and management. Clin Sports Med, 20: 299–320

Frank CB (2004) Ligament structure, physiology and function. J Musculoskel Neuron Interact, 42: 199–201

Hayes DW, Brower RL, John KJ (2001) Articular cartilage: Anatomy, injury and repair. Clin Podiatr Med Surg, 18: 35–53

Harvey C (2005) Wound healing. Orthop Nurs, 24: 143–159

Hildebrand KA, Gallant-Behm CL, Kydd AS, Hart DA (2005) The basics of soft-tissue healing and general factors that influence such healing. Sports Med Arthrosc Rev, 13: 136–144

Jarvinen TAH, Jarvinen TLN, Kaariainen M, Kalimo H, Jarvinen M (2005) Muscle injury: Biology and treatment. Am J Sports Med, 33: 745–764

Johnstone CC, Farley A (2005) The physiological basics of wound healing. Nurs Stand, 19: 59–65

Khan KM, Cook JL, Bonar F, Harcourt P, Astrom M (1999) Histopathology of common tendinopathies: Update and implications for clinical management. Sports Med, 27: 393–406

La Stayo PC, Winters KM, Hardy M (2003) Fracture healing: Bone healing, fracture, management, and current concept to the hand. J Hand Ther, 16: 81–93

Li J, Zhang YP, Kirsner RS (2003) Angiogenesis in wound repair: Angiogenic growth factors and the extracellular matrix. Micros Res Tech, 60: 107–114

Li WW, Talcott KE, Zhai AW, Kriger EA, Li, VW (2005) The role of therapeutic angiogenesis in tissue repair and regeneration. Adv Skin Wound Care, 18: 491–500

Mandelbaum B, Waddell D (2005) Etiology and pathophysiology of osteoarthritis. Orthop, 28: S207–S214

Phillips AM (2005) Overview of the fracture healing cascade. Int J Care Inj, 365: S5–S7

Rummler LS, Gupta R (2004) Peripheral nerve repair: A review. Curr Opin Orthop, 15: 215–219

Sevier TL, Wilson JK, Helfst RH, Stover SA (2000) Tendinitis: A critical review. Crit Rev Phys Med Rehab Med, 12: 119–130

Sharma P, Maffulli N (2005) Tendon injury and tendinopathy: Healing and repair. J Bone Joint Surg (Am), 87: 187–202

Tonnesen MG, Feng X, Clark RA (2000) Angiogenesis in wound healing. J Investig Dermatol Symp Proc, 5: 40–46

Walsh DA (2007) Pathophysiological mechanisms of angiogenesis. Adv Clin Chem, 44: 187–221

Wernig A, Schafer R, Knauf U, Mundegar RR, Zweyer M, Hogemeier O, Martens UM, Zimmermann S (2005) On the regenerative capacity of human skeletal muscle. Artif Org, 29: 192–198

Whitney JD (2005) Overview: Acute and chronic wound. Nurs Clin North Am, 40: 191–205

Woo SLY, Debski RE, Zeminski J, Abramowitch SD, Chan Saw, SS, Fenwick JA (2000) Injury and repair of ligaments and tendons. Annu Rev Biomed Eng, 2: 83–118

Woo SLY, Thomas M, Chan Saw SS (2004) Contribution of biomechanics, orthopaedics and rehabilitation: The past, present and future. Surg J R Coll Surg Edinb Irel, 2: 125–136

Chapters of Textbooks

Carrilero LP, Hamming M, Nelson BJ, Taylor DC (2013) Muscle and tendon injury and repair. In: ASMS's Sports Medicine: A Comprehensive Review. O'Connor FG, Casa DJ, Davis BA, St-Pierre P, Sallis RE, Wilder RP (Eds). Lippincott Williams & Wilkins, Baltimore, pp 51–58

Clancy WG (1990) Tendon trauma and overuse injuries. In: Sports-Induced inflammation: Clinical and Basic Science Concepts. Leadbetter WB, Buckwalter JA, Gordon SL (Eds). American Academy of Orthopaedic Surgeons, Park Ridge, pp 609–618

Delforge G (2002a) Hemorrhage and hemostasis. In: Musculoskeletal Trauma: Implications for Sports Injury Management. Human Kinetics, Champaign, pp 21–26

Delforge G (2002b) Soft connective tissue repair. In: Musculoskeletal Trauma: Implications for Sports Injury Management. Human Kinetics, Champaign, pp 29–52

Delforge G (2002c) Therapeutic implications: Scar formation and maturation. In: Musculoskeletal Trauma: Implications for Sports Injury Management. Human Kinetics, Champaign, pp 87–114

Delforge G (2002d) Fracture healing. In: Musculoskeletal Trauma: Implications for Sports Injury Management. Human Kinetics, Champaign, pp 117–131

Denegar CR (2000) Tissue injury, inflammation and repair. In: Therapeutic Modalities for Athletic Injuries. Human Kinetics, Champaign, pp 28–45

Dhawan A, Karas V, Cole BJ (2013) Articular cartilage injury. In: ASMS's Sports Medicine: A Comprehensive Review. O'Connor FG, Casa DJ, Davis BA, St-Pierre P, Sallis RE, Wilder, RP (Eds). Lippincott Williams & Wilkins, Baltimore, pp 30–38

Eby SA, Jenkins JG, Buchner EJ (2013) Nerve injury. In: ASMS's Sports Medicine: A Comprehensive Review. O'Connor FG, Casa DJ, Davis BA, St-Pierre P, Sallis RE, Wilder RP (Eds). Lippincott Williams & Wilkins, Baltimore, pp 45–50

Frank CB, Shrive NG (1994) Ligament. In: Biomechanics of the Musculoskeletal System. Nigg BM, Herzog W (Eds). John Wiley & Sons, New York, pp 106–132

Herzog W (1994) Muscle. In: Biomechanics of the Musculoskeletal System. Nigg BM, Herzog W (Eds). John Wiley & Sons, New York, pp 154–190

Herzog W, Loitz B (1994) Tendon. In: Biomechanics of the Musculoskeletal System. Nigg BM, Herzog W (Eds). John Wiley & Sons, New York, pp 133–153

LaRose CR, Guanche CA (2013) Bone injury and fracture healing. In: ASMS's Sports Medicine: A Comprehensive Review. O'Connor FG, Casa DJ, Davis BA, St-Pierre P, Sallis RE, Wilder, RP (Eds). Lippincott Williams & Wilkins, Baltimore, pp 39–44

Leadbetter WB (2001) Soft-tissue athletic injury. In: Sports Injury: Mechanisms, Prevention and Treatment, 2nd ed. Fu FH, Stone DA (Eds). Lippincott Williams & Wilkins, Philadelphia, pp 839–888

Martinez-Hernandez A (1994) Repair, regeneration, and fibrosis. In: Pathology, 2nd ed. Rubin E, Farber JL (Eds). Lippincott Williams & Wilkins, Philadelphia, pp 31–64

Martinez-Hernandez A, Amenta PS (1990) Basic concepts in wound healing. In: Sports-Induced Inflammation. Leadbetter WB, Buckwalter JA, Gordon SL (Eds). American Academy of Orthopaedic Surgeons, Park Ridge, pp 132–178

Norris C (2004) Healing. In: Sports Injuries: Diagnosis and Management, 3rd ed. Norris C (ed). Butterworth-Heinemann, Edinburg, pp 29–60

Textbooks

Belanger AY (2009) Therapeutic Electrophysical Agents: Evidence Behind Practice. Lippincott Williams & Wilkins, Baltimore

Hess CT (2005) Clinical Guide: Wound Care, 5th ed. Lippincott Williams & Wilkins, Philadelphia

Key K (2012) A Simple Guide to Lymphatic System and Lymphatic Diseases. Kindle Edition. Amazon Digital Services

Leadbetter WB, Buckwalter JA, Gordon SL (1990) Sports-Induced Inflammation. American Academy of Orthopaedic Surgeons, Park Ridge, IL

O'Connor FG, Casa DJ, Davis BA, St-Pierre P, Sallis RE, Wilder RP (2013) ASMS's Sports Medicine: A Comprehensive Review. Lippincott Williams & Wilkins, Baltimore

Salter RB (1999) Textbook of Disorders and Injuries of the Musculoskeletal System, 3rd ed. Lippincott Williams & Wilkins, Baltimore

Sussman C, Bates-Jensen B (2012) Wound Care: A Collaborative Practice Manual for Health Professionals, 4th ed. Lippincott Williams & Wilkins, Baltimore

Chapter 4

Pain Following Soft-Tissue Pathology

Chapter Outline

Learning Objectives

Remembering: List and describe the categories and dimensions of pain.
Understanding: Compare the categories of pain and the various pain assessment tools.
Applying: Apply and score the VAS, SF-MPQ, and the PDI tools.
Analyzing: Explain the process of pain modulation.
Evaluating: Formulate the relationship between the different categories of pain and the various available pain therapies.
Creating: Discuss the future of pain management.

I. CONCEPT, DEFINITION, AND PUZZLE

The word *pain* comes from the Latin word *poena,* meaning "punishment." The concept of pain as a form of punishment for sinful activity is as old as humankind. For example, Christians long believed that pain during childbirth was a consequence of Eve's sin that was transferred to women directly by God (Parris, 2003). Pain is undoubtedly the main reason people seek treatment from health professionals (Turk et al., 2011). The International Association for the Study of Pain (IASP) defines *pain* as "an unpleasant sensory and emotional experience associated with actual or potential tissue damage, or described in terms of such damage" (www.iasp-pain.org). This definition highlights the duality of pain as a physiologic and psychological experience. Pain is a physiologic event within the body that depends on its subjective recognition or perception by the individual, or on the person's psychological awareness of it, in order to exist. It also highlights the fact that pain can arise from both actual and perceived tissue damage, meaning that pain can occur in the absence of tissue damage although the experience may be described as if the damage had occurred. The essence of the puzzle of pain, as stated by Melzack and Wall (2008), is that injury may occur without pain, and pain without injury. For Melzack and Wall, the critical question is this: Does the brain examine just a specific message ascending along specific fibers, or does it monitor *all* input and make a decision based on the activity in all fibers? The answer to this question represents the key to the puzzle of pain (Melzack et al., 2008).

II. THRESHOLD VERSUS TOLERANCE

Although no one likes pain, this unique sensation is nonetheless essential to our survival, serving as our body's final line of self-awareness and protection against pathology and harmful environments (Strong et al., 2002; Sikes, 2004). Pain usually helps tissue healing by preventing us from further aggravating our pathologic and painful conditions. It is important to distinguish between pain threshold and pain tolerance level. *Pain threshold* is defined as the minimum intensity of a stimulus that is perceived as painful (www.iasp-pain.org). *Pain tolerance level,* on the other hand, is defined as the maximum intensity of a pain-producing stimulus that a subject is willing to accept in a given situation (www.iasp-pain.org). A patient's pain tolerance threshold is most important in that it influences the decision about whether or not to seek treatment.

III. ACUTE VERSUS CHRONIC

Humans present with two major types of pain: acute and chronic (Turk et al., 2011). Table 4-1 presents key characteristics that distinguish acute pain from chronic pain. *Acute pain* practically always signals tissue damage, whereas chronic pain may or may not be associated with tissue damage. Acute pain serves a crucial biologic purpose, which is to protect the patient from further aggravating his or her pathology. *Chronic pain,* on the other hand, not only serves no biologic purpose but very often imposes several psychological, emotional, and socioeconomic stresses on the patient him- or herself, on his or her family, and on society in general (i.e., through the patient's lack of productivity).

TABLE 4-1 ACUTE VERSUS CHRONIC PAIN

Acute	Chronic
Sudden	Gradual
Related to tissue damages	Poorly related to tissue damages
Lasts days to weeks	Lasts months to years
Localized	Diffuse and/or referred
Limited to physical signs and symptoms	Often associated with psychological, emotional, or social distress
Serves biologic purpose (self-protection)	Serves no biologic purpose
Normal use of therapy	Often related to abusive use of therapy
Normal pain behavior	Often abnormal pain behavior
No pain-compounding factors	Pain response may be compounded by economic or legal problems
Good response to treatment	Poor/limited response to treatment
Encompasses the unpleasantness of past injury and the hope for future recovery	Encompasses a sense of helplessness, hopelessness, and meaningless
Monodisciplinary approach	Multidisciplinary approach

Acute pain, if not properly assessed, treated, and managed, can become chronic pain. Chronic pain, unfortunately, is prevalent and very often difficult to treat and manage.

IV. PAIN CATEGORIES

Before addressing the anatomic and physiologic aspect of pain, it is important to identify and briefly describe the major categories of pain in humans. Figure 4-1 illustrates the broad spectrum of pain, which revolves around four categories of pain: nociceptive, neuropathic, psychogenic, and carcinogenic (Derasari, 2003).

A. NOCICEPTIVE

Nociceptive pain is pain that arises from actual or threatened damage to nonneural tissue and is due to the activation of nociceptors (www.iasp-pain.org). This term

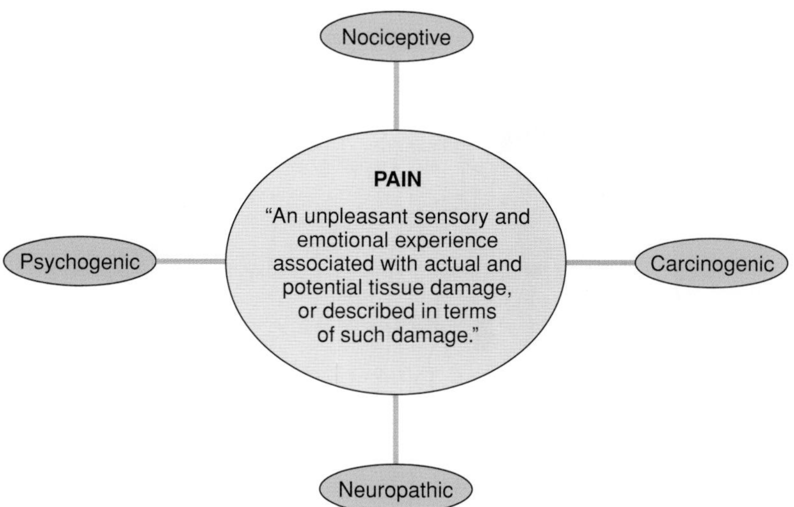

FIGURE 4-1 Categories of pain.

is designed to contrast with neuropathic pain (see later discussion). *Nociceptors* are high-threshold sensory receptors of the peripheral somatosensory nervous system that are capable of transducing and encoding noxious stimuli (www.iasp-pain.org). A *noxious stimulus* is a stimulus that is damaging or threatens damage to normal tissues. A *nociceptive stimulus* is an actual or potential tissue-damaging event transduced and encoded by nociceptors (www.iasp-pain.org). Nociceptive pain is subdivided into two categories: somatic and visceral.

1. Somatic

Somatic pain stems from the activation of nociceptors found in most body tissues, with the exception of neural tissue, which has none. Nociceptors, labeled as pain receptors, are mainly present in tissues such as skin, muscle, tendon, ligament, and bone. Somatic pain is the most prevalent category of pain and results primarily from pathologies caused by injuries, chronic diseases, and surgical interventions (i.e., postoperative pain). It is commonly described as normal pain because the sensation felt (pain) usually matches the noxious nature of the stimulus. For example, if one touches a very hot source or surface with a finger, a severe burning pain is perceived. This is a classic example of somatic pain. Somatic pain is the subcategory of nociceptive pain *most frequently* treated with electrophysical agents (EPAs).

2. Visceral

Visceral pain results from the activation of nociceptors found in the viscera (Derasari, 2003; Bielefeld et al., 2006). Disease, rather than injury, is the most common cause of such pain. Visceral pain is frequently perceived as referred pain, meaning that pain is perceived at some distance from the site of the affected organ. Referred visceral pain rests on a phenomenon called *viscerosomatic convergence* (Galea, 2002; Bielefeld et al., 2006). The reason for this convergence is the lack of a dedicated sensory pathway to the brain for information concerning the internal organs. It is proposed that sensory neurons from the viscera connect to the brain via a sensory pathway that carries information from the skin and muscles. As a result, the brain interprets the nociceptive input that originates from the diseased organs as also coming from these soft tissues. Angina is a perfect example of referred pain. Angina, a pain originating from the heart due to poor oxygen supply, is very often perceived as a pain in the left part of the chest and sometimes in the left arm and hand, which corresponds to the cutaneous segments supplied between the third cervical level (C3) and the fifth thoracic level (T5). Cardiac pain is thus referred to this cutaneous zone because the heart is derived from the mesoderm in the neck and upper thoracic area, with the result that nociceptive afferents from the heart enter the spinal cord through the dorsal roots C3–T5, rather than lower down (Galea, 2002). Visceral pain differs significantly from somatic pain in that it is a referred, diffuse, and poorly localized type of pain, often associated with strong psychological and emotional responses (Bielefeld et al., 2006). Not all viscera are sensitive to pain. For example, many diseases of the lungs, kidneys, and liver are painless until abnormal functioning becomes severe, whereas a relatively minor lesion in viscera such as the bladder, the stomach, or the ureters can produce excruciating pain. Visceral nociceptors are similar to those associated with somatic pain, in that they respond to mechanical (overstretching, distension) and chemical (inflammation) stimuli. Figure 4-2 illustrates pain locations commonly associated with several human viscera. This figure clearly shows the true referred nature of pain in many viscera—for example, heart pain felt in the left arm. Therapeutic EPAs are *rarely* used to modulate visceral pain.

B. NEUROPATHIC

Neuropathic pain is pain caused by a lesion or a disease of the somatosensory nervous system (Devor, 2006; www.iasp-pain.org). It is often characterized, especially when it has become chronic, by an array of abnormal painful sensations

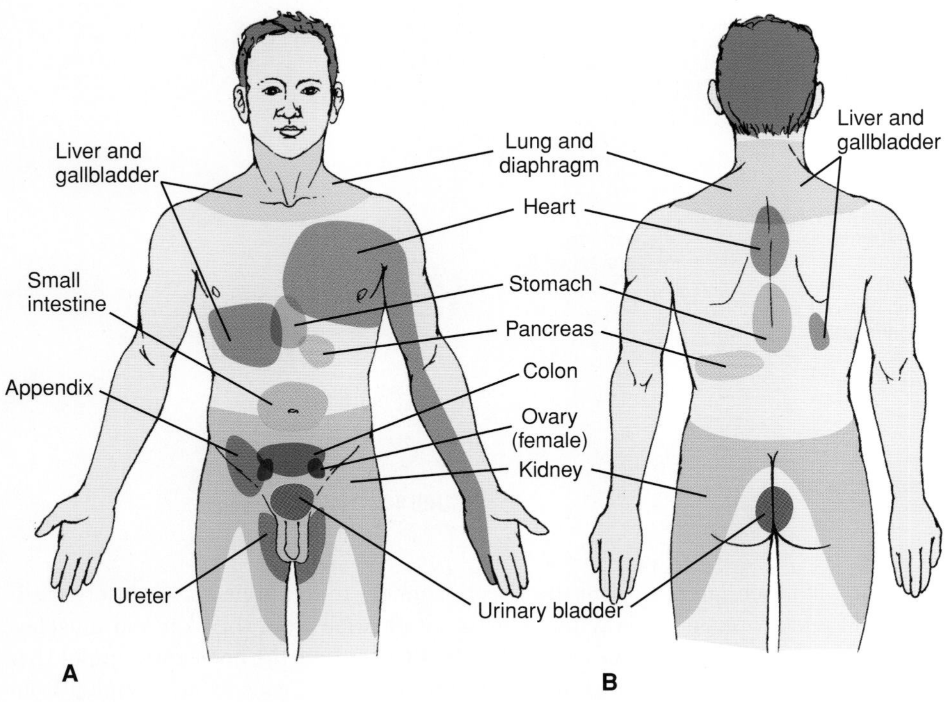

FIGURE 4-2 Visceral pain: anterior (**A**) and posterior (**B**) views of pain referred from viscera.

such as allodynia (pain due to a stimulus that does not normally provoke pain) and hyperalgesia (increase in pain from a stimulus that normally provokes pain). Neuropathic pain is subdivided into two categories: peripheral and central.

1. Peripheral

Peripheral pain results from the pathologic functioning of the peripheral nervous system—namely, sensory and motor nerves (Derasari, 2003; Devor, 2006). Injury and disease to peripheral nerves are common causes of such pain.

2. Central

Central pain relates to the pathologic functioning of the central nervous system—namely, the spinal cord, the medulla, the brainstem, and the brain (Derasari, 2003; Boivie, 2006). Disease is the common cause of such pain. Central pain may start almost immediately after occurrence of the malfunction, or it may be delayed for up to several years, as seen in many cases of stroke, multiple sclerosis, and Parkinson's disease. Therapeutic EPAs are *frequently* used to modulate peripheral pain. They are, however, *seldom* used to modulate central pain.

C. PSYCHOGENIC

As its name implies, psychogenic pain originates from nonorganic psychological sources (Flor et al., 2006). In a broad sense, it refers to pain complaints that are best understood in psychological rather than biomedical terms (Turk et al., 2011). For example, the origin of pain is assumed to be of psychogenic nature when pain complaints cannot be objectively confirmed, are judged to be disproportionate to objectively determined pathology, or are unresponsive to appropriate physical treatments (Flor et al., 2006). Psychogenic pain is complex in that it is frequently associated with emotional, cognitive, and behavioral responses (Flor et al., 2006). This type of pain is best managed with therapeutic interventions other than EPAs because it is caused by sources other than organic pathology. Its management is therefore *beyond* the use of therapeutic EPAs.

D. CARCINOGENIC

Carcinogenic pain, or cancer-related pain, is caused by the presence of cancerous pathology (nonmalignant or malignant tumor) anywhere in the body (Mantyh, 2006). This pain is unique in that in addition to often being severe, the pathology underlying this pain may also have a significant impact on both the quality of life and the survival of the patient (Mantyh, 2006). Coverage of carcinogenic pain is beyond the scope of this textbook because it is practically never treated using EPAs. When EPAs are used, it is more than often in the context of palliative care. Because of its severity, the effective management of carcinogenic pain requires the use of powerful pharmacologic (narcotic) painkillers delivered orally, or by means of patches or implanted pumps, in addition to radiotherapy and oncologic surgery.

V. PAIN DIMENSIONS

Pain is one of the most complex phenomena to study in the field of health care because of its strong subjective component and multidimensional aspect (Melzack et al., 2008; Turk et al., 2011). There is a consensus among researchers and clinicians that pain, as illustrated

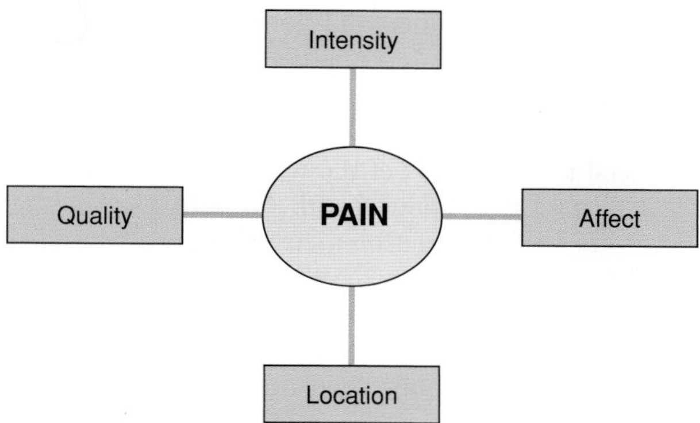

FIGURE 4-3 Dimensions of pain.

in Figure 4-3, is essentially a four-dimensional phenomenon that refers to its (1) intensity, (2) quality, (3) affect, and (4) location (see McMahon et al., 2006; Melzack et al., 2008; Turk et al., 2011; Jensen et al., 2011).

A. INTENSITY

The first dimension of pain relates to its intensity or evaluative aspect. Pain intensity may be defined as how much a person hurts (Jensen et al., 2011). Intensity is the dimension of pain most frequently assessed by clinicians. There is a linear trend between the level of pain intensity, treatment delivery, and discharge. In most cases, the more intense the pain, the more aggressive the treatment delivery and the less rapid the discharge. Inversely, the lesser the pain is, the less aggressive the treatment and the more rapid the patient's discharge.

B. QUALITY

The second dimension of pain concerns its quality or sensory aspect. It refers to the specific physiologic sensations associated with pain. It reveals how the person feels or senses the pain (e.g., burning, itching). This dimension is very informative in determining the cause or nature of pain.

C. AFFECT

The affective dimension of pain is very complex because it relates to the degree of emotional arousal—that is, the changes in action readiness caused by the sensory experience of pain (Jensen et al., 2011). Pain affect is a mental state triggered by an implicit or explicit appraisal of threat. In chronic pain, the emotional aspects can come to dominate the clinical picture (Jensen et al., 2011). This pain dimension is very important to clinicians and helps them determine the extent to which the patient is emotionally affected by his or her pain condition. This information can help to make a better choice of pain therapy—a psychological versus somatic approach, for example.

D. LOCATION

Pain location is defined as the perceived location(s) of pain sensation that patients experience on or in their bodies. Assessing pain location is important because the numbers of locations and sites indicated by the patients may be related to physical and psychological functioning (Jensen et al., 2011).

VI. THE EXPERIENCE OF SOMATIC PAIN

A. EXPERIENCING PAIN

Of all categories of pain (see Fig. 4-1), nociceptive somatic pain is by far the most prevalent. To focus on how patients experience such pain is central considering the fact that several EPAs are used to manage this type of pain. So how do patients experience or feel pain from soft-tissue pathology resulting from injury, trauma, surgical incision, or disease? The experience of pain can be described as a process, illustrated in Figure 4-4, made of five distinct and successive physiologic phases: transduction, peripheral transmission, modulation, central transmission, and perception (Dahl et al., 2006). The first phase, transduction, originates at the level of the nociceptors within soft tissues. The last phase, perception, takes place at the level of the cerebral cortex or brain. Before considering each of these pain

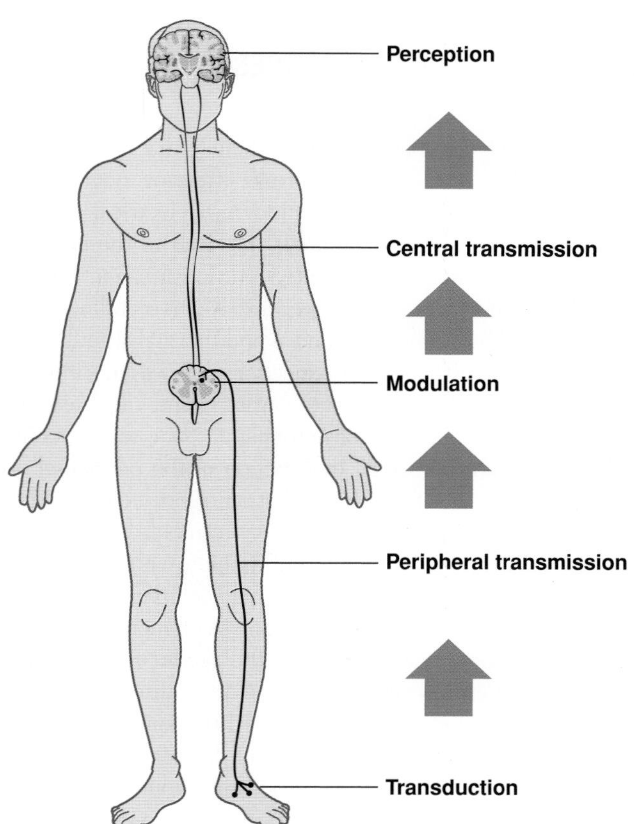

FIGURE 4-4 Physiologic phases leading to the experience of nociceptive pain.

perception phases, it is important to define, and further characterize the term *nociceptor,* because nociceptive pain begins with its activation. The word *nociceptor* is derived from the Latin word *nocere,* meaning "to harm." There is a consensus in the scientific literature to designate free nerve endings as pain receptors or nociceptors (McMahon et al., 2006). Most nociceptors have a high stimulation or activation threshold and, as a result, do not respond to everyday stimuli (Mense et al., 2001; Mense, 2003). This means, for example, that the nociceptors in our skin are not activated when we are sitting (compression of the gluteal skin area) or that muscle nociceptors are not activated when we are walking (muscle fiber contraction and elongation). Only when their activation thresholds are exceeded is a noxious stimulus message generated. Nociceptors respond to intense mechanical, thermal, and chemical stimuli capable of damaging the tissues surrounding them. Stimuli that activate nociceptors are called *noxious stimuli.* Cutaneous mechanoreceptors, such as Meissner and Pacinian corpuscles and Merkel tactile disks, provide us with the senses of touch, pressure, and vibration. Cutaneous thermoreceptors provide our thermal sense for detecting heat (Ruffini corpuscles) and cold (Krause end bulbs). It is important to always keep in mind that *pain threshold* is the level of noxious stimulus required to alert the individual to a potential threat to tissue. *Pain tolerance,* on the other hand, is a measure of how much pain a person can or will withstand (Sikes, 2004). Both pain threshold and pain tolerance can vary greatly between individuals.

B. PAIN PERCEPTION PROCESS

1. Transduction Phase

Transduction is the phase of converting energy (i.e., of mechanical, thermal, and chemical forms) affecting nociceptors at the site and around the wound into electrical energy, which generates action potentials that lead to the production of nerve impulses. As stated previously, pain initially develops in nociceptors, the specialized nerve endings that are activated by strong mechanical and thermal stimuli, and by chemical substances produced and released (inflammatory response) in the tissue at the wound site. Readers should note that in cases of neuropathic pain, transduction originates from the overall dysfunction of the peripheral or central system, not from the activation of nociceptors. This transduction, or conversion, of energy results from a change in the nociceptor's structural confirmation with the formation of pores (ionic channels) within its cell membrane. Ion exchanges in and out of the nociceptor's cell membrane generate action potentials leading to the production of nerve impulses, which will subsequently be transmitted along specialized sensory afferent fibers toward the spinal cord. For transduction to occur, the quantum of physical energy available at the tissue injury site must be large enough, or intense enough, to exceed the nociceptor's membrane threshold of activation, because most nociceptors are dormant—that is, they do not respond to light and moderate stimuli.

2. Peripheral Transmission Phase

The peripheral transmission phase includes the propagation or transmission of nerve impulses generated as a result of transduction from the nociceptors to the spinal cord. The terminal ends of the nociceptors—that is, the free nerve endings—connect with the spinal cord through two distinct afferent sensory nerve fibers: A-delta fibers and C fibers (Wright, 2002; Weisberg et al., 2006). The noxious message, now coded in nerve impulses, is transmitted to the dorsal horn of the spinal cord along these two afferent sensory fibers, whose cell body (neuron) resides in the dorsal root ganglia. Impulse transmission in the A-delta fibers occurs more rapidly than in the C fibers (approximately 15 m/s vs. 1 m/s) because the axons of the former are lightly myelinated (larger in diameter), whereas those of the latter are unmyelinated (smaller in diameter). A-delta fibers conduct mechanical as well as thermal noxious stimuli. C fibers, on the other hand, conduct mechanical, thermal, and chemical noxious stimuli. These nerve fibers are sustained by first-order neurons located in the dorsal root ganglia.

3. Modulation Phase

Modulation is the third phase leading to the experience of pain. This phase is characterized by a diminution, suppression, or amplification of pain (hence the word *modulation*). Research has shown that pain modulation occurs because of the action of nociceptive nerve impulses on the spinal gating system located in the dorsal horn of the spinal cord (McMahon et al., 2006). Because pain modulation reflects the action of our own thoughts and emotions, it is logical that the two remaining phases, central transmission (fourth phase) and perception (fifth phase), are addressed before the modulation phase.

4. Central Transmission Phase

Central transmission is the phase that encompasses the ascending transmission, or projection, of nociceptive nerve impulses, generated by the spinal pain-transmitting neurons, also referred to as T neurons, along the spinal cord and through the anterolateral system (ALS) and the lower brain and cortex areas (Dostrovsky et al., 2006). There are two types of T neurons: nociceptive specific (NS) and wide dynamic range (WDR), both located in the dorsal horn of the spinal cord (Rubertone et al., 2005). Both NS and WDR neurons are referred to as second-order neurons.

a. Anterolateral System

Nerve impulses are first transmitted centrally—from the spinal cord and up to the medulla, pons, and midbrain—along the axons of the anterior and lateral portions (or bundles) of the ALS. They are then transmitted through the ALS to various subcortical areas directly involved in the detection and modulation of pain, such as the thalamus, the reticular formation, the limbic system, the nucleus raphe magnus (NRM), and the periaquaductal gray matter (PAG) (see Galea, 2002; Dostrovsky et al., 2006).

The ALS is composed of several specific pathways or tracts: the spinothalamic tract, the spinoreticular tract, the spinomesencephalic tract, and the spinohypothalamic-limbic tract (Rubertone et al., 2005). These pathways serve different functions. The *spinothalamic tract* is the primary nociceptive pathway within the ALS, carrying discriminative aspects of pain such as type and location (Rubertone et al., 2005). The *spinoreticular tract* is linked to the motivational, emotional, and unpleasant aspects of pain (Rubertone et al., 2005). The *spinomesencephalic tract* is associated with the sensorimotor integration of pain, which includes motor reflex responses to pain (Rubertone et al., 2005). Finally, the *spinohypothalamic-limbic tract* is involved in the tissue autonomic responses following pain (Rubertone et al., 2005). Nociceptive message ascends along the ALS tracts, from the spinal cord, ipsilaterally and contralaterally, to a number of subcortical sites, bilaterally (Rubertone et al., 2005).

b. Subcortical and Cortical Neurons

After the long axons in the ALS system have made their synaptic contact with the subcortical neurons (third-order neurons), a new set of nerve impulses is then generated by those neurons along their own axons. These nerve impulses, carrying the nociceptive message from the subcortical areas, are finally transmitted to the cortical neurons (fourth-order neurons) for pain perception to finally occur. There is an enduring notion in the field of pain-related studies that the lateral thalamus is involved in discriminative pain (i.e., location and intensity), whereas the medial thalamus is linked to its motivational and emotional aspects (Dostrovsky et al., 2006).

5. Perception Phase

Perception—the fifth and final phase—relates first to the detection of pain and subsequently to the determination of its meaning and relevance (Bushnell et al., 2006). It is during this crucial phase that nociception (the organic aspect) finally becomes pain (the cognitive aspect). It is also during this phase that pain is processed. There is evidence from brain imaging and electrophysiologic studies that different cortical regions may be preferentially involved in different aspects of the complex experience of pain (Bushnell et al., 2006; Melzack et al., 2008). Most evidence suggests that the somatosensory cortex is more important for the perception of spatial and temporal features, such as the location and duration of pain, whereas the limbic and paralimbic regions are more important for the emotional and motivational aspects of pain (Bushnell et al., 2006). As soon as we perceive pain, we try to modulate it downward—that is, we attempt to diminish or suppress it by acting on it ourselves or by seeking the help of health practitioners. Unfortunately, pain can also be modulated up, or amplified, through a cascade of biologic mechanisms and cognitive/emotional responses.

VII. SOMATIC PAIN MODULATION

A. THE SPINAL GATING SYSTEM

There is a consensus in the literature that the modulation of pain requires peripheral or central interventions on the classic spinal pain gating system originally proposed by Melzack and Wall (1965, 2008). According to the gate control theory, pain is perceived only if the spinal gate is open. It thus follows that to suppress the perception of pain, we need therapeutic interventions designed to **close** this gate.

1. Dorsal Horn

Figure 4-5 is a simplified schematic representation of the revised gate control theory (Melzack et al., 2008). The

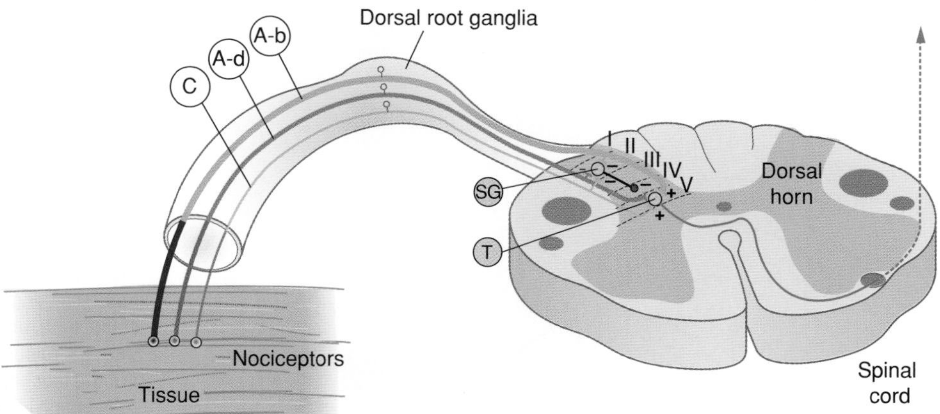

FIGURE 4-5 Schematic representation of the spinal gate control theory of pain. This gating system occurs at the level of the pain-transmitting neurons (T neurons [*T*]) and is under the powerful inhibitory action trigger by the neurons contained in the substantial gelatinosa (*SG*). Nociceptors buried in tissues are connected to the spinal cord through the larger A-beta (*A-b*) and A-delta (*A-d*) and smaller C afferent sensory (*C*) fibers, whose neurons (first order) are located in the dorsal root ganglia. These three fibers make synaptic contact with both the inhibitory neurons located in the SG and T neurons (second order) located deeper in the dorsal horn of the spinal cord.

figure shows a cross-sectional view of the spinal cord with its dorsal and ventral horns made of gray matter and surrounded by white matter. The gating system is located in the dorsal horn, more precisely within Rexed anatomic laminae II and V. The gating effect (open or closed) occurs after physiologic interaction between the inhibitory neurons located in the substantia gelatinosa (SG) and the pain-transmitting neurons (T) located deeper in the dorsal horns.

2. A and C Afferent Nerve Fibers

Figure 4-5 also illustrates a schematic representation of the neurologic connections between the gating system located in the spinal cord and the peripheral tissues containing nociceptors. Nociceptors are shown attached to the large-diameter A-beta (mechanoreceptors) fibers, smaller-diameter A-delta fibers, and smaller-diameter C fibers. These three afferent sensory fibers, whose cell bodies or neurons (first-order neurons) are located in the dorsal root ganglia, are shown making their excitatory (+) and inhibitory (–) synaptic contacts with the inhibitory neurons of the SG and the T neurons, respectively.

B. PERIPHERAL MODULATION

Based on the spinal gating mechanism, it logically follows that to close the gate (to suppress pain), a greater neural activity must be present in the *larger* A-beta mechanosensitive afferent fibers as opposed to the neural activity in the *smaller* A-delta and C fibers. A greater neural activity along the A-beta fibers will activate or excite (+) the inhibitory neurons within the SG. Those neurons will then induce a net and powerful inhibitory effect (–) on the pain-transmitting (T) neurons, causing the gate to close, thus suppressing pain. How can the suffering patient or the treating clinician provoke such a large neural activation along the A-beta fibers by acting on the periphery—that is, at the injury site and surrounding areas?

1. Mechanical Modulation

The patient can decrease some of his or her pain, as illustrated in Figure 4-6A, simply by rubbing or massaging the skin area over and around the site of the lesion. This action preferentially activates the mechanoreceptors attached to A-beta fibers, as illustrated by the larger

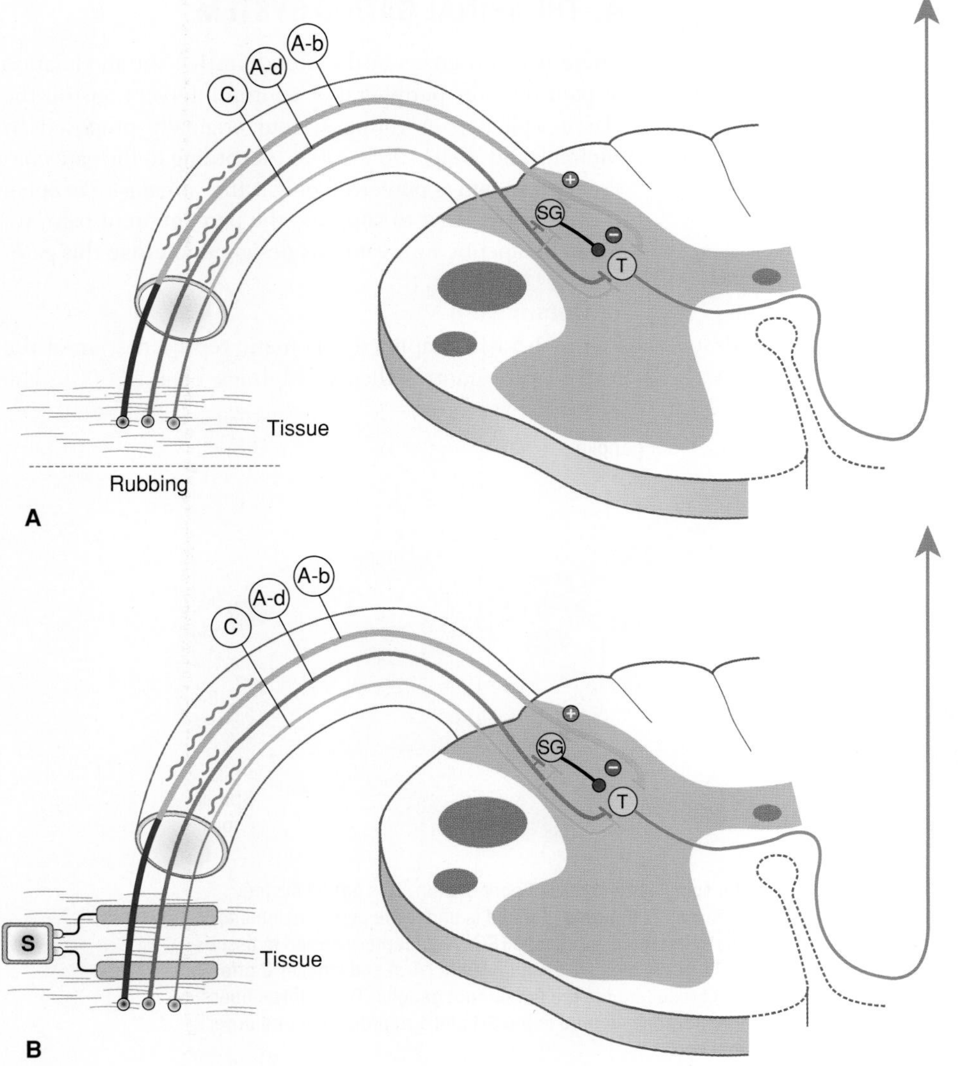

FIGURE 4-6 Schematic representation of two peripheral interventions resulting in the closing of the spinal gate, or pain suppression, through T neuron inhibition. Shown are the mechanical activation of A-beta (*A-b*) nerve fibers by rubbing the skin (**A**), and electrical activation of the same nerve fibers with an electrical stimulator (*S*) connected to a pair of surface electrodes (**B**). *C,* C afferent sensory fibers; *A-d,* A-delta nerve fibers; *SG,* substantial gelatinosa; *T,* T neurons.

number of nerve impulses (squiggles) along them, which leads to pain modulation. A common intervention of humans when experiencing relatively intense somatic pain is to immediately rub or massage the painful body area.

2. Electrical Modulation

Practitioners can also activate these mechanoreceptors by using a transcutaneous electrical nerve stimulator (TENS), as shown in Figure 4-6B. The purpose of this intervention is to electrically, yet preferentially, activate the A-beta fibers by using a pair of electrodes positioned over or around the painful area. The use of electrical stimulation to suppress pain falls into the broad field of electroanalgesia or TENS therapy (see Chapter 14).

C. CENTRAL MODULATION

Research has shown that the brain not only senses pain but can also exert a powerful suppressing or amplifying modulating effect on it (see McMahon et al., 2006; Melzack et al., 2008; Turk et al., 2011). Two supraspinal, or central pain-modulating, systems are described in the scientific literature: the descending endogenous opiate system (DEOS) and the cortical system (CS). Figure 4-7 offers a simplified schematic representation of these two central pain-modulating systems.

1. Descending Endogenous Opiate System

The DEOS exerts a *descending* (from central to spinal level) inhibitory effect (closing the gate) on the spinal pain-transmitting neurons (T neurons) by releasing endogenous opiate, morphinelike substances known as endorphins into the bloodstream and cerebrospinal fluid (Fig. 4-7A). The DEOS originates primarily from neurons located in the PAG and the NRM areas, both located in the midbrain. The powerful pain-relieving effect of opioids (from the term *opium,* the juice extracted from the poppy seeds of the *Papaver somniferum* plant) has been known for centuries in medicine (Melzack et al., 2008). Of all opioid drugs available, morphine is still the gold standard for opioid pain therapy (Schug et al., 2006). Scientific evidence supporting the existence of this endogenous opiate system in humans is found in the results of studies using naloxone, which is a powerful morphine antagonist (Fields et al., 2006).

2. Cortical System

The CS refers to the patient's cognitive (thoughts) and emotional responses to painful events and situations. As its name implies, this system is located in the brain cortex, above the DEOS, as illustrated in Figure 4-7B. Research has shown that the CS can express its inhibitory action on the spinal gate by directly activating (+) the DEOS, which then inhibits (−) pain by acting on the T neurons. In other words, activation of the CS triggers the excitation of the DEOS, which then closes the gate, thus suppressing pain. Research also suggests that the CS can also inhibit the spinal gating system simply with positive modification of the patient's thoughts and emotional response to pain (Sikes, 2004; Fields et al., 2006a). In other words, events and situations in which the patient is distracted (thoughts), takes control of himself or herself, or feels reassured that the pain is not that harmful (emotions) can lead to a decrease of pain (Sikes, 2004; Fields et al., 2006a). Practitioners should always remember that patients who focus on and worry about their pain too much (cognitive) or who express excessive anger, anxiety, frustration, and hopelessness about it (emotional) will inhibit their CS, which may further amplify their pain (Sikes, 2004; Craig, 2006; Fields et al., 2006a).

D. PAIN HYPERSENSITIVITY

The pain perception system described earlier, with its five physiologic phases, must be sensitive enough to detect harmful or nociceptive stimuli, thus warning us early enough so that we can protect ourselves from harmful situations. But what happens when our nociceptive pain system becomes hypersensitive to pain after injury and disease? A common clinical example is the increased perception of pain in the hours and days after the injury (acute pain) from nonnoxious stimuli (such as a light pressure) applied over and around the

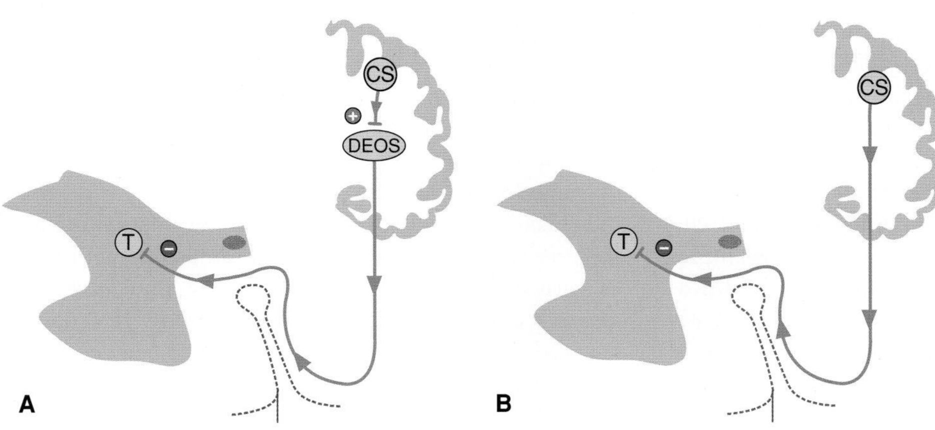

FIGURE 4-7 (**A**) Schematic representation of the descending endogenous pain system (*DEOS*) and (**B**) cortical system (*CS*). *T,* T neurons.

tissue injury site. Another example is this same increase in pain, this time months after the injury has occurred (chronic pain), with the application of the same non-noxious stimuli at the site of injury. Research has shown that this hypersensitivity arises because our pain system has increased its sensitivity to noxious stimuli when it relays pain messages to the brain (Mense, 2003; Meyer et al., 2006). Pain hypersensitivity takes two forms. First, pain thresholds are lowered so that stimuli that would normally not produce pain are now perceived as painful; this is known as allodynia. Second, pain responsiveness is increased so that noxious stimuli now produce an exaggerated pain; this is known as hyperalgesia. Pain hypersensitivity is an adaptive response that helps the healing process by ensuring minimal contact with, and minimal use of, the injured tissues until healing is complete. Pain hypersensitivity is thus present in acute pain after tissue injury and disease, and plays a useful role, although we may experience more pain as a result of it.

E. MECHANISMS BEHIND PAIN HYPERSENSITIVITY

Two mechanisms are proposed in the scientific literature to explain pain hypersensitivity: peripheral and central sensitization. *Sensitization* is defined as an increase responsiveness of nociceptive neurons to their normal input and/or recruitment of a response to normally subthreshold inputs (Mense, 2003; Meyer et al., 2006; www.iasp-pain.org).

1. Peripheral Sensitization

Peripheral sensitization takes place at the peripheral level—that is, at the level of the nociceptors buried in the tissues. It is defined as an increased responsiveness and reduced threshold of nociceptive neurons in the periphery to the stimulation of their receptive fields (Mense, 2003; www.iasp-pain.org). Peripheral sensitization is very closely associated with the presence of tissue inflammation, as discussed later. Peripheral or nociceptor sensitization arises primarily from the action of chemicals released (sensitizing chemical cocktail) by the damaged cells within and around the site of the lesion during the postinjury inflammatory phase. The release of these inflammatory chemicals, such as bradykinin, prostaglandins, substance P, and other chemicals, in the vicinity of the nociceptors triggers the process of pain transduction, the first physiologic phase in the experience of pain. Peripheral sensitization contributes to pain hypersensitivity found in both acute and chronic pain. For example, pain hypersensitivity to heat stimuli after sunburn, when the normally warm water from the shower feels burning hot over the sunburned area, is an example of acute pain hypersensitivity. In such a case, inflammatory chemicals directly activate the nociceptors until the damaged tissue has been repaired. Once the tissue has healed, acute pain theoretically ends. Because the duration of healing varies, the duration of acute pain will also vary, but the presence or absence of pain is usually tightly linked to the healing process. An example of peripheral sensitization in chronic pain is the presence of an ongoing degenerative disease that continually activates or sensitizes nociceptors, as in the case of arthritis, when chronic inflammation (rheumatoid arthritis) or increasing tissue damage (osteoarthritis) results in severe chronic pain when the affected joints are moved.

2. Central Sensitization

Central sensitization is one of the first steps in the transition from acute to chronic muscle pain (Mense, 2003). It is defined as an increased responsiveness of nociceptive neurons in the central nervous system or subthreshold afferent input (www.iasp-pain.org). Sometimes, pain persists long after the biologic healing process is completed or the amount of pain perceived by the patient is much greater than the detectable tissue damage would seem to suggest. This is chronic pain that extends beyond the normal course of injury or illness. This type of chronic pain may be explained by the central sensitization mechanism, which is characterized by an increase in the excitability of neurons within the spinal cord. An example may be pain hypersensitivity to mechanical stimuli (such as gently bending forward), felt for months after a mild episode of back pain, for which the patient has received appropriate and timely treatments. Central sensitization is believed to be a manifestation of abnormal sensory processing within the central nervous system (i.e., neural plasticity affecting synaptic organization). It is as if the pain system has increased its gain (i.e., becomes more sensitive) such that a previously normal innocuous stimulus is now perceived as a noxious stimulus despite the absence of tissue damage and peripheral sensitization. Neuroplastic changes (neuroplasticity), such as sprouting of spinal afferent fibers and the formation of new synaptic contacts within the dorsal horns, have to be considered important steps in the transition from acute to chronic pain (Mense, 2003). Central sensitization is responsible for tactile allodynia (when light brushing of the skin causes pain) and for the enlargement of the painful area (when pain extends to adjacent nonoriginally damaged tissues or areas); both responses often are observed in cases of chronic pain. Both peripheral and central sensitizations are observed in somatic, neuropathic, and visceral pain. The main conclusion reached by Mense (2003) on the topic of sensitization is the importance of abolishing acute pain as early and effectively as possible to prevent central nervous alterations (central sensitization). If a patient has already developed alterations in the nociceptive system, treatment will be difficult and long lasting because these alterations resolve very slowly.

VIII. PAIN ASSESSMENT TOOLS AND SCORING

Although pain is a highly personal and subjective phenomenon, it can nevertheless be assessed objectively with various standardized scales or tools for patients of all ages (see Turk and Melzack, 2011). Because pain is the primary symptom leading most people to seek the attention of health care providers, it is now considered by many clinicians as the fifth vital sign, together with heart rate, respiration rate, blood pressure, and body temperature. Like all sensations, pain is both a physiologic and a psychological phenomenon (Melzack et al., 2008). Like all of the other vital signs, it must be assessed so that adequate therapeutic interventions can be used to reduce or alleviate it. If the study of pain in people is to have a scientific foundation, it is essential to assess it (Melzack et al., 2008; Turk et al., 2011). The measurement of pain is important (1) to determine pain intensity, quality, and duration; (2) to aid in diagnosis; (3) to decide on appropriate therapy; and (4) to evaluate the relative effectiveness of different therapies (Katz et al., 1999; Melzack et al., 2006). Despite the subjective nature of pain, researchers and clinicians use several standardized and valid tools to assess pain in patients of all ages. To review all of them is beyond the scope of this chapter. Interested readers are directed to Turk and Melzack (2011) for a thorough review of pain assessment tools and scoring. The purpose of this section, therefore, is to present some of those assessment tools commonly used to assess the dimensions of somatic pain, in patients of all ages, following soft-tissue pathology. Figure 4-8 illustrates a framework related to the use of pain assessment tools to assess the intensity, quality, affect, location, and disability caused by somatic pain. As stated by Melzack and Katz (2006), to make the topic of pain a science, we must not only assess it but also measure or score it.

A. PAIN INTENSITY TOOLS

1. Infant Pain

Several tools are described in the literature to assess pain in infants, which includes newborns and preverbal children up to 3 years old (see Duhn et al., 2004; McGrath et al., 2006; Ruskin et al., 2011). There is a consensus among experts that the best way to assess pain in infants is to assess their behavioral responses to pain, such as vocalization, facial expressions, and body movements. Because EPAs are rarely used to treat infants, only a brief description of two of those pain assessment tools is presented: the Neonatal Facial Coding System (NFCS) and the Postoperative Pain Measure for Parents (PPMP).

a. Neonatal Facial Coding System

The NFCS requires that practitioners first observe the face of the infant experiencing pain and then compare and score the facial responses against a set of 10 standard facial actions or expressions. Coding or scoring may be done live at the infant's bedside or later in the office after videotaping the infant's face (Grunau et al., 1987; Grunau et al., 1998). Proper training is necessary before using this tool.

b. Postoperative Pain Measure for Parents

The PPMP is a checklist of 15 behavioral actions that the suffering infant may or may not display when visually observed for a given period of time (Chambers et al., 1996; Chambers et al., 2003). Parents and practitioners can use this tool at the infant's bedside. The PPMP is easy

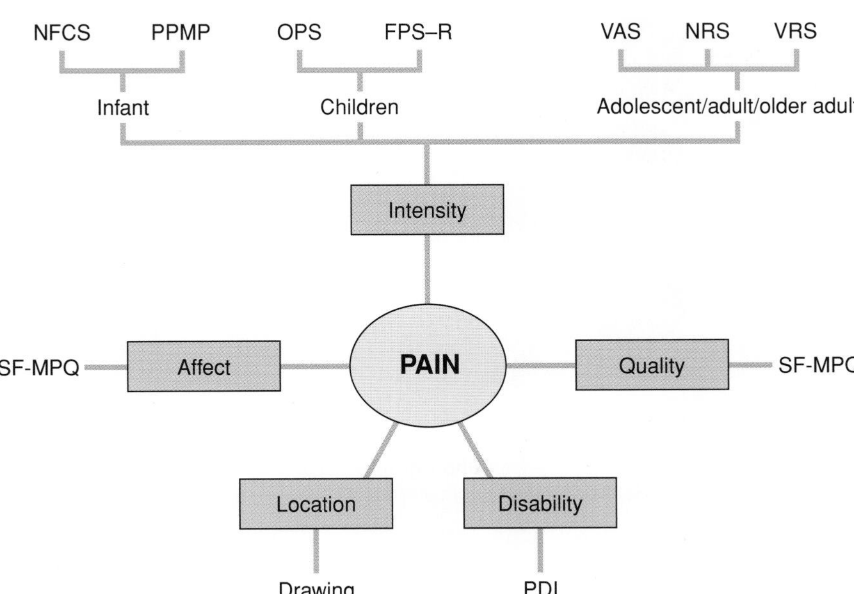

FIGURE 4-8 Framework of pain assessment tools. NFCS, Neonatal Facial Coding System; PPMP, Postoperative Pain Measure for Parents; OPS, Oucher Pain Scale (OPS); FPS–R, Faces Pain Scale–Revised; VAS, Visual Analogue Scale; NRS, Numerical Rating Scale; VRS, Verbal Rating Scale; SF-MPQ, Short-Form McGill Pain Questionnaire; PDI, Pain Disability Index.

to use and score and provides both parents and the treating clinicians with a valid assessment of the infant's pain. In summary, these two pain assessment tools measure the infant's overall pain intensity as perceived by the practitioner or parents. They do not assess and measure, as shown later, the other dimensions of pain.

2. Children

Measuring pain in children between 4 and 12 years of age presents a major challenge to practitioners (McGrath et al., 2006; Ruskin et al., 2011). Although using verbal self-report is considered the gold standard in human pain assessment, all self-reported measures have intrinsic limitations. According to McGrath and Unruh (2006), reliable and valid behavioral scales should be used instead of verbal self-reports to assess pain in children. Some of the most common tools to assess pain in children are the Oucher Pain Scale (OPS) and the Faces Pain Scale–Revised (FPS–R). These two tools make use of face-type scales because they are easy to understand by children, regardless of their cognitive and verbal development. Facial expressions are important, because they are relatively free of learning biases and represent the child's response to invasive and noxious events (Craig et al., 2006).

a. Oucher Pain Scale

The OPS, illustrated in Figure 4-9, is a variant of the many face scales described in the literature and is designed to

Oucher Pain Scale

Directives: The Oucher pain scale consists of two separate vertical scales; a numerical scale for older children and a photographic scale for younger children. *For younger children only.* Point to the face that shows how much you hurt now. *For older children only.* Put an X on the line beside the number that best represents how much you hurt now.

OUCHER

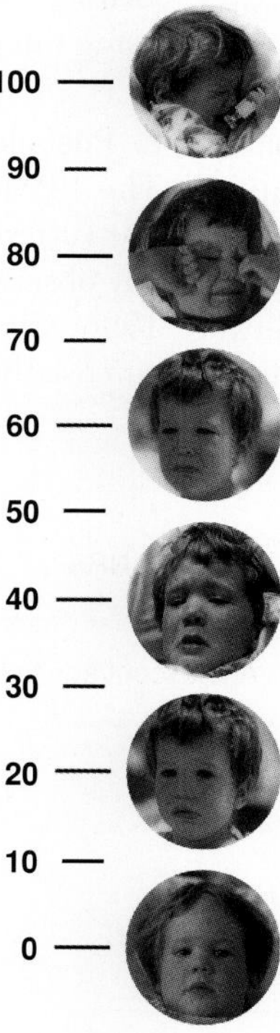

Scoring

Numerical Scale
Ranked from 0-100

Photographic Scale
Ranked for the bottom starting with 0-5

FIGURE 4-9 The Oucher Pain Scale. (From the Caucasian version of the Oucher, developed and copyrighted by Judith E. Beyer, PhD, RN. With permission.)

The Faces Pain Scale Revised

Directives: These faces show how much something can hurt. This face *(point to leftmost face)* shows no pain. The faces show more and more pain *(point to each from left to right)* up to this one *(point to the rightmost face)* – it shows very much pain. Please point to the face that shows how much you hurt *(right now)*.

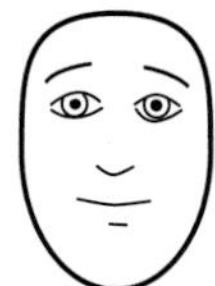
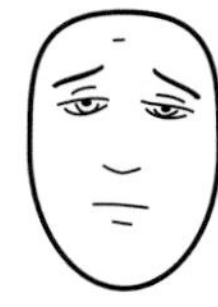
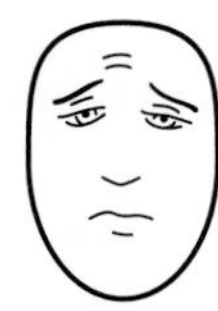
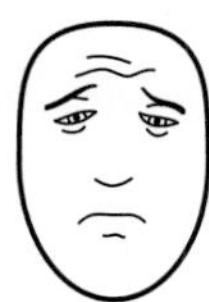
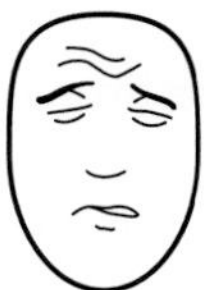
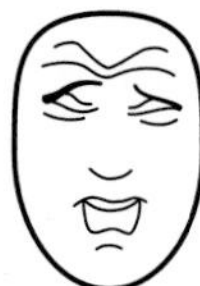

Scoring

Ranked from left to right, starting with 0, 2, 4, 6, 8, and 10

FIGURE 4-10 The Faces Pain Scale–Revised. (From Hicks CL, von Baever CL. Soafford P. van Koriaar I, Goodenough B. The Faces Pain Scale-Revised; Toward a common metric in pediatric pain measurement. Pain 2001; 93:173–183; scale adapted from Bieri D, Reeve R, Champion GD, Addicoat L, Ziegter J. The Faces Pain Scale for the self-assessment of the severity of pain experienced by children: Development, initial validation and preliminary investigation for ratio scale properties. Pain 1990:41:139–150. Used by permission of the International Association for the Study of Pain and the Pain Research Unit. Sydney Children's Hospital, Randwick, NSW 2031, Australia.)

measure pain intensity in children 4 to 12 years of age (Beyer, et al., 1992; Beyer et al., 1998; Beyer et al., 2005). The tool is displayed in a poster format and consists of a vertical numerical scale (0–100) on the left and six photographs of children in varying degrees of pain positioned vertically to the right. Variants of the Caucasian OPS version presented in this figure have been designed and validated for African American and Hispanic children (Beyer et al., 1998). The young child is asked to point, with a finger, to the face that best matches how much he or she is hurting now. The older child is asked to put an X on the line, beside the number, that best represents how much he or she is hurting now. The tool is scored using either a numerical (x/100) or photographic scale (x/5).

b. The Faces Pain Scale–Revised

The Faces Pain Scale–Revised, illustrated in Figure 4-10, also assesses the intensity of children's pain (Bieri et al., 1990). This tool consists of six faces expressing different levels of pain intensity, ranging from *no pain* to *very much pain* (Hicks et al., 2001). The child is ask to point, with his or her finger, to the picture that best describes his or her current level of pain. The examiner scores this tool by reporting the number associated with the photograph identified by the suffering child on a scale ranging from 0 to 10.

3. Adolescents, Adults, and Older Adults

Three pain assessment tools, each illustrated in Figure 4-11, are commonly used to assess pain intensity with adolescents, adults, and older adult patients: the Visual Analogue Scale (VAS), the 101-point Numerical Rating Scale (NRS-101), and the 5-point Verbal Rating Scale (VRS-5).

a. Visual Analogue Scale

The VAS is considered one of the most common and reliable pain intensity assessment tools (Turk et al., 2011). It is a self-reported measurement consisting of a horizontal line with extreme anchors of *no pain* to *as bad as it could be*. The horizontal line represents a continuum of pain intensity and is 10 cm long. The patient is asked to mark on the line the current level of pain. Caution is advised when using the VAS with older patients because increasing age has been associated with a higher frequency of incomplete or unscorable responses (Bird, 2005; Gagliese et al., 2006). Compared with younger adults, older people may be more reluctant to report painful stimuli. Moreover, pathologic conditions that are painful to young adults may in older patients produce only behavioral changes such as confusion, restlessness, aggression, anorexia, and fatigue (Gagliese et al., 2006). Pain intensity is scored on a scale of 10 (x/10). The larger the score, the more severe the pain.

b. The 101-Point Numerical Rating Scale

The NRS-101 tool is a numerical variant of the VAS that uses numbers from 0 to 100 (thus, 101 numbers to choose from) to rate the pain. The patient is asked to write a number that best represents the current level of pain. The more intense the pain, the larger the number. Scoring is expressed as a percentage.

Visual Analog Scale (VAS)

Directives: Using the vertical line, please mark on the line below your current level of pain.

No pain ________________________________ Pain as bad as it could be

The 101-point Numerical Rating Scale (NRS – 101)

Directives: Please indicate on the line below the number between 0 and 100 that best describes your pain now. A zero (0) means no pain, and a one hundred (100) means pain as bad as it could be. Please write only one number.

____

The 5-point Verbal Rating Scale (VRS – 5)

Directives: Please place an X beside the pain adjective below that best describes your current level of pain.

(_____) Mild

(_____) Discomforting

(_____) Distressing

(_____) Horrible

(_____) Excruciating

FIGURE 4-11 The Visual Analog Scale, the 101-Point Numerical Rating Scale, and the Five-Point Verbal Rating Scale. (Adapted from Jensen MP, Karoly P, Braver S (1986). The measurement of clinical pain intensity: A comparison of six methods. Pain, 27:117–126. With permission.)

c. The Five-Point Verbal Rating Scale

The VRS-5 is a verbal variant of both the VAS and the NRS-101 tools. It uses five adjectives describing pain, and each adjective is assigned a blank bracket. The patient is asked to select which of the five adjectives best represents the current level of pain by putting an X in its corresponding bracket. Practitioners can choose to verbalize these adjectives aloud to the patient, or ask the patient to read them off the sheet of paper, before making the selection. Scoring is on a scale of four (x/4).

B. PAIN QUALITY AND AFFECT TOOLS

One of the best and most commonly used tools to assess both the quality (sensory) and affect (affective) dimensions of pain is the Short-Form McGill Pain Questionnaire (SF-MPQ). This well-known pain assessment tool is a three-dimensional tool because it measures the quality and affect of pain as well as its intensity. This pain questionnaire, illustrated in Figure 4-12, is a shorter version of the original McGill Pain Questionnaire (MPQ) developed by Ronald Melzack (1975). Melzack developed the short form in an attempt to make his multidimensional tool more attractive to practitioners and patients who did not have the time to use the original MPQ version. The SF-MPQ takes approximately 10 minutes to administer after instructions are given to the patient. This self-report contains 11 sensory (quality) and 4 affective (affect) descriptors rated on a scale of 0 to 3. It also contains the VAS and the Present Pain Index (PPI), both of which measure the intensity of pain. The SF-MPQ is not intended to replace the original MPQ (Katz et al., 2011), but simply to provide an alternative when clinical time is a

Short Form McGill Pain Questionnaire (SF-MPQ)

Directives: *For the sensory and affective dimension only.* From the set of pain descriptors or words below, please select the words that best describe your pain now and for each of these words, rate the intensity of that particular quality of pain by putting a circle around the appropriate number. If a word does not correspond to your pain, please circle the number 0. *For the intensity dimension only.* VAS; Visual Analog Scale: Using a vertical line please mark, on the line below, your current level of pain. PPI; Present Pain Index: Please place an X beside the pain adjective below that best describes your current level of pain.

	None	Mild	Moderate	Severe
Sensory dimension:				
Throbbing	0	1	2	3
Shooting	0	1	2	3
Stabbing	0	1	2	3
Sharp	0	1	2	3
Cramping	0	1	2	3
Gnawing	0	1	2	3
Hot-Burning	0	1	2	3
Aching	0	1	2	3
Heavy	0	1	2	3
Tender	0	1	2	3
Splitting	0	1	2	3
Affective dimension:				
Tiring-Exhausting	0	1	2	3
Sickening	0	1	2	3
Fearful	0	1	2	3
Punishing-Cruel	0	1	2	3

Intensity dimension:

VAS No pain ________________________ Worst possible pain

PPI		
No pain	0	________
Mild	1	________
Discomforting	2	________
Distressing	3	________
Horrible	4	________
Excruciating	5	________

FIGURE 4-12 The Short-Form McGill Pain Questionnaire. (From Melzack R (1987) The Short-Form McGill Pain Questionnaire. Pain, 30: 191–197. With permission.)

concern. The patient is asked to fill the questionnaire by following the directives with regard to each section of the questionnaire. The questionnaire may be filled out by the patient independently or with the practitioner's assistance. This powerful assessment tool indicates which pain dimension is dominant in the patient, thus helping clinicians to determine the best type of pain therapy to use. For example, a pain profile with a high intensity score (VAS = 8.5), a high quality score (30/33), and a low affect score (3/12) is indicative of a pathology likely to benefit more from physical therapeutic interventions, such as the use of drugs, EPAs, and possibly surgery. Inversely, a pain profile revealing a high affective score (11/12), a low quality score (8/33), and a moderate intensity score (VAS = 5) will guide the clinician toward using a cognitive/psychological type of intervention instead of a physical intervention. Moreover, the patient's pain intensity score (VAS) and present pain intensity (PPI) score, if measured, would further help practitioners in gauging the acuity of pain and the potency of his or her therapeutic interventions. This textbook highly recommends the use of this tool, particularly in cases of chronic pain.

C. PAIN LOCATION TOOL

Assessing pain location is important in helping clinicians to better locate and diagnose the cause of pain and can aid in visualizing pain when it is felt at multiple sites on the body. Figure 4-13 shows four body diagrams that can be used by practitioners and patients to assess the location of pain. Practitioners score the number of sites and visually appreciate the pain areas in relation to the pain condition under treatment.

D. PAIN DISABILITY TOOL

One of the most important aspect of pain is the disability it may cause to the individual in his or her daily life (Tait et al., 1987; Jerome et al., 1991; Gauthier et al., 2011). The Pain Disability Index (PDI) tool shown in Figure 4-14 provides an insight into the degree to which pain interferes with normal functioning in a wide range of chronically painful conditions. The PDI assesses perceived disability related to seven dimensions of life: family and home responsibilities, recreation, social activity, occupation, sexual behavior, self-care (e.g., taking a shower, getting dressed, driving), and life support activity (e.g., eating, sleeping, breathing). Each dimension is rated by the patient on an 11-point scale (from 0 being no disability to 10 being total disability). The patient's overall score provides the treating clinician additional insight into what activities are more disabling to the patient because of his or her pain. This tool provides the patient's total disability index (total PDI score) and apprises the clinician of the nature of activities that most disable the patient (i.e. physical, self-care, or life supporting). The total disability index is marked out of 70 (x/70).

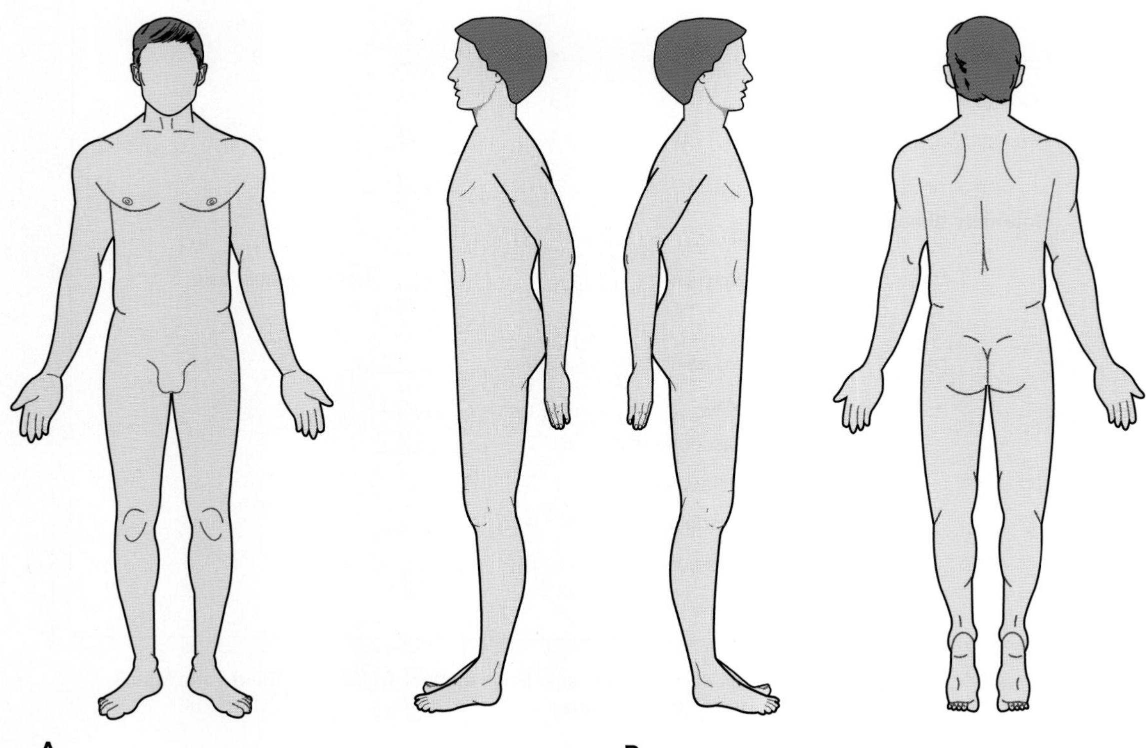

FIGURE 4-13 Assessment of pain location on the body. **A:** Front and left side view. **B:** Right side and back view.

Pain Disability Index

Directives: The rating scales below are designed to measure the degree to which several aspects of your life are presently disrupted by pain. In other words, we would like to know how much your pain is preventing you from doing what you would normally do, or from doing it as well as you normally would. Respond to each category by indicating the overall impact of pain in your life, not just when the pain is at its worst. For each of the seven categories of live activity listed, please circle the number on the scale, which describes the level of disability you typically experience. A score of 0 means no disability at all, and a score of 10 signifies that all of the activities in which you would normally be involved have been totally disrupted or prevented by your pain.

1. *Family/Home Responsibilities.* This category refers to activities related to the home or family. It includes chores and duties performed around the house (i.e., yard work) and errands or favors for other family members (i.e., driving the children to school).

0 1 2 3 4 5 6 7 8 9 10
No disability — Total disability

2. *Recreation.* This category includes hobbies, sports, and other similar leisure time activites.

0 1 2 3 4 5 6 7 8 9 10
No disability — Total disability

3. *Social Activity.* This category refers to activities, which involve participation with friends and acquaintances other than family members. It includes parties, theater, concerts, dining out, and other social functions.

0 1 2 3 4 5 6 7 8 9 10
No disability — Total disability

4. *Occupation.* This category refers to activities that are part of or directly related to one's job. This includes non-paying jobs as well, such as that of a housewife or volunteer worker.

0 1 2 3 4 5 6 7 8 9 10
No disability — Total disability

5. *Sexual Behavior.* This category refers to the frequency and quality of one's sex life.

0 1 2 3 4 5 6 7 8 9 10
No disability — Total disability

6. *Self-Care.* This category includes activities, which involve personal maintenance and independent daily living (i.e., taking a shower, driving, getting dressed, etc.).

0 1 2 3 4 5 6 7 8 9 10
No disability — Total disability

7. *Life-Support Activity.* This category refers to basic life supporting behaviors such as eating, sleeping, and breathing.

0 1 2 3 4 5 6 7 8 9 10
No disability — Total disability

FIGURE 4-14 The Pain Disability Index. (Adapted from Tait RC, Pollard CA, Margolis RB, Duckro PN, Krause SJ (1987). The pain disability index: Psychometric and validity data. Arch Phys Med Rehab, 68: 438–441. With permission.)

IX. ASSESSMENT OF PATIENTS WITH LIMITED ABILITY TO COMMUNICATE

The gold standard in the field of clinical pain assessment is the verbal self-report (Turk et al., 2011). There is a consensus that pain in patients with limited ability to communicate due, for example, to age, intellectual disability, head injury, and dementia, is often underassessed and undertreated (Hadjistavropoulos et al., 2011). The diverse causes that can lead to communication impairments could also affect the way pain is experienced and expressed. Newborns and infants, up to 3 years of age have very limited ability to communicate their pain. Consequently, facial tools (see Fig. 4-9), as opposed to self-report tools, are routinely used to assess pain in this patient's population. Many adolescents, adults, and older people with limited ability to communicate are still capable of self-reporting pain despite the presence of cognitive impairment (Hadjistavropoulos et al., 2011). Caution is advised, however, when using self-reports with such patients because the experience of pain may not be completely described. There has been a proliferation of tools designed to assess pain among older adults with limited communication due to various forms of dementia (Hadjistavropoulos et al., 2011). One such tool, presented in Figure 4-15, is the Pain Assessment Checklist for Seniors with Limited Ability to Communicate (PACSLAC) originally developed by Fuchs-Lacelle and Hadjistavropoulos (2004). Scoring the subscales is derived by counting the checkmarks in each column. A total pain score is generated by summing all four subscale totals (Hadjistavropoulos et al., 2011).

X. SPECTRUM OF PAIN MANAGEMENT

Health care systems, as well as all caregivers, have an obligation to provide comfort, and thus adequate pain management, to all suffering human beings. This is why pain is now considered as the fifth vital sign, requiring the same level of attention that caregivers provide when facing dysfunctions of the other classic vital signs (body temperature, blood pressure, heart rate, respiration rate). In other words, when pain is present, clinicians are obliged to respond accordingly and provide adequate management. To address all of the complexity of pain management is beyond the scope of this textbook. Clinicians must always keep in mind that the ultimate goal of any therapeutic intervention is to maximize the patient's quality of life by minimizing suffering while maximizing function and productivity. Although total abolishment of pain is a legitimate therapeutic goal, it is often an unrealistic one, especially when caregivers deal with chronic pain. Figure 4-16 presents an overview of the broad spectrum of therapeutic tools that clinicians use today to manage pain. This spectrum can be divided into two approaches: pharmacologic and nonpharmacologic. It is very important to always keep in mind that pain management is based on the severity of pain perceived by the patient, not on the extent of biologic damages caused to his or her body (Melzack et al., 2008).

A. PHARMACOLOGIC APPROACH

No one will dispute that the most common therapeutic strategy to manage pain is pharmacotherapy or the use of drugs (Unruh, 2002; Wright et al., 2002; Katz et al., 2005; Melzack et al., 2008). This approach involves the use of nonopioid, opioid, and adjuvant drugs. The nonpharmacologic approach, on the other hand, rest on the use of several therapies, including EPAs.

1. Nonopioid Drugs

Nonopioid drugs include analgesic agents and nonsteroidal anti-inflammatory drugs (NSAIDs). These drugs are routinely used by patients themselves (e.g., over-the-counter drugs such as acetaminophen [Tylenol] and ibuprofen [Advil]) and by treating physicians (e.g., prescription drugs such as celecoxib [Celebrex] and diclofenac sodium [Voltaren]) to manage mild to moderate acute or chronic pain. If used for a relatively prolonged period, these drugs can cause side effects such as gastric irritation and ulceration depending on their strength. What constitutes a prolonged period varies between patients and ranges usually from a few weeks to a few months.

2. Opioid Drugs

Therapeutic narcotics are used when nonopioid drugs fail to provide adequate pain relief. Opioid drugs, such as hydromorphone (Dilaudid) and oxycodone (OxyContin), are strictly under a physician's control. Narcotics have a much greater pain-suppressing potency than nonopioid drugs and may give rise to physical dependence and addiction. If taken for a relatively long period, opioids can cause serious side effects such as nausea, dizziness, sleepiness, and, in some cases, physical dependence and addiction.

3. Adjuvant Drugs

The term *adjuvant* implies that a drug is given in addition to, or in conjunction with, an opioid drug to potentiate its analgesic effect. Adjuvant drugs are also under the control of physicians. They are designed primarily to treat disorders or symptoms often associated with pain, such as depression (antidepressants), epilepsy (anticonvulsants), anxiety (antianxiolytics), and muscle spasm and spasticity (muscle relaxants). Studies have shown that the use of these adjuvant drugs, in combination with opioid drugs, can lead to significantly greater pain relief, especially in severe cases of chronic pain (Curatolo et al., 2002; Unruh, 2002; Wright et al., 2002).

Pain Assessment Checklist for Seniors with Limited Ability to Communicate (PACSLAC)

Indicate with a checkmark, which of the items on the PACSLAC occurred uring the period of interest. Scoring the sub-scales is derived by counting the checkmarks in each column. To generate a total pain sum all sub-scale totals.

Facial expression	Present
Grimacing	
Sad look	
Tighter face	
Dirty look	
Change in eyes (squinting, dull, bright, increased eye movements)	
Frowning	
Pain expression	
Grim face	
Clenching teeth	
Wincing	
Open mouth	
Creasing forehead	
Screwing up nose	

Activity/body movement	Present
Fidgeting	
Pulling away	
Flinching	
Restless	
Pacing	
Wandering	
Trying to leave	
Refusing to move	
Thrashing	
Decreased activity	
Refusing medications	
Moving slow	
Impulsive behaviors (Repeat movements)	
Uncooperative/resistance to care	
Guarding sore area	
Touching/holding sore area	
Limping	
Clenching fist	
Going into fetal position	
Stiff/rigid	

Social/personality/mood	Present
Physical aggression (e.g. pushing people and/or objects, scratching others, hitting others, striking, kicking).	
Verbal aggression	
Not wanting to be touched	
Not allowing people near	
Angry/mad	
Throwing things	
Increased confusion	
Anxious	
Upset	
Agitated	
Cranky/irritable	
Frustrated	

Other (physiological changes/eating sleeping changes/vocal behaviors)	Present
Pale face	
Flushed, red face	
Teary eyed	
Sweating	
Shaking/trembling	
Cold clammy	
Changes in sleep routine (please circle 1 or 2) 1) Decreased sleep 2) Increased sleep during the day	
Changes in appetite (please circle 1 or 2) 1) Decreased appetite 2) Increased appetite	
Screaming/yelling	
Calling out (i.e. for help)	
Crying	
A specific sound of vocalization for pain "ow," "ouch"	
Moaning and groaning	
Mumbling	
Grunting	
Total checklist score	

FIGURE 4-15 The pain assessment checklist for seniors with limited ability to communicate—PACSLAC. (The PACSLAC may not be reproduced without permission. For permission to reproduce the PACSLAC contact the worldwide copyright holders (thomas.hadjistavropoulos@uregina.ca). The developers of the PACSLAC specifically disclaim any and all liability arising directly or indirectly from use or application of the PACSLAC. Use of the PACSLAC may not be appropriate for some patients and the PACSLAC is not a substitute for a thorough assessment of the patient by a qualified health professional. The PACSLAC (like all other related observational tools for seniors with dementia) is a screening tool and not a definitive indicator of pain. As such, sometimes it may incorrectly signal the presence of pain and, other times, it may fail to identify pain. As such, it should be used by qualified health care staff within the context of their broader knowledge and examination of the patient.)

B. NONPHARMACOLOGIC APPROACH

The pharmacologic treatment of pain is not a panacea, and when it fails to provide adequate relief, other pain management approaches are used (Fig. 4-16).

1. Physical Therapies and Electrophysical Agents

A common therapeutic approach for most painful conditions is the combination of physical therapies (e.g., therapeutic exercises, mobilizations, manipulations) mixed with EPAs. The use of EPAs covered in this textbook presents a

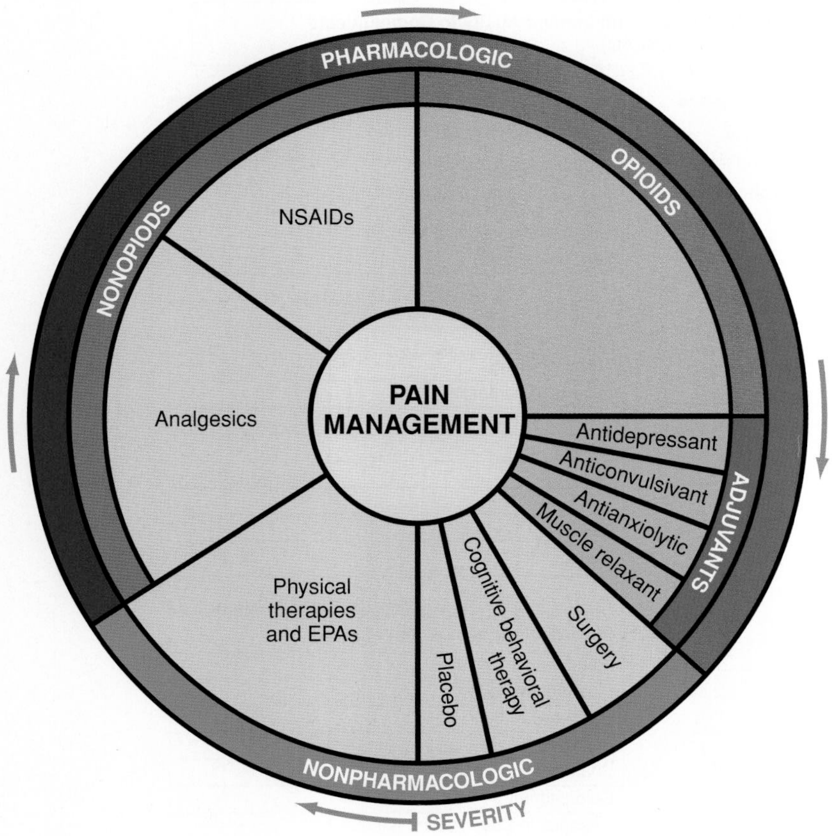

FIGURE 4-16 Spectrum of pain management. EPAs, electrophysical agents.

major advantage over the pharmacologic approach, in that they have no known side effects. However, EPAs also have a major disadvantage, in that their pain-suppressing potency is often weaker and shorter-lasting than that associated with drugs. Because the pain-suppressing potency of some EPAs, like the use of TENS, may be comparable with that of nonopioid drugs, EPAs appear to be an adequate alternative to nonopioid drugs for the management of mild to moderate postsurgical, somatic, and neuropathic pain (Barlas et al., 2006). This is especially true for those patients whose health status (specifically, their stomach, liver, and kidney function) is compromised and can be further aggravated by taking nonopioid drugs. EPAs are also appealing to those health-conscious patients whose preference is to use pain therapeutics with minimal side effects first, leaving the door open to take drugs later if necessary. This approach, combined with the use of nonopioid drugs, is frequently used for the management of light to moderate pain.

2. Surgery

When pain increases in severity and becomes chronic, surgery becomes a therapeutic option. Because of its highly invasive and potentially life-threatening nature, surgery is usually restricted to cases where the other therapies have failed to cure the organic pathology or failed to provide adequate pain relief. The aim of surgery is to repair pathologic tissues and organs and often involves partial or total ablation of such tissues. For obvious reasons, pharmacotherapy is always used postsurgically to alleviate surgical pain. Acceptable long-term control of pain is rarely achieved by surgery (Melzack et al., 2008).

3. Cognitive Behavioral Therapy

When pain has become chronic and characterized by a strong psychogenic component, psychotherapy, in the form of cognitive behavioral therapy, can be of significant help to those patients whose chronic pain has led them to present significant psychological and emotional distress, leaving them unable to experience adequate pain relief or to adequately cope with their pain. The concept behind this therapy relates to the way that patients think about things affecting how they feel emotionally. This therapy focuses on present thinking, behavior, and communication rather than on past experiences and is oriented toward problem solving. Psychotherapy may be the first choice of treatment for those patients who have refused drugs and who just cannot get adequate pain relief by using them. It may also be the treatment of choice for those patients suffering from chronic pain who have had enough of the side effects caused by their medications. Psychotherapeutic and cognitive interventions are used primarily in cases of severe chronic organic and nonorganic pain.

4. Placebo Therapy

The field of pain management cannot end without touching on the important and controversial topic of placebo analgesia, because, in some circumstances, placebo treatments can be as effective as real treatment to suppress pain (Roche, 2002; Fields et al., 2006b). Among all symptoms related to pathologies, pain appears to be the most common symptom known to respond to placebo therapy (Roche, 2002). Some believe that the word *placebo* is derived from the Latin verb *placere,* meaning "to please," whereas others believe it comes from the Latin stem *placebit,* meaning "it will please" (Roche, 2002; Fields et al., 2006b). Regardless of its source, common to the origin of this word is its pleasing aspect for the patient. The meaning of placebo analgesia is the patient's expectation of effectiveness of the therapeutic intervention that he or she is receiving (Fields et al., 2006b). There is a body of evidence to suggest that the hope for pain relief and the suggestion that such a relief will come are critical parameters in the generation of placebo analgesia (Fields et al., 2006b). Placebo analgesia may be seen as a demonstration of the body's natural tendency to reduce pain—a demonstration that is activated by psychological mechanisms such as conditioning and expectancy (Roche, 2002). Placebo analgesia is therapeutically desirable. It is a pain-suppressing response that can be triggered by positive verbal expectations and motivational attitudes and the reduction of anxiety and stress. Placebo analgesia is closely associated with the management of pain using psychotherapy. Opposite to a placebo response is the nocebo response. *Nocebo* is the patient's expectation that his or her treatment is ineffective or that it will make the pain worse (Fields et al., 2006b). Two meta-analyses conducted by Hrobjartsson and Gotzsche (2001, 2004) have shown little evidence to support the claim that when placebo therapies had a positive therapeutic response, it was for the continuous management of pain, thus giving support to the concept of placebo analgesia. Research has shown that both placebo and nocebo responses can significantly affect the outcome of pain therapy. Just as the placebo effect works by making the patient believe that he or she will get better, the nocebo effect can serve to make the patient worse. If the patient expects pain relief, he or she will present a placebo analgesia response regardless of whether a real treatment, a placebo treatment, or no treatment is administered. In contrast, if the patient expects that no relief will be obtained or that the pain may get worse, then a nocebo response will manifest itself. In closing, it is very important to remind clinicians one more time that the ultimate goal of pain management is not to try to abolish pain at all costs but, rather, to maximize the patient's quality of life, function, and productivity by minimizing it.

C. OVERLAPPING PAIN THERAPIES

The spectrum of pain therapies (Fig. 4-16) is linked to the severity of pain experienced by the patient. The proposed action mechanisms behind each of these therapies are listed in Table 4-2. Practically speaking, the management of mild to moderate acute pain often begins with physical therapies mixed with EPAs (e.g., thermotherapy, cryotherapy, TENS) and may include nonopioid drugs. If pain increases in severity and duration to become severe and chronic, then opioid drugs, with or without adjuvant drugs, are introduced in the pain management plan. If this severe and chronic pain is determined to be related to tissue damage, whether it be nociceptive (somatic, visceral) or carcinogenic in nature, surgery (tissue repair or ablation) may be considered. Note that surgery is rarely used for the management of neuropathic pain, whether it be peripheral or central in nature (Melzack et al., 2008). If this severe and chronic pain is determined to be predominantly psychogenic in nature, then psychotherapy, in the form of cognitive behavioral therapy, is added to the therapeutic plan. What about the place of placebo therapy? Although placebo therapy is positioned at the end of the pain severity scale in Figure 4-16, readers should take into consideration that its therapeutic effect can operate anywhere in the timeline of pain severity and treatment. Moreover, it is capital to realize that the pain therapies presented in Figure 4-16 often overlap with each other at any time during therapy, depending on the pain condition presented by the patient. For example, we may have a patient suffering from moderate to acute pain treated with a regimen of therapeutic exercises, EPAs, and NSAIDs. Another case may be a patient suffering from

TABLE 4-2 THERAPEUTICS FOR PAIN MANAGEMENT

Therapeutics	Proposed Action Mechanisms
Physical therapies +/– electrophysical agents	Counter irritation Modulate spinal gate control
Nonopioids	Alter injured tissue chemistry Modulate spinal gate control
Opioids	Alter spinal cord and brain chemistry Modulate spinal and central gate control
Adjuvants	Alter brain chemistry Decrease depression, anxiety, and spasm
Surgery	Pathologic tissue repair and/or ablation
Cognitive behavioral therapies	Alter state of mind
Placebo	Self-induced alteration of state of mind Soothing effect

severe chronic pain treated with a regimen of opioid plus adjuvant (antidepressant) drugs combined with cognitive behavioral therapy. In summary, the management of pain is a highly personal affair that requires both adequate pain assessment and regular monitoring.

XI. THE BOTTOM LINE

- Pain is defined as an unpleasant sensory and emotional experience associated with actual or potential tissue damage, or described in terms of such damages.
- The puzzle of pain revolves around the fact that pain may occur without injury and injury without pain.
- Pain may be acute, serving a biologic purpose, or chronic, serving no useful purpose.
- Pain may be categorized as nociceptive, neuropathic, psychogenic, or carcinogenic.
- Pain is a four-dimensional process revolving around its intensity, quality, affect, and location.
- The process of pain perception involves five phases: transduction, peripheral transmission, modulation, central transmission, and perception.
- Pain is modulated via the opening or closing of the gate control process located in the spinal cord, which is influenced by ascending (from tissue up to the spinal cord) and descending inputs (from the brain down to the spinal cord).
- All dimensions of pain (intensity, quality, affect, location), including disability, can be assessed and scored using a variety of tools in infants, children, adolescents, adults, and older adults.
- Pain can be assessed and scored in patients with limited communication by using facial tools, as well as specialized checklists.
- The spectrum of pain management rests on two approaches: pharmacologic and nonpharmacologic.
- The pharmacologic approach rests on the use of nonopioid, opioid, and adjuvant drugs.
- Nonpharmacologic approaches include physical therapies with or without EPAs, surgery, and cognitive behavioral therapy.
- Placebo therapy is very important in the context of pain management and should be encouraged and monitored.
- Effective pain management often implies the overlapping of several therapies.
- The management of pain is highly personal, requiring adequate assessment and regular monitoring.

XII. CRITICAL THINKING QUESTIONS

Clarification: What is meant by pain, categories of pain, and pain modulation?

Assumptions: You assume that pain has dimensions and that it is possible to assess and score each of them. How do you justify making that assumption?

Reasons and evidence: The perception, or experience, of nociceptive pain implies the fulfillment of five distinctive physiologic phases. How did this come to be?

Viewpoints or perspectives: You agree with the consensus that pain can be objectively and quantitatively assessed and scored. What would someone who disagrees with you say?

Implications and consequences: You state that pain modulation occurs peripherally and centrally. What are you implying?

About the question: Is it possible to effectively modulate pain without the use of drugs? Why do you think I ask this question?

XIII. REFERENCES

Articles

Beyer J, Denyes M, Villarruel A (1992) The creation, validation, and continuing development of the Oucher: A measurement of pain intensity in children. J Pediat Nurs, 7: 335–346

Beyer JE, Knott C (1998) Construct validity estimation of the African-American and Hispanic versions of the Oucher scale. J Pediat Nurs, 13: 20–31

Beyer JE, Turner SB, Jones L, Young L, Onikul R, Bohaty B (2005) The alternate forms reliability of the Oucher pain scale. Pain Manag Nurs, 6:10–17

Bieri D, Reeve R, Champion GD, Addicoat L, Ziegler J (1990) The Faces Pain Scale for the self-assessment of the severity of pain experienced by children: Development, initial validation and preliminary investigation for ratio scale properties. Pain, 41:139–150

Chambers CT, Finley GA, McGrath PJ, Walsh TM (2003) The parent's postoperative pain measure: Replication and extension to 2–6 year-old children. Pain, 105: 437–443

Chambers CT, Reid GJ, McGrath PJ, Finley GA (1996) Development and preliminary validation of a postoperative pain measure for parents. Pain, 68: 307–313

Fuchs-Lacelle S, Hadjistavroupoulos T (2004) Development and preliminary validity of the pain assessment checklist for seniors with limited ability to communicate (PACSLAC). Pain Manage Nurs, 5: 37–49

Grunau RVE, Craig KD (1987) Pain expression in neonates: Facial action and cry. Pain, 28: 395–410

Grunau RE, Oberlander T, Holsti L, Whitfield MF (1998) Bedside application of the Neonatal Facial Coding System in pain assessment of premature neonates. Pain, 76: 277–286

Hicks CL, von Baeyer CL, Spafford P, van Korlaar I, Goodenough, B (2001) The Faces Pain Scale-Revised: Toward a common metric in pediatric pain measurement. Pain, 93: 173–183

Jensen MP, Karoly P, Braver S (1986) The measurement of clinical pain intensity: A comparison of six methods. Pain, 27: 117–126

Jerome A, Gross RT (1991) Pain disability index: Construct and discriminant validity. Arch Phys Med Rehabil, 72: 920–922

Katz J, Melzack R (1999) Measurement of pain. Surg Clin North Am, 79: 231–252

Katz WA, Rothenberg R (2005) Treating the patient in pain. J Clin Rheumatol, 11: S16–S28

Melzack R. (1987) The short-form McGill Pain Questionnaire. Pain, 30: 191–197

Melzack (1975) The McGill pain questionnaire: Major properties and scoring methods. Pain, 1: 277–299

Melzack R, Wall PD (1965) Pain mechanism: A new theory. Science, 150: 971–979

Mense S (2003) The pathogenesis of muscle pain. Cur Pain Headache Rep, 7: 419–425

Tait RC, Pollard CA, Margolis RB, Duckro PN, Krause SJ (1987) The pain disability index: Psychometric and validity data. Arch Phys Med Rehabil, 68: 438–441

Review Articles

Bird J (2005) Assessing pain in older people. Nurs Stand, 19: 45–52

Curatolo M, Sveticic G. (2002). Drug combinations in pain treatment: A review of the published evidence and a method for finding the optimal combination. Best Pract Res Clin Anaesthesiol, 16: 507–519

Duhn LJ, Medves JM (2004) A systematic integrative review of infant pain assessment tools. Adv Neonatal Care, 4: 126–140

Hrobjartsson A, Gotzsche PC (2001) Is the placebo powerless? An analysis of clinical trials comparing placebo with no treatment. New Engl J Med, 344: 1594–1602

Hrobjartsson A, Gotzsche PC (2004) Is the placebo powerless? Update of a systematic review with 52 new randomized trials comparing placebo with no treatment. J Intern Med, 256: 91–100

Chapters of Textbooks

Barlas P, Lundeberg T (2006) Transcutaneous electrical nerve stimulation and acupuncture. In: Wall and Melzack's Textbook of Pain, 5th ed. McMahon S, Koltzenburg M (Eds). Churchill Livingstone, Edinburg, pp 583–590

Bielefeld K, Gebhart G (2006) Visceral pain: Basic mechanism. In: Wall and Melzack's Textbook of Pain, 5th ed. McMahon S, Koltzenburg M (Eds). Churchill Livingstone, Edinburg, pp 721–736

Boivie J (2006) Central pain. In: Wall and Melzack's Textbook of Pain, 5th ed. McMahon S, Koltzenburg M (Eds). Churchill Livingstone, Edinburg, pp 1057–1074

Bushnell MC, Apkarian AV (2006) Representation of pain in the brain. In: Wall and Melzack's Textbook of Pain, 5th ed. McMahon S, Koltzenburg M (Eds). Churchill Livingstone, Edinburg, pp 107–124

Craig KD (2006) Emotions and psychobiology. In: Wall and Melzack's Textbook of Pain, 5th ed. McMahon S, Koltzenburg M (Eds). Churchill Livingstone, Edinburg, pp 231–239

Craig KD, Prkachin KM, Grunau RE (2011) The facial Expression of Pain. In: Handbook of Pain Assessment, 3rd ed. Turk DC, Melzack R (Eds). The Guildford Press, New York, pp 117–133

Dahl JB, Kehlet (2006) Post-operative pain and its management. In: Wall and Melzack's Textbook of Pain, 5th ed. McMahon S, Koltzenburg M (Eds). Churchill Livingstone, Edinburg, pp 635–651

Devor M (2006) Response of nerves to injury in relation to neuropathic pain. In: Wall and Melzack's Textbook of Pain, 5th ed. McMahon S, Koltzenburg M (Eds). Churchill Livingstone, Edinburg, pp 909–927

Derasari MD (2003) Taxonomy of pain syndromes. In: Pain Medicine: A Comprehensive Review, 2nd ed. Prithvi Raj P (Ed). Mosby, St-Louis, pp 17–22

Dostrovsky JO, Craig AD (2006) Ascending projection systems. In: Wall and Melzack's Textbook of Pain, 5th ed. McMahon S, Koltzenburg M (Eds). Churchill Livingstone, Edinburg, pp 187–203

Flor H, Turk DC (2006) Cognitive and learning aspects. In: Wall and Melzack's Textbook of Pain, 5th ed. McMahon S, Koltzenburg M (Eds). Churchill Livingstone, Edinburg, pp 241–258

Fields Hl, Basbaum AI, Heinricher MM (2006a) Central nervous system mechanisms of pain modulation. In: Wall and Melzack's Textbook of Pain, 5th ed. McMahon S, Koltzenburg M (Eds). Churchill Livingstone, Edinburg, pp 125–142

Fields HL, Price DD (2006b) Placebo analgesia. In: Wall and Melzack's Textbook of Pain, 5th ed. McMahon S, Koltzenburg M (Eds). Churchill Livingstone, Edinburg, pp 361–367

Gagliese L, Melzack R (2006) Pain in the elderly. In: Wall and Melzack's Textbook of Pain, 5th ed. McMahon S, Koltzenburg M (Eds). Churchill Livingstone, Edinburg, pp 1169–1180

Galea MP (2002) Neuroanatomy of the nociceptive system. In: Pain: A Textbook for Therapists. Strong J, Unruh AM, Wright A, Baxter GD (Eds). Churchill Livingstone, Edinburg, pp 13–41

Gauthier LR, Gagliese LA (2011) Assessment of Pain in Older Persons. In: Handbook of Pain Assessment, 3rd ed. Turk DC, Melzack R (Eds). The Guildford Press, New York, pp 242–259

Hadjistavropoulos T, Breau LM, Craig KD (2011) Assessment of Pain in Adults and Children with Limited Ability to Communicate. In: Handbook of Pain Assessment, 3rd ed. Turk DC, Melzack R (Eds). The Guildford Press, New York, pp 260–280

Jensen MP, Karoly P (2011) Self-Report Scales and Procedures for Assessing Pain in Adults. In: Handbook of Pain Assessment, 3rd ed. Turk DC, Melzack R (Eds). The Guildford Press, New York, pp 19–44

Katz J, Melzack R (2011) The McGill Pain Questionnaire. In: Handbook of Pain Assessment, 3rd ed. Turk DC, Melzack R (Eds). The Guildford Press, New York, pp 45–66

Mantyh PW (2006) Cancer pain: Causes, Consequences and Therapeutic Opportunities. In: Wall and Melzack's Textbook of Pain, 5th ed. McMahon S, Koltzenburg M (Eds). Churchill Livingstone, Edinburg, pp 1087–1097

McGrath PJ, Unruh AM (2006) Measurement and assessment of paediatric pain. In: Wall and Melzack's Textbook of Pain, 5th ed. McMahon S, Koltzenburg M (Eds). Churchill Livingstone, Edinburg, pp 305–315

Melzack R, Katz J (2006) Pain assessment in adult patients. In: Wall and Melzack's Textbook of Pain, 5th ed. McMahon S, Koltzenburg M (Eds). Churchill Livingstone, Edinburg, pp 291–304

Meyer RA, Ringkamp M, Campbell JN, Raja SN (2006) Peripheral mechanisms of cutaneous nociception. In: Wall and Melzack's Textbook of Pain, 5th ed. McMahon S, Koltzenburg M (Eds). Churchill Livingstone, Edinburg, pp 3–34

Parris WC (2003) The history of pain medicine. In: Pain Medicine: A Comprehensive Review, 2nd ed. Prithvi Raj P (Ed). Mosby, St-Louis, pp 3–6

Roche PA (2002) Placebo analgesia—friend not foe. In: Pain: A Textbook for Therapists. Strong J, Unruh AM, Wright A, Baxter GD (Eds). Churchill Livingstone, Edinburg, pp 81–97

Rubertone JA, Barbe M (2005) Wound healing and pain. In: Modalities for Therapeutic Interventions. Michlovitz SL, Nolan TP (Eds). FA Davis Co., pp 15–40

Ruskin DA, Amaria KA, Warnock FF, McGrath PA (2011) Assessment of Pain in Infants, Children, and Adolescents. In: Handbook of Pain Assessment, 3rd ed. Turk DC, Melzack R (Eds). The Guildford Press, New York, pp 213–241

Sikes RW (2004) The physiology and psychology of pain. In: Therapeutic Modalities, 3rd ed. Starkey C (Ed). FA Davis Co, Philadelphia, pp 29–54

Schug SA, Gandham N (2006) Opioids: Clinical use. In: Wall and Melzack's Textbook of Pain, 5th ed. McMahon S, Koltzenburg M (Eds). Churchill Livingstone, Edinburg, pp 443–457

Unruh (2002) Generic principles of practice. In: Pain: A Textbook for Therapists. Strong J, Unruh AM, Wright A, Baxter GD (Eds). Churchill Livingstone, Edinburg, pp 151–167

Weisberg J, Deturk W (2006) Pain. In: Integrated Physical Agents in Rehabilitation, 2nd ed. Hecox B, Andemicael Mehreteab T, Weisberg J, Sanko J (Eds). Prentice Hall, Upper Saddle River, pp 57–71

Wright A (2002) Neurophysiology of pain and pain modulation. In: A Textbook for Therapists. Strong J, Unruh AM, Wright A, Baxter GD (Eds). Churchill Livingstone, Edinburg, pp 43–64

Wright A, Benson HAE, O.Callaghan J (2002) Pharmacology of pain management. In: A Textbook for Therapists. Strong J, Unruh AM, Wright A, Baxter GD (Eds). Churchill Livingstone, Edinburg, pp 307–324

Textbooks

Melzack R, Wall PD (2008) The Challenge of Pain, 2nd ed. Penguin Books Ltd, New York

Mense S, Simons DG (2001) Muscle Pain. Understanding Its Nature, Diagnosis and Treatment. Lippincott Williams & Wilkins, Philadelphia

McMahon S, Koltzenburg M (2006) Wall and Melzack's Textbook of Pain, 5th ed. Churchill Livingstone, Edinburg

Strong J, Unruh AM, Wright A, Baxter GD (2002) Pain: A Textbook for Therapists. Churchill Livingstone, Edinburg

Turk DC, Melzack R (2011) Handbook of Pain Assessment, 3rd ed. The Gilford Press, New York

Internet Resource

www.iasp-pain.org: International Society for the Study of Pain

Chapter 5

Purchase, Electrical Safety, and Maintenance

Chapter Outline

Learning Objectives

Remembering: List each of the eight steps in purchasing electrophysical agents. Describe the genesis and nature of a micro- and a macroelectrical shock.

Understanding: Compare each step in relation to the whole process of purchasing. Explain the operating mechanism behind a GFCI receptacle.

Applying: Show how each step contributes to the whole purchasing process. Show how a macroshock can be prevented when line-powered devices are used.

Analyzing: Explain the significance of each step. Distinguish between standard three-wire and GFCI electrical receptacles.

Evaluating: Create a mock purchase order based on the eight-step approach. Formulate the possible physiologic consequences resulting from the flow of a 1A alternating leakage current through the thoracic area of a patient via his or her two hands.

Creating: Construct a practical guideline related to the purchase and electrical safety related to the use of line-powered electrophysical agents. Elaborate a rescue plan in the event of a severe macroshock and electrocution in your clinical setting.

I. THE PURCHASING PROCESS

Most practitioners who use electrophysical agents (EPAs) on a regular basis inevitably will be confronted with the task of advising on or preparing a purchase order to either renew existing agents or acquire new ones. The purchase of EPAs can be a pleasant experience or can easily turn into a frustrating exercise. Because a large variety of models and related accessories are available, potential buyers must learn how to navigate this market properly. To complicate matters further, they also must choose among a substantial number of manufacturers and distributors, as well as learn how to deal with sales representatives who, one after another, will display their best marketing efforts to sell their own line of equipment. To facilitate the purchasing process, the American Physical Therapy Association (APTA) annually updates and publishes a comprehensive directory of companies and distributors in the United States that supply rehabilitation products, including EPAs. This directory, which bears the name of *Buyer's Guide,* is available online (www.apta.org) and represents an excellent source of information for guiding the purchase of most EPAs discussed in this textbook. To make the purchasing process of EPAs a pleasant, satisfactory, and cost-effective experience for clinicians, the following eight-step approach is recommended.

II. EIGHT-STEP APPROACH TO PURCHASING ELECTROPHYSICAL AGENTS

Although the purchase of EPAs is unavoidable, nowhere in other EPA textbooks can practitioners find guidance in making this necessary process pleasant and cost-effective. This chapter fills the gap. Table 5-1 presents a eight-step approach to purchasing EPAs. This approach begins with information gathering and ends with the signing of the purchase order. It stresses the importance of good communication, the use of adequate terminology, and the use of written as opposed to verbal communication.

III. ELECTRICAL HAZARDS

A. ELECTRICAL SHOCK

Electricity is a ubiquitous source of energy that can be fatal to human beings. Electrical shocks, although rare in the field of health care, represent a serious occupational hazard for both patients and clinicians operating line-powered EPAs. To be unaware of or to overlook the dangers associated with electricity increases one's vulnerability and risk of becoming a victim of a fatal electrical shock (see Geddes et al., 2006; OSHA, 2012; Cadick et al., 2012).

B. LINE- VERSUS BATTERY-POWERED DEVICES

The majority of EPAs covered in this textbook are powered by a line source of electricity whereas the remainder are powered using batteries. A *line-powered device* is powered by a building's conventional power-line voltage, which in North America is characterized by a 60-Hz alternating current (AC) delivered between 110 and 125 V. A *battery-powered device,* on the other hand, is powered by a battery source, characterized by the delivery of a continuous direct current (DC) at a relatively low voltage, such as 9 V.

C. DANGERS OF LINE-POWERED DEVICES

The flow of an unwanted 60-Hz AC in the body, referred to as a leakage current, can cause an electrical shock that can induce mild, moderate, severe, and sometimes lethal physiologic responses, depending on its amplitude, duration of flow, and path of flow. A *leakage current* is defined as any loss of current from a line-powered device, usually resulting from breaks in the insulation system (chassis and power cord). In other words, a leakage current is an unwanted current that leaks out from the intended pathway because of defective insulation, often caused by excessive wear, tear, and misuse of the device. Using line-powered devices is dangerous because passage of this 60-Hz alternating leakage current in the body, if it is of sufficient amplitude and duration, can depolarize motor nerves, thus inducing light to strong involuntary muscle contractions. Because fused tetanus (i.e., maximum tetanic muscle contraction) occurs in most human muscles at frequencies between 40 and 60 Hz, the passage of this 60-Hz alternating leakage current can definitely cause such a physiologic muscle response. Is leakage current from a battery-powered (DC) device as dangerous as that originating from a line-powered device? The answer is no. Battery-powered devices are safe because the continuous 0-Hz direct leakage current, regardless of its amplitude and duration, is incapable of causing nerve depolarization and thus is unable to induce electrically evoked muscle contraction.

D. PHYSIOLOGIC TISSUE DAMAGE

There is undisputed evidence to show that when a 60-Hz alternating leakage current **larger than 5 mA** passes through the body (see later discussion), the individual is exposed to a variety of unwanted physiologic responses, such as tetanic muscle contraction and tissue burn, which may cause minor to severe body injuries, including death. The victim (operator or patient) may display minimal to extremely violent tetanic muscle contractions, ranging from the classic "can't let go" contraction (forearm muscles) to respiratory arrest (intercostal muscles) to cardiac arrest (ventricle/heart fibrillation) to, at worst,

TABLE 5-1	EIGHT-STEP APPROACH TO PURCHASING ELECTROPHYSICAL AGENTS
Step	**Rationale**
1. Research, gather, and review technical information.	The best tool available to research electrophysical agent (EPA) equipment is the American Physical Therapy Association's online *Buyer's Guide* and Web sites. The last thing that practitioners should do is rely too heavily on the word of sales representatives who, logically, will do their best to convince you of the "merits" of their company's equipment. Focus on choice of models, prices, availability, warranty, and delivery terms, including any special features you are looking for.
2. Make sure that everyone speaks the same technical language.	Now that your research information is completed, the second step is to contact some distributors through their head offices or sales representatives. The field of therapeutic EPAs is highly technical, as exemplified by this textbook. Too often, major confusion arises because you, the users, and the sales representatives simply are not speaking the same language when discussing the technical features of the EPAs that you are interested in purchasing. One of the best ways to minimize such confusion is for both sides to use recommended terminology. The more standardized and accurate the technical terminology used, the better will be the verbal exchanges and written correspondence between you and sales representatives. Use the terminology found in this text to facilitate this step.
3. Assess the need for portable versus cabinet devices.	The third step is to determine whether you need portable (battery-powered) or cabinet-type (line-powered) EPAs. This assessment should be based on your patient clientele. Portable devices are preferable when you need greater mobility in providing therapy to patients, wherever they might be—in hospital wards, department rooms, outdoor fields, or at home. A key disadvantage of this type of equipment is the supply and maintenance of batteries. A key advantage is that they require minimal floor space and are easy to store after use. Cabinet devices are preferable when a large number of patients need to be treated on a daily basis, which implies the frequent use of agents. A key advantage is that no battery is needed. A key disadvantage is that more floor space is needed.
4. Inquire about business credentials.	The fourth step involves inquiring about the business credentials of manufacturers, distributors, and sales representatives. Wise consumers never make blind purchases; they want to know, before making a purchase, whether the product, the company, the distributor, and the sales representative all have solid credentials. Do not be afraid to ask questions about credentials. The manufacturers' credentials are based on the quality of the equipment manufactured as well as on the terms and duration of the warranty provided. Keep in mind that manufacturers do not have the same quality control and warranty policies. The distributors' and sales representatives' credentials are based on the quality of the services they offer before, during, and—most importantly—after the purchase is made and the warranty has expired. Do not hesitate to draw on the experience of your colleagues, and that of colleagues working in other clinical settings, with regard to this subject. Ask the sales representatives where their repair and parts centers are located and their current hourly rate for a repair. In addition, inquire about the terms related to the shipping of equipment to the repair centers. Finally, ask for written documents regarding the terms of the warranty, and the distributor's own policies and procedures for services offered, both during the warranty period and after the warranty expires.
5. Ask for at least two written price quotations.	This step addresses the all-important issue of purchasing price. As is common in the field of health care, the cost of EPAs can vary greatly from one distributor to the next. Therefore, asking for at least two quotations, from two different distributors, can only guide you better toward a cost-effective purchase. Each quotation must be written and must include the price of each item, all taxes and shipping charges that apply, and other related costs such as customs fees if you are buying from a foreign distributor. Beware of verbal quotes over the phone! Remember that quality and service have a price of their own. In the long run, you will never regret purchasing a quality piece of equipment from a reputable manufacturer, distributor, and sales representative.
6. Consider purchasing the equipment on a trial basis.	Purchasing equipment on a trial basis is preferable but, unfortunately, not always possible. Doing so will give you the opportunity to test it in your academic or clinical settings. It will also give you time to have a qualified technician inspect it for compliance with the manufacturer's listed specifications and safety standards.
7. Consider purchasing a post-warranty maintenance and/or service contract.	Some distributors may offer a post-warranty maintenance or service contract for 1 year or longer, at a fixed annual price, which may or may not include parts, labor, and shipping costs. Ask your sales representative for more details. You may choose to give your maintenance business to local electronics repair shops. Remember, however, that these local shops may have a hard time obtaining replacement parts to make the necessary repairs, which may lead to a significant delay before you can use the equipment again.
8. Establish a deadline for delivery.	This last step, if forgotten, can lead to a fair degree of frustration for you, the buyer. Before signing any purchase order, think of adding a clause regarding the delivery date that your distributor must meet for complete delivery, to your working site, of all items purchased. This clause will likely prevent excessive delay in the delivery of your equipment. Discuss with your sales representative the consequences to the distributor if this deadline is not respected. To avoid any misunderstandings, put these delivery deadline terms in writing before putting your signature at the bottom of the purchase order.

death by electrocution. This 60-Hz AC passing through the body can also cause light to severe tissue burn injuries, because heat is produced when the current flows through the resistance offered by the tissues. Burn injuries caused by an electrical shock are located primarily at the skin surface (external) level rather than in the deeper tissues (internal), because skin tissue offers much greater resistance to current flow than deeper, moist tissues. Internal burn injuries are likely to be more substantial if the skin, in contact with the live, faulty electrical source, is wet. Wet skin presents much less resistance to electrical current than dry skin and, as a result, decreases the natural protection that dry skin offers against internal burn injuries. Note that even if the victim survives cardiorespiratory failure, the damages caused by internal burn injuries to the neurovascular system are often the cause of death a few hours or days following an electrical shock.

E. FACTORS DETERMINING THE EXTENT OF BODY INJURY

The extent of body injury caused by the passage of an electrical shock depends on three key factors: leakage current amplitude, duration of flow within the body, and the path of flow through the body.

1. Leakage Current Amplitude

There is a consensus that the maximum 60-Hz leakage AC amplitude that can safely flow though the human chest area is 5 mA. Leakage currents will cause microshocks, and possibly lethal macroshocks, depending of their amplitudes. Leakage currents smaller than 5 mA produce microshocks, which are harmless to humans. Leakage currents larger than 5 mA, on the other hand, produce macroshocks, which can trigger the cascade of harmful physiologic responses discussed earlier. Thus, the larger the leakage current amplitude, the larger the macroshock, and the more damaging and deadly the body injuries will be.

2. Duration of Current Flow

For body injuries to occur, the duration of flow of the leakage current must also be sufficiently long. It is logical to say that the longer the duration of current flow into the body (from seconds to minutes), the more severe the body damages will be.

3. Path of Flow Through the Body

The path of leakage current flow through the thoracic region, via both arms, is potentially much more dangerous and deadly because of the risk of depolarizing vital tissues, such as the vagus and phrenic nerves, than a path of flow from one arm to the trunk and leg, and finally to earth. This is why touching the chassis or power cord of a live line-powered EPA device with two hands, as opposed to one hand, always represents a greater risk of suffering from a potentially deadly macroshock.

4. Practical Meaning

First, practitioners must always remember that it is the magnitude of the leakage current (larger than 5 mA)—not the magnitude of voltage (e.g., 120 V) nor current amplitude (e.g., 1 A) powering the device—which is responsible for electrical shocks that cause body damages. Second, one must always remember that a large leakage current (e.g., 400 mA), flowing for only 2 seconds, causes much less tissue damage and is much less dangerous than a weaker leakage current (e.g., 25 mA) flowing for 45 seconds. Third, always recall that the danger of a leakage current is determined by the path of flow it takes in the body, which means that a leakage current flowing through a sensitive area, such as the thorax, may interfere with the functioning of life-sustaining organs, causing death.

IV. GENESIS OF AN ELECTRICAL SHOCK

A. GROUND-FAULT PATHWAY

An electrical shock occurs when the victim's hand(s) or other body parts contact a leakage source of electrical current, thus providing a path for this current to go to the ground. For this to occur, a ground-fault pathway must be present. A ground fault is described as an unintentional electrical path between a source of current and a grounded surface. It occurs when current leaks to the ground from the line-powered device's hardware—in other words, when the line-powered AC escapes from the device to travel through the victim's body to earth. The leakage current that results from the ground fault is what causes a micro- or a macroshock.

B. DEVICE ELECTRICAL INSULATION BREAKDOWN

The main cause of a leakage current is a break or failure in the device's hardware electrical insulation, often due to abuse of the device and/or to a lack of regular electrical maintenance. Faulty insulation of the live wire within the power cord is a common example that results from abusive or careless use (e.g., pulling on and walking over the cable). Another example is a live chassis caused by a break in the internal device's electrical insulation system due to repeated mechanical vibrations and shocks sustained by the device over time.

C. BODY AS PATHWAY

If the patient's or operator's body provides the path for the leakage current to flow to the ground, one or both will be the victim of an electrical shock that can cause burn injuries, respiratory/cardiac arrest, and, potentially, death by electrocution, as discussed previously.

V. PROTECTION AGAINST ELECTRICAL SHOCKS

A. THE GFCI RECEPTACLE

The ideal and easiest way to protect against a macroshock is to plug each line-powered EPA device into a ground-fault circuit interrupter (GFCI) receptacle or outlet, as opposed to the standard three-wire receptacles found practically everywhere in clinics, hospitals, and homes. Figure 5-1 shows the most common type of GFCI receptacle, which is characterized by its Reset and Test buttons, as well as the standard three-wire receptacle.

B. THE GFCI OPERATING MECHANISM

The GFCI receptacle is designed to protect both patient and operator from severe to fatal electrical shocks. It does so by constantly monitoring the flow of the 60-Hz AC from the device to the circuit interrupter and back, thus detecting any loss or leakage of the current. Its purpose is to detect ground faults. GFCIs are designed to cut off electrical power to the device, within a fraction of a second, if a leakage current greater than 5 mA (the safe limit for the human thoracic region) is present, therefore preventing any harmful or deadly injuries. In other words, plugging line-power devices into GFCI receptacles prevents the operator and patient from being exposed to a potentially lethal leakage current. Unfortunately, the GFCI can malfunction, so there is a need for periodic testing of functionality.

C. TESTING THE GFCI RECEPTACLE

All GFCIs are mounted with Test and Reset buttons (see Fig. 5-1A). These buttons are used to quickly test the receptacle to see if it is working properly. To test a GFCI, plug a regular lamp into the receptacle and turn the light on. Now, press the Test button; the Reset button should immediately pop out, and the light should go out. This indicates that the GFCI is working properly. Press the Reset button to restore power to the outlet. If the Reset button pops out but the light is still on, the GFCI is incorrectly wired. If the Reset button does not pop out, the GFCI receptacle is defective and should be replaced immediately. It is recommended that all GFCIs be tested once a month.

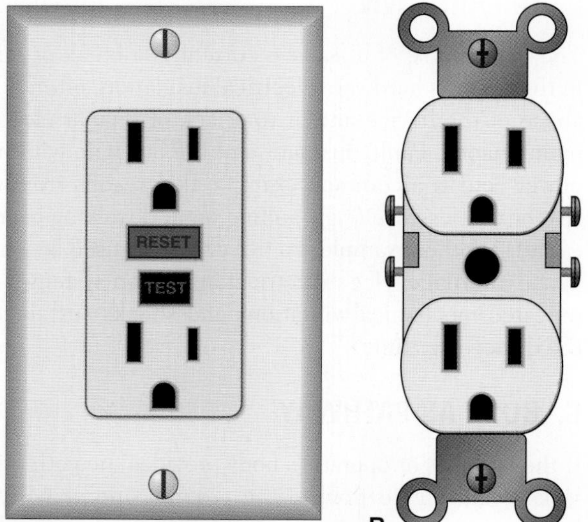

FIGURE 5-1 Ground-fault circuit interrupter (**A**) and standard three-wire electrical (**B**) receptacles.

VI. PREVENTION, OPERATIONAL SAFETY, AND MAINTENANCE

The adoption of the following preventive, operational safety, and maintenance measures is one of the best ways to prevent the genesis of electrical shocks when working with line-powered EPAs.

A. PREVENTIVE MEASURES

The prevention of electrical shocks begins with two preventive measures: safe wall electrical receptacle and line-powered device electrical certification. First, replace all standard three-wire receptacles (Fig. 5-1B) on walls with GFCI receptacles (Fig. 5-1A). Three-wire receptacles provide a true ground connection to the earth, but they offer no protection against harmful leakage currents passing through the body. Their purpose is to protect the equipment—not the users—against a sudden flow of large leakage currents. The U.S. National Electrical Code requires that in all health facilities, electrically line-powered devices and accessories be plugged into GFCI receptacles or outlets to ensure their safe use in areas where water is omnipresent. Wet skin, as opposed to dry skin, presents less resistance to current flow, thus overexposing the person to macroshocks when working in a wet environment, such as in a hydrotherapy unit. This textbook urges all operators of line-powered EPAs to **always** plug their devices into GFCI outlets to ensure maximum protection against electrical shocks. Second, ensure that the seal of a reputable testing laboratory, such as the Underwriters Laboratories, is on the device's chassis before using it. This seal certifies that the device has a maximum leakage current of less than 1 mA, which is considered to be absolutely safe to humans. If any of your older devices do not have this seal, take them to a qualified technician for a complete inspection and upgrade in order to bring all line-powered EPA devices into compliance with currently recognized electrical safety standards.

B. OPERATIONAL SAFETY MEASURES

Adopting proper operational safety measures is another good way to prevent an electrical shock. First, always read the manufacturer's brochure regarding safety measures and manipulation of the line-powered device before using it for the first time. Second, always disconnect the device by gripping and pulling its plug, not its power cord. Make sure that the plug remains firmly seated in the socket and that the tines of the plug are not visible. Never use extension cords. Third, instruct all patients **never** to touch a line-powered device—whether it be on or off—including its knobs, power cord, cables, and electrodes. In addition, educate patients about how to shut off the device in case of an emergency or major discomfort and how to call for help when needed during treatment sessions. Fourth, post visible signs on the entry doors or walls adjacent to the treatment areas to warn patients, visitors, and staff that they are entering areas in which electrical, electromagnetic, and acoustic fields of radiation are being generated. As well, post a visible sign on the same entry doors to alert those persons wearing electronic implants, such as a cardiac pacemaker, or carrying electronic devices, such as a cellular phone, not to enter this area without receiving full authorization by an attending clinician. Finally, use battery-powered devices over line-powered devices for home therapy, because a leakage DC current is harmless (no motor nerve depolarization is possible) compared with a 60-Hz leakage AC. Before recommending the use of a line-powered device for home therapy, make sure that the patient's home is equipped with at least one GFCI receptacle, and instruct the patient to plug the device *only* into that receptacle.

C. MAINTENANCE MEASURES

Adopting regular maintenance measures can only help to minimize the occurrence of an electrical shock. First, do weekly visual inspections to check the integrity of the device's basic components and accessories such as knobs, power cords, plugs, cables, and electrodes. Second, have a qualified technician inspect, repair, and calibrate all line-powered EPAs used in the facility at least once a year, or whenever a problem is suspected. Ask the repair technician to place a sticker on the chassis of each line-powered device that shows the date of its last inspection, repair, and calibration. Third, keep an inspection/repair/calibration log for each EPA used in your facility. Finally, designate one clinician, from among those practicing with line-powered EPAs, as the clinician in charge for all matters relating to the functioning and maintenance of these devices. This person's role is one of prevention and central information gathering to ensure proper and timely communication between users and maintenance technicians about safety and maintenance issues for all line-powered equipment. Of course, his or her role is **not** to be held fully responsible if an electrical hazard occurs.

VII. IMMEDIATE PROCEDURES FOLLOWING A SEVERE MACROSHOCK

A. BACKGROUND

The occurrence of a severe macroshock during treatment can be catastrophic. What to do immediately after witnessing such an electrical accident? Described below is a hypothetic scenario, which exemplified the procedures that you—the rescuer—may want to follow. **The following procedures must not be interpreted in any way, shape, or form as containing any legal statement or advice.** Readers must refer to legal counsel in their own country for any legal advice relating to this topic. Users of line-powered EPAs are reminded to *always* apply the procedures approved in their own facility if an electrical macroshock occurs before applying the procedures described below. Only when no such procedures are stipulated should practitioners adopt and expand on those listed below.

B. SCENARIO AND PROCEDURES

Let us consider the following hypothetic scenario. Your clinic is located 10 minutes away from a major hospital. Your line-powered ultrasound device, plugged into a standard three-wire receptacle (see Fig. 5-1B), is ready to use. Your patient, a graceful 67-year-old woman, in a courteous effort to help you move the device closer to the treatment table, grabs the device's power cord with both hands. An unfortunate break of insulation in this power cord causes her to be victim of a severe electrical shock, manifested by violent "can't let go" forearm muscle contractions. She falls on the floor, unconscious, unable to let go of the faulty power cord. What should you do to rescue this patient? Table 5-2 lists immediate and sequential procedures that should ensure proper management of this electrical incident. Crucial to the success of this delicate rescue operation is to stop the current to the device **before** attending to the patient.

C. A LESSON TO BE LEARNED

The unfortunate incident narrated in the scenario could have been prevented if only the ultrasound device would have been plugged into a GFCI as opposed to a standard three-wire receptacle. In such a case, no current would have flown into the power cord, because the GFCI outlet would have detected the ground-fault pathway (leakage current) caused by the break in the power cord electrical insulation, thus switching off the electrical power supply to the device. The operator would have realized that something was wrong because he or she would not have been able to switch on the ultrasound device. Finally, a quick look by the operator

TABLE 5-2	IMMEDIATE PROCEDURES FOLLOWING A SEVERE MACROSHOCK
Procedures	**Rationale**
FIRST: Stop the Current Flow	**Before touching the patient, you, the rescuer, must stop the origin of the leakage current—that is, the 60-Hz AC powering the device.** This is achieved by pulling the power cord plug (safe insulation through its thick rubber coating), *not the cord* (faulty insulation), out of the wall electrical receptacle or outlet. If you fail to disconnect the device from the electrical outlet before touching or attending to the patient, you will be exposed to the same electrical shock, thus becoming the second victim.
SECOND: Attend to the Patient	With the faulty power cord disconnected, immediately attend to the patient by checking vital signs (i.e., measuring the carotid pulse and monitoring the respiratory rate). If the vital signs are absent or very weak, call immediately for emergency help and begin cardiopulmonary resuscitation (CPR) maneuvers. All clinicians using line-powered EPA devices *must* be knowledgeable in both the theory and practice of CPR.
THIRD: Arrange the Patient's Transfer	When vital signs are reestablished to the point at which the patient can breathe regularly without assistance, plan for immediate transfer to the nearest hospital for a full medical examination. If the electrical shock occurs at the hospital, arrange for the patient to be taken immediately to the emergency department. You, the rescuer, should plan for such a transfer even if the victim's vital signs were maintained after the electrical shock. Because of the possible legal and delayed fatal consequences of an electrical shock, it is in the best interests of both the victim and the rescuer that a physician conducts a complete physical examination of the victim immediately after or within hours of an electrical shock.
FOURTH: Secure the Faulty Equipment	After the victim's departure from the scene, the rescuer should immediately secure all faulty equipment related to the event so that no one else can access the equipment. Instruct all colleagues not to touch or use this equipment until further notice from you or the facility's administrative team.
FIFTH: File an Incident Report	You, the rescuer, should report in writing to the administrative authorities the nature of the incident and all the circumstances surrounding it. Either the rescuer or another person directly involved with the incident should create a device incident file. Because you were involved in the incident, you may be asked to testify in court if the victim launches a lawsuit; therefore, you should be kept informed about the evolution of the case. You can help to ensure a proper resolution of the incident by working in collaboration with the facility's administrative authorities.

at the GFCI receptacle would have indicated that the Reset button had popped out, indicating the occurrence of an electrical problem.

VIII. THE BOTTOM LINE

- The purchase and maintenance of EPAs are integral parts of clinical practice.
- The purchase of EPAs can be a pleasant and cost-effective experience if enough time and effort are devoted to researching information, speaking the proper technical language, assessing needs, inquiring about business credentials, asking for written quotations, considering the warranty and maintenance plan, and establishing a deadline for delivery.
- Electrical shocks, although rare in health care practice, still represent a major occupational hazard for both patients and operators of line-powered EPA devices.
- The passage of a 60-Hz alternating leakage current through the thorax of a person could cause serious body injuries, including death by electrocution.
- It is the magnitude of the leakage current—not its voltage—that is responsible for body injuries.
- To cause serious body damage, a leakage current must be greater than 5 mA, flow for a certain period, and pass through the thoracic area.
- Electrical insulation breakdown is the major cause of leakage current.
- The ideal way to protect against macroshock and potential deadly body damage, including death by electrocution, is to plug all line-powered devices into GFCI receptacles.
- GFCI receptacles should be tested on a monthly basis.
- The best way to prevent and minimize the occurrence of macroshock is to adopt and apply preventative, operational safety, and maintenance measures.
- All users of line-powered EPA devices must be knowledgeable in the field of cardiopulmonary resuscitation.
- The occurrence of a severe macroshock may have serious legal consequences.
- Knowing what to do immediately after the occurrence of a macroshock may have life or death consequences for both operator and patient.

IX. CRITICAL THINKING QUESTIONS

Clarification: What is meant by having a pleasant, cost-effective, and satisfactory purchasing experience? What is an electrical shock, and what is the difference between a microshock and a macroshock?

Assumptions: You have assumed that it is important to inquire about the business credentials of manufacturers, distributors, and sales representatives when purchasing EPAs. You have also assumed that the genesis of an electrical shock can be prevented if users of line-powered EPAs take adequate measures. How do you justify making these assumptions?

Reasons and evidence: The effective and cost-related process of purchasing something requires preliminary research and processing of key information. Why are these precautions necessary? GFCI receptacles are designed to prevent the flow of a leakage current capable of generating a macroshock. How does this happen?

Viewpoints or perspectives: You agree with the consensus that purchasing EPAs should include many, if not all, of the eight steps proposed in this chapter. You also agree with the viewpoint that users of line-powered EPAs should take and apply regular preventive, operational, and maintenance measures even though death by electrocution when using such EPAs is extremely rare. What would someone who disagrees with you say?

Implications and consequences: You state that the effective purchase of EPAs is not as easy as one may think. What are you implying? You also state that the first thing to do before attending to the victim of a macroshock is to unplug the device from the wall receptacle. What are the possible consequences if the rescuer fails to do this first?

About the question: Does your clientele have anything to do with the types of EPAs you plan to purchase? Why is it important for the rescuer to follow all procedures described in this chapter if someday his or her patient receives a severe macroshock during the application of a line-powered EPA? Why do you think I ask these questions?

X. REFERENCES

Textbooks

Cadick J, Capelli-Schellpfeffer M, Neitzel D, Windfield A (2012) Electrical Safety Handbook, 4th ed. McGraw-Hill Professional, Columbus

Geddes LA, Roeder RA (2006) Handbook of Electrical Hazards and Accidents, 2nd ed. Lawyers & Judges Publishing Co, Tucson

Occupational Safety and Health Administration (OSHA) (2012) Controlling Electrical Hazards. OSHA 3075. Policy Reference Services, Washington

Internet Resource

www.apta.org: American Physical Therapy Association Online Buyer's Guide

Chapter 6

Therapeutic Spectrum, Selection, and Indication

Chapter Outline

Learning Objectives

Remembering: List the cardinal signs and symptoms, and their respective causes, associated with acute soft-tissue pathology.

Understanding: Compare the choice of electrophysical agents and related therapeutic interventions used during the first, second, and third stages of tissue healing.

Applying: Show how the application of electrophysical agents benefits the healing process of soft tissues.

Analyzing: Explain the differences among the therapeutic goals for each stage of healing.

Evaluating: Explain how the judicious and timely use of electrophysical agents may benefit soft-tissue healing.

Creating: Discuss the future spectrum of electrophysical agents for the treatment of soft-tissue pathology.

I. THERAPEUTIC SPECTRUM

The electrophysical agents (EPAs) covered in this textbook have a broad therapeutic spectrum that can affect several components of the International Classification of Functioning, Disability, and Health (ICF) disablement model, such as body structures and functions, activities, and participation (see Chapter 1). They make up, with the use of medication, surgery, therapeutic exercises, mobilizations, and manipulations, the overall spectrum of physical therapeutics for the management of soft-tissue pathology (Belanger 2002, 2009). Table 6-1 presents the therapeutic spectrum associated with the EPAs covered in this text. It shows that EPAs can affect pain and several soft-tissue structures and functions—namely edema, joint motion restriction, muscle spasm, muscle weakness and atrophy, and dermatosis, as well as wound, bone, and tendon healing. Also presented in this table are the groups of EPAs that are likely to affect each of the mentioned structures and functions. For example, it shows that for the management of pain, practitioners may chose to apply cryotherapy, thermotherapy, hydrotherapy, shortwave diathermy, transcutaneous electrical nerve stimulation, or iontophoresis. Another

TABLE 6-1 THERAPEUTIC SPECTRUM

Body Structure and Function	Electrophysical Agent
Pain	Cryotherapy Thermotherapy Hydrotherapy Shortwave diathermy Transcutaneous electrical nerve stimulation Iontophoresis
Edema	Cryotherapy Hydrotherapy Limb compression
Joint motion restriction	Thermotherapy Shortwave diathermy Neuromuscular electrical stimulation Spinal traction Continuous passive motion Ultrasound
Muscle spasm	Cryotherapy Thermotherapy Shortwave diathermy Spinal traction
Muscle weakness/ atrophy	Neuromuscular electrical stimulation
Dermatosis	Ultraviolet
Wound healing	Electrical stimulation for tissue healing and repair Thermotherapy Low-level laser therapy Hydrotherapy
Bone healing	Ultrasound Extracorporeal shock wave therapy
Muscle, tendon and ligament healing	Low-level laser therapy Ultrasound Extracorporeal shock wave therapy

example may be that for bone healing where ultrasound may be applied. For tendon healing, other agents, such as low-level laser therapy and extracorporeal shock wave therapy, may be considered.

II. JUDICIOUS SELECTION AND TIMELY APPLICATION

The judicious selection and timely application of one EPA over another is closely related to the phases of the healing process (see Chapter 3). To judiciously select an EPA is to select the one that will best enhance the current healing phase of the pathologic tissue. To use it in a timely fashion means to apply the EPA during the period of time in which it will yield optimal results. For example, there is a consensus in the field that the application of cryotherapy immediately after an acute soft-tissue injury is the most judicious choice that practitioners can make to control the signs and symptoms associated with the first (hemostasis) and second (inflammatory) phases of healing.

III. FRAMEWORK FOR SELECTION

How can practitioners achieve more judicious selection and timely application of EPAs? This chapter proposes to use the *three-stage intervention framework* presented in Box 6-1. This framework rests on the four basic phases of soft-tissue healing, which are discussed at length in Chapter 3. Injury and disease are the primary causes of soft-tissue pathology. Wounds may present in their acute, subacute, or chronic state. How can practitioners differentiate between these three levels of wound acuity? Generally speaking, the more acute the wound, the more pronounced the signs and symptoms related to the hemostatic and inflammation phases of soft-tissue healing. Because the judicious and timely use of EPAs is closely related to the presence and magnitude of these signs and symptoms, it is important to briefly describe them. The acronym *RCTDSA* stands for six signs and symptoms commonly observed in acute and subacute types of soft-tissue pathologies. It includes redness (*r*ubor) and heating (*c*alor) of the skin overlying the wound, coupled with edema (*t*umor) and pain (*d*olor). Often associated with these four cardinal signs and symptoms are two additional clinical manifestations: muscle spasm (*s*) triggered by pain (the vicious pain/spasm circle) and abnormal function (*a*), the latter being the result of tissue damage causing pain, spasm, and edema.

A. FIRST STAGE: CONTROLLING BLEEDING AND INFLAMMATION

It is well established in the scientific literature that if the bleeding and inflammatory responses are not properly controlled following soft-tissue injury, satisfactory wound healing may be delayed and in some circumstances is unlikely to occur (see Chapter 3). Thus, the first stage of therapeutic intervention after acute tissue damage is to control the hemostatic and inflammatory reactions taking place at the wound site (see Box 6-1). The therapeutic goals are therefore to minimize wound bleeding, secondary tissue damage, edema, pain, and muscle spasm. The evidence from the scientific literature presented in this textbook shows that a broad spectrum of EPAs can be used to meet the therapeutic goals associated with this first stage of intervention.

BOX 6-1 FRAMEWORK FOR ELECTROPHYSICAL AGENT SELECTION

FIRST STAGE: CONTROLLING BLEEDING AND INFLAMMATION

Key Physiologic Events

Soft-tissue damage causes bleeding, which triggers a cascade of cellular and chemical responses that lead to blood clotting and a complex inflammatory response necessary for wound healing.

THERAPEUTIC GOALS	SELECTION
• Minimize wound bleeding.	✓ Cryotherapy, only if applied immediately or within the first few minutes post injury
• Minimize secondary tissue damage.	✓ Cryotherapy, only if applied within the first 24–48 hours post injury ✓ Iontophoresis (anti-inflammatory drugs)
• Minimize edema.	✓ Cryotherapy ✓ Limb compression ✓ Cryo-hydrotherapy
• Minimize pain and muscle spasm.	✓ Cryotherapy ✓ Transcutaneous electrical nerve stimulation ✓ Iontophoresis (analgesic drugs)

SECOND STAGE: ENHANCING REPAIR TISSUE PROLIFERATION AND FORMATION

Key Physiologic Events

Angiogenesis and fibroplasia are initiated, leading to the proliferation and formation of immature repair tissue at the wound site.

THERAPEUTIC GOALS	SELECTION
• Promote angiogenesis and fibroplasia.	✓ Thermotherapy ✓ Thermo-hydrotherapy ✓ Shortwave diathermy ✓ Ultrasound ✓ Extracorporeal shock wave therapy ✓ Low-level laser therapy ✓ Electrical stimulation for tissue healing and repair
• Minimize pain.	✓ Transcutaneous electrical nerve stimulation
• Optimize wound contraction.	✓ Continuous passive motion ✓ Spinal traction

THIRD STAGE: ENHANCING REPAIR TISSUE REMODELING, MATURATION, AND FUNCTION

Key Physiologic Events

Immature repair tissue remodels, gradually matures, and heals, in most cases, as functional repair tissue.

THERAPEUTIC GOALS	SELECTION
• Enhance tissue repair.	✓ Ultrasound ✓ Low-level laser therapy ✓ Extracorporeal shock wave therapy
• Enhance tissue strength/elasticity.	✓ Continuous passive motion ✓ Spinal traction
• Enhance tissue function.	✓ Neuromuscular electrical stimulation

1. Minimizing Wound Bleeding

The use of cryotherapy (Chapter 8) can minimize wound bleeding *only* if applied immediately after the injury—that is, within seconds and minutes of the injury (Knight, 1995). Remember that blood clotting is a very rapid physiologic phenomenon designed to minimize hemorrhaging. Therefore, applying cryotherapy hours after injury has very limited effect on wound bleeding.

2. Minimizing Secondary Tissue Damage

Cryotherapy, if applied within the first 24 to 48 hours following soft-tissue damage, can significantly minimize secondary tissue damage. Research has shown that primary tissue damage (dead cells) may lead to significant secondary tissue damage involving the viable cells located within the immediate vicinity of the wound, through enzymatic and metabolic changes (see Knight, 1995). To minimize secondary tissue damage, therefore, is to restrict total tissue damage. The lesser the total amount of tissue damage, the smaller the wound size at the site of injury. The smaller the wound, the faster and better the tissue repair process. Cryotherapy, when used in conjunction with other therapeutic interventions, such as rest and protection (i.e., the use of canes, splints, or slings), can further minimize secondary tissue damage. The delivery of anti-inflammatory drugs at the wound site, using iontophoresis (Chapter 16), is another EPA that practitioners can use to minimize secondary tissue damage (see Box 6-1).

3. Minimizing Edema

Swelling is the enlargement of a tissue or organ resulting from edema, which is the accumulation of fluids in the interstitial spaces. Cryotherapy can reduce edema at the wound site if applied within the first 24 to 48 hours post injury. It does this by minimizing secondary tissue damage (Knight, 1995). Minimizing secondary damage reduces the amount of free proteins in the wound vicinity, which in turn leads to less edema formation. Edema prevention and reduction can be further enhanced if cryotherapy is used with other therapeutic interventions, such as elevation and compression. Limb compression therapy (Chapter 18) and cryo-hydrotherapy (Chapter 9) can also be used to minimize the formation of post-injury edema.

4. Minimizing Pain and Muscle Spasm

Pain is always, and muscle spasm is occasionally, associated with soft-tissue pathology. Pain results from the chemical activation, triggered by the inflammatory response, of nociceptors buried within the tissues located near the wound (Chapter 4). Muscle spasm results from the vicious pain–spasm cycle, the role of which is to minimize pain by restricting joint movement. Cryotherapy can reduce pain by acting as a counterirritant stimulus (cold over pain) or by acting on pain nerve fibers (reducing/blocking nerve conduction). It can reduce muscle spasm by decreasing pain (less pain, less muscle spasm). Transcutaneous electrical nerve stimulation (TENS) (Chapter 14) can be used to modulate pain through its action on the endogenous opiate and gate systems. The use of analgesic drug iontophoresis is also indicated during this first stage of intervention to modulate pain.

B. SECOND STAGE: ENHANCING REPAIR TISSUE PROLIFERATION AND FORMATION

The second stage of intervention refers to enhancing repair tissue proliferation and formation (see Box 6-1). The objective is to enhance blood flow and cellular metabolism. During this stage, the therapeutic goals are to promote angiogenesis and fibroplasia while minimizing pain and optimizing wound contraction.

1. Promoting Angiogenesis and Fibroplasia

The proliferation and formation of repair tissues rest on a cascade of interrelated physiologic events. *Angiogenesis,* the formation of new blood vessels, and *fibroplasia,* the laying down of repair tissues, are both key processes that are optimized by increased blood flow and metabolism at the wound site. Many EPAs can be used to achieve these responses or therapeutic goals. The judicious choices are agents that are capable of inducing superficial and deep thermal vasodilation effects in soft tissues, such as thermotherapy (Chapter 7), thermo-hydrotherapy (Chapter 9), shortwave diathermy (Chapter 10), ultrasound (Chapter 20), and extracorporeal shock wave therapy (Chapter 21). Other EPAs that can be used during this healing stage include low-level laser therapy (Chapter 11) and electrical stimulation for tissues healing and repair (Chapter 15).

2. Minimizing Pain and Optimizing Wound Contraction

Decreasing pain (if still present) can best be achieved with TENS (Chapter 14) or with any other thermal agents listed previously. Wound contraction may be enhanced with the application of continuous passive motion therapy (Chapter 19) in cases of pathology to the upper and lower limbs, or with spinal traction therapy (Chapter 17) in cases of pathology to the spinal column. These last two EPAs can induce the necessary mechanical tensile stress on maturing repair tissue.

C. THIRD STAGE: ENHANCING REPAIR TISSUE REMODELING, MATURATION, AND FUNCTION

As the immature repair tissue gives way to mature and, hopefully, functional tissue, another set of therapeutic goals and therapeutic EPAs must be introduced. The goals during this third stage of intervention are to encourage optimal remodeling and maturation of these newly formed tissues or to optimize function (see Box 6-1). Remodeling and maturation may be enhanced with ultrasound (Chapter 20), low-level laser therapy (Chapter 11), and extracorporeal shock wave therapy (Chapter 21). The promotion of maturation and function can also be enhanced with spinal traction therapy (Chapter 17) and continuous passive motion therapy (Chapter 19). Finally, the enhancement of repair tissue strength and endurance may also be achieved by means of neuromuscular electrical stimulation therapy (Chapter 13). When the repair tissue is mature and strong enough, the use of all mentioned EPAs is replaced by active functional training and conditioning exercise programs, with the aim of returning the patient to home, leisure, sport, and work activities.

IV. PRESENT AND FUTURE MANAGEMENT OF SOFT-TISSUE PATHOLOGY

Today's approach to the therapeutic management of soft-tissue pathology is to use conservative treatments, such as therapeutic exercises, manual therapy, and EPAs, and more invasive treatments, such as medication and surgery. With the rapid advancement of science in the field of soft-tissue repair, tomorrow's therapeutic approach should differ drastically from that of today. The following are just a few examples of therapeutic interventions or therapies that may well become common in the next decade. For example, research has shown that a well-regulated growth factor cascade is important for the orderly progression of steps in the wound healing process. Injection of growth factors in patients suffering from soft-tissue injury may thus be beneficial. Research in tissue engineering opens the door for replacing injured tissue with tissue constructed in vitro for subsequent implantation in vivo that has similar structural, physiologic, and mechanical properties. The ability to deliver genes to the cells to improve soft-tissue healing outcomes is another therapeutic approach that may be beneficial to millions of patients. Stem cell therapy is perhaps the most exciting of all potential treatments. Injecting stem cells into damaged tissue may significantly contribute to the repair and regeneration of soft-tissue pathology by optimizing the healing process.

V. THE BOTTOM LINE

- EPAs have a broad therapeutic spectrum that can affect several components of the ICF disablement model.
- To judiciously select an EPA is to select the one that will best enhance the current healing phase of the pathologic tissue.
- To use the EPA in a timely fashion means to apply the agent during the period in which it will yield optimal results.
- The selection of one agent over another is guided by a three-stage intervention framework that rests on the four basic phases of soft-tissue healing.
- Several agents may be used concomitantly to maximize each of the stages of healing.
- EPAs primarily are used for the management of pain, edema, muscle spasm, muscle weakness and atrophy, and joint motion restriction, as well as for the enhancement of wound, tendon, muscle, ligament, and bone healing.

VI. CRITICAL THINKING QUESTIONS

Clarification: What is meant by judicious selection and timely application of EPAs based on a three-stage intervention framework?

Assumptions: You assume that acute soft-tissue pathology can be identified based on cardinal signs and symptoms. How do you justify this assumption?

Reasons and evidence: The use of cryotherapy, with or without other therapeutic interventions, is a judicious choice during the first stage of soft-tissue repair. Why?

Viewpoints or perspectives: You agree with the suggestion that closely monitoring the presence and magnitude of some of the cardinal signs and symptoms may be one of the best methods for determining the healing phase of soft tissue. What would someone who disagrees with you say?

Implications and consequences: The therapeutic effects of EPAs are best maximized when applied in conjunction with other therapeutic interventions. What are you implying?

About the question: Is today's therapeutic approach to the management of soft-tissue pathology viable for many years to come? Why do you think I ask this question?

VII. REFERENCES

Textbooks

Belanger AY (2002) Evidence-Based Guide to Therapeutic Physical Agents. Lippincott Williams & Wilkins, Baltimore

Belanger AY (2009) Therapeutic Electrophysical Agents: Evidence Behind Practice, 2nd ed. Lippincott Williams & Wilkins, Baltimore

Knight KL (1995) Cryotherapy in Sports Injury Management. Human Kinetics, Champaign, IL

PART II

Thermal Agents

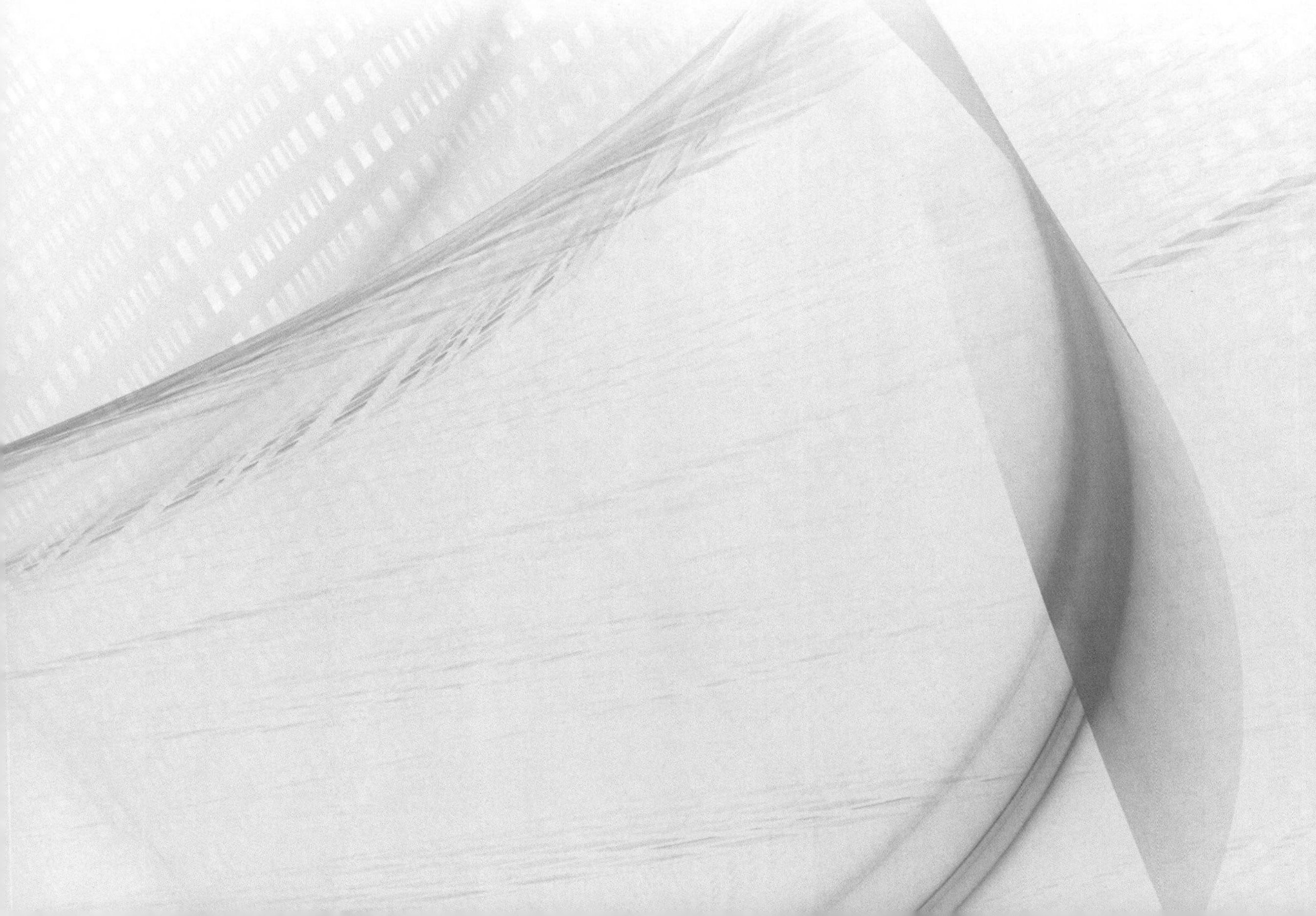

Chapter 7

Thermotherapy

Chapter Outline

Learning Objectives

Remembering: List the basic considerations associated with the application of thermotherapy using hot pack, paraffin bath, and Fluidotherapy.

Understanding: Summarize the physiologic and therapeutic effects of hot pack, paraffin bath, and Fluidotherapy. Compare the heat transfer properties and thermal responses of these three thermal agents. Explain the meaning of $T°_{ag\text{-}s}$ and $T°_{b\text{-}a}$. Explain the difference between heat and temperature.

Applying: Show how to record $T°_{ag\text{-}s}$ and $T°_{b\text{-}a}$ using a noncontact portable thermometer. Demonstrate how to conduct and score the skin sensory discrimination test.

Analyzing: Compare the thermophysical properties (specific heat and thermal conductivity) of hot pack (water), paraffin bath (paraffin wax), and Fluidotherapy (air).

Evaluating: Judge the advantage or benefit of complementing the qualitative approach to thermal dosimetry with a quantitative approach.

Creating: Predict the future of thermotherapy in the field of physical medicine and rehabilitation sports therapy based on its current strength of evidence and therapeutic effectiveness.

I. FOUNDATION

A. DEFINITION

Thermotherapy is defined as the application of heat sources, called *thermal agents,* over skin surface areas for heating superficial and deep soft tissues. This chapter focuses on the use of three thermal agents, namely hot pack, paraffin bath, and Fluidotherapy. Hot pack and paraffin bath deliver *moist* heat to flat body areas and distal upper and lower extremities. Fluidotherapy, on the other hand, delivers *dry* heat to both the upper and lower extremities.

B. HOT PACK

Figure 7-1 shows a typical commercial hot pack, commercial pack cover, and hydrocollator unit filled with hot water and used to store and heat the packs. Packs and covers come in various shapes and sizes to accommodate most body areas. Hydrocollator units, mounted with their hydrostatic water temperature controllers, also come in different sizes that accommodate small to large numbers of packs.

C. PARAFFIN BATH

Figure 7-2 illustrates a typical thermostatically regulated bath filled with a mixture of paraffin and mineral oil. Accessories related to paraffin bath therapy are shown, such as wrapping mittens and a brush assembly.

D. FLUIDOTHERAPY

Fluidotherapy uses a fluidized bed of organic particles, thus the term *fluido,* for the delivery of heat to soft tissues. Figure 7-3 illustrates a Fluidotherapy device and a container filled with cellulose particles. The device allows those finely divided particles to circulate around the treated area by a warm air current, creating a fluidlike medium.

E. HEAT WRAPS

In addition to the use of hot pack, paraffin bath, and Fluidotherapy, thermotherapy today is also delivered safely and effectively at home, using a variety of over-the-counter, easy-to-use, and reusable heat wraps. Figure 7-4 displays a heat wrap that draws moisture from air, retains it in 100% cotton covers, and then releases heat.

F. RATIONALE FOR USE

The rationale for hot pack, paraffin bath, and Fluidotherapy is to provide practitioners with thermal agents capable of generating moist and dry heat and distributing it to superficial and deep soft tissues. The agents also allow clinicians to heat large body surface areas (hot pack) and difficult-to-reach body areas such as fingers and toes (paraffin bath and Fluidotherapy).

II. BIOPHYSICAL CHARACTERISTICS

A. PRINCIPLES AND CONCEPTS

The biophysics of hot pack, paraffin bath and Fluidotherapy is based on the principles and concepts related to thermodynamics—the branch of physics concerned with the relationship between heat and other form of energy. Generally speaking, thermotherapy rests on heat transfer from the agent to the biologic tissues. To better understand the biophysics behind thermotherapy, the concepts related to the first and second law of thermodynamics, heat versus temperature, heat transfer modes, specific heat capacity, and thermal conductivity are discussed next. Note that the same biophysical principles and concepts apply to the use of cryotherapy (Chapter 8) and hydrotherapy (Chapter 9).

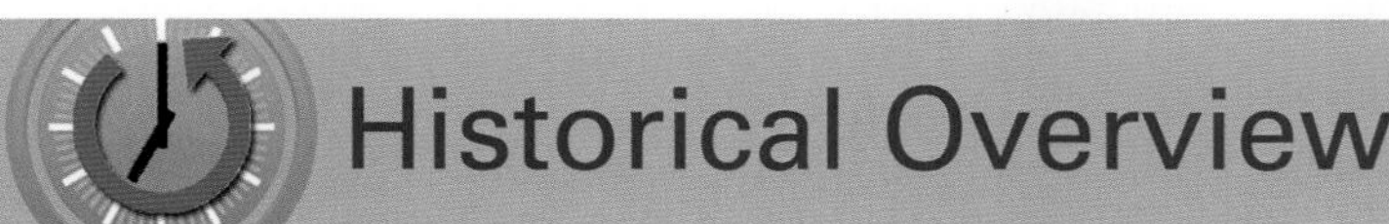

The literature suggests that the therapeutic use of hot packs was introduced during the mid-1950s by Hollander et al. (1949), Horvath et al. (1949), and Erdman et al. (1956). It also indicates that paraffin bath therapy was first used in the early part of the 20th century by De Sanfort (1915), Humphris (1920), Portmann (1926), Zeiter (1939), and Stimson et al. (1958). Fluidotherapy® is a trademarked name coined in 1973 by an American chemical engineer named Ernest Henley. Unimpressed by the capacity of existing moist thermal therapeutic agents, such as hot pack and paraffin bath therapy to deliver heat to soft tissues, Henley sought to develop a new dry thermal agent that would transfer a greater quantity of heat to superficial and deep soft tissues (Henley, 1991). Drawing on his engineering knowledge of the good thermal conductivity of fluidized beds for heat transfer in industry, Henley adapted the industrial concept of fluidization to the field of therapeutics.

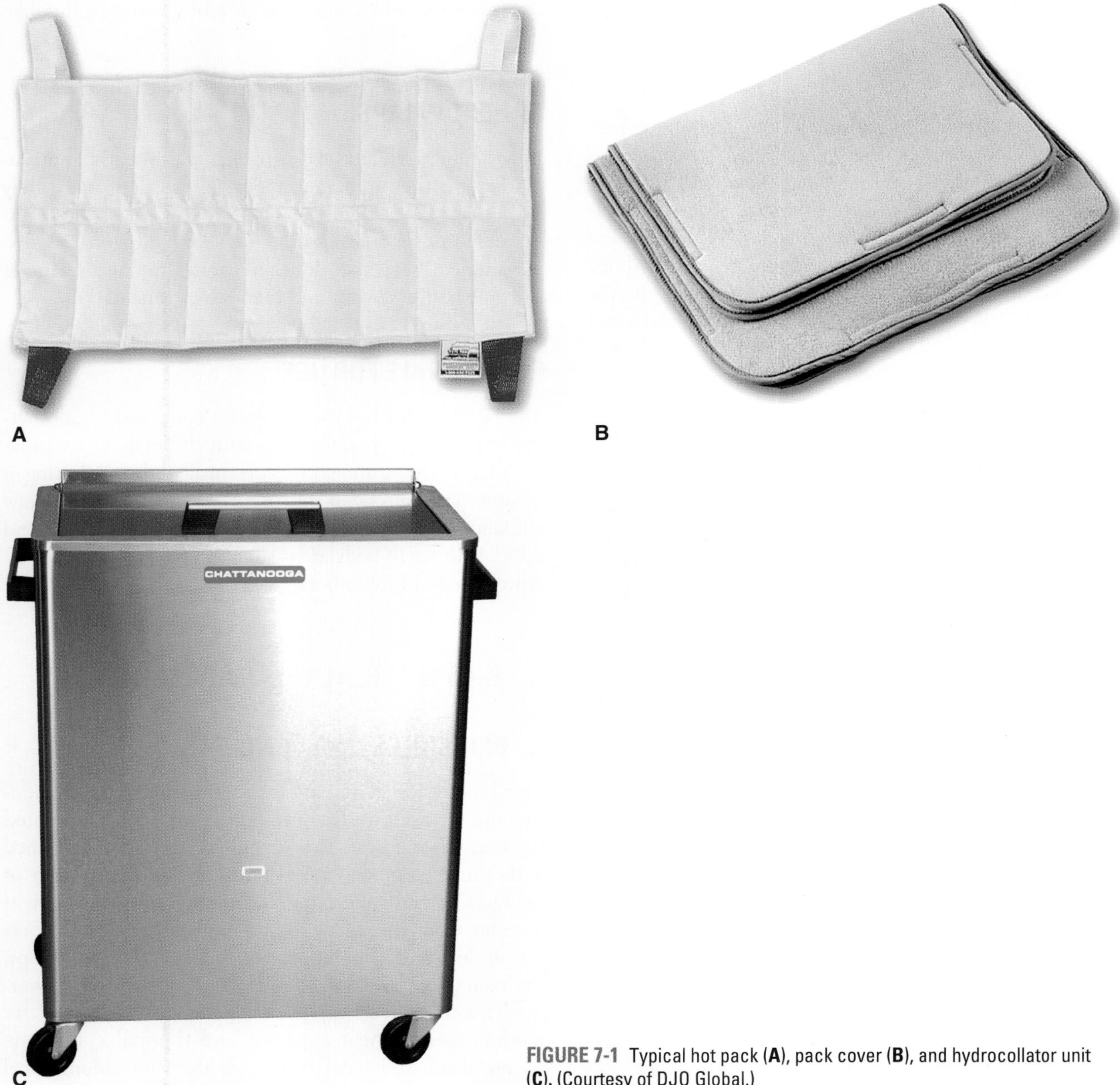

FIGURE 7-1 Typical hot pack (**A**), pack cover (**B**), and hydrocollator unit (**C**). (Courtesy of DJO Global.)

B. FIRST AND SECOND LAWS OF THERMODYNAMICS

The first law, called *law of conservation of energy,* states that energy cannot be created nor destroyed; it only changed from one form into another or transferred from one object to another. Let us consider the use of hot pack. During application, the thermal energy stored in the hot pack is transferred to both the targeted soft tissue and to the air surroundings both of them. This means that thermal energy was neither created nor destroyed; it was simply transferred from the hot pack to the soft tissue and surroundings. The second law stipulates that heat energy transfer always occur in one direction only, i.e., from the warmest to the coldest substance. For example, the heat contained in paraffin wax, which is greater than that of the target soft tissue, is transferred to the latter during therapy.

C. HEAT VERSUS TEMPERATURE

The concept of heat and temperature are often confused. Although related to each other, they are different. *It is critical to remember that heat is energy and that temperature is a measure of it.* Heat is the total kinetic energy, or molecular motion, of a substance. The greater the molecular motion of a substance, the more heat it contains. The heat energy of a substance depends on three elements: the speed of its particles (its kinetic energy), the number of particles (its mass), and the capacity of its particles to store heat (its specific heat capacity). Temperature is the measurement of the average kinetic

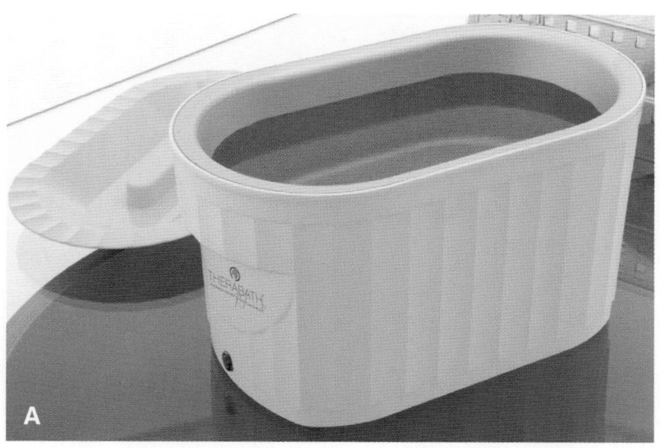

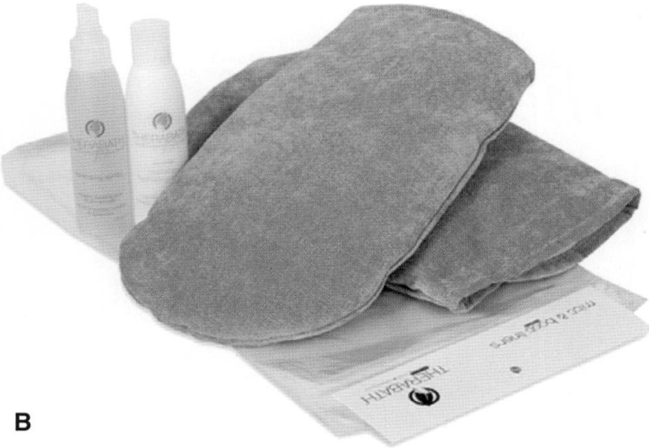

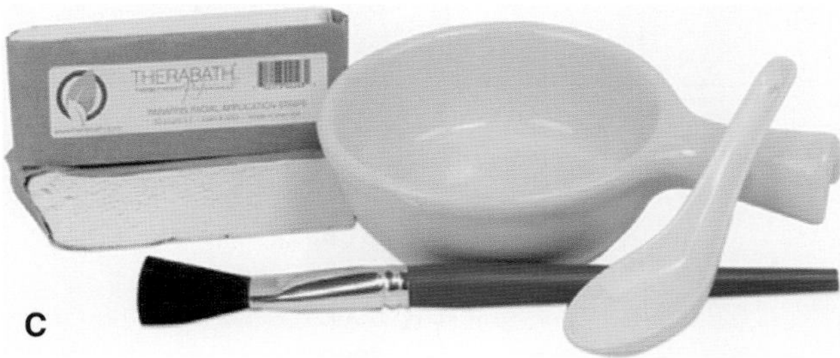

FIGURE 7-2 Typical paraffin bath (**A**) with related accessories such as wrapping mittens (**B**) and brushing assembly (**C**). (Courtesy of WR Medical Electronics.)

energy of a substance. The greater the amount of heat in a substance, the higher its temperature. Temperature depends on one element—the speed of particles (kinetic energy). Thus, the greater the kinetic energy of a substance, the higher its temperature. Keep in mind that *cold* is the absence of heat, whereas *coldness* is the sensation produced by a substance that has less heat or is at lower temperature. It is correct to state that the greater the amount of heat (or kinetic energy) within a thermal agent, the higher its temperature. Now is it correct to say that of two hot packs with the same temperature, say 70°C (158°F), the one with the larger mass (1,500 g vs. 1,000 g) will contain a greater amount of heat than the other? The answer is yes because the amount of heat (q) a material or substance possesses is directly related to its mass, as evidenced by the formula $q = m \times \Delta t° \times c$, where m is the mass of the hot pack in this case. Therefore, by analogy, there is more heat in a

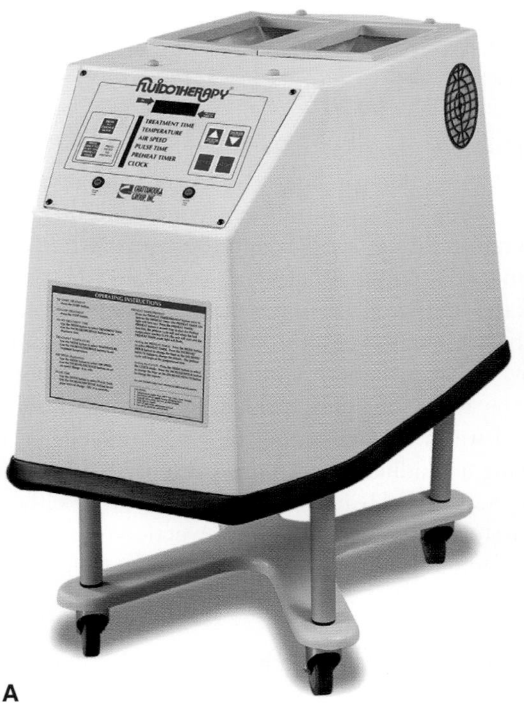

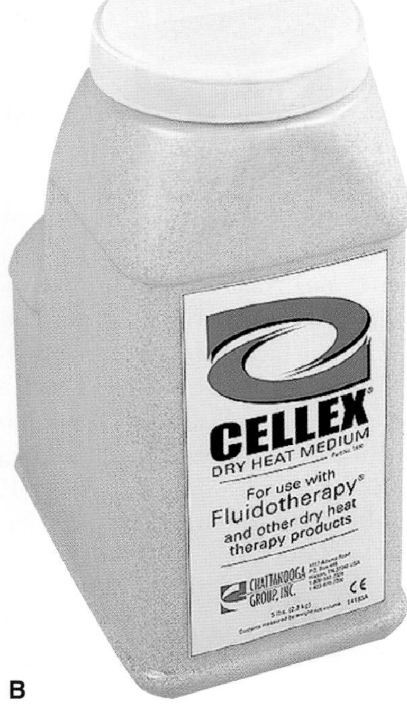

FIGURE 7-3 Typical Fluidotherapy device (**A**) shown with a container of fine organic particles of cellulose (**B**). (Courtesy of DJO Global.)

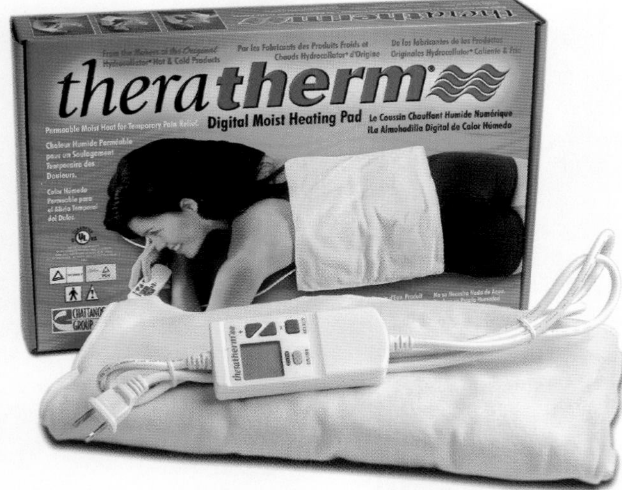

FIGURE 7-4 Commercial reusable heat wrap. (Courtesy of DJO Global.)

full kettle of boiled water (i.e., more mass or molecules of water) than in a single cup of boiled water, although the boiled water is 100°C (212°F) in both cases. Clinically speaking, practitioners should always select a larger hot pack over a smaller one, even if both have the same temperature, when the therapeutic purpose is to deliver more heat to the soft tissues per unit of time. This is simply because the larger pack contains more heat than the smaller pack.

D. HEAT TRANSFER MODES

Heat transfer between two substances, as illustrated in Figure 7-5, can occur through four different modes: conduction, convection, radiation, and evaporation. The result is that heat can be added (thermotherapy and thermohydrotherapy) or removed (cryotherapy and cryohydrotherapy) from the soft tissues.

1. Conduction Mode

Conduction occurs through the physical contact between two solid substances of different temperatures (see Fig. 7-5A). Conduction always occurs from the warmest to the coldest substance (see arrows in the figure). In thermotherapy, the higher kinetic energy of the warmer substance (the agent) increases, by conduction, the lower kinetic energy of the colder substance (tissue) through microscopic molecular collisions. The resulting heat added to the tissue increases its temperature. In cryotherapy, the higher kinetic energy of the warmer substance (tissue) increases, by conduction, the lower kinetic energy of the colder substance (the agent) through the same mechanism. The tissue thus loses heat, whereas the cryoagents gain heat. In hydrotherapy, the heat transfer is also achieved by conduction with the colder or warmer water in contact with the skin.

2. Convection Mode

Convection occurs through physical contact between a gaseous or fluid medium (such as air and water) and

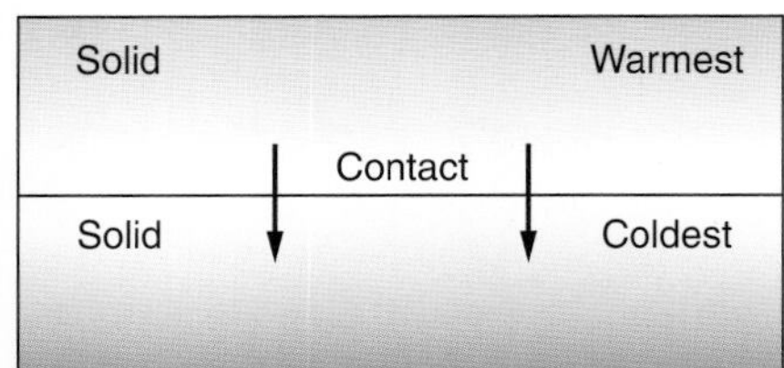

A Conduction

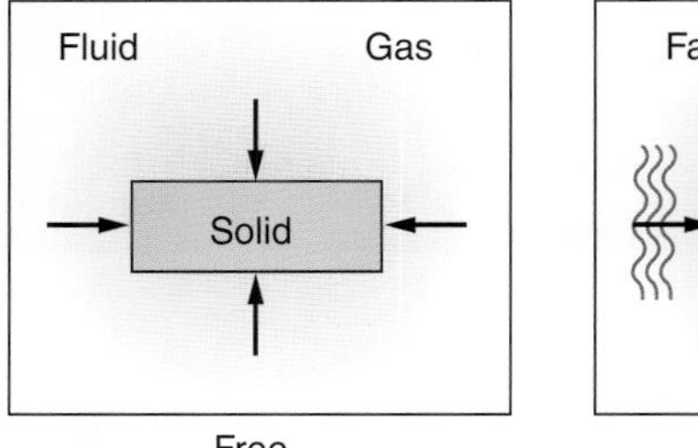

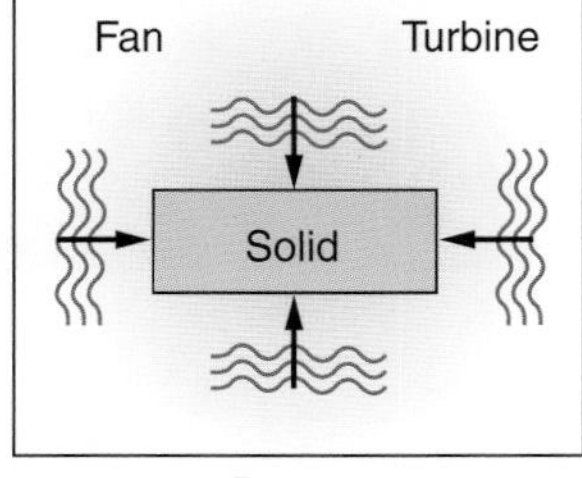

B Convection

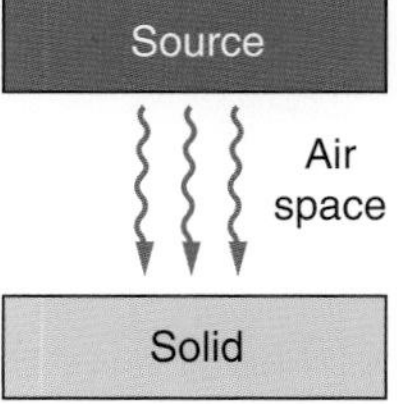

C Radiation

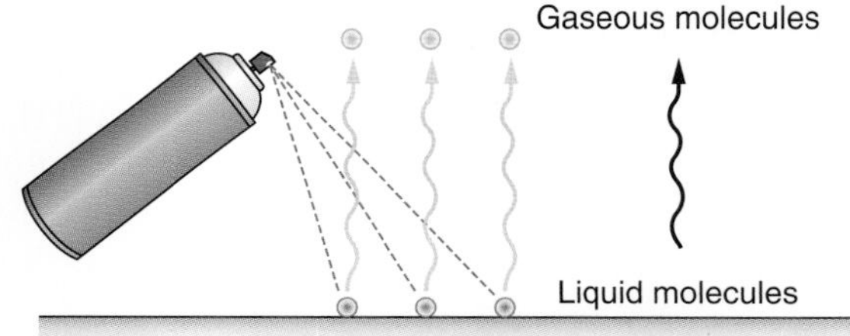

D Evaporation

FIGURE 7-5 Modes of heat transfer: conduction (**A**), convection (**B**), radiation (**C**), and evaporation (**D**).

a solid substance, both at different temperatures (see Fig. 7-5B). Convection can be free or forced. *Free convection* is the heating of the solid substance induced solely by the temperature difference between the two substances. *Forced convection,* on the other hand, is caused when the motion of the fluid or gas is imposed externally by means of a fan (Fluidotherapy) or a turbine (hydrotherapy). Fluidotherapy uses convection combined with fluidization, which is the result of finely divided particles, activated by a flow of warm air, to acquire the characteristics of a fluid causing a fluidlike effect on the exposed skin surface (Henley, 1991). Hydrotherapeutic agents use either free (still water) or forced (turbine) convection to transfer their energy to tissues.

3. Radiation

Radiation is the propagation of energy in the form of rays or waves. It occurs in the air space between the emitting source and the absorbing solid (Fig. 7-5C). The use of shortwave diathermy (Chapter 10) is a good example of heat transfer by radiation.

4. Evaporation

The fourth and final mode of heat transfer, *evaporation,* refers to the transformation, as illustrated in Figure 7-5D, of a liquid to a gaseous state (Sekins et al., 1990). For example, when a vapocoolant is sprayed on the skin, as is the case with cryotherapy (Chapter 8), the liquid molecules vaporize from the skin surface. The heat to produce this transition is extracted from the skin tissue, which is thus cooled. In other words, if part of a liquid evaporates, it cools the liquid remaining behind because it must extract heat of vaporization from that liquid in order to make the change from liquid to gaseous state.

E. SPECIFIC HEAT (c)

Specific heat, designated by the letter c, is defined as the capacity of a substance to store heat (Sekins et al., 1990). It corresponds to the heat input in calories (cal) required to increase the temperature of 1 g of a substance by 1°C. Specific heat (c) equals heat input (cal)/mass (g) × temperature (°C). Its unit is commonly expressed as cal/g°C. The specific heat (c) value of water is 1, because a heat input of 1 cal is needed to increase 1 g of pure water by 1°C at 15°C (1 c = 1 cal/(1 g × 1°C). Thus, the higher the specific heat of a substance, the higher its capacity to store heat.

F. THERMAL CONDUCTIVITY (k)

Thermal conductivity, designated by the letter k, is defined as the capacity of a substance to conduct heat (Sekins et al., 1990). It is the quantity of heat (cal) that passes in a unit of time (sec), through a unit area (cm) of a substance whose thickness is unity, when its opposite faces differ in temperature by 1°C. Its unit is commonly expressed as cal/sec-cm°C. The higher the thermal conductivity of a substance, the better its ability to conduct heat.

G. THERMOPHYSICAL PROPERTIES

Table 7-1 presents the specific heat capacity (c) and thermal conductivity (k) values of some materials and biologic tissues, including water. This table shows that water, at any given temperature, stores or holds approximately 2 times more heat than paraffin oil (1.00 vs. 0.45) and conducts heat approximately 2.5 times more rapidly than paraffin oil (1.42 vs. 0.59). It also shows that air, when compared with water, stores approximately 4 times less heat (0.24 vs. 1.00) and conducts heat approximately 70 times more slowly (0.02 vs. 1.42). What is the clinical significance of this table?

TABLE 7-1 THERMOPHYSICAL PROPERTIES OF MATERIALS AND BIOLOGIC TISSUES AT 25°C

Properties	Specific Heat (c)[a]	Thermal Conductivity (k)[b]
Units	**cal/g°C**	**cal/sec-cm°C × 10^3**
Aluminum	0.22	487.00
Rubber	0.48	0.37
Air	0.24	0.02
Paraffin oil	0.45	0.59
Ice	0.46	5.28
Water	**1.00**	**1.42**
Muscle	0.90	1.53
Skin	0.90	0.90
Subcutaneous fat	0.55	0.45
Blood	0.87	1.31
Bone	0.38	2.78

[a]c = The intrinsic capacity of a substance to hold, or store, heat at a given temperature. It is the capacity of a substance to store heat per unit of mass per degree Celsius.
[b]k = The intrinsic capacity of a substance to transmit, or conduct, heat. It is the quantity of heat transmitted in a unit of time through a unit area of a substance whose thickness is unity, when its opposite surfaces differ in temperature by 1°C.
Source: Adapted with permission from Sekins KM, Emery AF (1990) Thermal science for physical medicine. In: Therapeutic Heat and Cold, 4th ed. Lehmann JF (Ed). Williams & Wilkins, Philadelphia, pp 62–112

H. CLINICAL SIGNIFICANCE

The concepts of specific heat and thermal conductivity scientifically explain many aspects related to the application of thermotherapy. As discussed later, these two concepts explain why patients can tolerate the application of a thermal agent at higher temperature than the others can. They also explain why subcutaneous fat acts as a thermal barrier between the skin and the deeper tissues.

1. Hot Pack Versus Paraffin Bath

Why is it that if you apply a hot pack of a given temperature over one hand and immerse the other hand in a paraffin bath of the same temperature, the hot pack feels hotter than the paraffin wax mixture? It is because the water absorbed in the hot pack holds or stores approximately 2 times more heat (higher specific heat capacity; c = 1.00 vs. 0.45) and conducts heat approximately 2.5 times faster (higher thermal conductivity; k = 1.42 vs. 0.59) than paraffin. Why is it that applying a hot pack at 50°C (122°F) directly over the skin will cause severe pain and burn, whereas applying paraffin wax of the same temperature will feel comfortable and not burn the skin? The answer, once again, lies in the fact that compared with water, paraffin has a much lower capacity to retain or store (c = 0.45 vs. 1.00) and conduct heat (k = 0.59 vs. 1.42) to the soft tissues.

2. Fluidotherapy Versus Paraffin Bath

Why is it that if you immerse one hand in a Fluidotherapy air chamber of a given temperature and the other in a paraffin bath of the same temperature, the paraffin bath feels hotter than the air chamber? It is because paraffin wax holds approximately 2 times more heat (c = 0.45 vs. 0.24) and conducts heat approximately 30 times faster (k = 0.59 vs. 0.02) than air.

3. Fluidotherapy Versus Hydrotherapy

Again, why is it that if you immerse one hand in a Fluidotherapy air chamber of a given temperature and apply a hot pack of the same temperature on your other hand, the hot pack feels much hotter than the air chamber? Once again, the answer rests with the fact that water holds approximately 4 times more heat (c = 1.00 vs. 0.24) and conducts heat approximately 70 times faster (k = 1.42 vs. 0.02) than air.

4. Subcutaneous Fat Versus Other Biologic Tissues

Now, why is it that subcutaneous fat, at any given temperature and when compared with skin and muscle, acts as a thermal insulator, or barrier, between the skin and the deeper tissues? Values from Table 7-1 shows that subcutaneous fat has the lowest specific heat capacity (c = 0.55) and thermal conductivity (k = 0.45) values. Clinically speaking, this means that subcutaneous fat is the tissue that holds and conducts heat the least. Because of its poor capacity to conduct heat, subcutaneous fat thus acts as a significant thermal barrier, preventing heat from reaching the deeper soft tissues.

III. THERAPEUTIC EFFECTS AND INDICATIONS

A. SUPERFICIAL VERSUS DEEP HEATING

Historically, thermotherapy has subjectively been classified as either superficial or deep in nature in several textbooks on electrophysical agents (EPAs). For example, readers have noticed that agents such as hot packs and paraffin baths are often classified as superficial heat. What does the evidence say about this classification? As shown in Table 7-2, there is sufficient scientific evidence to suggest that such a classification is no longer justified and should be abandoned because all three thermal agents can induce both superficial and deep thermal effects (from skin to joint capsule) on healthy human tissues.

B. THERMOPHYSIOLOGIC EFFECTS

Figure 7-6 illustrates the proposed physiological and therapeutic effects of thermotherapy. Firstly, there is

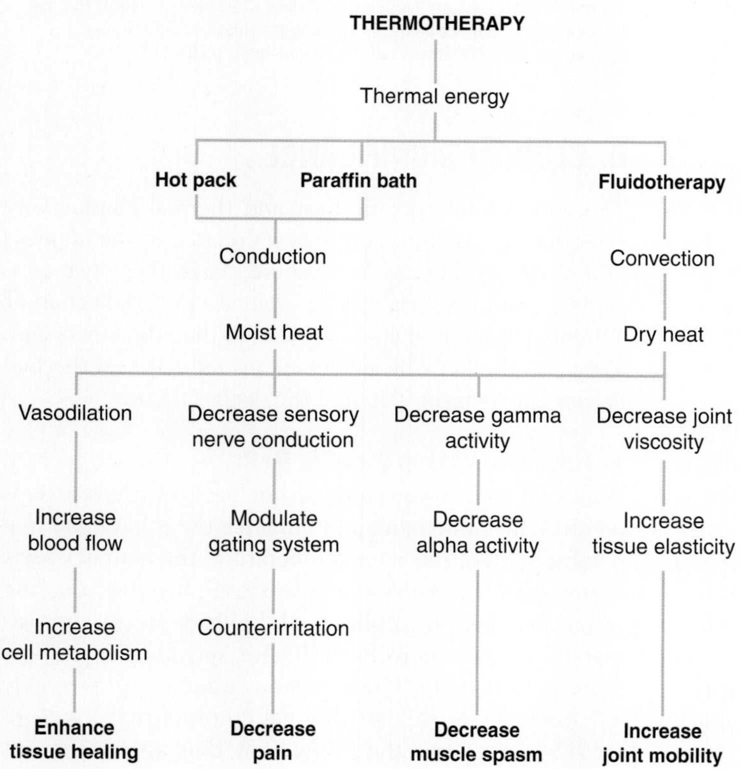

FIGURE 7-6 Proposed physiologic and therapeutic effects of thermotherapy delivered using hot pack, paraffin bath, and Fluidotherapy.

TABLE 7-2 PHYSIOLOGIC EFFECTS OF THERMOTHERAPY ON HEALTHY SUBJECTS

Source	Experimental Results
Abramson et al., 1964	Hot pack over forearm; increases skin temperature by an average of about 12°C, and subcutaneous fat and muscle temperature by 6°C and 3°C, respectively.
Lehmann et al., 1966	Hot pack over thigh area; increases skin surface temperature by 10°C and soft tissue temperature by 2°C at a depth of 3 cm.
Henrickson et al., 1984	Hot pack over hamstring muscle area; no significant increase in muscle length
Lentell et al., 1992	Hot pack over shoulder area; increases ROM
Taylor et al., 1995	Hot pack over hamstring muscle area; no significant increase in muscle length
Draper et al., 1998	Hot pack over triceps surae area; additive effect of ultrasound therapy for increasing the triceps surae muscle temperature
Knight et al., 2001	Hot pack over triceps surae area; increases ankle dorsiflexion ROM
Cosgray et al., 2004	Hot pack over hamstring muscle area; no change in hamstring length
Robertson et al., 2005	Hot pack over triceps surae area; increases ankle dorsiflexion ROM
Borrell et al., 1977	Paraffin bath over hand and foot; increases muscle temperature by an average of 4.5°C and joint capsule temperature by 7.5°C.
Borrell et al., 1980	Fluidotherapy over hands and feet; increase muscle temperature by an average of 5.2°C, and joint capsule temperature by 9°C.
Kelly et al., 2005	Fluidotherapy over the upper arm; increase skin temperature and decrease the distal latency of the superficial radial sensory nerve
Draper et al., 2008	Thermal wrap causes an average temperature increase of 3°C in the quadriceps muscle and knee joint capsule.

ROM, range of motion.

undeniable evidence to show that heat absorption causes vasodilation, which in turn increases blood flow and cell metabolism thus enhancing soft tissue healing. Secondly, heating stimulates sensory nerve conduction leading to decrease pain via modulation of the gating system and the counterirritation effect. The irritant stimuli, here, is the thermal sensation that decrease pain by diverting attention to that it produces. Thirdly, heating decreases gamma motoneuron activity, which in turn decrease alpha motoneuron activity leading to decrease muscle spasm. Fourthly, heating of deeper tissues alters the viscoelastic properties of muscles and tendons, and decreases joint viscosity, thus enhancing joint mobility (Nakano et al., 2012).

C. TARGET TEMPERATURE WINDOW

Scientific evidence suggests that to optimize the clinical effectiveness of thermotherapy, critical levels of soft tissue heating must be achieved following the application of thermal agents (see Lehmann et al., 1990). What are the soft tissue target temperature levels that need to be reached to accomplish the physiologic and therapeutic effects? Figure 7-7 illustrates evidence from the literature suggesting that the *optimal* therapeutic temperature window for thermotherapy may be between 40° and 45°C (104° and 113°F). According to classical work on thermotherapy by Lehmann and coworkers (1990), if a vigorous, or optimal, physiologic response is to be produced, it is necessary to elevate the tissue temperature, at the site of injury or disease, to the highest maximally tolerated temperature, which should range from 40° to 45°C (104° to 113°F). For Lehmann et al. (1990), elevating soft tissue temperature above 45°C (113°F) will cause tissue damage, whereas elevating tissue temperature below 40°C (104°F) will produce a suboptimal or milder physiologic response.

1. Skin Heating

Is it possible to increase human skin temperature to the optimal range of the therapeutic window by using thermal agents? The answer is yes. The body of evidence reviewed in this chapter indicates that increasing the skin temperature to such a temperature range is possible and easily achievable when proper dosimetry and

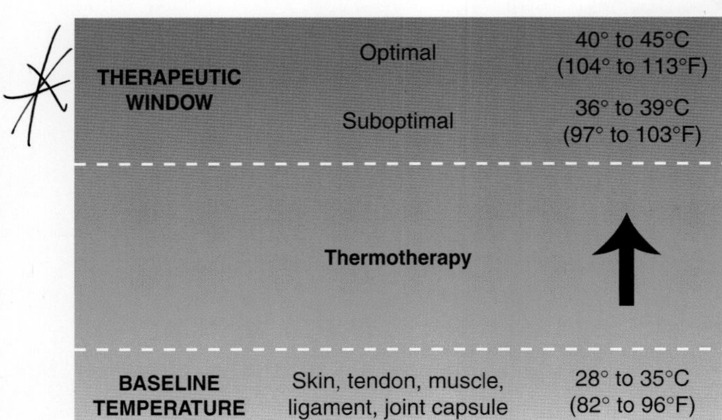

FIGURE 7-7 Thermotherapy therapeutic window.

application protocol are used (see Table 7-2). Unfortunately, the skin, when compared to deeper tissues such as muscles, tendons, ligaments, or joint capsules, is rarely the targeted tissue when the time comes to use thermotherapy.

2. Muscle, Tendon, Ligament, and Joint Capsule Heating

Is it possible to elevate the temperature of targeted deeper tissues, all covered by a layer of subcutaneous fat, to the optimal range of the therapeutic window using thermal agents? The answer is yes in certain cases and no in others. Theoretically speaking, it may all depend on which body areas these thermal agents are applied, the magnitude of the dose used (see later discussion), and whether or not the deeper tissues within the treatment areas are covered with either thick or thin layers of subcutaneous fat. For example, the answer is yes if one applies a thermal agent with a high temperature differential or dose (see later discussion) over the area of the feet where the adiposity, or skinfold, is at its lowest value. The answer is no if one applies the same thermal agent over the back area of a patient who is overweight or obese, in whom adiposity may be excessive.

3. Suboptimal Versus Optimal Heating

The goal of thermotherapy is to increase deep soft tissue temperatures within the therapeutic temperature window (see Fig. 7-7). The theoretical therapeutic rationale is that the warmer soft tissues, the better the physiologic and therapeutic effects. Results in Table 7-2 show that it is possible, by using hot pack, paraffin bath, or Fluidotherapy, to elevate the temperatures of human muscles and joint capsules within the suboptimal range of up to 40°C (104°F). To elevate the temperature of deeper tissues within the optimal range of above 40°C (104°F) may be very difficult to do. Why? First, the ability of thermal agents to heat up deep soft tissues is limited by the skin's nociceptive response to thermal stimulus. There is evidence to show that above 45°C (113°F), human skin nociceptors are activated, causing thermal pain that will become intolerable as skin temperature further increases. Second, the thickness of subcutaneous fat, which has poor thermal conductivity, also poses a problem (see Table 7-1). During thermotherapy, thermal energy is transferred from the warmest to the cooler areas. This practically means that the heat of the warmest area (thermal agent) is first transferred to the cooler skin tissue. As the skin gets warmer than the deeper tissues, heat is further transferred from the skin, through the subcutaneous fat, to those cooler deeper tissues. Because subcutaneous fat acts as a thermal barrier, it becomes practically impossible to elevate the temperature of deeper soft tissues to the optimal range of the therapeutic thermal window without causing intolerable pain and possibly skin damage (burn).

D. RESEARCH-BASED INDICATIONS

The search for evidence behind the use of thermotherapy, displayed in the *Research-Based Indications* box, led to the collection of 28 English peer-reviewed human clinical studies. The methodologies and criteria used to assess the strength of evidence and therapeutic effectiveness are described in Chapter 2. As indicated in the box, the strength of evidence is ranked as *moderate* for rheumatoid/osteoarthritic conditions and neck/back/shoulder pain. Analysis is *pending* for the remaining health conditions because fewer than five studies could be collected. Over all conditions, the strength of evidence behind the use of thermotherapy is determined to be *moderate* and its therapeutic effectiveness *substantiated* for only two conditions, namely rheumatoid/osteoarthritic conditions and neck/back/shoulder pain. Only two clinical studies could be found on the use of Fluidotherapy.

IV. DOSIMETRY

A. QUALITATIVE VERSUS QUANTITATIVE

The practice of evidence-based thermotherapy, cryotherapy (Chapter 8), and hydrotherapy (Chapter 9) requires that practitioners objectively and quantitatively assess the thermal dose delivered to the tissues, and well as the amount of thermal heating added or extracted to the exposed tissues following the application of thermal agents. To simply ask the patient about his or her perceived thermal sensation during or after treatment—still routinely done by the very large majority of practitioners today—is practical but unfortunately no longer acceptable as the sole source of dosimetry. No one will argue that it is important for practitioners to know the patient's perception of heat caused by the agent during therapy. However, what does this qualitative or subjective information tell you, as clinicians, about the thermal dose delivered and the amount of heat added or withdrawn to the

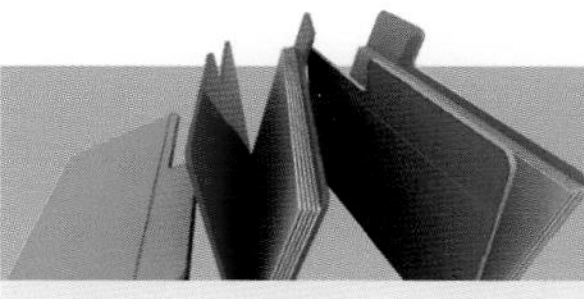

Research-Based Indications

THERMOTHERAPY

Health Condition	Benefit—Yes Rating	Benefit—Yes Reference	Benefit—No Rating	Benefit—No Reference
Rheumatoid/ osteoarthritic conditions	I	Dellhag et al., 1992 (pb)		
	I	Harris et al., 1955 (pb)		
	II	Hawkes et al., 1985 (pb)		
	II	Yung et al., 1986 (pb)		
	II	Bromley et al., 1994 (pb)		
	II	Williams et al., 1986 (hp)		
	II	Myrer et al., 2011 (pb)		
	II	Cetin et al., 2008 (hp)		
Strength of evidence: Moderate **Therapeutic effectiveness:** Substantiated				
Neck/back/ shoulder pain	II	Landen, 1967 (hp)	II	Garra et al., 2010 (hp)
	II	Cordray et al., 1959 (hp)		
	II	Miller et al., 1996 (hp)		
	II	Nuhr et al., 2004 (hw)		
	II	Mayer et al., 2005 (hw)		
	II	Nadler et al., 2002 (hw)		
	II	Nadler et al., 2003a (hw)		
	II	Nadler et al., 2003b (hw)		
Strength of evidence: Moderate **Therapeutic effectiveness:** Substantiated				

Health Condition	Benefit—Yes Rating	Benefit—Yes Reference	Benefit—No Rating	Benefit—No Reference
Fewer Than 5 Studies				
Hand scleroderma	I	Sandqvist et al., 2004 (pb)		
	II	Pils et al., 1991(pb)		
	III	Mancuso et al., 2009 (pb)		
Second stage of labor—pain	II	Dahlen et al., 2009 (hp)		
	II	Dahlen et al., 2007 (hp)		
Trigger point pain	II	McCray et al., 1984 (hp)		
Poliomyelitis	II	Fountain et al., 1960 (hp)		
Burn contracture	II	Head et al., 1977 (pb)		
Traumatic hand injury	II	Hoyrup et al., 1986 (pb)		
Sickle cell anemia	II	Alcorn et al., 1984 (fl)		
Podiatric conditions	III	Valenza et al., 1979 (fl)		
Strength of evidence: Pending **Therapeutic effectiveness:** Pending				
ALL CONDITIONS **Strength of evidence:** Moderate **Therapeutic effectiveness:** Substantiated				

hp, hot pack; pb, paraffin bath; fl, Fluidotherapy, hw, heat wrap.

soft tissues? *Nothing*. Now, how can practitioners move from qualitative to quantitative dosimetry?

B. TEMPERATURE MEASUREMENT

The goal of this textbook is to bring objective quantification to the art and science of heat transfer between the thermal agent and the exposed soft tissues after therapy. To do so, actual temperature measurements need to be taken using reliable thermometers before and after applications. This quantitative approach is meant to complement, not replace, the traditional qualitative dosimetric approach described earlier and still practiced today by most practitioners.

1. Temperature Differential

The quantitative approach proposed in this text is based on measuring two temperature differentials by using a portable and noncontact thermometer. The first temperature differential is the difference between the temperature of the agent (ag) and that of the skin (s) surface overlying the treated area before the application; this differential is

TABLE 7-3	QUANTITATIVE THERMAL DOSIMETRIC EXAMPLE		
Treatment	**Agent Temperature ($T°_{ag}$)**	**Skin Temperature ($T°_{s}$)**	**Dose ($T°_{ag\text{-}s}$)**
Before (b)	54°C (130°F)	30°C (86°F)	**24°C (44°F)**
After (a)	—	40°C (104°F)	—
Actual heating ($T°_{b\text{-}a}$)		**+10°C (+18°F)**	

designated as $\mathbf{T°_{ag\text{-}s}}$. The second temperature differential is that between the skin surface temperature before (b) and after (a) treatment; this differential is designated as $T°_{b\text{-}a}$. What is the clinical significance of these two measurements? Measurement of $\mathbf{T°_{ag\text{-}s}}$ quantifies the therapeutic thermal dose delivered to the soft tissues. It reflects the agent's potential capacity to induce a thermal response in the exposed soft tissues. The larger the temperature difference between the agent and the skin surface before treatment, the greater the capacity of the agent to elevate the temperature of soft tissues. Measurement of $T°_{b\text{-}a}$, on the other hand, quantifies the actual thermal skin change induced by the thermal agent at the end of treatment. To illustrate this proposed quantitative approach, let us look at the following dosimetric example.

2. Dosimetric Example

As mentioned previously, the objective approach complements the subjective approach described earlier by assigning numbers (temperature scores) to the patient's qualitative thermal assessment, which are often represented by words such as mild, moderate, high, vigorous, or intense heat. In the example presented in Table 7-3, the thermal agent temperature is measured at 54°C (130°F) and the exposed skin at 30°C (86°F) before application; thus, the thermal dose ($T°_{ag\text{-}s}$) delivered to the tissue was 24°C (44°F). Immediately after application, the skin temperature is measured at 40°C (104°F). The delivery of this dose created an actual skin surface heating ($T°_{b\text{-}a}$) of +10°C (+18°F) immediately after treatment. In other words, the thermal dose in this example added (hence the plus sign) heat to the exposed soft tissues, raising the exposed skin temperature from 30° to 40°C (86° to 104°F). In this example, the elevation of skin temperature by 10°C (18°F) corresponds to the patient's perception of heat being high.

3. Temperature Measurement Protocol

How difficult is it to take these measurements? Is it time consuming? Is it expensive? What type of thermometer is needed? Practitioners will discover, as discussed next, that taking these temperature measurements is simple, not time consuming, and requires only a reliable, accurate, and low-cost noncontact thermometer.

a. Thermometer

Recommended is the use of a portable noncontact thermometer, such as the one illustrated in Figure 7-8. These newer noncontact, portable, and low-cost infrared surface thermometers are now available on the market at a relatively low cost (less than $200). A significant advantage of using noncontact as opposed to contact-type thermometers is that these thermometers quickly, accurately, and safely measure the surface temperature of the skin without contacting its surface, thus eliminating the risk of damaging or contaminating the skin treatment area. The thermometer's optic sensors emit, reflect, and transmit infrared energy, which is collected and focused onto a deflector. The device then translates this optic energy into a temperature reading, which is digitally displayed on its screen. Because infrared rays are invisible, the thermometer is mounted with a nontherapeutic class II laser pointer. The focused laser beam is used only for aiming or pointing purposes.

b. Measurement Taking

Noncontact thermometers are very easy to use. As illustrated in Figure 7-9, the practitioner aims the laser beam at the surface of the thermal agent or the exposed skin

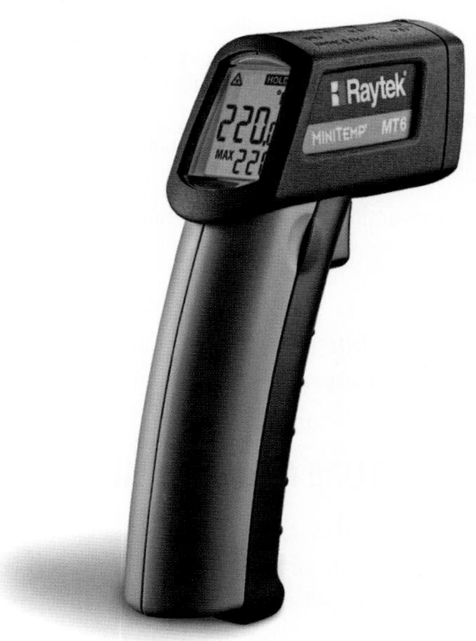

FIGURE 7-8 Typical noncontact, portable thermometer. (Courtesy of Raytek Corp.)

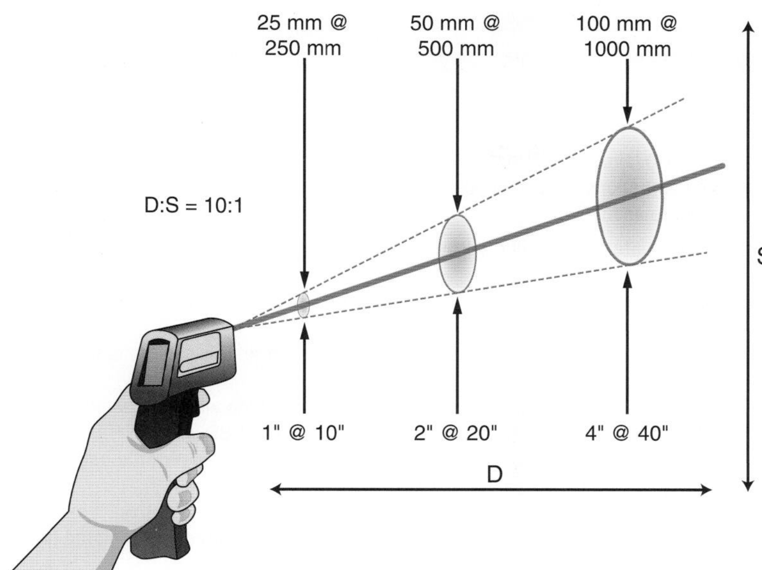

FIGURE 7-9 Noncontact infrared thermometer's optimal thermal ranges and laser sighting. D:S, distance to spot size ratio. (Courtesy of Raytek Corp.)

surface, pulls the trigger, and reads the current surface temperature (°C or °F) in less than 1 second. It is that simple. When taking a measurement with this type of noncontact thermometer, be sure to consider the distance to spot size ratio (D:S ratio) and the field of view. The type of infrared thermometer featured in Figure 7-9 is intended for close-range targets with a D:S ratio of 10:1. This means that this thermometer measures a minimum target area of 2.5 cm (1 in) in diameter from a distance of approximately 25 cm (10 in), and has a 10 cm (4 in) target measurement area at a distance of 100 cm (40 in). So the farther away the thermometer is from the surface of the thermal agent or skin, the larger the agent and skin areas from which the temperature is taken. Therefore, to standardize the measurement of both $T°_{ag\text{-}s}$ and $T°_{b\text{-}a}$ within and between treatment sessions, practitioners must *always* keep the D:S ratio constant and *always* aim at the same spot on the thermal agent and exposed skin. Failure to do so will lead to unreliable temperature measurements within and between sessions.

C. IMPORTANCE OF SKIN THERMAL DISCRIMINATION TESTING

There is unanimity in the literature and clinical community that the **safe** delivery of any thermal dose must begin with the conduct of a skin thermal discrimination test, which assesses the patient's ability to perceive thermal stimuli. The rationale for such a test is to prevent thermal skin damage caused by the high doses. Patients with impaired skin sensory discrimination abilities are at greater risk of not reporting accurately what their skin is really experiencing during the application of thermal agents. An impaired ability to discriminate thermal stimuli may have serious consequences to patients, who could suffer effects ranging from a mild to severe skin damage. Although all educators and practitioners know that conducting such a test is mandatory before considering thermal agents, *nowhere* in current published textbooks on therapeutic EPAs can students and practitioners find guidelines to help in conduction of such a test. The following test protocol fills that gap. Table 7-4 outlines the proposed testing procedures and scoring method associated with skin thermal discrimination testing. Five levels of skin sensory heat and cold discrimination are recommended in order to discriminate between thermal stimuli that are normally perceived by healthy individuals, with intact skin, as either very cold, cold, neutral, warm, or hot. Human skin is composed of two distinct layers of cells: the epidermis and the dermis. Within the *dermis* are buried specialized sensory receptors, which allow an individual to sense and discriminate levels of pain (*nociceptors*), heat and cold (*thermoreceptors*), and touch and pressure (*mechanoreceptors*). Testing skin discrimination for heat and cold allows practitioners to test both the patient's thermal and nociceptive capabilities to distinguish between warm and hot and between cold and very cold stimuli. As shown in Table 7-4, scoring is based on the total number of positive responses. Test scores may range between 5 and 0, indicating normal, slightly impaired, moderately impaired, severely impaired, or totally impaired thermal skin discrimination. The higher the score, the safer the application should be. To facilitate the selection of one thermal agent over another, comparison of key considerations, in addition to advantages and disadvantages, are presented in Table 7-5.

D. PREDICTING DEEPER THERMAL CHANGES

Measuring the actual skin surface temperature change ($T°_{b\text{-}a}$) following therapy, as described earlier, does not reveal the extent of the thermal changes that occur in the deeper tissues. To quantify deeper tissue thermal changes

TABLE 7-4	SKIN THERMAL DISCRIMINATION TESTING AND SCORING
Step	**Rationale and Procedure**
1. Prepare test probes.	This protocol recommends testing for five levels of thermal perception: very cold, cold, neutral (room temperature), warm, and hot. Recommendations as to the making of probes and temperature ranges associated with each thermal probes are as follows: • *Very cold:* Use a glass tube filled with water. Store it in the freezer compartment of a cold unit; range: –5° to 0°C (23° to 32°F). • *Cold:* Use another glass tube filled with water. Store it in the refrigerator compartment of a cold unit; range: 10° to 13°C (50° to 55°F). • *Neutral:* Use a third glass tube filled with water. Store it in a small bucket of water left at room temperature; range: 20° to 22°C (68° to 72°F). • *Warm:* Use a fourth glass tube filled with water. Store it in a small bucket of water into which a custom thermal element is plunged to keep the bucket water warm; range: 33° to 35°C (91° to 95°F). • *Hot:* Use a fifth glass tube filled with paraffin wax. Hook it to the wall of a thermoregulated paraffin bath unit; range: 51° to 54°C (124° to 129°F).
2. Position the patient.	Position the patient in a comfortable manner while explaining the general purpose and procedures related to the skin testing session.
3. Inspect the skin.	Expose the skin area to be treated, and visually inspect this area to determine the integrity of the skin.
4. Blind the patient.	Cover the patient's eyes so that he or she cannot see which testing probes are being used. Make sure that thermal discrimination is done through the skin, not through the eyes.
5. Randomly apply the probes.	Apply the five test probes one at a time, in a random fashion, and with a constant, light pressure over the designated area of skin. Keep the probe in contact with the skin for approximately 10–15 seconds—long enough for the patient to fully appreciate the thermal sensation. Wait 60 seconds between each application. Repeat applications until all five probes are used. The test, done only once prior to the first application, should take less than 10 minutes.
6. Record patient's responses.	After maintaining the test probe in place for 10–15 seconds, ask the patient if he or she perceives the probe as being very cold, cold, neutral, warm, or hot. Repeat for each probe.
7. Record test results.	Determine whether the patient's response to each test probe is positive or negative. A positive response is recorded when the patient's response matches the probe used. For example, a test result would be recorded as positive if the patient answers "neutral" when the probe that was just applied over the skin was at room temperature. Conversely, the test will be recorded as negative if the patient answers "neutral" after the application of a cold test probe.
8. Score the test.	The patient's score is established, as shown below, on the basis of the number of test probes positively identified. The maximum score is 5/5, and the minimum score is 0/5. Scores of 5/5 and 4/5 are interpreted as normal and slightly impaired skin thermal sensation, respectively; both scores pose no restriction to application. A score of 3/5 is interpreted as moderately impaired thermal skin discrimination; precautions are advised when using thermal agents with these patients. Scores of 2/5 and 1/5 are interpreted as severely impaired and pose a risk if thermal agents are applied. Finally, a score of 0/5 is interpreted as totally impaired thermal skin discrimination and calls for contraindication to all thermal therapeutic electrophysical agents.

in patients following thermotherapy, practitioners must use needle probe thermometers, such as those used in research settings. In such studies, each of these needle probes is positioned in different layers of soft tissue, such as within muscles, tendons, ligaments, and joint capsules. The use of needle-probe thermometers is, without a doubt, unsuitable for clinical practice because very few patients, if any, will volunteer to have them inserted in their different tissue layers after routine application of thermotherapy. Thus, surface skin temperature measurement is the only acceptable clinical alternative. Is there a relationship or correlation between skin thermal changes and thermal changes occurring in the deeper soft tissues? To date, the strength of the relationship between skin temperature and deeper tissues temperature is still unknown. The results of Jutte et al. (2001), who found a weak relationship between skin temperature change and deep tissue temperature changes following the application of cryotherapy on 15 healthy subjects, do not rule out the possibility that such a relationship may be stronger. Overall, experimental studies on humans using multineedle thermometers implanted at various depths

TABLE 7-5 COMPARATIVE CONSIDERATIONS FOR THERMOTHERAPY

Consideration	Hot Pack	Paraffin Bath	Fluidotherapy
Heat type	Moist	Moist	Dry
Temperature range	70° to 76°C (158° to 169°F)	51° to 54°C (124° to 129°F)	43° to 52°C (110° to 126°F)
Heat transfer	Conduction	Conduction	Convection
Heating pattern	Declining over time	Declining over time	Constant over time
Coupling medium	Commercial terrycloth cover or layers of towels	*Intact skin:* None is needed. *If minor or superficial wound present:* Cover with sterile gauze.	None
Body application	Primarily over flat and large body areas	Primarily over irregular body areas such as the extremities (wrist/hand; ankle/foot)	Over the upper and lower limbs, unilaterally or bilaterally
Application duration	~20 min	~30 min	~30 min
Advantages	Inexpensive Easy home therapy	Inexpensive Easy home therapy Circumferential heat distribution	Requires no water plumbing or toweling Circumferential heat distribution Free limb movement during therapy Controlled and stable temperature during treatment
Disadvantages	Requires water plumbing and toweling Radial heat distribution No limb movement allowed No control over temperature during therapy	Requires toweling No limb movement allowed No control over temperature during therapy	Very expensive Treatment limited to upper and lower limbs Bulky device requiring appropriate floor space Clinic-based therapy only

in soft tissues tend to reveal the following trend: Keeping the duration of application identical, the greater the dose—that is, the skin temperature differential between the agent and the skin area being treated ($T°_{ag\text{-}s}$)—the greater the skin thermal changes, and consequently, the greater the thermal changes in the deeper tissues. Awaiting further research on this topic, this textbook subscribes to this trend by assuming that measuring thermal skin change is a reasonable clinical predictor of deeper tissue thermal changes induced by the thermal agent.

E. HOT PACK DOSIMETRIC FACTORS

The thermal dose of a hot pack rests on the following four parameters: size of the pack, temperature differential between the agent and the skin ($T°_{ag\text{-}s}$), application duration, and coupling thickness. The larger the size (or mass) of the pack for any given temperature, the more heat will be conducted or transmitted to the treated area. The higher the $T°_{ag\text{-}s}$, the greater the heating potential of the thermal agent. Hot packs are kept in water-thermoregulated units, at a temperature range of 70° to 76°C (158° to 169°F) is maintained. Clinicians should never assume that the temperature of the hot pack they used yesterday with their patient is at the same temperature today. They should also never assume that the hot pack they just pulled out of the hydrocollator unit is exactly at the temperature indicated on the hydrocollator thermometer, unless they are certain that this hot pack was immersed in the unit for at least 30 minutes prior to usage. Recommended treatment duration is approximately 20 minutes (Lehmann et al., 1990). Lehmann and coworkers demonstrated that maximum heating of soft tissues was achieved after approximately 20 minutes of application and that repeated applications every 10 minutes did not increase soft tissue temperature any further. Finally, hot pack (water) must *never* be applied directly over the skin surface because their high heat content (specific heat) and heat conduction (thermal conductivity) can easily cause a skin burn. A coupling medium, such as layers of towels or pack cover, is therefore, always required.

F. PARAFFIN BATH DOSIMETRIC FACTORS

The thermal dose associated with paraffin bath is determined by setting the following three parameters: temperature differential between the agent and the skin ($T°_{ag-s}$), application duration, and method of application. The higher the $T°_{ag-s}$ value, the greater the heating potential of the paraffin bath. The temperature of the paraffin mixture (ag) can be read directly on the thermometer attached to the bath (or by using the portable infrared thermometer), and the skin temperature (s) is obtained using an infrared thermometer. The paraffin mixture temperature is usually maintained in the thermoregulated bath between 51° and 54°C (124° and 129°F). The recommended application duration is 30 minutes. Paraffin bath is applied using one of these three methods: (1) dipping with continuous immersion, (2) dipping with wrapping, and (3) brushing with wrapping.

G. FLUIDOTHERAPY DOSIMETRIC FACTORS

Fluidotherapy dosage is determined by setting the following parameters on the device's console. Set the desired temperature, which normally ranges between 43° and 52°C (110° and 126°F) and the desired particle agitation or speed value, which ranges from 0% to 100% (in 5% increments). The combined effect of air temperature and agitation of particles in the device's chamber causes the phenomenon of fluidization on the exposed limb. Recommended duration is approximately 20 minutes. Fluidotherapy delivers dry heat using forced convection. Energy transfer takes place through forced movements, or agitation, of heated air and cellulose particles in the unit chamber, which together are circulated around the body part during treatment. A limb immersed in a fluidized bed of a higher temperature than itself will experience a heat transfer rate many times greater than it would if immersed in a warm airbed alone (Borrell et al., 1977, 1980; Henley, 1991). This is because the heated particles make physical contact with the immersed limb, thus enhancing the heat transfer.

V. APPLICATION, CONTRAINDICATIONS, AND RISKS

Prior to considering the application of hot pack, paraffin bath, and Fluidotherapy, practitioners must first check for contraindications, consider the risks, and then go through key application steps and procedures designed to optimize treatment safety, efficacy, and effectiveness.

APPLICATION, CONTRAINDICATIONS, AND RISKS

Thermotherapy

IMPORTANT: Because skin thermal damage is always a possibility with the application of thermotherapy, skin thermal discrimination testing MUST BE CONDUCTED PRIOR to the first application. The description and scoring of this test are documented in Table 7-4. Shown, as examples, are applications of hot pack (Fig. 7-10), paraffin bath (Fig. 7-11) and Fluidotherapy (Fig. 7-12).

ALL AGENTS

STEP	RATIONALE
1. Check for contraindications.	*Over skin area where sensation to heat is severely impaired*—cutaneous burn
	Over a cancerous area—enhance tumor growth and metastasis
	Over thrombophlebitic area—dislodge blood clot, which may then circulate into the vessels of vital organs, causing serious circulatory problems and possibly death
	Over a hemorrhagic area—additional bleeding caused by increased blood flow
	Over the abdominal, pelvic, and low back areas of pregnant women (hp)—teratogenic effects on fetal development and growth caused by increased local or systemic maternal body temperature
	Over acute and severe inflammatory conditions—worsen the condition by aggravating the inflammatory response through increased blood flow resulting from heat application
	In patients who are confused and unreliable—complications during therapy that reduce treatment effectiveness

STEP	RATIONALE
2. **Consider the risks.**	*Over an area of impaired blood circulation*—may cause tissue overheating because the treated area will not be able to cope with the demand for additional and cooler blood flow during treatment *In patients presenting with severe cardiac insufficiency*—may not being able to cope with the increased cardiac demand triggered by the heat-induced increase in blood circulation. Periodic monitoring of vital signs is advised during and after therapy. *Over superficial closed and open wounds, including grafted or burn wounds (pb)*—may break down the immature burn scars and grafts (Head et al., 1977). To minimize this risk, Burns et al. (1987) proposed the following brushing with wrapping method: (1) Keep the paraffin mixture at a constant 47°C (117°F); (2) cover the open wound with a nonadherent, sterile gauze before applying the paraffin; (3) begin to wax the wound and surrounding area using the brushing with wrapping method; and (4) wrap the waxed area in paper or cloth and wait 15–20 minutes. *Over superficial closed and open wounds, including grafted or burn wounds (hp)*—may break down the immature repair tissue. To minimize the risk, first cover the wound surface with nonadherent, sterile gauze and then add the necessary insulation through additional layers of toweling before applying the hot pack. *Over body areas with superficially located metal implants (hp, pb)*—may cause internal soft tissue burns because metals absorb and conduct heat well. Use caution when applying hot pack and paraffin over such body areas. *On hand motor skills and reaction time*—may delay reaction time and decrease tapping speed in healthy subjects. Inform patients that their hand motor skills may be impaired for a few hours following therapy. *In cases of systemic infectious diseases*—may increase core body temperature, which may increase fever *In the presence of flammable anesthetics (fl)*—may cause explosion

HOT PACK

STEP	PROCEDURE
1. **Check for contraindications.**	See All Agents section.
2. **Consider the risks.**	See All Agents section.
3. **Position and instruct patient.**	Ensure comfortable body positioning. Inform patient that he or she should feel a heating sensation during therapy.
4. **Prepare treatment area.**	Apply hot pack over bare skin or over a thin layer of clothing. All open wounds must be covered with sterile gauze.
5. **Select hot pack type.**	Select the pack that best matches the geometry of the treated area. Make sure that the hydro collator unit is plugged into a GFCI receptacle.
6. **Determine and measure dose ($T°_{ag-s}$).**	Select the dose that can induce the desired physiologic and therapeutic effects in the targeted tissue. Dose should be high enough to elevate the targeted tissue temperature within the suboptimal/optimal therapeutic window (Fig. 7-7). Immediately after removing the hot pack from the hydrocollator, and just before wrapping and applying it over the exposed skin area, measure the dose—that is, the temperature differential between the agent and the skin surface ($T°_{ag-s}$) over which it is applied.

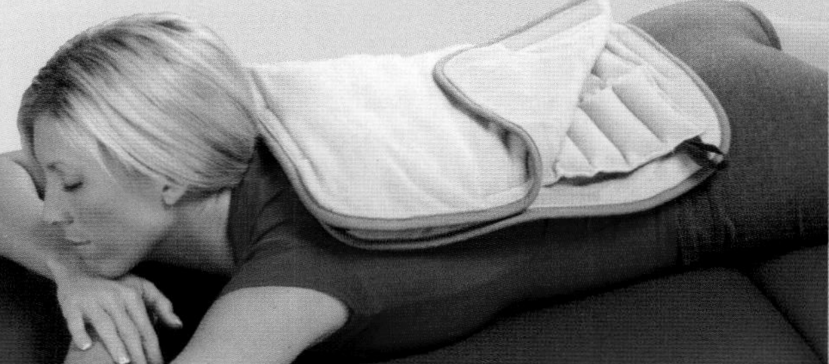

FIGURE 7-10 Application of hot pack. (Courtesy of DJO Global.)

STEP	PROCEDURE
7. Wrap up and secure the pack.	Use a commercial terrycloth wrap or layers of toweling. Keep wrapping thicknesses to a minimum for optimal tissue heating. Secure the pack with elastic bandages or towels.
8. Apply treatment.	Apply for approximately 20 minutes. Check the patient after 5 minutes of application to ensure thermal comfort. If necessary, adjust the thickness of coupling by adding or removing layers of toweling to ensure maximal heating.
9. Measure thermal skin heating ($T^{\circ}_{b\text{-}a}$).	Immediately after removing the hot pack, measure the exposed skin temperature and then calculate the differential before and after treatment ($T^{\circ}_{b\text{-}a}$). Question the patient on the level of heat that he or she has perceived during treatment.
10. Conduct post-treatment procedures.	Inspect the treated area, and record any adverse reaction. Reddening of the skin is normal after thermotherapy. Unwrap the hot pack, and put it back into the hydrocollator unit. Put towels into the wash. Hang the pack cover to dry.
11. Ensure post-treatment equipment maintenance.	Follow manufacturer recommendations. Immediately report defects or malfunctions to technical maintenance staff.

 View **online videos** for more details.

PARAFFIN BATH

STEP	PROCEDURE
1. Check for contraindications.	See All Agents section.
2. Consider the risks.	See All Agents section.
3. Position and instruct patient.	Ensure comfortable body positioning. Instruct the patient not to move the treated body part during treatment, because this may crack the wax coating and cause air to enter, thus cooling the treatment area. Inform the patient that he or she should feel a heating sensation during therapy. In addition, instruct not to touch the walls of the bath.
4. Prepare treatment area. 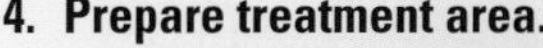	Remove clothing and jewelry. Cleanse the exposed skin with water and soap, or rubbing alcohol, to remove impurities. Shave excessive hair if necessary. All open wounds must be covered with sterile gauze.
5. Prepare the paraffin bath.	Plug unit into a GFCI receptacle. Put the mixture of paraffin wax and mineral oil into the bath. Turn the thermostatic control switch on to heat the mixture to the desired temperature.
6. Select the application method.	There are three methods to choose from: • *Dipping with continuous immersion:* Perform 7–10 consecutive dips in the bath, waiting a few seconds between each dip for each wax coating to harden. Immediately after the last coating, redip the treated body part into the bath for a continuous immersion period of 30 minutes. • *Dipping with wrapping:* Perform 7–10 consecutive dips in the bath, waiting a few seconds between each dip for each wax coating to harden. Immediately after the last coating, wrap the treated body part in a plastic liner and then put it into a towel or commercial wrapping mitten or sock. Keep the wrapping on for 30 minutes. • *Brushing with wrapping:* Apply 7–10 layers of paraffin wax onto the treated body area with a brush, waiting for a few seconds in between until each layer hardens. Cover or wrap the treated body part with a plastic liner, towel, or commercial wrapping mitten or sock.

FIGURE 7-11 Application of paraffin bath. (Courtesy of WR Medical Electronics.)

STEP	PROCEDURE
7. Determine and measure dose ($T°_{ag\text{-}s}$).	Select the dose that can induce the desired physiologic and therapeutic effects in the targeted tissue. The dose should be high enough to increase the targeted tissue temperature within the suboptimal/optimal therapeutic window. Just prior to application, read the temperature of the paraffin wax mixture either from the built-in bath thermometer or from the portable infrared thermometer. Measure the dose—that is, the temperature differential between the agent and the skin surface ($T°_{ag\text{-}s}$) over which it is applied.
8. Apply treatment.	Apply for approximately 30 minutes. Check the patient after 5 minutes of application to ensure thermal comfort.
9. Measure thermal skin heating ($T°_{b\text{-}a}$).	At the end of the treatment, unwrap the body segment and peel off the paraffin coat. Measure the exposed skin temperature and then calculate the differential before and after treatment ($T°_{b\text{-}a}$). Question the patient on the level of heat that he or she perceived during treatment.
10. Conduct post-treatment procedures.	Inspect the exposed treatment area, and record any adverse reactions. Put the cover over the bath until further use. Add new paraffin–oil mixture if needed. Discard the used plastic liner and paraffin mixture.
11. Ensure post-treatment equipment maintenance.	Follow manufacturer recommendations. Immediately report defects or malfunctions to technical maintenance staff.

View **online video** for details.

FLUIDOTHERAPY

STEP	PROCEDURE

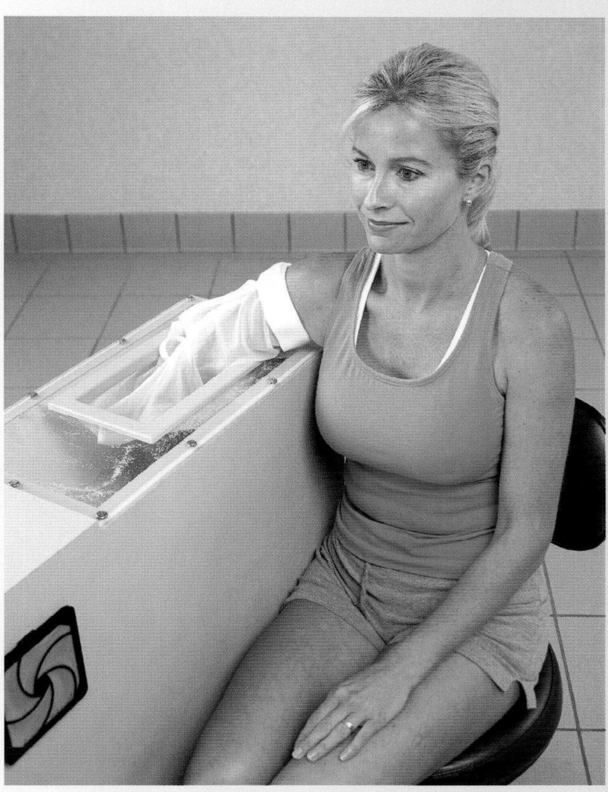

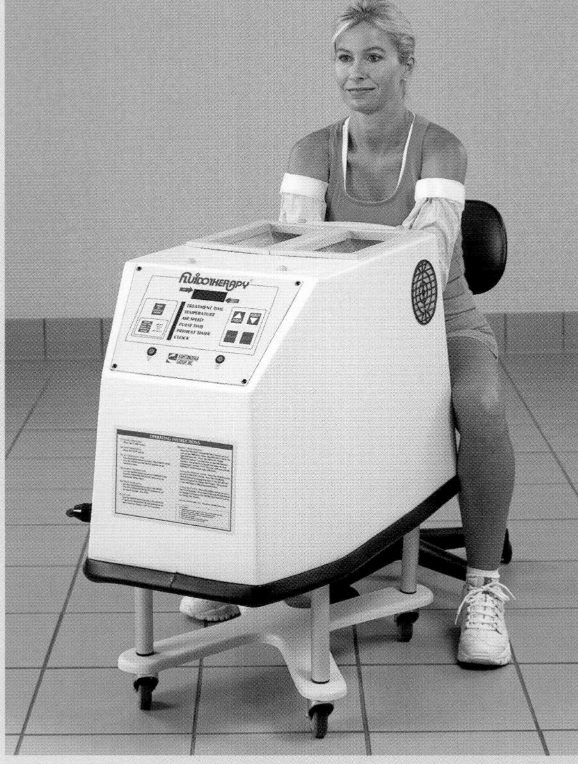

FIGURE 7-12 Application of Fluidotherapy. (Courtesy of DJO Global.)

STEP	PROCEDURE
1. Check for contraindications.	See All Agents section.
2. Consider the risks.	See All Agents section.
3. Position and instruct patient.	Ensure comfortable body positioning. Inform the patient that he or she should feel a heating sensation during therapy. Inform that movement of the treated body segment is allowed during treatment. In all cases, the patient sits in front of the device and then immerses his or her bare upper or lower limb into the unit chamber.
4. Prepare treatment area.	Remove clothing and jewelry. Cleanse the exposed skin with water and soap, or rubbing alcohol, to remove impurities. Shave excessive hair if necessary. All open wounds must be covered with sterile gauze.
5. Prepare patient and device for treatment.	Contrary to hot pack and paraffin bath therapy, which deliver moist heat to small/large flat body surfaces and to the extremities (ankle/feet, wrist/hands), Fluidotherapy devices delivers dry heat to the entire upper (arm, forearm, wrist, and hand) and lower (thigh, leg, ankle, and foot) limbs. Plug device into a GFCI receptacle. Put the cellulose particles into the device's chamber. Place the treated body segment though the portal of the device. Secure the portal's sleeve to prevent particles from escaping the chamber. Ensure that all entry ports are sealed properly.
6. Determine and measure dose ($T°_{ag\text{-}s}$).	Select the dose that can induce the desired physiologic and therapeutic effects in the targeted tissue. Dose should be high enough to increase the targeted tissue temperature within the suboptimal/optimal therapeutic window. Set the desired temperature and agitation speed. Read the operating temperature from the device's console and the skin temperature from the portable infrared thermometer. Measure the dose—that is, the temperature differential between the agent and the skin surface ($T°_{ag\text{-}s}$) over which it is applied.
7. Apply treatment.	Apply for approximately 30 minutes. Check the patient after 5 minutes of application to ensure thermal comfort. Instruct the patient to exercise or not exercise the treated limb during therapy. The treated body part may or may not be manipulated, or mobilized, by the treating clinician during the application.
8. Measure skin thermal heating ($T°_{b\text{-}a}$).	At the end of treatment, ask the patient to slowly remove his or her body segment from the device's chamber. Immediately after, measure the treated skin temperature, and calculate the differential before and after treatment ($T°_{b\text{-}a}$). Question the patient on the level of heat that he or she has perceived during treatment.
9. Conduct post-treatment procedures.	Inspect the exposed treatment area, and record any adverse reaction. Add new cellulose particles to the device's chamber if needed.
10. Ensure post-treatment equipment maintenance.	Follow manufacturer recommendations. Immediately report defects or malfunctions to technical maintenance staff.

View **online video** for details.

hp, hot pack; pb, paraffin bath; fl, Fluidotherapy.

CASE STUDIES

Presented are three case studies summarizing the concepts, principles, and applications of thermotherapy discussed in this chapter. Case Study 7-1 addresses the use of hot pack for low back pain affecting a middle-aged man. Case Study 7-2 is concerned with the application of paraffin bath for rheumatoid arthritis affecting a senior sedentary woman. Case Study 7-3 relates to the application of Fluidotherapy for upper extremity joint stiffness and pain caused by chronic osteoarthritis affecting an older adult woman. Each case is structured in line with the concepts of evidence-based practice (EBP), the International Classification of Functioning, Disability, and Health (ICF) disablement model, and SOAP (*s*ubjective, *o*bjective, *a*ssessment, *p*lan) note format (see Chapter 2 for details).

CASE STUDY 7-1: LOW BACK PAIN

EVIDENCE-BASED CLINICAL DECISION MAKING PROTOCOL

1. Formulate the Case History

A 48-year-old male accountant suffering from subacute low back pain consults for treatment. His back pain first appeared 2 weeks earlier while lifting a heavy box of documents from the floor of his office. He went to see his physician on the following day and left with a prescription for analgesic agents as well as anti-inflammatory and muscle relaxant drugs. Battling chronic gastric problems for years, this patient wants to stop his drug treatment and replace it with a more conservative treatment. He has no history of back pain. The patient is wearing a pacemaker. Physical examination reveals a man who is underweight for his height. It further reveals moderate pain over the entire bilateral low back area as well as a light paravertebral muscle spasm causing difficulty with prolonged sitting at work. There is no neurologic sign, and spinal range of motion (ROM) is within normal range. The patient has reduced his work schedule from 5 to 4 days a week. His goals are to resume prolonged sitting and full-time work without having to take medication.

2. Outline the Case Based on the ICF Framework

LOW BACK PAIN		
BODY STRUCTURES AND FUNCTIONS	**ACTIVITIES**	**PARTICIPATION**
Low back pain	Difficulty with prolong sitting	Difficulty with work
Paravertebral muscle spasm		

PERSONAL FACTORS	ENVIRONMENTAL FACTORS
Middle-aged man	Stressful work
Professional character	Team work
University educated	

3. Outline Therapeutic Goals and Outcome Measurements

GOAL	OUTCOME MEASUREMENT
Decrease pain	Visual Analogue Scale (VAS)
Decrease muscle spasm	Manual palpation
Eliminate drug intake	Drug diary
Improve sitting time and resume full-time work	Modified Oswestry Low Back Pain Questionnaire

4. Justify the Use of Thermotherapy Based on the EBP Framework

PRACTITIONER'S EXPERIENCE	RESEARCH-BASED EVIDENCE	PATIENT'S EXPECTATION
Very experienced in thermotherapy	*Strength:* Moderate	No opinion on thermotherapy
Has used thermotherapy in previous cases	*Effectiveness:* Substantiated	Just wants to return to full-time work
Believes that thermotherapy can be beneficial		

5. Outline Key Intervention Parameters

- **Treatment base:** Private clinic
- **Thermal agent:** *Hot pack.* Considering that this patient is lean (thin fat layer), heat transfer between the hot pack and the paravertebral musculature should be maximized. Shortwave diathermy (Chapter 10) is contraindicated because the patient wears a pacemaker. Ultrasound (Chapter 20) is excluded considering the disproportion between the small soundhead size and the much larger symptomatic treatment area.
- **Application protocol:** Follow the suggested application protocol in *Application, Contraindications, and Risks* box for hot pack, and make the necessary adjustments for this case.
- **Patient's positioning:** Lying prone
- **Application site:** Over the symptomatic lower back area
- **Hot pack size:** 38 × 60 cm (15 × 24 in)
- **Coupling medium:** Terrycloth wrap (2 cm)
- **Application duration:** 20 minutes
- **Dosage ($T°_{ag\text{-}s}$):** 38° ± 5°C (100° ± 4°F)
- **Treatment frequency:** Daily; 5 days a week
- **Intervention period:** 8 days
- **Concomitant therapies:** Regimen of back mobilization, flexibility, and strengthening exercises

6. Report Pre- and Post-Intervention Outcomes

OUTCOME	PRE	POST
Pain (VAS score)	6/10	1/10
Paravertebral muscle spasm	Present	Absent
Drug intake	8 pills/day	0
Functional status (Oswestry score)	30%	0%

7. Document Case Intervention Using the SOAP Note Format

S: Middle-aged healthy male Pt presents subacute low back pain leading to difficulty with prolonged sitting and full-time work.

O: *Test:* Normal thermal discrimination test (5/5). *Intervention:* Hot pack applied over the lower back area; Pt lying prone; dosage ($T°_{ag\text{-}s}$): 38° ± 5°C (100° ± 4°F); treatment schedule: daily, 5 days/week, for 8 days; application duration: 20 minutes. *Pre–post comparison:* Pain decrease (VAS score 6/10 to 1/10), disappearance of muscle spasm, elimination of drugs, and return to normal functional status.

A: No adverse effect. Treatment very well tolerated. Pt very pleased with the results.

P: No further treatment required. Pt discharged. If a similar back pain episode recurs, Pt is advised to use an over-the-counter heat wrap or bag before consulting again or relying on medication.

CASE STUDY 7-2: RHEUMATOID ARTHRITIS

EVIDENCE-BASED CLINICAL DECISION MAKING PROTOCOL

1. Formulate the Case History

A 65-year-old woman with a long history of moderate rheumatoid arthritis consults for treatment. Physical examination reveals painful walking, bilateral ankle joint and toe stiffness, light toe deformity, and chapped and dry skin on the feet and ankles. Examination of the upper limbs reveals adequate wrist and hand function. She is under the regular care of her rheumatologist, who has prescribed analgesic and anti-inflammatory drugs for her condition. She wears regular shoes and rubs an over-the-counter cream on her feet and ankles daily to soften her skin. She is concerned about her reduced and declining ability to walk and perform activities of daily living (ADLs). She is also concerned about the increasing side effects of her medication. Her goals are to reduce drug intake while keeping her mobility. Her favorite social activity is to visit and chat with her friends who live at a walking distance from her home. Her preference is definitively for a home treatment, considering her reduced walking ability and the fact that she has no personal and easy access to public transportation to facilitate any hospital or clinic displacements. She heard from a good friend about the possibility of using home paraffin bath therapy for her arthritic condition. She is convinced that this conservative therapy may help her condition.

2. Outline the Case Based on the ICF Framework

RHEUMATOID ARTHRITIS		
BODY STRUCTURES AND FUNCTIONS	**ACTIVITIES**	**PARTICIPATION**
Ankle pain	Difficulty with walking	Difficulty with social visiting
Ankle joint stiffness	Difficulty with ADLs	
Reduced ankle range of motion (ROM)		
Chapped and dry skin		

PERSONAL FACTORS	ENVIRONMENTAL FACTORS
Elderly woman	Social
Housewife	Friend and family oriented
Retired	

3. Outline Therapeutic Goals and Outcome Measurements

GOAL	OUTCOME MEASUREMENT
Decrease pain	101-point Numerical Rating Scale (NRS-101)
Increase ROM	Goniometry
Improve skin texture	Visual observation
Improve functional status	Arthritis Impact Measurement Scale (AIMS)

4. Justify the Use of Thermotherapy Based on the EBP Framework

PRACTITIONER'S EXPERIENCE	RESEARCH-BASED EVIDENCE	PATIENT'S EXPECTATION
Experienced in thermotherapy	*Strength:* Moderate	Convinced that thermotherapy will work
Has used thermotherapy occasionally in previous cases	*Effectiveness:* Substantiated	
Believes that thermotherapy may be beneficial		

5. Outline Key Intervention Parameters

- **Treatment base:** Home
- **Thermal agent:** *Paraffin bath*. This agent is expected to significantly heat the muscles and periarticular joint structures of the ankle, foot, and toe joints, and to hydrate and soften the skin overlying these joints. Deep heating of these periarticular structures is expected to reduce ankle and toe joint stiffness by decreasing joint viscosity, thus improving walking ability. The irregular surfaces associated with the ankles, feet, and toes are ideal body areas for the application of paraffin bath therapy, transmitting heat to entire cutaneous surfaces. The fact that this elderly patient prefers a home therapy approach, and strongly believes that paraffin bath therapy can improve her condition, are other reasons behind the selection of this agent over any other thermal agents. Finally, this patient is alert, able to follow instructions, and has adequate upper limb mobility and function to operate a paraffin bath at home. Considering the reduced mobility and age of this patient, a home treatment approach is used. The recommendation is for the patient to rent a paraffin bath for a month. The first four treatments are delivered by the practitioner at home. During these visits, the patient is instructed about how to use the unit, how to do proper maintenance, and how to maximize safety during application. She is also instructed about how to mobilize her ankle and toes after therapy.
- **Application protocol:** Follow the suggested application protocol in *Application, Contraindications, and Risks* box for paraffin bath, and make the necessary adjustments for this case.
- **Patient's positioning:** Sitting
- **Application site:** Over the ankle and foot areas
- **Application method used:** Dipping with continuous immersion
- **Dosage ($T°_{ag\text{-}s}$):** 20° ± 2°C (68° ± 2°F)
- **Treatment frequency:** Daily; 7 days a week
- **Intervention period:** 21 days
- **Concomitant therapies:** Regimen of ankle and foot self-mobilizing exercises

6. Report Pre- and Post-Intervention Outcomes

OUTCOME	PRE	POST
Ankle pain (NRS-101 score)	70	20
Ankle ROM (dorsi-plantarflexion)	Deficit of 30 degrees	Deficit of 10 degrees
Skin texture	Chapped and dried	Normal
Functional status (AIMS score)	30	10

7. Document Case Intervention Using the SOAP Note Format

S: Elderly female Pt presents chronic rheumatoid arthritis over bilateral ankle and foot causing pain and difficulty with ADLs and social activities.

O: *Test:* Normal thermal discrimination (4/5). *Intervention:* Home-based paraffin bath applied over ankle and foot bilaterally; bath plugged into a GFCI receptacle; Pt sitting; dosage ($T°_{ag\text{-}s}$): 20° ± 2°C (68° ± 2°F); method of application: dipping with continuous immersion; treatment schedule: daily, 7 days/week, for 21 days. *Pre–post comparison:* Pain decrease (NRS-101 70 to 20), increased ankle ROM (deficit 30 to 10 degrees), normal skin texture, and return to normal functional status (AIMS 30 to 10).

A: No adverse effect. Treatment very well tolerated. Pt very pleased with the results.

P: No further treatment required. Pt advised to use paraffin bath therapy to control future rheumatoid flares, pain, or discomfort and to optimize functional activities.

CASE STUDY 7-3: ARTHRITIC JOINT ANKYLOSIS WITH OPEN WOUND

EVIDENCE-BASED CLINICAL DECISION MAKING PROTOCOL

1. Formulate the Case History

A 69-year-old woman who is diabetic presents with a history of chronic osteoarthritis causing bilateral hand, wrist, and elbow pain and ankylosis in addition to a recalcitrant open wound over the right wrist. Her main complaints are pain and joint stiffness, which cause difficulty with personal hygiene, ADLs, and carrying shopping bags. The open wound is slow to heal. Her preference is to receive dry heat therapy. Her goal is to maximize upper extremity function.

2. Outline the Case Based on the ICF Framework

ARTHRITIC JOINT ANKYLOSIS WITH OPEN WOUND		
BODY STRUCTURES AND FUNCTIONS	**ACTIVITIES**	**PARTICIPATION**
Bilateral hand, wrist, and elbow pain	Difficulty with personal hygiene Difficulty with ADLs	Difficulty with shopping
Bilateral hand, wrist, and elbow joint stiffness		

PERSONAL FACTORS	ENVIRONMENTAL FACTORS
Elderly woman	Housewife
Widow	

3. Outline Therapeutic Goals and Outcome Measurements

GOAL	OUTCOME MEASUREMENT
Decrease pain	Visual Analogue Scale (VAS)
Decrease joint stiffness	Goniometry
Improve upper extremity function	AIMS

4. Justify the Use of Thermotherapy Based on the EBP Framework

PRACTITIONER'S EXPERIENCE	RESEARCH-BASED EVIDENCE	PATIENT'S EXPECTATION
Minimal experience with Fluidotherapy	*Strength:* Weak	Believes that therapy will help
Believes that Fluidotherapy can be beneficial	*Effectiveness:* Pending	

5. Outline Key Intervention Parameters

- **Treatment base:** Hospital
- **Thermal agent:** *Fluidotherapy—upper extremity unit.* This agent is used because it can induce thermal effect simultaneously to both upper extremities, from the elbow to the fingers.
- **Application protocol:** Follow the suggested application protocol in *Application, Contraindications, and Risks* box for Fluidotherapy, and make the necessary adjustments for this case.
- **Patient's positioning:** Sitting
- **Application site:** Bilaterally over hand, wrist, and elbow with gauze applied over the open wound
- **Operating mode:** Continuous
- **Operating temperature:** 48°C (118°F)
- **Air agitation speed:** 75% of maximum
- **Application duration:** 30 minutes
- **Dosage ($T°_{ag-s}$):** 18° ± 2°C (32° ± 4°F)
- **Treatment frequency:** 3 times per week
- **Intervention period:** 4 weeks
- **Concomitant therapies:** Manual joint mobilization by practitioner during therapy. Home regimen of self-joint mobilization.

6. Report Pre- and Post-Intervention Outcomes

OUTCOME	PRE	POST
Pain (VAS score)	5/10	2/10
Joint stiffness (average deficit)	Finger: Deficit of 30% Wrist: Deficit of 20% Elbow: Deficit of 12%	Finger: Deficit of 10% Wrist: Deficit of 8% Elbow: Deficit of 5%
Functional status (AIMS score)	35	10

7. Document Case Intervention Using the SOAP Note Format

S: Older adult diabetic woman presents with upper extremity joint stiffness caused by chronic osteoarthritis with a small open wound over the R wrist leading to pain and difficulty with ADLs and shopping.

O: *Test:* Normal thermal discrimination test (4/5). *Intervention:* Fluidotherapy applied bilaterally over the upper extremities; Pt sitting; dosage ($T°_{ag\text{-}s}$): 18° ± 2°C (32° ± 4°F); application duration: 20 minutes; treatment schedule: 3 days/week for 4 weeks. *Pre–post comparison:* Pain decrease (VAS score 5/10 to 2/10); decrease joint stiffness deficit (finger by 20%; wrist by 12%; elbow by 7%); improved UE functional status AIMS score 35 to 10).

A: No adverse effect

P: No further treatment required. Pt discharged and advised to do her home therapeutic regimen daily.

VI. THE BOTTOM LINE

- Thermotherapy is the exchange of heat energy between warmer thermal agents and cooler exposed soft tissues for therapeutic purposes.
- Thermotherapy follows the first and second laws of thermodynamics. First, heat energy is never lost or gained during application; it is exchanged or transferred between the thermal agent and the exposed soft tissue. Second, heat energy transfer always occurs from the warmest to the coldest substances.
- Heat is energy and temperature is a measurement of it. Two thermal agents with similar temperature, but different mass, will not have the same heat energy.
- Heat transfer during thermotherapy occurs through conduction (hot pack and paraffin wax) and convection (Fluidotherapy).
- Specific heat (c) is the ability of a substance to store or hold heat, and thermal conductivity (k) the ability of this substance to conduct heat.
- Both specific heat and thermal conductivity explain why different thermal agents, all having the same temperature, may or may not be well tolerated by patients.
- The therapeutic goal with thermotherapy is to increase soft tissues temperature from its baseline to its optimal therapeutic window, which ranges between 40° to 45° C (104° to 113° F).
- Thermotherapy is used mainly to modulate pain and to enhance the proliferative and maturation/repair phases of soft tissue healing.
- The conduct of skin thermal discrimination testing is mandatory prior to the first application of thermotherapy.
- In the context of evidence-based practice, qualitative dosimetry is no longer acceptable has the sole source of dosimetric information. Quantitative dosimetry, based on reliable agent and skin temperature measurements, is required.
- Adopting quantitative dosimetry in day-to-day practice is neither complicated, time consuming and expensive to do.
- Because subcutaneous fat acts as a major thermal barrier between the skin and deeper soft tissues, higher dosages are required with overweight and obese patients.
- All line-powered thermal agents should be plugged into GFCI receptacles to prevent the occurrence of macroshock.
- The overall research-based indications gathered from human clinical trials shows the strength of evidence behind thermotherapy (hot pack, paraffin bath and Fluidotherapy) to be moderate and its level of therapeutic effectiveness substantiated.

VII. CRITICAL THINKING QUESTIONS

Clarification: What is meant by $T°_{ag\text{-}s}$ and $T°_{b\text{-}a}$ temperature differentials? What is meant by skin thermal discrimination testing?

Assumptions: Because they are classified as superficial thermal agents, many of your colleagues assume that hot pack and paraffin baths can only induce a heating effect in superficial soft tissues. How can you verify or disprove this assumption? You have assumed that it is important to measure $T°_{ag\text{-}s}$ and $T°_{b\text{-}a}$. How do you justify making that assumption?

Reasons and evidence: What leads you to believe that the subcutaneous fat layer, compared with other soft tissues, is the greatest thermal barrier? A colleague tells you that the hot pack treatment she just gave was perceived by her patient as moderately hot at the end of treatment. A few minutes later, another colleague tells you that the hot pack she just gave to her patient induced an actual skin temperature elevation of 12°C (21°F) and that heating sensation was felt as high. Which of these two verbal reports is more meaningful clinically? Why?

Viewpoints or perspectives: How would you respond to a colleague who says that there is no difference between the concepts of heat and temperature, and thus whatever agent has the highest temperature is always the hottest? How would you respond to a colleague who says that taking these two temperature differential measurements ($T°_{ag-s}$ and $T°_{b-a}$) is a waste of time and that simply asking the patient if he or she perceived the thermal treatment just received as mild, moderate, or intense is just as good an approach to assessing soft tissue temperature changes after treatment? You agree with the consensus that skin sensory thermal discrimination testing must be scored not only qualitatively but also quantitatively. What would someone who disagrees with you say?

Implications and consequences: What generalizations can you make about the use of hot pack, paraffin bath, and Fluidotherapy based on the scientific evidence available? You tend to agree with the assumption that one can reasonably predict the temperature changes in the deeper tissues if the temperature changes at the skin surface are known. What are you implying? You state that it is important to discriminate between a slightly, moderately, severely, and totally impaired test result when considering the application of thermal agents. What are you implying?

About the question: Why is it important to measure the temperature differential between the agent and the skin ($T°_{ag-s}$) overlying the treatment area before treatment, and the temperature differential of the skin overlying the treatment area before and immediately after treatment ($T°_{b-a}$)? Is it true that recording temperature measurements from the thermal agent and the treated skin surface requires a sophisticated and expensive thermometer and that the recording protocol is complicated and lengthy? Can therapeutic thermal agents be used with a patient who has an impaired skin sensory discrimination test? Why do you think I ask these questions?

VIII. REFERENCES

Articles

Abramson DI, Tuck S, Chu LS, Agustin C (1964) Effects of paraffin bath and hot fomentation on local tissue temperatures. Arch Phys Med Rehab, 45: 87–94

Alcorn R, Bowser R, Henley EJ, Holloway V (1984) Fluidotherapy and exercise in the management of sickle cell anemia: A clinical report. Phys Ther, 64: 1520–1522

Borrell RM, Henley EJ, Ho P, Hubbell MK (1977) Fluidotherapy: Evaluation of a new heat modality. Arch Phys Med Rehab, 58: 69–71

Borrell RM, Parker R, Henley EJ, Masley D, Repinecz M (1980) Comparison of in vivo temperatures produced by hydrotherapy, paraffin wax treatment and Fluidotherapy. Phys Ther, 60: 1273–1276

Bromley J, Unsworth A, Haslock I (1994) Changes in stiffness following short- and long-term application of standard physiotherapeutic techniques. Br J Rheumatol, 33: 555–561

Burns SP, Conin TA. (1987) The use of paraffin wax in the treatment of burns. Physiother Can, 39: 258–260

Cetin N, Aytar A, Atalay A, Akman NM (2008) Comparing hot pack, short-wave diathermy, ultrasound, and TENS on isokinetic strength, pain, and functional status of women with osteoarthritic knees: A single-blind, randomized, controlled trial. Am J Phys Med Rehabil, 87: 443–451

Cordray YM, Krusen EM (1959) Use of hydrocollator packs in the treatment of neck and shoulder pains. Arch Phys Med Rehab, 39: 105–108

Cosgray NA, Lawrance SE, Mestrich JD, Martin SE, Whalen RL. (2004). Effect of heat modalities on hamstring length: A comparison of pneumatherm, moist hot pack, and a control. J Orthop Sports Phys Ther, 34: 377–384

Dahlen HG, Homer CS, Cooke M, Upton AM, Nuun R, Brodick B (2007) Perineal outcomes and maternal comfort to the application of perineal warm packs in the second stage of labor: A randomized controlled trial. Birth, 34: 282–290

Dahlen HG, Homer CS, Cooke M, Upton AM, Nuun R, Brodick B (2009) Soothing the ring of fire: Australian women's and midwives' experiences of using perineal warm packs in the second stage of labor. Midwifery, 25: e39–e48

Dellhag B, Wollersjö I, Bjelle A (1992) Effect of hand exercise and wax bath treatment in rheumatoid arthritis patients. Arthritis Care Res, 5: 87–92

De Sanfort B. (1915). Keritherapy: New method of thermal treatment by means of paraffin. M Press, 100: 556, 580

Draper DO, Harris ST, Shulties S, Durrant E, Knight KL, Ricard M (1998) Hot-packs and 1-MHz ultrasound treatments have an additive effect on muscle temperature increase. J Athl Train, 33: 21–24

Draper DO, Hopkins TJ (2008) Increased intramuscular and intracapsular temperature via ThermaCare Knee Wrap application. Med Sci Monit, 14: 7–11

Erdman WJ, Stoner EK (1956) Comparative heating effects of moistaire and hydrocollator hot packs. Arch Phys Med Rehab, 37: 71–74

Fountain FP, Gersten JW, Sengir O (1960) Decrease in muscle spasm produced by ultrasound, hot packs, and infrared radiation. Arch Phys Med Rehab, 41: 293–297

Garra G, Singer AJ, Leno R, Taira BR, Gupta N, Mathaikutty B, Thode HJ (2010) Heat and cold packs for neck and back strain: A randomized controlled trial of efficacy. Acad Emerg Med, 17: 484–489

Harris R, Millard JB (1955) Paraffin-wax baths in treatment of rheumatoid arthritis. Ann Rheum Dis, 14: 278–282

Hawkes J, Care G, Dixon JS, Bird HA, Wright V (1985) Comparison of three physiotherapy regimens for hands with rheumatoid arthritis. Br Med J, 291: 1016

Head MD, Helms PA (1977) Paraffin and sustained stretching in the treatment of burns contracture. Burns, 4: 136–139

Henrickson AS, Fredriksson K, Persson I, Pereira R, Rostedt Y, Westlin N (1984) The effect of heat and stretching on the range of hip motion. J Orthop Sports Phys Ther, 13: 110–115

Hollander JL, Horvath SM (1949) Influence of physical therapy procedures on intra-articular temperature of normal and arthritic subjects. Am J Med Sci, 218: 543–548

Horvath SM, Hollander JL (1949) Intra-articular temperature as measure of joint reaction. J Clin Invest, 28: 469–473

Hoyrup G, Kjorvel L (1986) Comparison of whirlpool and wax treatments for hand therapy. Physiother Can, 38: 79–82

Humphris FH (1920) Melted paraffin wax bath. Br Med J, 2: 397–399

Jutte LS, Merrick MA, Ingersoll CD, Edwards JE (2001) The relationship between intramuscular temperature, skin temperature and adipose thickness during cryotherapy and rewarming. Arch Phys Med Rehab, 82: 845–850

Kelly R, Beehn C, Hansford A, Westphal KA, Halle JS, Greathouse DG (2005) Effect of Fluidotherapy on superficial radial nerve conduction and skin temperature. J Orthop Sports Phys Ther, 35: 16–23

Knight CA, Rutledge CR, Cox ME, Acosta M, Hall SJ (2001) Effect of superficial heat, deep heat, and active exercises warm-up on the extensibility of the plantar flexors. Phys Ther, 81: 1206–1214

Landen BR (1967) Heat or cold for the relief of low back pain? Phys Ther, 47: 1126–1128

Lehmann JF, Silverman DR, Baum BA, Kirk NL, Johnson VC (1966) Temperature distribution in the human thigh produced by infrared, hot pack and microwave applications. Arch Phys Med Rehab, 47: 291–299

Lentell G, Hetherington T, Eagan J, Morgan M (1992) The use of thermal agents to influence the effectiveness of a low-load prolonged stretch. J Orthop Sports Phys Ther, 16: 200–207

Mancuso T, Poole JL (2009) The effect of paraffin and exercise on hand function in persons with scleroderma: A series of single case studies. J Hand Therapy, 22: 71–78

Mayer JM, Ralph L, Look M, Erasala JL, Matheson LN, Mooney V (2005) Treating acute low-back pain with continuous low-level heat wrap therapy and/or exercise: A randomized controlled trial. Spine, 5: 395–403

McCray RE, Patton NJ (1984) Pain relief at trigger points: A comparison of moist heat and shortwave diathermy. J Orthop Sports Phys Ther, 5: 175–178

Miller M, Wirth M, Rockwood C (1996) Thawing the frozen shoulder: The "patient" patient. Orthopedics, 19: 849–853

Myrer JW, Johnson AW, Mitchell UH, Measom GJ, Fellingham GW (2011) Topical analgesic added to paraffin enhances paraffin bath treatment of individual with hand osteoarthritis. Dis Rehabil, 33: 467–474

Nadler SF, Steiner DJ, Erasala GN, Hengehold DA, Hinkle RT, Beth Goodale M, Abeln S, Weingand KW (2002) Continuous low-level heatwrap therapy provides more efficacy than ibuprofen and acetaminophen for acute low back pain. Spine, 27: 1012–1027

Nadler SF, Steiner DJ, Petty SR, Erasala GN, Hengehold DA, Weingand KW (2003a) Overnight use of continuous low-level heatwrap therapy for relief of low back pain. Arch Phys Med Rehab, 84: 335–342

Nadler SF, Steiner DJ, Erasala GN, Hengehold DA, Abeln SB, Weingand KW (2003b) Continuous low-level heatwrap therapy for treating acute nonspecific low back pain. Arch Phys Med Rehab, 84: 329–334

Nuhr M, Hoerauf K, Bertalanfty A, Bertalanfty P, Frickey N, Gore C, Gustorff B, Kober A (2005) Active warming during emergency transport relieves acute low back pain. Spine, 15: 1499–1503

Pils K, Graninger W, Sadil F (1991). Paraffin hand bath for scleroderma. Phys Med Rehab, 1: 19–21

Portmann U (1926) Electrically heated paraffin bath. Phys Ther, 44: 333–336

Robertson VJ, Ward AR, Jung P (2005) The effect of heat on tissue extensibility: A comparison of deep and superficial heating. Arch Phys Med Rehab, 86: 519–825

Sandqvist G, Akesson A, Eklund M (2004) Evaluation of paraffin bath treatment in patients with systemic sclerosis. Dis Rehabil, 26: 981–987

Stimson CW, Rose GB, Nelson PA (1958) Paraffin bath as thermotherapy: An evaluation. Arch Phys Med Rehab, 39: 219–227

Taylor BF, Waring OA, Brashear TA (1995) The effects of therapeutic application of heat or cold followed by static stretch on hamstring muscle length. J Orthop Sports Phys Ther, 21: 283–286

Valenza J, Rossi C, Parker R, Henley EJ (1979) A clinical study of a new heat modality: Fluidotherapy. J Am Podiatr Assoc, 69: 440–442

Williams J, Harvey J, Tannenbaum H (1986) Use of superficial heat versus ice for the rheumatoid arthritic shoulder: A pilot study. Physiother Can, 38: 8–13

Yung P, Unsworth A, Haslock I (1986) Measurement of stiffness in the metacarpophalangeal joint: The effects of physiotherapy. Clin Phys Physiol Meas, 7: 147–156

Zeiter WJ (1939) Clinical application of the paraffin bath. Arch Phys Ther, 20: 469–472

Review Article

Henley EJ (1991) Fluidotherapy. Crit Rev Phys Rehab Med, 3: 173–195

Nakano J, Yamabayashi C, Scott A, Reid WD (2012) The effect of heat applied with stretch to increase range of motion: A systematic review. Phys Ther Sport, 13: 180–188

Chapters of Textbooks

Lehmann JF, De Lateur BJ (1990) Therapeutic heat. In: Therapeutic Heat and Cold, 4th ed. Lehmann JF (Ed). Williams & Wilkins, Baltimore, pp 417–581

Sekins KM, Emery AF (1990) Thermal science for physical medicine. In: Therapeutic Heat and Cold, 4th ed. Lehmann JF (Ed). Williams & Wilkins, Baltimore, pp 62–112

Chapter 8

Cryotherapy

Chapter Outline

Learning Objectives

Remembering: Describe the various cryoagents that practitioners use to deliver cryotherapy.

Understanding: Explain the biophysical principles and concepts underlying the use of cryotherapy for managing soft tissue pathologies.

Applying: Demonstrate how to apply the different cryoagents.

Analyzing: Organize the proposed physiologic and therapeutic effects of cryotherapy.

Evaluating: Judge the strength of evidence and therapeutic effectiveness behind the use of cryotherapy for managing soft tissue pathologies.

Creating: Estimate the value and place of cryotherapy for the management of soft tissue pathology.

I. FOUNDATION

A. DEFINITION

Cryotherapy, derived from the Greek word *cryos* meaning cold, is defined as the use of surface cryoagents to lower soft tissue temperature for therapeutic purposes. Cryotherapy cools soft tissues by withdrawing heat, not by adding cold, to them. Practitioners can choose from a wide variety of cryoagents to deliver cryotherapy. This chapter focuses on the most commonly used cryoagents, namely ice pack, ice bag, ice cup, icicle, vapocoolant, and controlled continuous cold unit with compression.

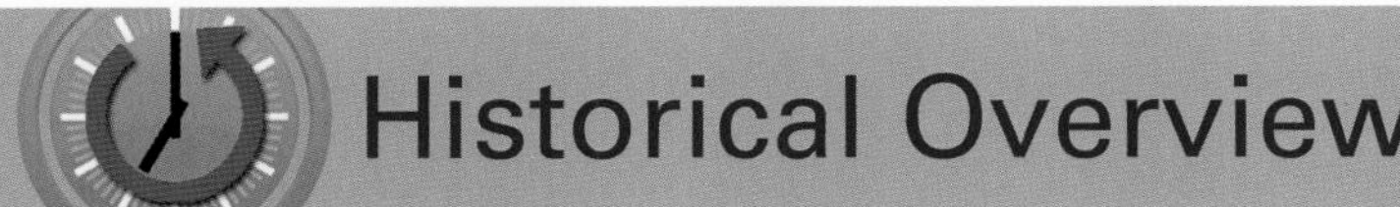

Historical Overview

Cryotherapy dates back to the ancient Greeks and Romans, who used snow and natural ice to treat a variety of health problems (Knight, 1995). During the mid-1950s, the clinical use of various cryoagents emerged under the leadership of physical therapists and athletic trainers for the treatment of various acute and subacute soft-tissue pathologies (Knight, 1995). Formal acceptance of cryotherapy by the health care mainstream came during the early 1960s after Grant (1964) and Hayden (1964) showed its benefits for the treatment of various musculoskeletal injuries in military populations. The results of their studies were important to the formal establishment and recognition of cryotherapy as an integral part of physical medicine, physical therapy, athletic therapy, and sports medicine.

B. CRYOAGENTS

Figure 8-1 illustrates a typical commercial gel pack and cooling unit, as well as commercial ice bags, an ice cup, an icicle, and vapocoolant spray. Homemade ice bags, ice cups, and icicles are also used. Figure 8-2 shows samples of controlled continuous cold units with compression. These units continuously pump cold water into a sleeve, cuff, or pad wrapped around the patient's limb while exerting compression on the wrapped body part. Readers will notice that contrary to most electrophysical textbooks, the use of water-based cryoagents such as whirlpool tubs and contrast baths, is covered in Chapter 9, which is dedicated to the practice of hydrotherapy. Table 8-1 lists the physical components and applicability of common cryoagents. Note that the cryobags can be filled with cubed, crushed, or wetted ice.

C. RATIONALE FOR USE

The therapeutic use of cryoagents relates primarily to the treatment of acute and subacute soft-tissue conditions,

TABLE 8-1 COMMON CRYOAGENTS

Agent	Physical Components	Applicability
Gel pack	Commercial mixture of water and antifreeze that forms a gel mixture and is enclosed in a flexible vinyl cover. Gel packs remain in a semisolid state despite being stored at below-freezing temperatures. Temperature should range between –5° and 0°C (23° and 32°F).	Available in different sizes and shapes. Reusable and relatively inexpensive. Used over relatively flat and large body areas.
Cubed-ice bag	Cubed ice in a commercial waterproof bag. Ice bag temperatures should range between 0° and 10°C (32° and 50°F).	Reusable and inexpensive. Used over relatively flat and large body areas.
Crushed-ice bag	Crushed ice into a commercial waterproof bag. Ice bag temperatures should range between 0° to 10°C (32° to 50°F).	
Wetted-ice bag	Mixture of cubed ice in a wet commercial waterproof bag. Ice bag temperatures should range between 0° and 10°C (32° and 50°F).	
Ice cup	Frozen water in a plastic or Styrofoam cup.	Reusable and inexpensive. Used over small and localized body areas.
Icicle	Frozen gel mounted on a plastic handle or wooden stick that is frozen in a water cup.	
Vapocoolant spray	Coolant liquid contained in a pressurized canister and activated manually by a valve.	Disposable when empty and relatively expensive. Used over localized body areas.
Controlled continuous cold unit with compression	Unit typically made of a cubed ice-water–filled cooler and a pad, cuff, or sleeve wrapped around the treated area, and an attaching hose system linking the cooler to the pad. Continuous flow of cold water is achieved by using a passive (gravity) or active (electrical pump) system. Compression is achieved by pressure exerted from the filled cuff that is wrapped around the treated segment.	Reusable and relatively more expensive. Used primarily postoperatively over body joints.

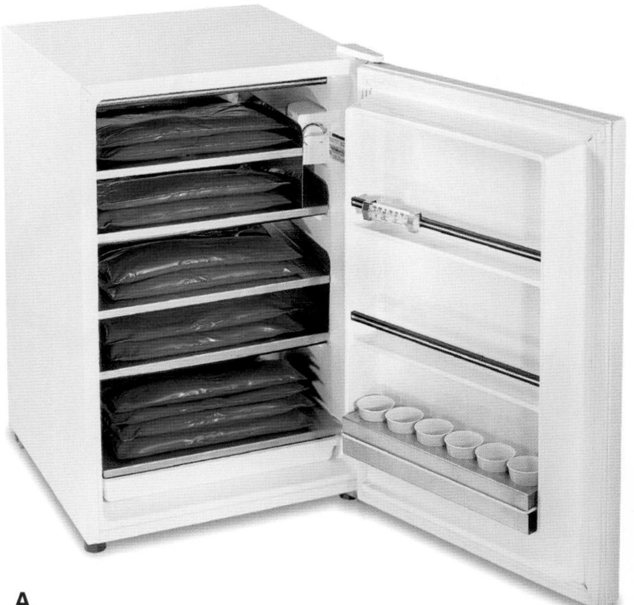

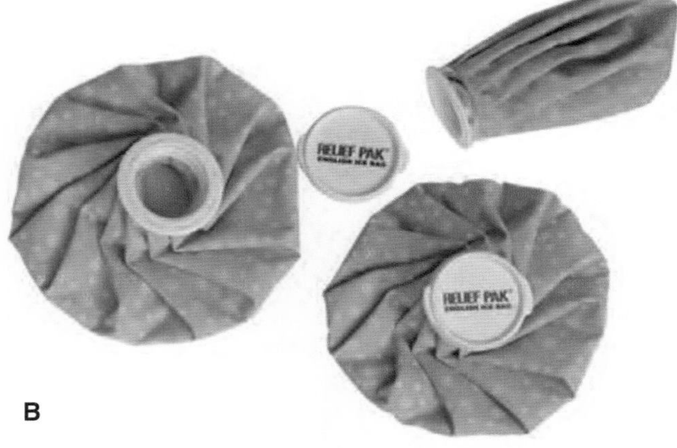

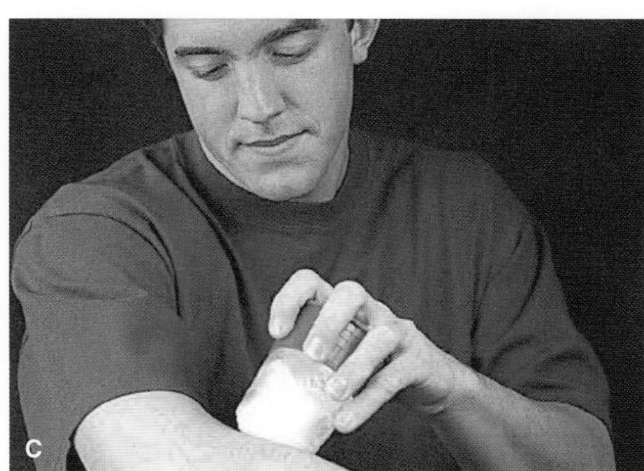

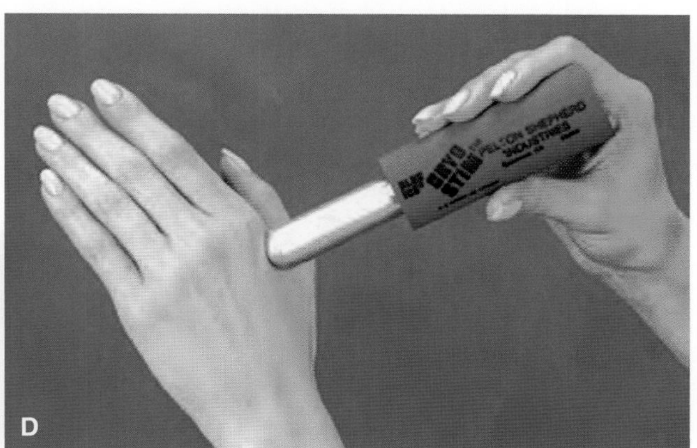

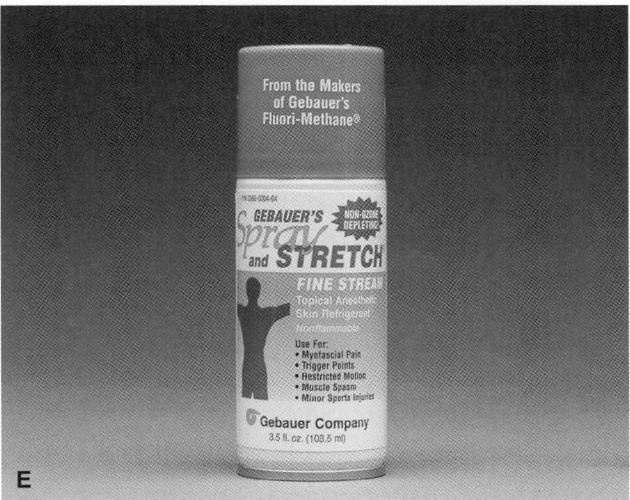

FIGURE 8-1 Common cryoagents. **A:** Commercial gel pack and storage cooling unit. **B:** Commercial ice bag to be filled with cubed, crushed or wetted ice. **C:** Ice cup. **D:** Icicle. **E:** Vapocoolant spray. (A: Courtesy of DJO Global; B–D: Courtesy of Best Priced Products; E: Courtesy of Gebauer Co.)

characterized by the two early phases of tissue repair: the hemostatic and inflammatory phases (see Chapter 2). It is hypothesized that by decreasing soft-tissue temperature, cryotherapy promotes the regulation of these two important phases, thus aiding in the process of tissue repair and recovery. Moreover, cooling other soft tissues, such as peripheral nerves, provides the rationale for using cryotherapy to manage pain and spasticity.

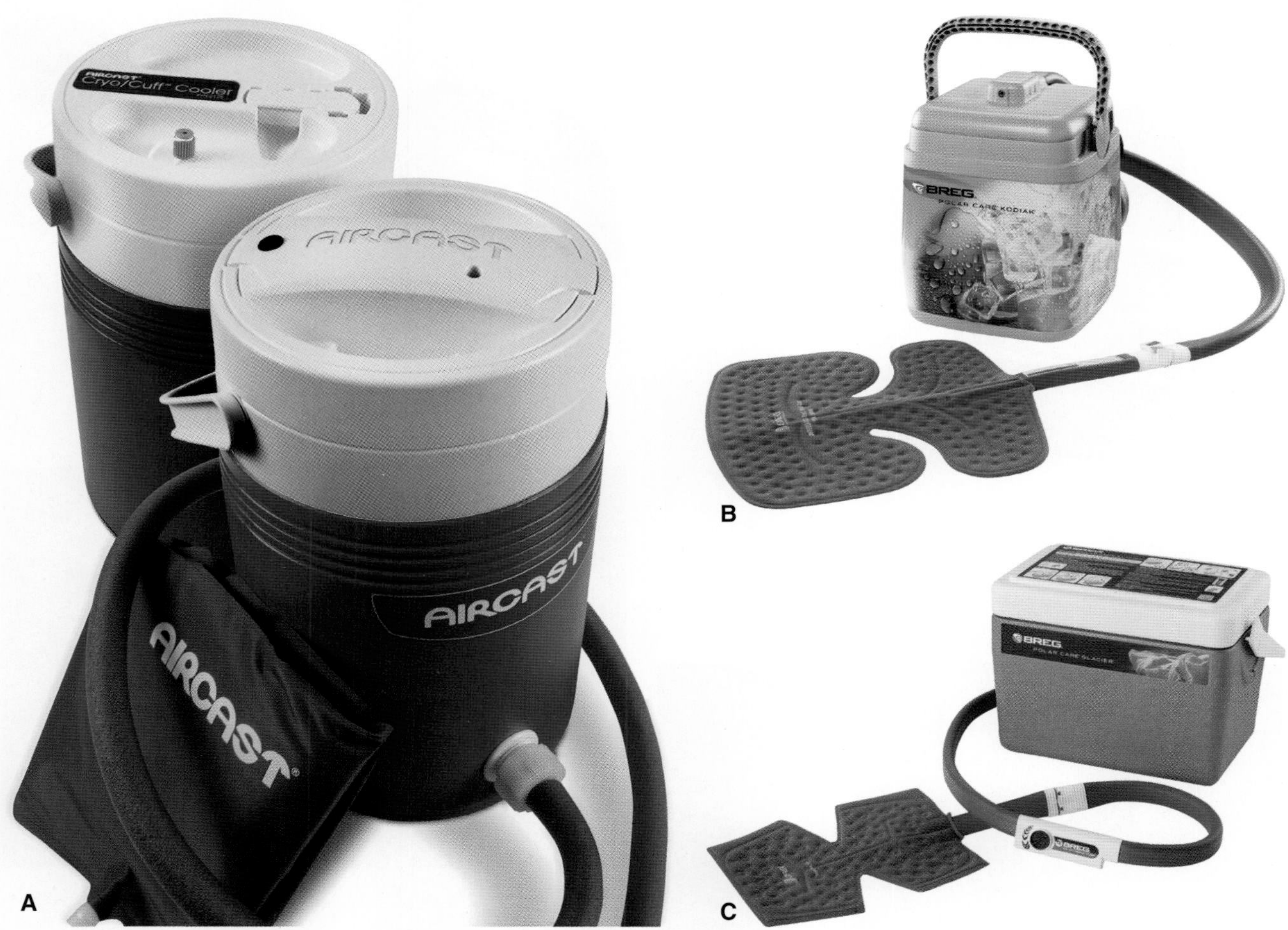

FIGURE 8-2 Typical controlled continuous cold units with compression. **A:** Passive (gravity) unit. **B:** Active (pump) unit without controlled temperature. **C:** Active (pump) unit with controlled temperature. Compression is achieved by the pressure exerted from the filled cuff, pad, or sleeve that is wrapped around the treated segment. Various shapes of pads, cuffs, and sleeves are available. (A: Courtesy of Aircast Global Corp.; B: Courtesy of Breg Inc.; C: Courtesy of Bledsoe Brace System.)

II. BIOPHYSICAL CHARACTERISTICS

A. PRINCIPLES AND CONCEPTS

The biophysics of cryotherapy rests on the concepts of heat absorption and heat transfer. The field of thermodynamics stipulates, as was the case for thermotherapy (see Chapter 7), that heat transfer is always unidirectional, occurring from the warmest to the coolest substance. Consequently, cryoagents cannot and do not transfer their coldness to the warmer soft tissues. Instead, the soft tissues themselves lose their heat to the cryoagents. In other words, the application of a cryoagent causes extraction of heat from soft tissues, thus cooling them for therapeutic purposes. The greater the amount of heat extracted by the cryoagent, the greater the cooling effect on the exposed soft tissues.

B. SUPERFICIAL VERSUS DEEP TISSUE COOLING

Superficial tissues, such as skin, cool down by losing heat to the cryoagents. Deeper tissues, such as muscles, tendons, ligaments, and joint capsules, cool in a similar fashion by losing their heat to the more superficial tissues that previously were cooled by the cryoagent (Merrick et al., 2003). Located in between the superficial and deep tissues is the subcutaneous fat tissue, which plays an important role in the process of heat transfer.

C. SUBCUTANEOUS FAT TISSUE

As stated earlier, deep tissue cooling can occur only if some of their heat is absorbed and lost to the cooler superficial tissues. Because cryotherapy is delivered through the skin, the process of heat transfer is inevitably influenced by the thickness of subcutaneous fat tissue that separates the deeper tissues from the skin in the treated area.

1. Fat Thermal Conductivity

As discussed in Chapter 7, the ability of a soft tissue to conduct heat is determined by its thermal conductivity (k). Subcutaneous fat ($k = 0.45$) conducts heat approximately two times less than skin ($k = 0.90$) and three times less than muscle (k = 1.53). This means that the thicker the subcutaneous layer, the greater the thermal barrier between superficial and deeper tissues.

2. Fat and Deep Tissue Cooling

There is strong experimental evidence to show that a significant inverse relationship exists between subcutaneous fat tissue thickness and the rate of intramuscular temperature change (Lowden et al., 1975; Johnson et al., 1979; Zemke et al., 1998; Myrer et al., 2001). This means that for any given cryoagent, the thinner the subcutaneous fat layer, the greater the rate and extent of deeper tissue cooling. In other words, the thinner the subcutaneous layer of fat, the easier it is for the deeper tissues to lose their heat to the cooler skin and subcutaneous fat tissues.

3. Fat and Application Duration

Experimental evidence also suggests a direct relationship between adipose thickness and required application duration or cooling time (Otte et al., 2002). This means that to cool deeper tissues covered by a thick subcutaneous fat layer, a longer application duration is required so that cooler superficial tissues can extract more heat from the warmer deep tissues. In other words, the greater the superficial tissue cooling, the greater the deep tissue cooling.

D. HEAT TRANSFER MODES

Heat transfer in cryotherapy occurs via two modes: conduction and evaporation. Heat transfer by *conduction* occurs when there is direct contact between the surface of the cryoagent and the skin surface over which it is applied (see Chapter 7). All cryoagents covered in this chapter, with the exception of vapocoolant spray, work by using this form of heat transfer. Heat transfer by *evaporation,* on the other hand, occurs through the conversion of a substance from a liquid to a vapor state (Sekins et al., 1990). For example, when the vapocoolant liquid spray hits the surface of the skin, the liquid is heated by the warm skin, thus changing its physical state from liquid to vapor. During this process of evaporation, the skin loses heat, resulting in its cooling.

III. THERAPEUTIC EFFECTS AND INDICATIONS

A. COOLING

The proposed physiologic and therapeutic effects of cryotherapy are presented in Figure 8-3. The initial and primary effect of cryotherapy is the cooling of soft tissues, which occurs usually within the first 20 minutes of application. As stated previously, soft tissue *cooling* is caused by the extraction, or withdrawal, of heat from the exposed tissue by the cryoagent. This cooling effect induces significant vascular and neural responses that may last as long as a few hours, or until full tissue rewarming occurs (see Knight, 1995; Adie et al., 2010; Markert, 2011; Knight et al., 2013a,b). The subsequent and secondary effect is *cold-induced vasodilation (CIVD).* This effect is the late or delayed response to tissue cooling, which, under some particular circumstances (intense cooling) and for some specific organs or body areas (such as the hand and foot, nail bed, elbow, lips, cheeks, ears, and nose) may prevent cold-induced tissue damage (see Daanen et al., 1997; Daanen, 2003).

1. Vasoconstriction, Blood Flow, and Cell Metabolism

Soft tissue cooling causes several physiologic effects, which may induce therapeutic responses that decrease blood flow, cell metabolism, secondary tissue damage, edema, pain, muscle spasm, and spasticity (see Fig. 8-3). The application of a cryoagent over a skin surface area triggers the reflex activation, or depolarization, of several sympathetic adrenergic nerve fibers. The depolarization of these nerve fibers leads to release of their neurotransmitter—norepinephrine—on the adrenergic receptors of smooth muscles surrounding blood vessels, which in turn causes a powerful reflex vasoconstriction. There is evidence to show that vasoconstriction decreases blood flow to soft tissues by reducing the lumen (or diameter) of blood vessels; the smaller the lumen, the less the amount of blood flowing per unit of time (Knight, 1995; Daanen, 2003). There is also evidence to show that reducing tissue temperature reduces cell metabolism, which in turn further reduces the tissue's oxygen requirement (Knight et al., 2013a,b).

2. Decrease Secondary Tissue Damage

Primary tissue damage refers to the cellular damages (dead cells) caused by injury or disease, found at the site of the wound. There is a consensus in the field of cryotherapy that the key therapeutic effect caused by the powerful reflex vasoconstriction described earlier decreases cell metabolism, as shown in Figure 8-3, which in turn will decrease secondary tissue damage (see Knight, 1995; Merrick, 2002; Knight et al., 2013a,b). *Secondary* tissue damage, on the other hand, refers to cellular damage previously caused to nondamaged or healthy cells within, and at the periphery of, the wound. Because soft tissues have a very limited time window during which they can survive ischemia (lack of blood) and hypoxia (lack of oxygen), the period of time that elapses between the moment of injury and the first application of cryotherapy is critical. There is a consensus that when applied as soon as possible after injury—that is, within the first 24 to 48 hours—cryotherapy makes a greater contribution to tissue repair by limiting the extent of secondary tissue damage (Knight, 1995; Knight et al., 2013a,b). When soft tissue temperatures are lowered, the rate of cellular metabolism is slowed

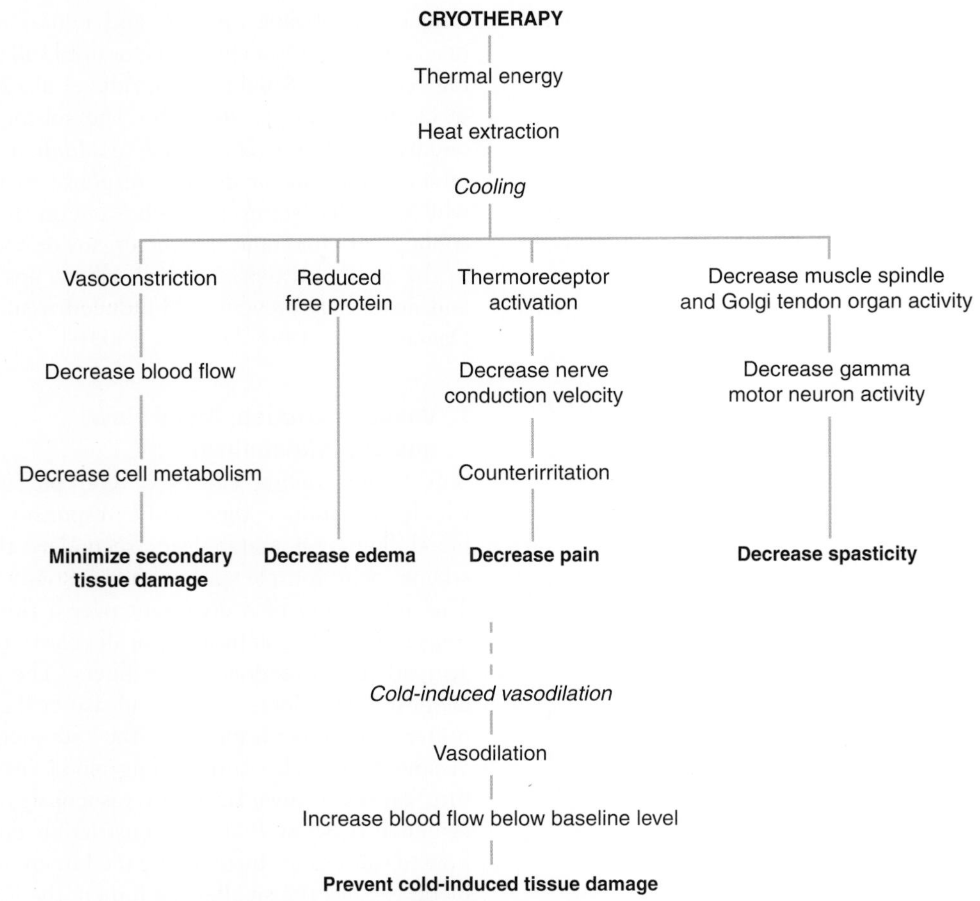

FIGURE 8-3 Proposed physiologic and therapeutic effects of cryotherapy.

down, and thus the oxygen requirement of local tissues is reduced. Consequently, cellular necrosis in tissues that are unaffected by the original injury may be minimized, which would limit the extent of necessary tissue repair (Knight, 1995; Knight et al., 2013a,b). In other words, when the metabolism of uninjured cells within the wound and of healthy or normal cells surrounding the wound is slowed down, their reliance on oxygen is reduced, which enables them to better face the temporary period of hypoxia caused by the impaired blood flow at the trauma site, or organ, that is affected.

3. Decrease Edema and Pain

Swelling is the enlargement of a tissue or organ resulting from edema, which is the accumulation of fluids in the interstitial spaces. Cryotherapy can decrease edema at the wound site if applied within the first 24 to 48 hours post injury. It does this, as illustrated in Figure 8-3, by minimizing secondary tissue damage (Knight et al., 2013a,b), which then decreases edema formation. Minimizing secondary damage reduces the amount of free proteins in the wound vicinity, which in turn leads to less edema formation. Cryotherapy also decreases pain through the following three physiologic processes. The first process, counterirritation, involves substituting one form of irritation (pain) with another form of irritation (cold). In other words, during cryotherapy, the sensation of pain is counteracted, or replaced, by the sensation of coldness, thus diminishing the patient's perception of pain. The second process, resulting from cooling, reduces the release of pain-sensitizing substances in the injured area, thus decreasing nociceptor sensitivity and pain (Allen, 2006). The third process relates to the transient reduction, or blocking, of the conduction velocity of pain nerve fibers.

4. Decrease Muscle Spasm and Spasticity

Cryotherapy can reduce the protective muscle spasm that follows injury by decreasing the pain–spasm–pain cycle. It can also decrease spasticity, or muscle tone, by decreasing the activity of the gamma motor neuron system, which is regulated by muscle spindle and Golgi tendon organ activity (Fig. 8-3). To sum up, cryotherapy is well known for its posttraumatic natural anti-inflammatory effects, which are to decrease some of cardinal signs of inflammation—namely, pain, secondary tissue damage, edema, and muscle spasm (Bleakley et al., 2010a).

B. COLD-INDUCED VASODILATION

CIVD is the secondary effect of cryotherapy that usually is observed with prolonged applications leading to soft tissue temperatures decreasing below 10°C (50°F).

It is defined as a vasodilation of cold-exposed blood vessels, in particular the arteriovenous anastomoses (AVAs) found in specific body areas, such as the hands and feet, and organs usually exposed without protection to cold, such as the lips, cheeks, ears, and nose (Daanen, 2003). This effect, which is discussed often in the field of cryotherapy and human exposure to cold, is still a subject of controversy (Daanen, 2003; Knight et al., 2013a) and, as a result, deserves further clarification. The main controversy is over the magnitude of vasodilation, and whether this physiologic response is strong enough to negate the main therapeutic purpose of cryotherapy, which is to cool soft tissues. This controversy stems from an early study by Clarke et al. (1958), which suggested that cryotherapy leads to a significant increase in blood flow that actually exceeds baseline values over time.

1. Hunting Response

Lewis (1930) was the first to observe CIVD. Experimentally measuring human finger temperatures during and after immersion in ice-cold water, Lewis observed cycles of increase and decrease in skin temperature, which he interpreted as cycles of vasoconstriction and vasodilation. To describe this cold-induced effect, he coined the term *hunting response,* hypothesizing that this cycling vascular effect was triggered by the release of a so-called H substance, similar in action to histamine at the site of injury. As pointed out by Knight (1995), many in the field have mistakenly inferred from Lewis's work that the magnitude of this CIVD response was large enough not only to reestablish the initial blood flow at the injury site (i.e., to reestablish the baseline level) but also to actually yield a net increase of warmer blood flow at this site, thus negating the cooling effect of cryotherapy. The clinical implication of this belief is that the application of cryotherapy should be brief to avoid such a late vasodilation. To answer these concerns, Knight and colleagues (1980, 1981) revisited this issue by replicating Lewis's original experiments in healthy humans.

a. Low-Magnitude Response

Knight and colleagues (1980, 1981) showed that the relatively small and irregular skin temperature changes measured by Lewis when the subject's fingers remained immobile in still (unstirred) ice-cold water were due to the formation of a "blanket" of warm water trapped around the fingers as the body part gave up heat to the water surrounding it. Stirring the ice water during the experiment, thus removing this blanket of warm water, led to smaller average temperature fluctuations, from a mean value of 2.1 ± 2°C (mean ± standard deviation) for unstirred water to a mean value of 1.6 ± 2°C for stirred water. Similar small and nonstatistically significant mean temperature changes (2°C) were also recorded by Daanen et al. (1997) in a similar study on healthy human subjects.

b. Little Physiologic Significance

The fact that measurement errors around the mean values (see previous discussion) are as large as the mean values themselves led Knight (1995) to conclude that these skin temperature changes of approximately 2°C after prolonged cold immersion have little physiologic and therapeutic significance. In other words, this CIVD, or hunting reaction, leads to only a small blood flow increase in the cooled tissues. CIVD is a complex response, which may be related to body core temperature. Daanen et al. (1997, 2003) showed that a cooler body core temperature in comparison to a warmer one before cold immersion is associated with decreased magnitude and frequency of the CIVD response. This finding contradicts the opinion of many who believe that the purpose of CIVD is to prevent excessive tissue cooling in victims suffering from hypothermia.

2. Blood Flow Changes

The effect of cryotherapy on human blood flow has been extensively studied since the release of Lewis's article in 1930, and the results provide evidence for a CIVD effect (see Bancroft et al., 1943; Greenfield et al., 1950; Duff et al., 1953; Clarke et al., 1958; Abramson et al., 1966; Aizawa et al., 1979; Ho et al., 1994). Together, the results of these studies reveal that this cyclic increase in blood flow, caused by late-induced vasodilation, always remains below baseline values, suggesting that the net effect of cryotherapy is one of vasoconstriction leading to soft-tissue cooling. Practitioners, therefore, need not be concerned that this CIVD response will negate the cooling effect of cryotherapy and should not limit cryotherapy application to short application durations.

3. Clinical Significance of Cold-Induced Vasodilation

Scientific evidence presented in this chapter strongly suggests that the purpose of CIVD, a genuine human physiological phenomenon, is to provide more warmed blood to specific body areas, such as the hands and feet, lips, cheeks, ears, and nose, which are often exposed to intense cold without protection (see Daanen, 2003). The net effect is to prevent cold-induced tissue damage, such as a frostnip or frostbite (Daanen, 2003). CIVD is presumed to be caused by a sudden decrease in the release of neurotransmitters from the sympathetic nerves to the muscular coat of the AVAs due to local cold (Daanen, 2003). AVAs, found primarily in the skin overlying the hands and feet as well as other organs such as lips, cheeks, ears, and nose, are specific thermoregulatory vascular structures that regulate blood flow in cold and hot conditions (Daanen, 2003). Finally, the present body of scientific evidence suggests that CIVD is more likely to occur when the extremities (hands and feet) are subjected to cryotherapy by means of immersion in cold water (see cryo-hydrotherapy discussion in Chapter 9). Practitioners can feel reassured that the presence of a CIVD response in the extremities (hands and feet), during and following cryotherapy, does not negate the prime cooling effect of this agent.

C. TARGET TEMPERATURE WINDOW

As is the case for thermotherapy (Chapter 7), scientific evidence suggests that to optimize the clinical effectiveness of cryotherapy, critical levels of soft tissue cooling must be achieved following the application of cryoagents (see Greenstein, 2007; Bleakley et al., 2010a,b). What are the soft tissue target temperature levels that need to be reached to accomplish the above physiologic and therapeutic effects? A review of animal and human research findings (Greenstein, 2007; Bleakley et al., 2010a,b) suggests that the *optimal* therapeutic temperature window for cryotherapy may be between 10° and 15°C (50° and 60°F). Figure 8-4 illustrates the therapeutic temperature window of cryotherapy. Practically speaking, to decrease soft-tissue temperatures within the suboptimal and optimal windows is the goal.

1. Skin Cooling

Is it possible to cool or reduce human skin to levels between 10°C (50°F) and 15°C (60°F) by using cryoagents? The answer is yes. The body of evidence reviewed in this chapter indicates that lowering the skin to such levels and below is easily achievable when the proper dosimetry and application protocol are used (see Lehmann et al., 1990, Greenstein, 2007; Bleakley et al., 2010a,b). Unfortunately, the skin tissue, when compared to the deeper tissues, is practically never the targeted soft tissue when the time comes to use cryotherapy.

2. Deeper Tissue Cooling

Is it possible to decrease the temperature of human deeper tissues, such as muscles, tendons, ligaments, and joint capsules, to levels within this the temperature window optimal range using cryoagents? The answer, as was the case with thermotherapy, may be yes *or* no. Theoretically speaking, it may all depend, once again, over which body areas these cryoagents are applied, the magnitude of dose used, and whether or not the exposed deeper tissues are covered with either thick or thin layers of subcutaneous fat. For example, the answer is yes if one applies a crushed-ice bag, with a high temperature differential or dose ($T°_{ag\text{-}s}$), over the hand area where the adiposity, or skinfold, is at its lowest value. The answer is no if one applies the same cryoagent over the thigh or back area of a patient who is overweight or obese. There appears to be a consensus in the cryotherapy literature that the lowest human muscle temperature ever recorded over the thigh area was 21°C (70°F), which is well above the optimal therapeutic window discussed earlier (Greenstein, 2007; Bleakley et al., 2010a,b).

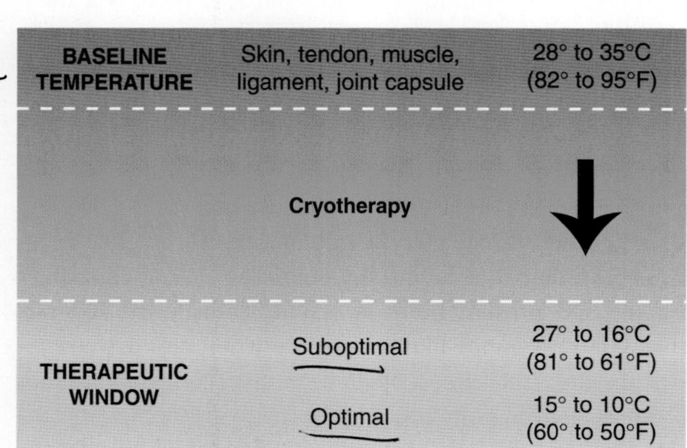

FIGURE 8-4 Cryotherapy thermal window.

3. Suboptimal Versus Optimal Cooling

Although decreasing temperature within the optimal window in the deeper tissues may be clinically very difficult to achieve, if not impossible, it does not mean that decreasing soft tissue temperatures within the suboptimal window range is therapeutically meaningless. It is fair to say, while awaiting further research on this very important subject, that the more tissue cooling practitioners can induce, the more important and beneficial will be the physiologic and therapeutic effects. It appears, based on the evidence, that it is much more difficult to extract heat from soft tissues than it is to add heat to them. Again, it is important to keep in mind that cryotherapy does not convey cold to tissues, because cold (the absence of heat) is not transferable. In contrast, tissues lose heat because they warm the cold agent. Following the same principle, deeper tissues lose heat to the more superficial cooled tissues. This practically means that the greater the extent of skin cooling achieved and maintained over time, the greater the cooling of deeper tissues, with deeper tissues losing more and more heat while trying to the warm the cooler skin.

D. RESEARCH-BASED INDICATIONS

The search for evidence behind the use of cryotherapy, displayed in the *Research-Based Indications* box shown earlier, led to the collection of 92 English peer-reviewed human clinical studies. The methodologies, as well as the criteria, used to assess the strength of evidence and therapeutic effectiveness are described in Chapter 2. As indicated, the strength of evidence is ranked as *strong* for postoperative knee arthroplasty and mixed postoperative musculoskeletal conditions, and as *moderate* for ankle sprain, spasticity, and joint, tendon, and muscle conditions, as well as for arthritic/rheumatoid conditions. Therapeutic effectiveness is found to be *conflicting* for postoperative knee arthroplasty and *substantiated* for all other mentioned conditions. Analysis is *pending* for the other remaining health conditions shown in the box because fewer than five studies could be collected. Over all conditions, the strength of evidence behind the use of cryotherapy is found to be *moderate* and its therapeutic effectiveness *substantiated*.

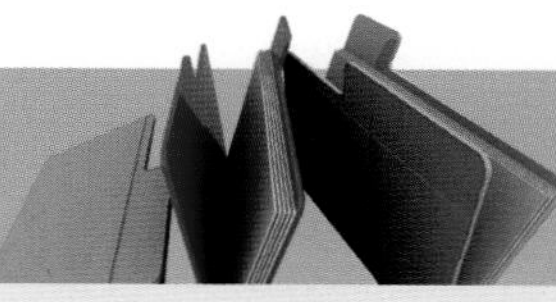

Research-Based Indications

CRYOTHERAPY

Health Condition	Benefit—Yes Rating	Benefit—Yes Reference	Benefit—No Rating	Benefit—No Reference
Postoperative knee arthroplasty	I	Ohkoshi et al., 1999	I	Daniel et al., 1994
	I	Martin et al., 2001	I	Dervin et al., 1998
	I	Barber et al., 1998	I	Edwards et al., 1996
	I	Cohn et al., 1989	I	Konrath et al., 1996
	I	Levy et al., 1993	I	Leutz et al., 1995
	I	Morsi, 2002	I	Scarcella et al., 1995
	I	Webb et al., 1998	I	Zaffagnini et al., 1998
	I	Bert et al., 1991	II	Walker et al., 1991
	II	Shelbourne et al., 1994	II	Healy et al., 1994
	II	Schroder et al., 1994	II	Ivey et al., 1994
	II	Woolf et al., 2008	II	Radkowsky et al., 2007
	II	Hecht et al., 1983	II	Smith et al., 2002
	II	Whitelaw et al., 1995		Gibbons et al., 2001
	II	Lessard et al., 1997		
	II	Sanchez-Inchausti et al., 2005		
	II	Kullenberg et al., 2006		

Strength of evidence: Strong
Therapeutic effectiveness: Conflicting

Health Condition	Benefit—Yes Rating	Benefit—Yes Reference	Benefit—No Rating	Benefit—No Reference
Ankle sprain	I	Sloan et al., 1989		
	II	Weston et al., 1994		
	II	Basur et al., 1976		
	II	Wilkerson, 1991		
	II	Wilkerson et al., 1993		
	II	Michlovitz et al., 1988		
	II	Hocutt et al., 1982		
	II	Pincivero et al., 1993		
	II	Cote et al., 1988		
	II	Bleakley et al., 2006		
	II	Stockle et al., 1997		
	III	Starkey (1976)		

Strength of evidence: Moderate
Therapeutic effectiveness: Substantiated

Health Condition	Benefit—Yes Rating	Benefit—Yes Reference	Benefit—No Rating	Benefit—No Reference
Spasticity	II	Price et al., 1993		
	II	Boes, 1962		
	II	Hedenberg, 1970		
	II	Knuttson, 1970a,b		
	II	Miglietta, 1973		
	II	Miglietta, 1964		
	II	DonTigny et al., 1962		
	II	Kelly, 1969		
	III	Hartvikksen, 1962		
	III	Basset et al., 1958		

Strength of evidence: Moderate
Therapeutic effectiveness: Substantiated

Health Condition	Benefit—Yes Rating	Benefit—Yes Reference	Benefit—No Rating	Benefit—No Reference
Mixed postoperative musculoskeletal conditions	I	Saito et al., 2004	I	Scarcella et al., 1995
	I	Singh et al., 2001		
	I	Osbahr et al., 2002		
	I	Speer et al., 1996		
	I	Brandner et al., 1996		
	I	Rembe, 1970		
	II	Schaubel, 1946		
	II	Showman et al., 1963		
	II	Scheffler et al., 1992		
	II	Barber, 2000		

Strength of evidence: Strong
Therapeutic effectiveness: Substantiated

Health Condition	Benefit—Yes Rating	Benefit—Yes Reference	Benefit—No Rating	Benefit—No Reference
Joint, tendon, and muscle conditions	II	Hayden, 1964		
	II	Grant, 1964		
	II	Modell et al., 1952		
	III	Lane, 1971		
	III	Kalenak et al., 1975		

Strength of evidence: Moderate
Therapeutic effectiveness: Substantiated

Health Condition	Benefit—Yes Rating	Benefit—Yes Reference	Benefit—No Rating	Benefit—No Reference
Arthritic/rheumatoid conditions	II	Halliday Pegg et al., 1969		
	II	Williams et al., 1986		
	II	Kirk et al., 1968		
	II	Clarke et al., 1974		
	II	Curkovic et al., 1993		

Strength of evidence: Moderate
Therapeutic effectiveness: Substantiated

Health Condition	Benefit—Yes Rating	Benefit—Yes Reference	Benefit—No Rating	Benefit—No Reference
Fewer Than 5 Studies				
Muscle spasm/ myofascial pain	II	Travell, 1952		
	II	Mennell, 1976		
	III	Nielsen, 1978, 1981		
Post-exercise delayed muscle soreness	I	Denegar et al., 1992	I	Yackzan et al., 1984
			I	Isabell et al., 1992
Neck/low back pain	II	Melzack et al., 1980		
	II	Landen, 1967		
	II	Travell, 1949		
Multiple sclerosis	II	Kinnman et al., 2000a		
	II	Kinnman et al., 2000b		
Postoperative cesarean/ laparoscopy			II	Amin-Hanjani et al., 1992
			I	Finan et al., 1993
Headache/migraine	II	Robbins, 1989		
	II	Diamond et al., 1986		
Post-fracture compartment pressure	II	Moore et al., 1977		
Trigeminal neuralgia	II	De Coster et al., 1993		
Myofascial masticatory pain	II	Burgess et al., 1988		
Post–carpal tunnel release	II	Hochberg, 2001		
Postoperative wrist arthroscopy	II	Meyer-Marcotty et al., 2011		

Strength of evidence: Pending
Therapeutic effectiveness: Pending

ALL CONDITIONS
Strength of evidence: Moderate
Therapeutic effectiveness: Substantiated

IV. DOSIMETRY

A. QUALITATIVE VERSUS QUANTITATIVE

As stated and discussed in Chapter 7 on thermotherapy, the practice of evidence-based cryotherapy requires that practitioners objectively and quantitatively assess the thermal dose delivered to the tissues, and well as the amount of heat extracted from the exposed tissues following the application of cryoagents. Considering that the rationale for quantitative dosimetry using cryotherapy is identical to that of thermotherapy and to avoid duplication, readers are referred to the material on this topic in the Dosimetry section in Chapter 7. To summarize, the temperature differential between the cryoagent (ag) and the exposed skin surface (s) is the dose ($T^{\circ}_{ag\text{-}s}$) delivered to soft tissues. This measurement is easily and rapidly done using a noncontact portable infrared thermometer. The larger the dose, the greater its capacity to cool soft tissues by extracting heat from them. The temperature differential between the exposed skin surface before (b) and after (a) treatment ($T^{\circ}_{b\text{-}a}$) represents the actual cooling of the skin caused by the dose. Let us consider the following example. Just prior to application, the temperature of a gel pack is measured at 5°C (41°F) and that of the exposed skin surface at 30°C (86°F). The thermal dose delivered ($T^{\circ}_{ag\text{-}s}$) thus equals 25°C (45°F), which represents the *potential* cooling effect of this gel pack. Immediately after treatment, the exposed skin temperature is measured at 12°C (54°F). The *actual* skin cooling effect ($T^{\circ}_{b\text{-}a}$) of this dose on the skin was –18°C (–32°F). Again, in the context of evidence-based practice (EBP), it is useful to ask the patient how cold the thermal agent feels against the body parts both during and after treatment, but it is better to supplement this qualitative information with actual temperature measurements. This text strongly encourages practitioners to supplement their qualitative approach to dosimetry with this suggested quantitative approach.

B. COOLING CHARACTERISTICS OF CRYOAGENTS

Is the ability of cryoagents to cool soft tissues the same? The answer is no. There is a consensus in the literature that cryoagents passing through a phase change—that is, *from a solid to a liquid form*—while cooling, regardless of their preapplication temperatures, are generally more effective in inducing faster and greater tissue cooling than those that do not (see Merrick et al., 2003; Kennet et al., 2007; Dykstra et al., 2009). For example, there is evidence to show that crushed-ice bags can induce greater cooling efficiency than gel packs (Kennet et al., 2007; Kanlayanaphotporn et al., 2005) or Liquid Ice (Leite et al., 2010). This is explained by the fact that contrary to crushed-ice packs, gel packs do not undergo phase change during treatment. There is also evidence to show that wetted-ice bags may be more effective than cubed- and crushed-ice bags, and that crushed ice may be more effective than cubed ice (Dykstra et al., 2009). Why? The greater effectiveness may be due to the fact that water has a much greater thermal conductivity (see Chapter 7) than air (1.42 vs. 0.02), which is found between the individual ice pieces within both cubed- and crushed ice. Both cubed- and crushed-ice use air to transfer thermal energy between the individual pieces of water, whereas wetted ice uses water to transfer the thermal energy within the bag or pack (Dykstra et al., 2009). To sum up, practitioners should select, when applicable, cryoagents that undergo phase changes during application for faster and greater soft tissue cooling.

C. COUPLING MEDIUM

The cryoagents covered in this chapter (see Table 8-1), with the exception of one, gel pack, can and should be applied **without** the use of a coupling medium—that is, directly over the bare skin area to maximize soft tissue cooling (Knight, 1995; Tsang et al., 1997; Janwantanakul, 2004). As discussed earlier, practitioners should always keep in mind that it may be very difficult to cool deeper soft tissues, and as a result, optimal thermal transfer is needed to lower tissues temperatures within the optimal range of the therapeutic window. Because commercially made gel packs are normally chilled to less than 0°C (32°F) before use, Knight (1995) recommends placing a layer of damp cloth between the pack and the exposed skin surface, and to limit its application to 30 minutes. Doing so will minimize the risk of causing cold-induced skin damage, such as frostnip and frostbite (Nadler et al., 2003; Janwantanakul, 2004). The use of cryoagents over dry/wet coupling media significantly reduces soft tissue cooling because of their insulation effect, thus reducing the overall effectiveness of cryotherapy (Lavelle et al., 1985; Belitsky et al., 1987; Culp et al., 1995; Metzman et al., 1996). Cryoagents may be applied over synthetic and plaster casts as well as over common bandages and dressings (Kaempffe, 1989; Metzman et al., 1996; Weresh et al., 1996; Okcu et al., 2006; Shibuya et al., 2007). In such cases, application duration needs to be significantly prolonged (for as long as 60 minutes) to significantly reduce soft tissue temperature. Compression of cryoagents with elastic wraps causes greater skin and intramuscular temperature changes when compared with no compression (Merrick et al., 1993; Tomchuk et al., 2010). The rule of thumb is that coupling media should be restricted as much as possible if the purpose is to obtain maximum deep tissue cooling within the shortest application duration. If coupling media are used, practitioners must either increase the dose ($T°_{ag\text{-}s}$) or increase the application duration to maximize cooling.

V. APPLICATION, CONTRAINDICATIONS, AND RISKS

Prior to considering the application of cryotherapy, practitioners must first check for contraindications, consider the risks, and then go through key application steps and procedures designed to optimize treatment safety, efficacy, and effectiveness. As is the case with the practice of thermotherapy (Chapter 7), there is unanimity in the literature and clinical community that safe application of all thermal electrophysical agents (EPAs), such as cryotherapy, must begin with the conduct of a skin thermal discrimination test that assesses the patient's ability to normally perceive such stimuli. To optimize treatment safety and effectiveness, the following tests are also recommended. A simple and effective prediagnostic test, the *ice-cube test,* is available to determine whether the patient suffers from cold urticaria, also referred to as cold hypersensitivity, or cold allergy (Harvey, 1992). This test, conducted before the first application, consists of massaging the skin with an ice cube for approximately 3 minutes. A normal reddish patch, or skin erythema, should occur over the massaged area within 5 minutes of the initiation of ice massage. If this reddish patch is replaced by a wheal (localized skin edema) that covers the tested surface area, the test is positive (Harvey, 1992). In this case, it is strongly recommended that the patient be referred to an allergist for confirmation of the diagnosis. Note that the skin redness observed during and after cryotherapy is a normal physiologic response to cold and, therefore, should not be interpreted as a sign of cold urticaria or CIVD. This reddening of the skin is caused by the increase in oxyhemoglobin concentration in the blood that results from the decrease in oxygen–hemoglobin dissociation that occurs at lower temperatures. The use of cryotherapy over the extremities requires adequate blood flow regulation to prevent tissue damage. Another simple and effective prediagnostic test to assess blood flow at these levels is the *nail bed test* (Starkey, 2004). This test, conducted before the first application, consists of exerting finger pressure over the nail bed of fingers or toes, which will flush out the blood, making the compressed nail bed area pale and white. Rapidly releasing the test finger pressure allows the blood to flush back into the nail bed, thus restoring its original reddish color. The test is positive if releasing pressure on the finger fails to restore the nail bed's original color within a few seconds, which suggests peripheral circulatory problems. Further comprehensive vascular assessment is thus required to determine if severe occlusive vascular disorder is present, in which case cryotherapy is contraindicated. In addition to local effects, cryotherapy may induce, in some patients, important systemic cardiovascular responses, including blood pressure changes. The diastolic and systemic blood pressure before, during, and after therapy should therefore be measured and monitored, especially for patients who have a history of cardiovascular or cardiorespiratory disorders, or both. Because the thickness of subcutaneous fat tissue at the treated area may significantly decrease the cooling of deeper soft tissues (Myrer et al., 2001), practitioners should measure skinfolds using a hand caliper before the first application of cryotherapy, especially in patients who are overweight or obese. Objective skinfold measurement will guide the dosimetry for treatment, helping practitioners to select appropriate temperature differentials or doses, as well as proper application methods and application durations. A survey by Nadler et al. (2003) revealed that of 362 complications documented by athletic trainers after the application of various EPAs, 42% of them were related to the use of cryotherapy. The most common complications were cold-induced allergic reaction (urticaria; $n = 86$), skin damage (frostnip to frostbite; $n = 23$), and intolerance to cold-induced pain ($n = 16$). These findings differ from those documented in the peer-reviewed literature, where most complications were related to cold-induced peripheral nerve injuries. The fact that no case of nerve injury was reported in this survey implies that either the respondents were well aware of this complication (i.e., they were fully prevented) or that such nerve injuries were underreported or missed during the course of assessing athletic injuries (Nadler et al., 2003). Although cryotherapy reduces the sensation of pressure, its use is not contraindicated as an analgesic before submaximal rehabilitative exercise programs (Rubley et al., 2003). Moreover, when supervising therapeutic exercise regimens, clinicians must recognize that cryotherapy may make joints stiffer and lessen the patient's sensitivity to position (Uchio et al., 2003). Finally, motor function may be enhanced after ankle joint cooling partly because of decreased residual pain, combined with facilitation of the motor neuron pools (soleus) that may have been affected by the joint injury (Hopkins et al., 2002).

APPLICATION, CONTRAINDICATIONS, AND RISKS

Cryotherapy

IMPORTANT: Because skin thermal damage is always a possibility with the application of cryotherapy, skin thermal discrimination testing MUST BE CONDUCTED PRIOR to the first application. The description and scoring of this test are documented in Table 7-4 of Chapter 7. Other tests, such as the ice-cube test and the nail bed test, are also recommended.

ALL AGENTS

STEP	RATIONALE
1. Check for contraindications.	*Over skin areas where sensation of cold is severely impaired*—cutaneous damage or burn (frostnip to frostbite) *In patients suffering from cold-induced urticaria (cold allergy) or cold hypersensitivity*—triggering local skin reactions, such as wheal or patches, or systemic allergic reactions, such as sneezing and dysphasia, in addition to moderate to severe itching (Day, 1974; Escher et al., 1992, Knight 1995) *In patients presenting with Raynaud's disease or phenomenon*—further enhancement of vasoconstrictive spasm, which, if prolonged, is likely to aggravate digital cyanosis and eventually lead to ischemic necrosis (Bolster et al., 1995) *In patients presenting with cryoglobulinemia*—aggravation characterized by the aggregation of serum proteins in the small distal vessels after cold applications, resulting in impaired blood circulation, possibly causing ischemia and, in the worst case, gangrene *In patients presenting with paroxysmal cold hemoglobinuria*—aggravation characterized by the undesirable release of hemoglobin in the urine, resulting from the rapid breakdown, or lysing, of many blood cells after cold applications *Over open dermal wounds*—further slowing or delaying the repair process because cold induces vigorous dermal vasoconstriction, reducing blood flow and metabolism *Over peripheral vascular disease areas*—further reducing the vascular supply to the area, caused by cold-induced vasoconstriction, leading to unnecessary pain and possible tissue necrosis. Conduct the nail bed test prior to therapy with patients who have a history of moderate to severe peripheral vascular disorders to determine if peripheral blood flow is adequate in the treated area. *In patients who are confused or unreliable*—complications during therapy, reducing treatment effectiveness

STEP	RATIONALE
2. Consider the risks.	*Over an area of impaired blood circulation*—risk of causing a frostnip or chilblain lesion, characterized by blanching of the skin, combined with a tingling and burning sensation (Knight, 1995). This skin lesion is temporary and reversible by slow and gentle rewarming of the exposed skin area (Knight, 1995). There is also a risk of causing a frostbite, which is characterized by the freezing of the skin and subcutaneous tissues (superficial), or the freezing of the skin, subcutaneous, muscle, and blood vessels (deep), if a very cold agent is applied directly over the skin for a prolonged and continuous period of time (Knight, 1995; Hoiness et al., 1998). Cases of frostbite due to the inadequate application of cryoagents have been reported (Quist et al., 1996; O'Toole et al., 1999; Graham, 2000; Cuthill et al., 2006; McGuire et al., 2006). *Over the thoracic area in patients with coronopathies*—risk of causing a reflex constriction of the coronary arteries. Seek the treating cardiologist's opinion, if necessary, before administering cryotherapy. *In hypertensive patients*—risk of inducing a transient increase of blood pressure when cooling larger areas and/or multiple sites. Continuous monitoring of blood pressure is advised both during and after treatment. Seek the treating cardiologist's opinion, if necessary, before administering cryotherapy. *In patients suffering from cardiovascular and cardiorespiratory disorders*—take blood pressure measurements, because cryotherapy may increase blood pressure beyond safe levels *Over superficial peripheral nerves*—risk of damaging peripheral nerve fibers causing transient neuropathies such as neurapraxia, axonotmesis, and neurotmesis (Drez et al., 1981; Parker et al., 1983; Collins et al., 1986; Green et al., 1989; Bassett et al., 1992; Malone et al., 1992; Covington et al., 1993; Moeller et al., 1997). Do not use compressive elastic bandages to secure cryoagents over superficial peripheral nerves. The evidence from the literature suggests that the compressive effect of the elastic bandage, not the cooling of the nerve per se, is what causes peripheral nerve damage (Knight, 1995). *In patients who are hemiplegic*—risk of producing myocardial ischemia (Lorenze et al., 1960) *In very young and very old patients*—risk of improper dosimetry and skin damage because of immature (in young patients) or impaired (in elderly patients) thermal regulation and difficulty to communicate cold sensation (in both young and elderly patients). Elderly patients have a decreased ability to maintain normal body thermoregulation because of their reduced ability to shiver and, thus, to produce heat (Leblanc et al., 1978) and because of their impaired vasoconstriction to conserve heat (Collins et al., 1977). *In patients who are overweight or obese*—risk of under dosage leading to inadequate tissue cooling. If the purpose is to maximize deep tissue cooling in the presence of a thick subcutaneous fat tissue, a longer application period is required. Skinfold measurements should be taken on patients who are overweight or obese to determine the proper application duration because the subcutaneous fat layer interferes with heat loss from deep tissues. The greater the skinfold thickness of the treated body area, the longer should be the application duration (Otte et al., 2002). A 25-minute application duration may be adequate for skinfolds of 20 mm or less; a 40-minute application is required to produce similar results in patients with skinfolds between 21 and 30 mm, and a 60-minute application is required for patients with skinfolds of 30–40 mm to produce similar results (Otte et al., 2002). *Position sense awareness*—risk of loosing this sense when returning patients to tasks requiring components of proprioceptive input immediately after cryotherapy applied over the stressed joint (Ingersoll et al., 1992; Isabell et al., 1992; La Riviere et al., 1994; Knight et al., 1994; Evans et al., 1995; Thieme et al., 1996; Tremblay et al., 2001; Costello et al., 2010; Khanmohammadi et al., 2011). *Compression with gel pack*—risk of causing frostbite (Knight, 1995). Compression of cryoagents against the skin surface produces significantly cooler temperatures at all tissue depths (Merrick et al., 1993).

GEL PACK/ICE BAG

STEP	PROCEDURE
1. **Check for contraindications.**	See All Agents section.
2. **Consider the risks.**	See All Agents section.
3. **Position and instruct patient.**	Ensure comfortable body positioning. Inform the patient that he or she should feel a light to vigorous cold sensation during therapy. Drape patients, if multiple cryoagents are used simultaneously, to prevent unnecessary heat loss and shivering during treatment.
4. **Prepare treatment area.**	Remove clothing and jewelry. Cleanse the exposed skin with water and soap, or rubbing alcohol, to remove impurities. Shave excessive hair if necessary. All open wounds must be covered with sterile gauze.
5. **Select the cryoagent.**	Choose between a commercial gel pack and a homemade ice bag. Select the pack or bag that best matches the geometry of the treated area.
6. **Determine and measure dose ($T°_{ag\text{-}s}$).**	Select the dose that can induce the desired physiologic and therapeutic effects in the targeted tissue. Dose should be high enough to decrease the targeted tissue temperature within the suboptimal/optimal therapeutic window. Immediately after removing the gel pack or ice bag from the cooling unit, and just before applying it over the exposed skin area, measure the dose—that is, the temperature differential between the agent and the skin surface ($T°_{ag\text{-}s}$) over which it is applied.
7. **Wrap up and secure the cryoagent.**	Only the gel pack requires the use of a coupling medium such as a commercial terrycloth wrap or layers of toweling. Keep wrapping thickness to a minimum for optimal tissue cooling. Secure the pack with towels. Ice bags should be applied directly over bare skin for maximum cooling effect.
8. **Apply treatment.**	Apply for approximately 10–20 minutes. Check the patient after 5 minutes of application to ensure thermal comfort. If necessary, adjust the thickness of coupling by adding or removing layers of toweling to ensure maximal cooling.
9. **Measure thermal skin cooling ($T°_{b\text{-}a}$).**	Immediately after removing the cryoagent, measure the exposed skin temperature and then calculate the differential before and after treatment ($T°_{b\text{-}a}$). Question the patient about the level of coldness that he or she has perceived during treatment.
10. **Conduct post-treatment procedures.**	Inspect the treated area, and record any adverse reaction. Reddening of the skin is normal after cryotherapy. Unwrap the gel pack, and put it back into the cooling unit. Homemade ice bags may be used again by putting them back into the cooling unit. Put towels into wash. Hang the pack cover to dry.
11. **Ensure post-treatment equipment maintenance.**	Follow manufacturer recommendations. Immediately report defects or malfunctions to technical maintenance staff.

View **online videos** for more details.

ICE CUP/ICICLE

STEP	PROCEDURE
1. **Check for contraindications.**	See All Agents section.
2. **Consider the risks.**	See All Agents section.
3. **Position and instruct patient.**	Ensure comfortable body positioning. Place towels around the treatment area to absorb dripping water and to wipe away water on the skin during treatment. Inform the patient that he or she should feel a vigorous cold sensation during therapy.

STEP	PROCEDURE
4. Prepare treatment area.	Remove clothing and jewelry. Cleanse the exposed skin with water and soap, or rubbing alcohol, to remove impurities. Shave excessive hair if necessary. Do not apply ice over open wounds.
5. Select the cryoagent.	Choose between a commercial or homemade ice cup or icicle.
6. Determine and measure dose ($T°_{ag\text{-}s}$).	Select the dose that can induce the desired physiologic and therapeutic effects in the targeted tissue. Dose should be high enough to decrease the targeted tissue temperature within the suboptimal/optimal therapeutic window. Just before applying it over the exposed skin area, measure the dose—that is, the temperature differential between the agent and the skin surface ($T°_{ag\text{-}s}$) over which it is applied.
7. Apply treatment.	Apply for 5–10 minutes, or until the patient experiences analgesia at the site of application. Rub the ice over the treated area by using small overlapping movements.
8. Measure thermal skin cooling ($T°_{b\text{-}a}$).	Immediately after treatment, measure the exposed skin temperature and then calculate the differential before and after treatment ($T°_{b\text{-}a}$). Question the patient about the level of coldness that he or she has perceived during treatment.
9. Conduct post-treatment procedures.	Inspect the exposed treatment area, and record any adverse reaction. For optimal hygiene, discard homemade ice cups and icicles.
10. Ensure post-treatment equipment maintenance.	Store a fair number of ice cups and icicles to accommodate your daily demand.

View **online video** for more details.

CONTROLLED CONTINUOUS COLD UNIT WITH COMPRESSION

STEP	PROCEDURE
1. Check for contraindications.	See All Agents section.
2. Consider the risks	See All Agents section.
3. Position and instruct patient.	Ensure comfortable body positioning. Inform the patient that he or she should feel a continuous cold sensation and compression during therapy.
4. Prepare treatment area.	Remove clothing and jewelry. Cleanse the exposed skin with water and soap, or rubbing alcohol, to remove impurities. Shave excessive hair if necessary. All open wounds must be covered with sterile gauze.
5. Select the cold unit.	Choose between the manual (gravity) and electrical (pump) controlled continuous cold flow units. Select the sleeve or wrap that best matches the treated area. Plug the electrical unit into a ground-fault circuit interrupter (GFCI) receptacle.
6. Prepare treatment area.	Cover the treated skin area with a stockinette and then wrap the cooling sleeve, or pad, around the area.
7. Determine and measure dose ($T°_{ag\text{-}s}$).	Select the dose that can induce the desired physiologic and therapeutic effects in the targeted tissue. Dose should be high enough to decrease the targeted tissue temperature within the suboptimal/optimal therapeutic window. Just before application, measure the temperature differential between the agent (mixture of ice cubes and water in the cooler) and the skin surface ($T°_{ag\text{-}s}$) over which it is applied. When applicable, preset the water temperature using the controller.

STEP	PROCEDURE
8. **Position the ice-water cooler.**	• *For the manually controlled continuous flow unit:* Place the cooler *above* the treated segment to ensure gravitational water flow. The passive recirculation of cold water into the cuff is done by elevating the water cooler above the treated segment, which allows gravity to pull water into the cuff. The continuous water flow is regulated by a manually operated valve. • *For the electrically controlled continuous flow unit:* Place the cooler at the level or proximity of the treated area to optimize the pumping action. Connect the cooler to the pad by using the hose system. The active controlled recirculation of cold water is achieved by an electrically powered pump.
9. **Apply treatment.**	These units primarily are used postoperatively when cryotherapy is needed continuously and for a longer period of time. Apply continuously for 1–8 hours depending on the condition. Ask the patient to pay particular attention to any unusual sensation, such as increase pain and burning. In addition, ask the patient to visually check his or her skin during therapy by lifting the edge of the pad with the fingers.
10. **Measure skin thermal cooling ($T°_{b-a}$).**	Immediately after treatment, measure the exposed skin temperature and then calculate the differential before and after treatment ($T°_{b-a}$). Question the patient about the level of coldness that he or she has perceived during treatment.
11. **Conduct post-treatment procedures.**	Remove the stockinette. Inspect the exposed treatment area, and record any adverse reaction. Drain the sleeve or pad.
12. **Ensure post-treatment equipment maintenance.**	Follow manufacturer recommendations. Immediately report defects or malfunctions to technical maintenance staff.

VAPOCOOLANT SPRAY

STEP	PROCEDURE
1. **Check for contraindications.**	See All Agents section.
2. **Consider the risks.**	See All Agents section.
3. **Position and instruct patient.**	Ensure comfortable body positioning. Inform the patient that he or she should feel brief and vigorous cold sensations during therapy, as well as mechanical muscle stretch.
4. **Prepare treatment area.**	Remove clothing and jewelry. Cleanse the exposed skin with water and soap, or rubbing alcohol, to remove impurities. Shave excessive hair if necessary. Do not use over open wounds.
5. **Locate and prepare treatment areas.**	Locate painful trigger points and myofascial areas.
6. **Apply treatment.**	Hold the vapocoolant can upright about 30 cm (12 in) from the skin and angled so that the spray hits the skin at about 90 degrees. Apply parallel sprays over the trigger point and along the related tight muscles. Repeat spray applications three to five times over the painful area, followed immediately by a series of manual passive muscle stretching exercises. It is important to remember that with this application, *stretch is the therapeutic action, whereas cold is the distraction.* Durations of each cold application may range between 30 and 90 seconds, whereas passive stretching exercises may range between 1 and 2 minutes. The number of applications will vary according to the acuity and severity of the condition under treatment. Ethyl chloride is a highly flammable and explosive pressurized liquid, possibly toxic to the environment and if inhaled. Fluori-Methane, in contrast, is nonflammable, nonexplosive, and nontoxic, but because it is made of chlorofluorocarbons, it represents a danger to the environment—destruction of the ozone layer. To eliminate all noted potential risks, the manufacturer has developed a third-generation vapocoolant spray. This spray is non–ozone depleting and can be used in facilities that restrict the use of flammable components.

STEP	PROCEDURE
7. **Conduct post-treatment procedures.**	Inspect the exposed treatment area, and record any adverse reaction.
8. **Ensure post-treatment equipment maintenance.**	Follow manufacturer recommendations.

CASE STUDIES

Presented are two case studies that summarize the concepts, principles, and applications of cryotherapy discussed in this chapter. Case Study 8-1 addresses the use of a wetted-ice bag for a traumatic ankle sprain affecting a young athletic man. Case Study 8-2 is concerned with the use of a controlled continuous cold unit with compression for postoperative anterior cruciate ligament (ACL) knee reconstruction in a middle-aged man. Each case is structured in line with the concepts of EBP, the International Classification of Functioning, Disability, and Health (ICF) disablement model, and SOAP (*s*ubjective, *o*bjective, *a*ssessment, *p*lan) note format (see Chapter 2 for details).

CASE STUDY 8-1: ACUTE ANKLE SPRAIN

EVIDENCE-BASED CLINICAL DECISION MAKING PROTOCOL

1. Formulate the Case History

A 20-year-old college football player who sustained a moderate right-ankle sprain approximately 20 minutes ago is referred for immediate treatment. Physical examination reveals all of the cardinal signs of an acute traumatic soft tissue lesion. There is no evidence of bone fracture or ligament rupture. A grade II inversion ankle sprain is suspected. The patient complains of pain at rest and particularly during ankle mobilization. He has difficulty bearing weight and walking. He is limping. This athlete is new to the team and the sports clinic. Questioned about his past experience with cryotherapy, he explains that sometimes a significant reddish patch over his exposed skin has occurred together with some kind of skin swelling. He adds that these skin reactions would go away a few hours after exposure to cryotherapy. There is a possibility that this patient may be allergic to cold. His goal is to return to play as soon as possible.

2. Outline the Case Based on the ICF Framework

ACUTE ANKLE SPRAIN		
BODY STRUCTURES AND FUNCTIONS	**ACTIVITIES**	**PARTICIPATION**
Ligament sprain	Difficulty with bearing weight	Unable to play football
Ankle pain	Difficulty with walking and running	
Ankle joint edema		

PERSONAL FACTORS	ENVIRONMENTAL FACTORS
Young healthy man	Recreational sport
Athletic character	Team play
College educated	Fitness and leisure

3. Outline Therapeutic Goals and Outcome Measurements

GOAL	OUTCOME MEASUREMENT
Decrease pain	Visual Analogue Scale (VAS)
Decrease edema	Volumetry
Improve functional activities	Patient-Specific Functional Scale (PSFS)

4. Justify the Use of Cryotherapy Based on the EBP Framework

PRACTITIONER'S EXPERIENCE	RESEARCH-BASED INDICATIONS	PATIENT'S EXPECTATION
Very experienced with cryotherapy	*Strength:* Moderate	Familiar with cryotherapy due to past sports-related injuries
Has used cryotherapy in previous cases	*Effectiveness:* Substantiated	Confident that cryotherapy will be beneficial
Strongly believes that cryotherapy will be beneficial		

5. Outline Key Intervention Parameters

- **Test:** As mentioned earlier, the patient may be allergic to cryotherapy. The ice-cube test is thus performed as a prediagnostic test. The result is negative. Further inquiries to the football team's physician reveal no additional element consistent with a diagnosis of cold urticaria. Cryotherapy is thus safe for this patient.
- **Treatment base:** Private clinic
- **Cryoagent:** *Wetted-ice bag* (bag filled with crushed ice and water). This agent appears to be the preferred agent because there is evidence behind its cooling and anti-inflammatory effects on soft tissues. The condition is acute, and cooling of soft tissues surrounding the site of injury is needed to minimize secondary tissue damage, which in turn will facilitate healing. The cryoagent, because applied within 1-hour post injury, is expected to regulate the inflammatory healing response by reducing tissue metabolism, thus minimizing secondary tissue damage as well as the cardinal signs and symptoms of inflammation. Such therapeutic effects are expected to promote healing by quickly promoting ankle mobility. The wetted-ice bag is chosen over the other cryoagents because of its higher ability to induce fast and deep cooling effects.
- **Application protocol:** Follow the suggested application protocol for ice bags in *Application, Contraindications, and Risks* box, and make the necessary adjustments for this case. Inform the patient that during treatment changes of sensation from cold to burning to aching and to numbness is likely to occur.
- **Patient's positioning:** Lying supine with the injured limb elevated
- **Application site:** Over the injured right lateral ankle area
- **Ice bag size:** 25 × 25 cm (10 × 10 in)
- **Coupling medium:** None
- **Application duration:** 20 minutes
- **Dosage ($T°_{ag\text{-}s}$):** –30°C ± 4°C (22°F ± 4°F)
- **Treatment frequency:** *First day:* Every 3 hours, except when sleeping. *Subsequent days:* Every 6 hours, except when sleeping.
- **Intervention period:** 5 days
- **Concomitant therapies:** Regimen of ankle protection (P), rest (R), compression (C), and elevation (E). In other words, the well-known therapeutic approach for acute soft tissue pathology in sports therapy, described as *PRICE*, is used in the present case. At rest (R), the affected lower limb is iced (I), kept elevated (E) and the ankle joint compressed (C) with an elastic bandage. During ambulation, the ankle joint is protected (P) using of a pair of crutches.

6. Report Pre- and Post-Intervention Outcomes

OUTCOME	PRE	POST
Pain (VAS score)	8/10	2/10
Swelling	15% larger than contralateral ankle	Normal
Functional activities (PSFS score)	3/10	8/10

7. Document Case Intervention Using the SOAP Note Format

S: Athletic healthy male Pt presents with painful acute R ankle sprain leading to difficulty with weight bearing, ambulation, and playing football.

O: *Test:* Normal thermal discrimination test (5/5); normal ice-cube test. *Intervention:* Wetted-ice bag applied over the lateral ankle area; Pt lying supine with injured limb elevated; dosage ($T°_{ag\text{-}s}$): −30°C ± 4°C (22°F ± 4°F); application duration between 10 and 20 minutes; treatment schedule: every 3–6 hours for 5 consecutive days. *Pre–post comparison:* Pain decrease (VAS 8/10 to 2/10), elimination of edema, and improved functional status (PSFS 3/10 to 8/10).

A: No adverse effect. Treatment well tolerated. Pt very pleased with the results.

P: No further treatment required. Full recovery is expected. Pt advised to gradually resume his regular football training schedule.

CASE STUDY 8-2: POSTOPERATIVE ANTERIOR CRUCIATE LIGAMENT KNEE RECONSTRUCTION

EVIDENCE-BASED CLINICAL DECISION MAKING PROTOCOL

1. Formulate the Case History

A 39-year-old male amateur soccer player was involved in a collision with another player during a match. The collision caused the complete rupture of the ACL of his right knee. He is referred for immediate postoperative treatment following ACL surgical reconstruction. Physical examination, done hours after surgery, reveals all of the signs of a traumatic inflammatory reaction caused by both the pathology (tissue damage) and the surgical procedure. Both feet and toes feel cooler than normal. Knee swelling is important. According to information in the file, this patient may have a history of a mild, and undiagnosed, occlusive peripheral vascular disorder particularly affecting his lower limbs. The patient is resting fully awake in his hospital bed awaiting further treatments. The knee is wrapped with surgical bandages. The surgeon prescribed the usual regimen of medication, which includes analgesic and anti-inflammatory drugs. The patient's immediate goals are to reduce pain, while taking the minimal number of pills, and then to resume weight bearing and free walking in his room as soon as possible. He is anxious to be discharged from the hospital to then receive treatment in a private sports clinic not far from his home. His later goals are to return, within the next few weeks, to his normal home and work activities. His ultimate goal is to one day be able to resume playing soccer.

2. Outline the Case Based on the ICF Framework

POSTOPERATIVE ANTERIOR CRUCIATE LIGAMENT KNEE RECONSTRUCTION		
BODY STRUCTURES AND FUNCTIONS	**ACTIVITIES**	**PARTICIPATION**
ACL rupture	Difficulty with weight bearing	Unable to work
Surgical wound	Difficulty with ambulation	Unable to play soccer
Knee pain	Difficulty with activities of daily living (ADLs)	
Knee joint edema		

PERSONAL FACTORS	ENVIRONMENTAL FACTORS
Middle-aged man	Active lifestyle
Friend and family oriented	Office work

3. Outline Therapeutic Goals and Outcome Measurements

GOAL	OUTCOME MEASUREMENT
Decrease pain	5-point Verbal Rating Scale (VRS-5)
Increase knee range of motion (ROM)	Goniometry
Minimize postoperative blood loss	Hemovac output (drainage volume)
Decrease drug intake	Daily log (pill count)
Improve functional status	Patient-Specific Functional Scale (PSFS)

4. Justify the Use of Cryotherapy Based on the EBP Framework

PRACTITIONER'S EXPERIENCE	RESEARCH-BASED INDICATIONS	PATIENT'S EXPECTATION
Experience in postoperative cryotherapy	*Strength:* Strong	Hopes that cryotherapy will be beneficial
Has used cryotherapy in similar cases	*Effectiveness:* Conflicting	Eager to receive cryotherapy
Believes that cryotherapy will be beneficial		

5. Outline Key Intervention Parameters

- **Test:** As mentioned earlier, this patient may be suffering from a mild case of peripheral vascular disorder affecting his lower limbs because his feet and toes are much cooler than normal. The nail bed test is performed on the big toe of both limbs. The result is negative. Cryotherapy is thus safe for this patient.
- **Treatment base:** Hospital
- **Cryoagent:** *Controlled continuous cold unit with compression.* The application of continuous cold therapy with compression, as opposed to the traditional periodic cold application without compression, appears as the preferred approach because of the extreme acuity of surgical wounds associated with ACL reconstruction. The continuous cooling and compression effects should minimize blood loss and regulate the inflammatory healing response by reducing tissue metabolism, thus minimizing secondary tissue damage as well as the cardinal signs and symptoms of inflammation, such as pain and edema. These therapeutic effects are expected to minimize blood loss and promote healing by quickly promoting knee mobility.
- **Application protocol:** Follow the suggested application protocol for controlled continuous cold with compression in *Application, Complications, and Risks* box, and make the necessary adjustments for this case. Inform the patient that cold application will last several hours per day for a few days and will be interrupted only for short periods of time. The cooling unit is applied in the surgical room immediately after tourniquet deflation.
- **Patient's positioning:** Lying supine with the injured limb elevated
- **Application site:** Around the knee joint
- **Coupling medium:** Sterile gauze dressing over surgical wound plus stockinette covering the entire knee joint
- **Knee pad:** Commercial cooling pad wrapped around the knee
- **Dosage ($T°_{ag\text{-}s}$):** In the present case, the cooling temperature in the pad was kept at 10° ± 2°C (50° ± 2°F) throughput the treatment period.
- **Application frequency and duration:** Cooling flow applied continuously postoperatively except for short periods for knee mobilization, weight bearing, and short walking.
- **Intervention period:** 6 days
- **Concomitant therapies:** Regimen of bedside knee mobilization, followed by short periods of knee mobilization, weight bearing, and short walking.

6. Report Pre- and Post-Intervention Outcomes

OUTCOME	PRE	POST
Pain (VRS score)	4—Horrible	2—Discomforting
Knee ROM	58 degrees	84 degrees
Blood loss (Hemovac)	—	700 mL loss; no blood transfusion needed
Drug intake	5 pills/day	2 pills/day
Functional status (PSFS score)	1/10	5/10

7. Document Case Intervention Using the SOAP Note Format

S: Middle-aged male Pt presents with postoperative right ACL knee reconstruction causing severe acute pain and inability with weight bearing and ambulation.

O: *Test:* Normal thermal discrimination test (5/5); normal nail bed test. *Intervention:* Active (electric) controlled continuous cold with compression applied over injured knee area; Pt lying supine with injured limb elevated; dosage ($T°_{ag\text{-}s}$): 10° ± 2°C (50° ± 2°F) throughout; sterile gauze over wound; stockinette over the knee that is covered by the knee pad; treatment schedule: continuous and daily for 6 days, except for short periods. *Pre–post comparison:* Cryotherapy (active controlled continuous cold with compression) applied concomitantly with short periods of knee mobilization, weight bearing, and short walking led to significant pain decrease (VRS 4 to 2), ROM increase (58 to 84 degrees), minimal blood loss (700 mL); decrease drug intake (5 to 2 pills a day), and enhanced functional status (1/10 to 5/10). Pt now walks with crutches.

A: Mild blood loss. Treatment well tolerated. Pt very pleased with the results.

P: Pt discharged from hospital. Referred to private clinic for further rehabilitation treatments until optimal functional status is achieved. Pt informed that a reconstructed ligament takes months to heal, so *gradual return* to ADLs is strongly advised. Prognosis for a possible return to recreational soccer is good.

VI. THE BOTTOM LINE

- Cryotherapy is the exchange of heat between cooler cryoagents and warmer soft tissues.
- Cryotherapy does not add cold to soft tissues; it extracts heat from them thus lowering their baseline temperatures.
- Cold is the absence of heat and temperature is a measurement of it.
- Heat exchange during cryotherapy occurs through conduction and evaporation.
- There is strong scientific evidence to show that cryotherapy can induce significant cooling effects on human superficial and deep soft tissues.
- Because subcutaneous fat acts as a major thermal barrier between the skin and deeper tissues, higher dosages are required with overweight and obese patients.
- The therapeutic goal with cryotherapy is to decrease soft tissues temperature within its therapeutic window, which ranges from 10 to 27°C (50° to 81°F).
- Repeated and/or continuous applications of cryotherapy sustains decreased temperature.
- Cryoagents that pass through a phase change from solid to liquid, such as wetted-ice, cubed-ice and crushed-ice, during application, regardless of their pre-application temperatures, are generally more effective in inducing faster and greater tissue cooling than those that do not.
- In the context of evidence-based practice, qualitative dosimetry is no longer acceptable has the sole source of dosimetry. Quantitative dosimetry based on reliable skin temperature measurements is required as a complement.
- Adopting quantitative dosimetry in the day-to-day practice is neither complicated, time consuming or expensive.
- Cryotherapy should be used immediately after trauma or injury to optimize its effects.
- Cold-induced vasodilation (CIVD) is no contraindication to the prolonged and continuous application of cryotherapy.
- Skin thermal discrimination testing is mandatory prior to the first application of cryotherapy.
- There is no consensus with respect to the best agent and method of application to use.
- All line-powered cryoagents should be plugged into GFCI receptacles to prevent macroshock.
- The overall body of research-based evidence reported in this chapter shows the strength of evidence behind cryotherapy to be *moderate,* and its level of therapeutic effectiveness *substantiated*.

VII. CRITICAL THINKING QUESTIONS

Clarification: What is meant by cryotherapy?

Assumptions: You assume that cryotherapy is effective in preventing secondary tissue damage following trauma. How do you justify that assumption?

Reasons and evidence: What leads you to believe that applying a cryoagent over the skin will cool deeper soft tissues such as muscle, tendons, ligaments, and joint capsules? If this is true, by which mechanism does cooling occur?

Viewpoints or perspectives: How would you respond to a colleague who says that the late CIVD effect should be avoided at all costs because it significantly diminishes the prime effect of cryotherapy, which is to cool soft tissues?

Implications and consequences: What are the implications of (a) applying a cryoagent using a coupling medium and (b) applying a cryoagent without a coupling medium over a body part that has a thick layer of adipose tissue?

About the question: Should practitioners who use cryotherapy not be concerned with the issue of cold urticaria and seriously concerned with frostbite and peripheral nerve injury? Why do you think I ask this question?

VIII. REFERENCES

Articles

Abramson DI, Chu LS, Tuck S, Lee SW, Richardson M (1966) Effect of tissue temperature and blood flow on motor nerve conduction velocity. JAMA, 198: 1082–1088

Aizawa Y, Shibata A, Tajiri M, Hirasawa Y (1979) Reflex vasoconstriction to a cold stimulus for non-invasive evaluation of neurovascular function in man. Jpn Heart, 20: 301–305

Amin-Hanjani S, Corcoran J, Chatwani A (1992) Cold therapy in the management of postoperative cesarean section pain. Am J Obstet Gynecol, 167: 108–109

Bancroft H, Edholm OG (1943) The effect of temperature on blood flow and deep temperature in the human forearm. J Physiol, 102: 5–20

Barber FA (2000) A comparison of crushed ice and continuous flow cold therapy. Am J Knee Surg, 13: 97–101

Barber FA, McGuire DA, Click S (1998) Continuous-flow cold therapy for outpatient anterior cruciate ligament reconstruction. Arthroscopy, 14: 130–135

Bassett FH, Kirkpatrick JS, Englehartd DL, Malone TR (1992) Cryotherapy-induced nerve injury. Am J Sports Med, 20: 516–518

Basset SW, Lake BM (1958) Use of cold applications in the management of spasticity. Phys Ther Rev, 38: 333–334

Basur RL, Shephard E, Mouzas GL (1976). A cooling method in the treatment of ankle sprains. Practitioner, 216: 708–711

Belitsky RB, Odam SJ, Hubley-Kozey C (1987) Evaluation of the effectiveness of wet ice, dry ice, and cryogen packs in reducing skin temperature. Phys Ther, 67: 1080–1084

Bert JM, Stark JG, Maschka K, Chock C (1991) The effect of cold therapy on morbidity subsequent to arthroscopic lateral retinacular release. Orthop Rev, 20: 755–758

Bleakley CM, McDonough SM, MacAuley DC, Bjordal J (2006) Cryotherapy for acute ankle sprains: A randomized controlled study of two different icing protocols. Br J Sports Med, 40: 700–705

Boes MC (1962) Reduction of spasticity by cold. J Am Phys Ther Assoc, 42: 29–32

Bolster MB, Maricq HR, Leff RL (1995) Office evaluation and treatment of Raynaud's phenomenon. Cleve Clin J Med, 62: 51–61

Brandner B, Munro L, Bromley LM, Hetreed M (1996) Evaluation of the contribution to postoperative analgesia by local cooling of the wound. Anaesthesia, 51: 1021–1025

Burgess JA, Sommers EE, Truelove EL, Dworkin SF (1988) Short-term effect of two therapeutic methods on myofascial pain and dysfunction of the masticatory system. J Prosthet Dent, 60: 606–610

Clarke GR, Willis LA, Stenner L, Nichols PJ (1974) Evaluation of physiotherapy in the treatment of osteoarthrosis of the knee. Rheumatol Rehab, 13: 190–197

Clarke RH, Hellon R, Lind A (1958) Vascular reactions of the human forearm to cold. Clin Sci, 17: 165–179

Cohn BT, Draeger RI, Jackson DW (1989) The effects of cold therapy in the postoperative management of pain in patients undergoing anterior cruciate ligament reconstruction. Am J Sports Med, 17: 344–349

Collins K, Storey M, Peterson K (1986) Peroneal nerve palsy after cryotherapy. Physician Sportsmed, 14(5): 105–108

Collins KJ, Dore C, Exton-Smith AN, Fox RH, McDonald IC, Woodward PM (1977) Accidental hypothermia and impaired temperature homeostasis in the elderly. Br Med J, 1(6057): 353–356

Cote DJ, Prentice WE, Hooker DN, Shields EW (1988) Comparison of three treatment procedures for minimizing ankle sprain swelling. Phys Ther, 68: 1072–1076

Covington DB, Bassett FH (1993) When cryotherapy injures. Physician Sportsmed, 21(3): 78, 82, 84, 93

Culp R, Taras J (1995) The effect of ice application versus controlled cold therapy on skin temperature when used with postoperative bulky hand and wrist dressings: A preliminary study. J Hand Ther, 8: 249–251

Curkovic B, Vitulic V, Babic-Naglic D, Durrigl T (1993) The influence of heat and cold on the pain threshold in rheumatoid arthritis. Z Rheumatol, 52: 289–291

Cuthill JA, Cuthill GS (2006) Partial-thickness burn to the leg following application of cold pack: Case report and results of a questionnaire survey of Scottish physiotherapists in private practice. Physiotherapy, 92: 61–65

Daanen HA, Van de Linde FJ, Romet TT, Ducharme MB (1997) The effect of body temperature on the hunting response of the middle finger skin temperature. Eur J Appl Physiol, 76: 538–543

Daniel DM, Stone ML, Arendt DL (1994) The effect of cold therapy on pain, swelling, and range of motion after anterior cruciate ligament reconstructive surgery. Arthroscopy, 10: 530–533

Day MJ (1974) Hypersensitive response to ice massage: Report of a case. Phys Ther, 54: 592–593

De Coster D, Bossuyt M, Fossion E (1993) The value of cryotherapy in the management of trigeminal neuralgia. Acta Stomatol Belg, 90: 87–93

Denegar CR, Perrin DH (1992) Effect of transcutaneous electrical nerve stimulation, cold, and a combination on pain, decreased range of motion, and strength loss associated with delayed muscle soreness. J Athl Train, 27: 200–206

Dervin GF, Taylor DE, Keene GC (1998) Effects of cold and compression dressings on early postoperative outcomes for the arthroscopic anterior cruciate ligament reconstruction patient. J Orthop Sports Phys Ther, 27: 403–406

Diamond S, Freitag FG (1986) Cold as an adjunctive therapy for headache. Postgrad Med, 79: 305–309

DonTigny RL, Shelton KW (1962) Simultaneous use of heat and cold in treatment of muscle spasm. Arch Phys Med Rehab, 43: 148–150

Drez D, Faust DC, Evans JP (1981) Cryotherapy and nerve palsy. Am J Sports Med, 9: 256–257

Duff F, Greenfield AD, Shepherd JT, Thompson ID, Whelan RF (1953) The response of vasodilator substances on blood vessels in fingers immersed in cold water. J Physiol, 121: 46–54

Dykstra JH, Hill HM, Miller MG, Cheatham CC, Micheal TJ, Baker RJ (2009) Comparisons of cubed ice, crushed ice, and wetted ice on intramuscular and surface temperature changes. J Athl Train, 44: 136–141

Edwards DJ, Rimmer M, Keene GC (1996) The use of cold therapy in the postoperative management of patients undergoing arthroscopic anterior cruciate ligament reconstruction. Am J Sports Med, 24: 193–195

Escher S, Tucker A (1992) Preventing, diagnosing, and treating cold urticaria. Physician Sportsmed, 20 (12): 73–84

Evans TA, Ingersoll C, Knight K, Worrell T (1995) Agility following the application of cold therapy. J Athl Train, 30: 231–234

Finan MA, Roberts WS, Hoffman MS, Fiorica JV, Cavanagh D, Dudney BJ (1993) The effects of cold therapy on postoperative pain in gynecologic patients: A prospective, randomized study. Am J Obstet Gynecol, 168: 542–544

Gibbons CE, Solan MC, Ricketts DM, Patterson M (2001) Cryotherapy compared with Robert Jones bandage after total knee replacement: A prospective randomized trial. Int Orthop, 25: 250–252

Graham CA (2000) Frozen chips: An unusual cause of severe frostbite injury. Br J Sports Med, 34: 382–384

Grant AE (1964) Massage with ice (cryokinetics) in the treatment of painful conditions of the musculoskeletal system. Arch Phys Med Rehab, 45: 233–238

Green GA, Zachazewski JE, Jordan SE (1989) Peroneal nerve palsy induced by cryotherapy. Physician Sportsmed, 17: 63–70

Greenfield AD, Shepherd JT (1950) A quantitative study of the response to cold of the circulation through the fingers of normal subjects. Clin Sci, 9: 323–334

Halliday Pegg SM, Littler TR, Littler MD (1969) A trial of ice therapy and exercise in chronic arthritis. Physiotherapy, 55: 51–56

Hartvikksen K (1962) Ice therapy in spasticity. Acta Neurol Scand, 38: 79–84

Harvey CK (1992) An overview of cold injury. J Am Podiatr Med Assoc, 82: 436–438

Hayden CA (1964) Cryokinetics in an early treatment program. J Am Phys Ther Assoc, 44: 940–943

Healy WL, Seidman J, Pfiefer B, Brown DG (1994) Cold compressive dressing after total knee arthroplasty. Clin Orthop, 299: 143–146

Hecht PJ, Bachmann S, Booth RE, Rothman RH (1983) Effects of thermal therapy on rehabilitation after total knee arthroplasty. Clin Orthop, 178: 198–201

Hedenberg L (1970) Functional improvement of the spastic hemiplegic arm after cooling. Scand J Rehab Med, 2: 154–158

Ho SS, Coel MN, Kagawa R, Richardson AB (1994) The effect of ice on blood flow and bone metabolism in knees. Am J Sports Med, 22: 537–540

Hochberg J (2001) A randomized prospective study to assess the efficacy of two cold-therapy treatments following carpal tunnel release. J Hand Ther, 3: 208–215

Hocutt JE, Jaffe R, Rylander CR, Beebe JK (1982) Cryotherapy in ankle sprains. Am J Sports Med, 10: 316–319

Hoiness PR, Hvaal K, Engebretsen L (1998) Severe hypothermic injury to the foot and ankle caused by continuous cryocompression therapy. Knee Surg Sports Traumatol Arthrosc, 6: 253–255

Hopkins JT, Stencil R (2002) Ankle cryotherapy facilitates soleus function. J Orthop Sports Phys Ther, 32: 622–627

Ingersoll CD, Knight KL, Merrick MA (1992) Sensory perception of the foot and ankle following therapeutic applications of heat and cold. J Athl Train, 27: 231–234

Isabell WK, Durrant E, Myrer W, Anderson S (1992) The effects of ice massage and exercise on the prevention and treatment of delayed onset muscle soreness. J Athl Train, 27: 208–217

Ivey M, Johnson RV, Uchida T (1994) Cryotherapy for postoperative pain relief following knee arthroplasty. J Arthroplasty, 9: 285–290

Janwantanakul P (2004) Different rate of cooling time and magnitude of cooling temperature during ice bag treatment with and without damp towel wrap. Phys Ther Sports, 5: 156–161

Johnson DJ, Moore S, Moore J, Oliver RA (1979) Effect of cold submersion on intramuscular temperature of the gastrocnemius muscle. Phys Ther, 59: 1239–1242

Kaempffe FA (1989) Skin surface temperature reduction after cryotherapy to a casted extremity. J Orthop Sports Phys Ther, 10: 448–450

Kalenak A, Medlar CE, Fleagle SB, Hochberg WJ (1975) Treating thigh contusions with ice. Physician Sportsmed, 3(3): 65–67

Kanlayanaphotporn R, Janwantanakul P (2005) Comparison of skin surface temperature during the application of various cryotherapy modalities. Arch Phys Med Rehabil, 86: 1411–1415

Kelly M (1969) Effectiveness of a cryotherapy technique on spasticity. Phys Ther, 49: 349–353

Kennet J, Hardaker N, Hobbs S, Selfe J (2007) Cooling efficiency of 4 common cryotherapeutic agents. J Athl Train, 42: 343–348

Khanmohammadi R, Someh M, Ghafarinejad F (2011) The effect of cryotherapy on the normal joint position sense. Asian J Sports Med, 2: 91–98

Kinnman J, Andersson T, Andersson G (2000a) Effect of cooling suit treatment in patients with multiple sclerosis evaluated by evoked potentials. Scand J Rehab Med, 32: 16–19

Kinnman J, Andersson T, Wetterquist L, Kinnman Y, Andersson U (2000b) Cooling suit for multiple sclerosis: Functional improvement in daily living? Scand J Rehab Med, 32: 20–24

Kirk JA, Kersley GD (1968) Heat and cold in the physical treatment of rheumatoid arthritis of the knee. Ann Phys Med, 9: 270–274

Knight KL, Aquino J, Johannes SM, Urban CD (1980) A re-examination of Lewis' cold-induced vasodilation in the finger and the ankle. J Athl Train, 15: 238–250

Knight KL, Elam JF (1981) Rewarming of the ankle, finger, and forearm after cryotherapy: Further investigation of Lewis' cold-induced vasodilation. J Can Athl Ther Assoc, 8: 17–18

Knight KL, Ingersoll CD, Trowbridge CA, Connolly TA, Cordovia ML, Hyink LL, Welch SM (1994) The effects of cooling the ankle, the triceps surae, or both on functional agility. J Athl Train, 29: 165–169

Knutsson E (1970a) On effects of local cooling upon motor functions in spastic paresis. Prog Phys Ther, 1: 124–131

Knutsson E (1970b) Topical cryotherapy in spasticity. Scand J Rehab Med, 2: 159–163

Konrath G, Lock T, Goitz H, Scheider J (1996) The use of cold therapy after anterior cruciate ligament reconstruction. A prospective, randomized study and literature study. Am J Sports Med, 24: 629–633

Kullenberg B, Ylipaa S, Soderlund K, Resch S (2006) Postoperative cryotherapy after total knee arthroplasty: A prospective study of 86 patients. J Arthroplasty, 21: 1175–1179

Landen BR (1967) Heat or cold for the relief of low back pain? Phys Ther, 47: 1126–1128

Lane LE (1971) Localized hypothermia for the relief of pain in musculoskeletal injuries. Phys Ther, 51: 182–183

La Riviere J, Osternig LR (1994) The effect of ice on joint position sense. J Sports Rehab, 3: 58–67

Lavelle BE, Snyder M (1985) Differential conduction of cold through barriers. J Adv Nurs, 10: 55–61

Leblanc J, Cote J, Dulac S, Dulong-Turcot F (1978) Effects of age, sex, and physiological fitness on responses to local cooling. J Appl Physiol, 44: 813–817.

Leite M, Ribeiro F (2010) Liquid Ice™ fails to cool the skin surface as effectively as crushed ice in a wet towel. Physioth Theory Pract, 26: 393–398

Lessard LA, Scudds RA, Amendola A, Vaz AA (1997) The efficacy of cryotherapy following arthroscopic knee surgery. J Orthop Sports Phys Ther, 26: 14–22

Leutz DW, Harris H (1995) Continuous cold therapy in total knee arthroplasty. Am J Knee Surg, 8: 121–123

Levy AS, Marmar E (1993) The role of cold compression dressings in the postoperative treatment of total knee arthroplasty. Clin Orthop, 297: 174–178

Lewis T (1930) Observations upon the reactions of the vessels of the human skin to cold. Heart, 15: 177–208

Lorenze EJ, Caroutonis G, DeRosa AJ (1960) Effect on coronary circulation of cold packs to hemiplegic shoulders. Arch Phys Med Rehab, 41: 394–399

Lowden BJ, Moore RJ (1975) Determinants and nature of intramuscular temperature changes during cold therapy. Am J Phys Med, 54: 223–233

Malone TR, Englehardt DL, Kirkpatrick JS, Basset FH (1992) Nerve injury in athletes caused by cryotherapy. J Athl Train, 27: 235–237.

Martin SS, Spinder KP, Tarter JW, Detwiler K, Petersen HA (2001) Cryotherapy: An effective modality for decreasing intra-articular temperature after knee arthroscopy. Am J Sports Med, 29: 288–291

McGuire DA, Hendricks SD (2006) Incidences of frostbite in arthroscopic knee surgery postoperative cryotherapy rehabilitation. J Arthros Relat Surg, 22: 1141–1146

Melzack R, Jeans ME, Stratford JG, Monks RC (1980) Ice massage and transcutaneous electrical stimulation: Comparison of treatment for low-back pain. Pain, 9: 209–217

Mennel J (1976) Spray-stretch for the relief of pain from muscle spasm and myofascial trigger points. J Am Podiatr Assoc, 66: 873–876

Merrick MA, Jutte LS, Smith ME (2003) Cold modalities with different thermodynamic properties produce different surface and intramuscular temperatures. J Athl Train, 38: 28–33

Merrick MA, Knight KL, Ingersoll CD, Potteiger JA (1993) The effects of ice and compression wraps on intramuscular temperatures at various depths. J Athl Train, 28: 236–245

Metzman L, Gamble JG, Rinsky LA (1996) Effectiveness of ice packs in reducing skin temperatures under casts. Clin Orthop, 330: 217–221.

Meyer-Marcotty M, Jungling O, Vaske B, Vogt PM, Knobloch K (2011) Standardized combined cryotherapy and compression using Cryo-Cuff after wrist arthroscopy. Knee Surg Sports Traumatol Arthrosc, 19: 314–319

Michlovitz S, Smith W, Watkins M (1988) Ice and high voltage pulsed stimulation in the treatment of acute lateral ankle sprains. J Orthop Sports Phys Ther, 9: 301–304

Miglietta O (1964) Electromyographic characteristics of clonus and influence of cold. Arch Phys Med Rehab, 45: 508–512

Miglietta O (1973) Action of cold on spasticity. Am J Phys Med, 52: 198–205

Modell W, Travel J, Kraus H (1952) Relief of pain by ethyl chloride spray. N Y State J Med, 52: 1550–1558

Moeller JL, Monroe J, McKeag DB (1997) Cryotherapy-induced common peroneal nerve palsy. Clin J Sports Med, 7: 212–216

Moore CD, Cardea JA (1977) Vascular changes in leg trauma. South Med J, 70: 1285–1286

Morsi E (2002) Continuous-flow cold therapy after total knee arthroplasty. Arthroplasty, 17: 718–722

Myrer JW, Myrer KA, Measom GJ, Fellingham GW, Evers SL (2001) Muscle temperature is affected by overlying adipose when cryotherapy is administered. J Athl Train, 36: 32–36

Nadler SF, Prybicien M, Malanga GA, Sicher D (2003) Complications from therapeutic modalities: Results of a national survey of athletic trainers. Arch Phys Med Rehab, 84: 849

Nielsen AJ (1978) Spray and stretch for myofascial pain. Phys Ther, 58: 567–569

Nielsen AJ (1981) Case study: Myofascial pain of the posterior shoulder relieved by spray and stretch. J Orthop Sports Phys Ther, 3: 21–26

Ohkoshi Y, Ohkoshi M, Nagasaki S, Ono A, Hashimoto T, Yamane S (1999) The effect of cryotherapy on intra-articular temperature and postoperative care after anterior cruciate ligament reconstruction. Am J Sports Med, 27: 357–362

Okcu G, Yercan HS (2006) Is it possible to decrease skin temperature with ice packs under cast and bandages? A cross-sectional, randomized trial on normal and swollen ankles. Arch Orthop Trauma Surg, 126: 668–673

Osbahr DC, Patrick W, Cawley PW, Speer KP (2002) The effect of continuous cryotherapy on glenohumeral joint and subacromial space temperature in the postoperative shoulder. J Arthrosc Rel Surg, 18: 748–754
O'Toole G, Rayatt S (1999) Frostbite at the gym: A case report of an ice pack burn. Br J Sports Med, 33: 278–279
Otte JW, Merrick MA, Ingersoll CD, Cordova ML (2002) Subcutaneous adipose tissue thickness alters cooling time during cryotherapy. Arch Phys Med Rehabil, 83: 1501–1505
Palmieri RM, Garrison JG, Leonard JL, Edwards JE, Weltman A, Ingersoll CD (2006) Peripheral ankle cooling and core body temperature. J Athl Train, 41: 185–188
Parker JT, Small NC, Davis PG (1983) Cold-induced nerve palsy. Athl Train, 18: 76
Pincivero D, Gieck J, Saliba E (1993) Rehabilitation of a lateral ankle sprain with cryokinetic and functional progressive exercise. J Sport Rehab, 2: 200–207
Price R, Lehmann JF, Boswell-Bessette S, Burleigh S, de Lateur BJ (1993) Influence of cryotherapy on spasticity at the human ankle. Arch Phys Med Rehab, 74: 300–304
Quist LH, Peltier G, Lundquist KJ (1996) Frostbite of the eyelids following inappropriate applications of ice compresses. Arch Ophthalmol, 114: 226
Radkowsky CA, Pietrobon R, Vail TP, Nunley JA, Jain NB, Easley ME (2007) Cryotherapy temperature differences after total knee arthroplasty: A prospective randomized trial. J Surg Orthop Adv, 16: 67–72
Rembe EC (1970) Use of cryotherapy on the postsurgical rheumatoid hand. Phys Ther, 50: 19–23
Robbins LD (1989) Cryotherapy for headache. Headache, 29: 598–600
Rubley MD, Denegar CR, Buckley WE, Newell KM (2003) Cryotherapy, sensation and isometric-force variability. J Athl Train, 38: 113–119
Saito N, Horiuchi H, Kobayashi S, Nawata M, Takaoka K (2004) Continuous local cooling for pain relief following total hip arthroplasty. J Arthroplasty, 19: 334–337
Sanchez-Inchausti G, Vaquero-Martin J, Vidal-Fernandez C (2005) Effect of arthroscopy and continuous cryotherapy on the intramuscular temperature of the knee. Arthroscopy, 21: 552–556
Scarcella JB, Cohn BT (1995) The effect of cold therapy on the postoperative course of total hip and knee arthroplasty patients. Am J Orthop, 24: 847–852
Schaubel HJ (1946) The local use of ice after orthopedic procedures. Am J Surg, 72: 711–714
Scheffler NM, Sheitel PL, Lipton MN (1992) Use of Cryo/Cuff for the control of postoperative pain and edema. J Foot Surg, 31: 141–148
Schroder D, Passler HH (1994) Combination of cold and compression after knee surgery. A prospective randomized study. Knee Surg Sports Traumatol Arthrosc, 2: 158–165
Shelbourne KD, Rubinstein RA, McCarrol JR, Weaver J (1994) Postoperative cryotherapy for the knee in ACL reconstruction surgery. Orthop Int Ed, 2: 165–170
Shibuya N, Schinke TL, Canales MB, Yu GV (2007) Effect of cryotherapy devices in the postoperative settings. J Am Podiatr Med Assoc, 97: 439–446
Showman J, Wedlick LT (1963) The use of cold instead of heat for the relief of muscle spasm. Med J Aust, 50: 612–614
Singh H, Osbahr DC, Holovacs TF, Cawley PW, Speer KP (2001) The efficacy of continuous cryotherapy on the postoperative shoulder: A prospective, randomized investigation. J Shoulder Elbow Surg, 10: 522–525
Sloan JP, Hain R, Pownall R (1989) Clinical benefits of early cold therapy in accident and emergency following ankle sprain. Arch Emerg Med, 6: 1–6
Smith J, Stevens J, Taylor M, Tibbey J (2002) A randomized, controlled trial comparing compression bandaging and cold therapy in postoperative total knee replacement surgery. Orthop Nurse, 21:61–66
Speer KP, Warren RF, Horowitz L (1996) The efficacy of cryotherapy in the postoperative shoulder. J Shoulder Elbow Surg, 5: 62–68
Starkey JA (1976) Treatment of ankle sprains by simultaneous use of intermittent compression and ice packs. Am J Sports Med, 41: 142–144
Stockle U, Hoffmann R, Schultz M, von Fournier C, Sudkamp NP, Haas N (1997) Fastest reduction of posttraumatic edema: Continuous cryotherapy or intermittent impulse compression? Foot Ankle Int, 18: 432–438
Thieme H, Ingersoll C, Knight K, Ozmun JC (1996) Cooling does not affect knee proprioception. J Athl Train, 31: 8–11
Tomchuk D, Rubbley MD, Holcomb WR, Guadagnoli M, Tarno JM (2010) The magnitude of tissue cooling during cryotherapy with varied types of compression. J Athl Train, 45: 230–237
Travell J (1949) Rapid relief of acute stiff neck by ethyl chloride spray. J Am Med Womens Assoc, 4: 89–95
Travell J (1952) Ethyl chloride for painful muscle spasm. Arch Phys Med Rehab, 32: 291–298
Tremblay F, Estephan L, Legendre M, Sulpher S (2001) Influence of local cooling on proprioceptive acuity in the quadriceps muscle. J Athl Train, 36: 119–123
Tsang KKW, Buxton BP, Guion WK, Joyner AB, Browder KD (1997) The effects of cryotherapy applied over various barriers. J Sports Rehab, 6: 343–354
Uchio Y, Ochi M, Fujihara A, Adachi N, Iwasa J, Sakai Y (2003) Cryotherapy influences joint laxity and position sense on healthy knee joint. Arch Phys Med Rehab, 84: 131–135
Walker RH, Morris BA, Angulo DL, Scheinder J, Colwell CW (1991) Postoperative use of continuous passive motion, transcutaneous electrical nerve stimulation and continuous cooling pad following total knee arthroplasty. J Arthroplasty, 6: 151–156
Webb JM, Williams D, Ivory JP, Day S, Williamson DM (1998) The use of cold compression dressings after total knee replacement: A randomized controlled trial. Orthopedics, 21: 59–61
Weresh MJ, Bennett GL, Njus G (1996) Analysis of cryotherapy penetration: A comparison of the plaster cast, synthetic cast, Ace wrap dressing, and Robert-Jones dressing. Foot Ankle Int, 17: 37–40
Weston M, Taber C, Casgranda L, Cornwall M (1994) Changes in local blood volume during cold gel pack application to traumatized ankles. J Orthop Sports Phys Ther, 19: 197–199
Whitelaw GP, DeMuth KA, Demos HA, Schepsis A, Jacques E (1995) The use of Cryo/Cuff versus ice and elastic wrap in the postoperative care of knee arthroscopy patients. Am J Knee Surg, 8: 28–30
Wilkerson GB (1991) Treatment of the inversion ankle sprain through synchronous application of focal compression and cold. J Athl Train, 26: 220–237
Wilkerson GB, Horn-Kingery HM (1993) Treatment of the inversion ankle sprain: Comparison of different modes of compression and cryotherapy. J Orthop Sports Phys Ther, 17: 240–246
Williams J, Harvey J, Tannenbaum H (1986) Use of superficial heat and ice for the rheumatoid arthritic shoulder: A pilot study. Physiother Can, 38: 3–13
Woolf SK, Barfield WR, Merrill KD, McBryde AM (2008) Comparison of a continuous temperature-controlled cryotherapy device to a simple icing regimen following outpatient knee arthroscopy. J Knee Surg, 21: 15–19
Yackzan L, Adams C, Francis KT (1984) The effects of ice massage on delayed muscle soreness. Am J Sports Med, 12: 159–165
Zaffagnini S, Iacono F, Petito A, Loreti I, Fu FH, Marcacci M (1998) Cryo/Cuff use after arthroscopic surgery: Effect on knee joint temperature. Am J Knee Surg, 11: 203–207
Zemke JE, Anderson JC, Guion WK (1998) Intramuscular temperature responses in the human leg to two forms of cryotherapy: Ice massage and ice bag. J Orthop Sports Phys Ther, 27: 301–307

Review Articles

Adie S, Naylor JM, Harris IA (2010) Cryotherapy after total knee arthroplasty. J Arthroplasty, 25: 709–715
Allen RJ (2006) Physical agents used in the management of chronic pain by physical therapists. Phys Med Rehabil Clin N Am, 17: 315–345
Bleakley CM, Davidson GW (2010a). Cryotherapy and inflammation: Evidence beyond the cardinal signs. Phys Ther Rev, 15: 431–435
Bleakley CM, Hopkins JT (2010b) Is it possible to achieve optimal levels of tissue cooling in cryotherapy? Phys Ther Rev, 15: 345–350
Bleakley CM, Costello JT, Glasgow PD (2013) Should athletes return to sport after applying ice? A systematic review of the effect of cooling on functional performance. Sports Med, 42: 69–87

Costello JT, Donnelly AE (2010) Cryotherapy and joint position sense in healthy participants: A systematic review. J Athl Train, 45: 306–316
Daanen HA (2003) Finger cold-induced vasodilation: A review. Eur J Appl Physiol, 89: 411–426
Greenstein G (2007) Therapeutic efficacy of cold therapy after intraoral surgical procedures: A literature review. J Periodontol, 78: 790–800
Markert SE (2011) The use of cryotherapy after a total knee replacement: A literature review. Orthop Nurse, 30: 29–36
Merrick MA (2002) Secondary injury after musculoskeletal trauma: A review and update. J Athl Train, 37: 209–217

Chapters of Textbooks

Knight KL, Draper DO (2013a) Cryotherapy beyond immediate care. In: Therapeutic Modalities: The Art and Science, 2nd ed. Lippincott Williams & Wilkins, Philadelphia, pp 211–235
Knight KL, Draper DO (2013b) Cryotherapy application for post-immediate care. In: Therapeutic Modalities: The Art and Science, 2nd ed. Lippincott Williams & Wilkins, Philadelphia, pp 236–251
Lehmann JF, De Lateur BJ (1990) Cryotherapy. In: Therapeutic Heat and Cold, 4th ed. Lehmann JF (Ed). Williams & Wilkins, Baltimore, pp 590–632
Sekins KM, Emery AF (1990) Thermal science for physical medicine. In: Therapeutic Heat and Cold, 4th ed. Lehmann JF (Ed). Williams & Wilkins, Baltimore, pp 62–112
Starkey C (2004) Thermal modalities. In: Therapeutic Modalities, 3rd ed. FA Davis, Philadelphia, pp 110–123

Textbook

Knight KL (1995) Cryotherapy in Sports Injury Management. Human Kinetics, Champaign, IL

Chapter 9

Hydrotherapy

Chapter Outline

Learning Objectives

Remembering: List and describe the three common delivery modes for hydrotherapy.

Understanding: Explain the intrinsic, thermal, and mechanical properties of water.

Applying: Demonstrate how to apply hydrotherapy using baths, tubs, tanks, and irrigator devices.

Analyzing: Organize the proposed physiologic and therapeutic effects of hydrotherapy.

Evaluating: Judge the strength of evidence and therapeutic effectiveness behind the use of hydrotherapy for managing soft tissue pathologies.

Creating: Estimate the value and place of hydrotherapy for the management of soft tissue pathology.

I. FOUNDATION

A. DEFINITION

Hydrotherapy is broadly defined as the use of water (*hydro*) for therapeutic purposes. Because water may be warmer or colder in relation to the patient's neutral or baseline skin temperature, hydrotherapy is further classified in this chapter as the application of *thermo-hydrotherapy* (warm water immersion), and *cryo-hydrotherapy* (cold water immersion). Hydrotherapy is delivered in three modes: bath/tub/tank/irrigator therapy, pool/aquatic

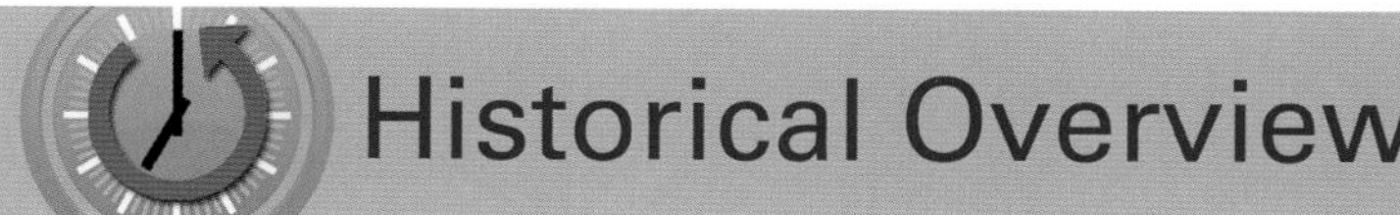

Historical Overview

Historical accounts suggest that hydrotherapy began in the era of water healing, which existed in Greece from 500 to 300 BC, during which time Hippocrates himself was reported to have used hot- and cold-water immersion baths to treat a wide variety of diseases (Baruch, 1920; Jackson, 1990; Irion, 1997). In the 17th century, Sir John Floyer is reported to have written the first treatise on hydrotherapy, entitled *An Inquiry Into the Right Use and Abuse of Hot, Cold, and Temperate Baths* (Irion, 1997). The 18th through 20th centuries saw a major increase in the use of water for therapeutic purposes. Hydrotherapy evolved from its traditional mode of body immersion in baths, tubs, and tanks to include two other modes known as pool/aquatic therapy and spa/balneotherapy.

therapy, and spa/balneotherapy. Table 9-1 lists key characteristics of each mode. The main difference between these three modes of hydrotherapy is the type of water used, i.e., tap water with or without therapeutic additives vs. tap water with chlorine alone vs. natural waters and muds. The focus of this chapter is on the delivery of hydrotherapy using the classic bath/tub/tank/irrigator modes found in most clinical settings around the world. The pool/aquatic therapy mode is beyond the scope of this chapter because the main therapeutic effects come from physical exercises and not from the effect of water. In other words, pool/aquatic therapy is an exercise-based treatment rather than a water-based or hydrotherapy-type treatment. The spa/balneotherapy mode is also beyond the scope of this chapter because the water type and mud used for therapy are found only in oceans or natural springs and thus are not commonly available in traditional clinical settings.

B. HYDROTHERAPY EQUIPMENT AND ACCESSORIES

The hydrotherapy mode covered in this chapter is subdivided into immersion and nonimmersion techniques. *Immersion* is delivered using various baths, tubs, and tanks and *nonimmersion* via manual water irrigators. Immersion equipments are movable or stationary and are fitted with drains and thermostatically controlled water valves. Nonimmersion equipments are portable and manually operated. Figure 9-1 shows common sitz bath, tubs, tanks, and lifting systems that facilitate a patient's access to and from tubs and tanks. It also shows accessories such as electrical turbines mounted on tubs and tanks. The use of disposable and inexpensive plastic liners prevents the risk of contamination while greatly facilitating sanitary maintenance of baths, tubs, and tanks. Figure 9-2 illustrates common nonimmersion manually pressured and pulsed water irrigators. Description and applicability of these hydroagents are presented in Table 9-2.

C. RATIONALE FOR USE

The rationale for the use of water for therapeutic purposes rests with its intrinsic cleansing, thermal, and mechanical properties, and that water is cheap and readily available in all clinical settings.

II. BIOPHYSICAL CHARACTERISTICS

The biophysics of hydrotherapy rests on the principles and concepts related to the intrinsic, thermal, and mechanical properties of water.

TABLE 9-1 HYDROTHERAPY MODES

Bath/Tub/Tank/Irrigator	Pool/Aquatic	Spa/Balneotherapy
Tap water alone or mixed with therapeutic additives	Tap water mixed with chlorine	Natural waters and mud with their own minerals
Bath, tub, tank, and irrigator	Full-size pool; customized pool	Ocean water and mud
Single patient only	Single as well as groups of patients	Single as well as groups of patients
Water-based treatment	Exercise-based treatment	Water-based treatment
Normal and damaged skin	Normal skin only	Normal skin only

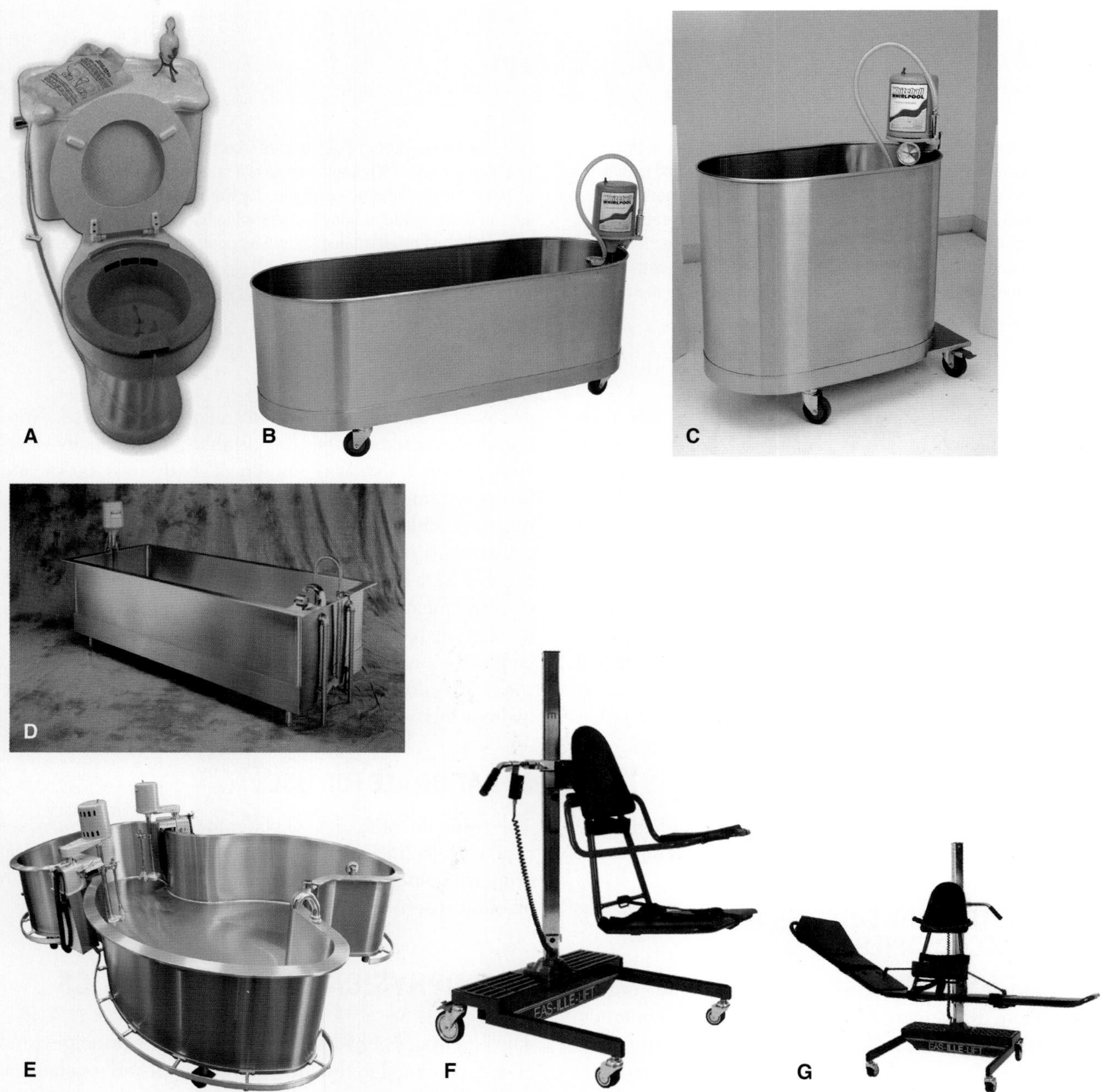

FIGURE 9-1 Typical immersion hydroagents and accessories. **A:** Sitz bath mounted on standard toilet bowl. **B:** Lo-Boy tub with turbine. **C:** Hi-Boy tub with turbine. **D:** Burn tank with turbine. **E:** Hubbard tank with turbines. **F, G:** Motorized patient-handling systems mounted with a chair or a stretcher. (A: Courtesy of Invacare Corporation; B–D: Courtesy of Whitehall Manufacturing; E: Courtesy of Colonial Medical Corp; F, G: Courtesy of Ferno Performance Pools.)

A. WATER INTRINSIC PROPERTIES

The intrinsic properties of water refer to its density, specific gravity, and viscosity.

1. Density (ρ)

Designated by the Greek letter ρ, the *density* of a substance, such as water, is the measure of how compactly its atoms and molecules are arranged together (Kreighbaum et al., 1996). Density is defined as mass (m) over volume (v)—that is, $\rho = m/v$. The more compactly arranged the molecules, the denser the substance. Because weight (w) is directly proportional to mass (weight = mass × gravity) and the measurement of weight is more readily available than that of mass, the concept of density can be substituted for weight density, such that weight density (ρ_w) equals weight (w) over volume (v). Common units of ρ_w are newton per liter (N/L), where 1 L equals 1,000 cc, and pound per cubic foot (lb/ft^3). The ρ_w of fresh water is 9.8 N/L or 62.4 lb/ft^3 (Kreighbaum et al., 1996).

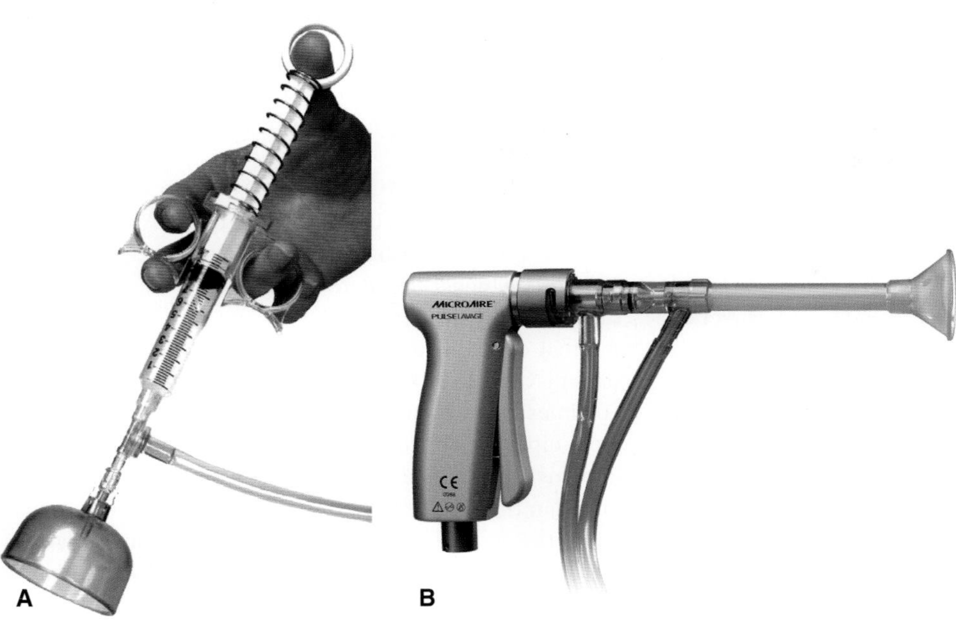

FIGURE 9-2 Typical nonimmersion water irrigation systems. **A:** Manually pressurized water irrigator. **B:** Pulse lavage with suction unit. (A: Courtesy of LMA North America, Inc.; B: MicroAire® Surgical Instruments, LLC.)

TABLE 9-2 COMMON HYDROAGENTS AND ACCESSORIES

Hydroagent	Description	Application and Temperature Range
	Immersion	
Sitz bath	Commercially designed plastic or stainless steel bath fitted with a gravity water irrigation system and placed over a conventional toilet bowl	Pelvic, genital, and buttock areas 22° to 38°C (72° to 100°F)
Contrast bath	Commercial bath made of two side-by-side stainless steel tanks. One tank is fitted with a heating element and the other tank with a cooling element, thus providing the desired contrasting temperatures. Each tank has a digital temperature indicator and controller. Two individual common plastic baths are often used as a substitute to commercial contrast baths.	Distal upper and lower limbs *Hot:* 40° to 45°C (104° to 113°F) *Cold:* 10° to 20°C (50° to 68°F)
Tubs	Commercially designed stainless steel tub fitted with a drain valve, a thermometer, and an electric turbine. The turbine can be adjusted to the desired pressure, height, and direction in relation to the treated body part. These tubs are commercialized under names such as Extremity, Hi-Boy, and Lo-Boy tubs.	*Extremity tub:* Distal extremities, including the elbows and knees 10° to 40°C (50° to 104°F) *Hi-Boy tub:* For partial-body immersion (from the waist down) *Lo-Boy tub:* For partial-body immersion (from the armpit down) 30° to 38°C (86° to 100°F)
Tank	See previous Tubs description. These tanks are commercialized under names such as burn tank and Hubbard tank.	For full-body immersion (from the neck down) 30° to 38°C (86° to 100°F)
Motorized patient-handling device	Movable hydraulic patient-handling device mounted with a chair or stretcher	To move and position patients over and into the tubs or tanks
	Nonimmersion	
Pressure water irrigation unit	Commercial manual unit made of a syringe connected to a flexible plastic infusion tube	To irrigate and debride open wounds
Pulse lavage with suction unit	Commercial air pressure and vacuum unit made of a gunlike handle and disposable flexible tubing and splash shields	To irrigate, debride, and suction open wounds

2. Specific Gravity (S_g)

The *specific gravity* (S_g) of a substance is the ratio of its weight density to the weight density of water (Kreighbaum et al., 1996). The specific gravity of water is unity, or 1, because its weight density, as a fluid, equals 9.8 N/L or 62.4 lb/ft^3, as stated earlier (S_g = 9.8 N/L/9.8 N/L = 1; 62.4 lb/ft^3/62.4 lb/ft^3 = 1). The flotation of a substance depends on its specific gravity. For example, if the weight density of an object or body segment is *less than or equal to* the weight density of water (i.e., $S_g \leq 1$), that object or body segment will float. In contrast, if its weight density is *greater* than the weight density of water (i.e., $S_g > 1$), then that object or body segment will sink. This is why a piece of wood (S_g = 0.79) will float but a piece of aluminum (S_g = 2.65) will sink if immersed in water. The specific gravity of the human body, which varies depending on the individual's somatotype and residual air volume in the lungs at immersion, is less than 1. As a result, the human body generally floats when totally immersed in water. The specific gravity of the human body is 0.97, which means that approximately 97% of the body surface is totally submerged in water and the remaining 3% is exposed to air.

3. Viscosity (v)

Designated by the Greek letter ν, the *viscosity* of a fluid refers to the ease with which it flows. Viscosity is caused by the chemical binding forces holding the fluid molecules together, such as the forces binding hydrogen (H_2) to oxygen (O) molecules to form water (H_2O). The stronger these chemical binding forces, the more viscous the substance. Viscosity is inversely influenced by temperature. The lower a fluid's temperature, the higher its viscosity. The viscous state of a fluid is commonly represented by its coefficient of viscosity (designated by the Greek letter η [eta]) and is expressed in units of pascal-second (Pa.s). The coefficient of viscosity of tap water at 20°C is 1.0×10^{-3} Pa.s.

B. WATER THERMAL PROPERTIES

The thermal properties of water relate to its specific heat and thermal conductivity.

1. Specific Heat (c)

As discussed in Chapter 7, the *specific heat* (designated by the letter c) of a fluid or material refers to its capacity to hold (store) heat (Sekins et al., 1990). Heat is defined as the total kinetic energy, or molecular motion, of a substance. To avoid duplication, readers may refer to Chapter 7 for more details on the concepts of specific heat and thermal conductivity. The specific heat value of water is 1 cal/g°C because a heat input of 1 calorie is needed to increase the temperature of 1 g of pure water at 15°C by 1°C. At any given temperature, water (c = 1.00) holds approximately two times more heat than paraffin oil (c = 0.45) and four times more than air (c = 0.24). In other words, a paraffin mixture contains approximately 50% less heat than water at the same temperature, which explains why patients can tolerate the former at a much higher temperature than the latter.

2. Thermal Conductivity (k)

Thermal conductivity (designated by the letter k) refers to the rate at which a substance conducts heat (Sekins et al., 1990). The higher the thermal conductivity of a substance, the better this substance performs as a heat conductor. The thermal conductivity value of water at 15°C is 1.42 cal/sec-cm°C. Water (k = 1.42) conducts heat approximately 70 times more rapidly than air (k = 0.02) and 2.5 times more rapidly than paraffin oil (k = 0.59). This explains why humans feel the heat contained in water much more rapidly than that in air or paraffin oil when all three elements are at the same temperature. The thermal conductivity of subcutaneous fat (k = 0.45) is approximately 50% that of the skin (k = 0.90) and approximately 30% that of skeletal muscle (k = 1.53). This makes subcutaneous fat a less effective heat conductor, or a better heat insulator, than skin and muscle. Thus, the thicker the layer of subcutaneous fat between skin and deeper soft tissues, the lesser the amount of heat that can be conducted from the skin to the deeper tissues during thermotherapy.

C. WATER MECHANICAL PROPERTIES

The mechanical properties of water refer to its hydrostatic pressure, buoyancy force, and drag force.

1. Hydrostatic Pressure (P)

Designated by the letter P, *hydrostatic pressure* is the pressure exerted by water on a submerged object or body part (Kreighbaum et al., 1996). According to Pascal's law, hydrostatic pressure is applied from all directions on the surface of the immersed object or body part and varies directly in relation to the depth of immersion. In other words, this law stipulates that the deeper an object is immersed in water, the greater is the water pressure exerted on it. Thus, the deeper the immersion, the greater the hydrostatic pressure exerted on the object or body part. Hydrostatic pressure (P) equals the amount of force (F) acting over a given area (A), or $P = F/A$. It is commonly expressed as newton per square meter (N/m^2), pounds per square inch (lb/in^2 or psi), or millimeter of mercury (mm Hg). Figure 9-3 shows the magnitude of hydrostatic pressure exerted on a given body part in relation to various water immersion depths. For example, an ankle joint immersed in water at a depth of 1.2 m (4 ft) theoretically experiences hydrostatic pressure of approximately 89.6 mm Hg (1.73 lb/in^2). To understand what these various pressures would feel like on the body, imagine how you feel when your arm is squeezed by a blood pressure cuff as your diastolic and systolic blood pressure is taken. Remember, as a reference point, that normal blood pressure values are approximately 80 over 120 mm Hg.

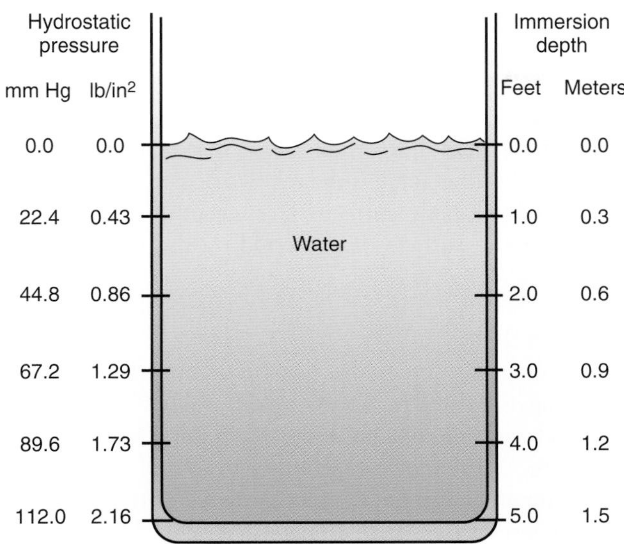

1 ft of water = 0.8826 in. of mercury (Hg) = 22.4 mm Hg

1 mm Hg = 0.0193 lb/in²; 1 psi = 51.8 mm Hg

FIGURE 9-3 Relationship between hydrostatic pressure and immersion depth.

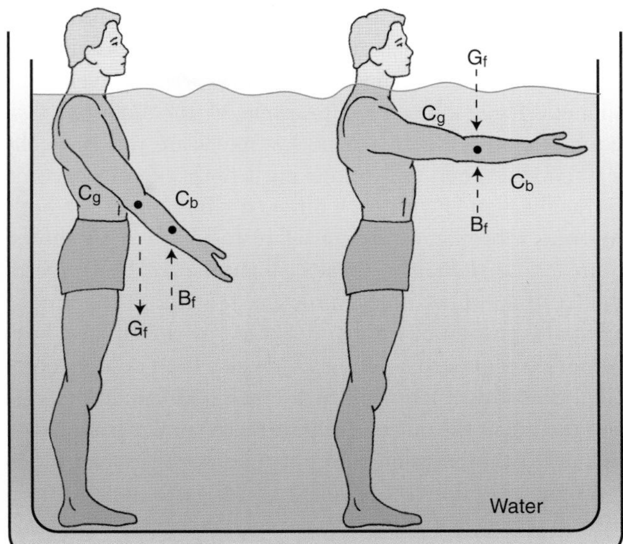

A

B

FIGURE 9-4 Buoyancy force (B_f) acting on its center of buoyancy (C_b) to lift or move upward the upper limb, which is itself pulled down by the gravitational force (G_f) acting on its center of gravity (C_g). **A:** When the two centers are vertically aligned with each other, and if B_f equals G_f, the upper limb will resume a stable resting position near the surface of the water. **B:** The buoyancy force may be resistive or assistive, depending on which direction the limb movement is taking place in the water.

2. Buoyancy Force

a. Archimedes' Principle

Buoyancy is a fluid force, as illustrated in Figure 9-4, that always acts vertically upward (Hall, 2006). This force generated by water is based on Archimedes' principle, which states that an object or body part, totally or partially immersed in a fluid, experiences an upward, buoyant force equal to the weight of the volume of fluid displaced by that object or body part (Kreighbaum et al., 1996). Buoyancy force (B_f) is calculated as the product of the displaced volume (V_d) and the fluid's weight density (ρ_w)—that is, $B_f = V_d \times \rho_w$ (Hall, 2006). For example, if a patient's upper limb has a volume of 0.3 L and that limb is completely submerged in water at 20°C, the buoyant force acting on it is equal to 2.94 N (2.94 N = 0.3 L × 9.8 N/L).

b. Weightlessness

Buoyancy force is an antigravitational force and, as such, induces a state of relative body weightlessness. The percentage of the body immersed in water directly affects the magnitude of the buoyancy force that induces this relative weightlessness. This explains why a patient suffering from a hip disorder may experience hip pain while standing on land (no buoyancy force acting) but much less pain when standing in water with approximately 70% of his or her body submerged (with buoyancy force acting) in water during hydrotherapy. Gravitational force (G_f) acts at the center of gravity (C_g), which is the center at which the object or body mass is concentrated (Kreighbaum et al., 1996; Hall et al., 1996). Buoyancy force, on the other hand, acts at the center of buoyancy (C_b). The center of buoyancy is the center of volume of the body displacing water, which is the point around which the body's volume is equally distributed (Hall, 2006).

c. Rotational Force

In humans, the volume centers (C_b) of the body and of each of its segments are not located at the same place as their mass centers (C_g), because the density related to each body part varies from one part to the next (Kreighbaum et al., 1996). Because weight acts at the center of gravity and buoyancy acts at the center of volume, a rotational effect, or torque, is created that rotates the body until it is positioned so that these two acting forces are vertically aligned (Hall, 2006). For example, if the body is positioned in water such that both centers are not vertically aligned, the body will rotate until both centers become vertically aligned with each other, at which point the body resumes a balanced position at rest. Figure 9-4A shows, from left to right, the vertical alignment of the C_g with the C_b of an upper limb immersed in water as the limb is gradually pushed upward and rotated by the B_f until both centers coincide. If B_f equals G_f when both centers coincide, then this upper limb will reach a balanced position and float near the surface. Figure 9-4B shows, from left to right, that the buoyancy force can be *assistive,* if acting in the same direction as the desired body movement, or *resistive,* if acting in the opposite direction from the desired movement.

3. Drag Force

The force exerted by water on a submerged and moving object or body segment is defined as the *drag force.* Drag is the force parallel to the direction of motion, but in the opposite direction. Drag force resists the movement of an object or body part in water. There are three different drag forces: surface drag, profile drag, and wave drag (Kreighbaum et al., 1996; Hall, 2006). They act together to exert a total drag force on the moving object or body part. Figure 9-5 illustrates these three drag forces acting together to resist the adduction movement of a lower limb, using as an example the sole of the foot of a patient floating supine near the surface of the water.

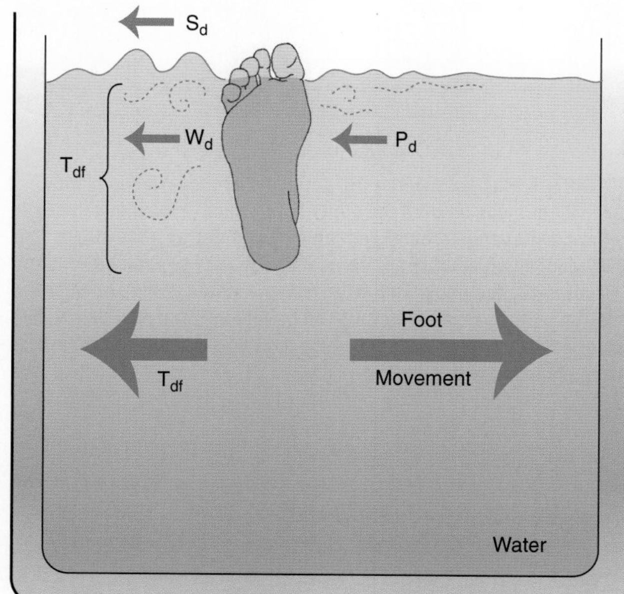

FIGURE 9-5 Surface drag (S_d), profile drag (P_d), and wave drag (W_d) force, which together form the total drag force (T_{df}) resisting the lower limb movement of a subject lying supine in the water. Shown is the front view of the lower limb (sole of the foot) performing an adduction movement near the surface of the water.

a. Surface Drag

Surface drag (S_d) force, also known as skin friction and viscous drag, is caused by friction between adjacent layers of water near the body part moving through water (Hall, 2006). One important factor that may increase or decrease this drag force is the relative degree of roughness of the moving body surface. The smoother the surface, the lesser the surface drag exerted on the moving body part.

b. Profile Drag

Profile drag (P_d) force, also known as form drag or pressure drag, is created by a pressure differential between the lead and rear sides of a body moving in water (Hall, 2006). This force is the major contributor to overall drag during most human and projectile motion in water (Hall, 2006). Two important factors that may increase or decrease this force are the body part's relative velocity with respect to water and the amount of the body part's surface area that is aligned perpendicular to the flow (Hall, 2006). Doubling the velocity of movement in water will quadruple the magnitude of the profile drag force. Doubling the surface area of the moving object or body part will also quadruple the magnitude of the profile drag.

c. Wave Drag

Wave drag (W_d) force is created by the generation of waves at the interface between two different fluids, such as water and air (Hall, 2006). Wave drag increases with the proximity of the moving body part from the water surface and with the velocity of that moving body part. Thus, the closer the body part from the surface of the water, and the faster the displacement of this body part in water, the greater the wave drag force exerted on that body part.

d. Total Drag Force

As shown in Figure 9-5, the total drag force (T_{df}) opposing the lower limb movement results from the grouped drag action exerted by the surface (S_d), profile (P_d), and wave (W_d) drag forces, where $T_{df} = S_d + P_d + W_d$.

D. WATER PRESSURE AND SUCTION FORCE

The use of nonimmersion commercial water irrigator and suction units rests on water pressure and suction force. The irrigation pressure delivered by the device should range between 4 and 15 psi. Pressures less than 4 psi (207 mm Hg) may not cleanse the wound adequately, and pressures greater than 15 psi (777 mm Hg) may cause trauma and drive bacteria in the wound tissue (Luedtke-Hoffmann et al., 2000).

E. ENERGY TRANSFER MODE

Thermal energy transfer between water and skin is achieved through conduction and convection (see Chapter 7 for details). Thermal transfer by convection far exceeds that achieved by conduction, because in most hydrotherapeutic applications, water always circulates around the treated body area as a result of passive and/or active movements and the use of electric turbines. A thin layer of insulation around and next to the skin, called *thermopane,* is formed when the immersed body part and the water stay still during treatment. In such cases, thermal energy transfer happens by conduction only. The thermopane is lost when body movement, the use of electric turbines, or both create water agitation or turbulence around the immersed body part. In such cases, the thermal energy transfer occurs primarily by convection.

F. CONTROL OVER WATER PROPERTIES

Practitioners have *no* control over the density, specific gravity, specific heat, and thermal conductivity of tap water used to deliver bath/tub/tank hydrotherapy. They have, however, *some* control over the following properties of water. Viscosity can be increased or decreased by varying water temperature. Hydrostatic pressure can be increased or decreased by varying the depth of immersion. Buoyancy force can be increased or decreased by varying the percentage of body immersion. Finally, total drag force can be increased or decreased by varying body movement velocity and body surface area or by the use of an electrical turbine. The setting of these water properties will establish the dosimetry that will be delivered to the patient in order to achieve the therapeutic goals.

III. THERAPEUTIC EFFECTS AND INDICATIONS

Figure 9-6 lists the proposed physiologic and therapeutic effects associated with the practice of hydrotherapy. Water is used for its thermal and mechanical effects on the body. The thermal effects of hydrotherapy are similar to, but much less pronounced than, those induced by

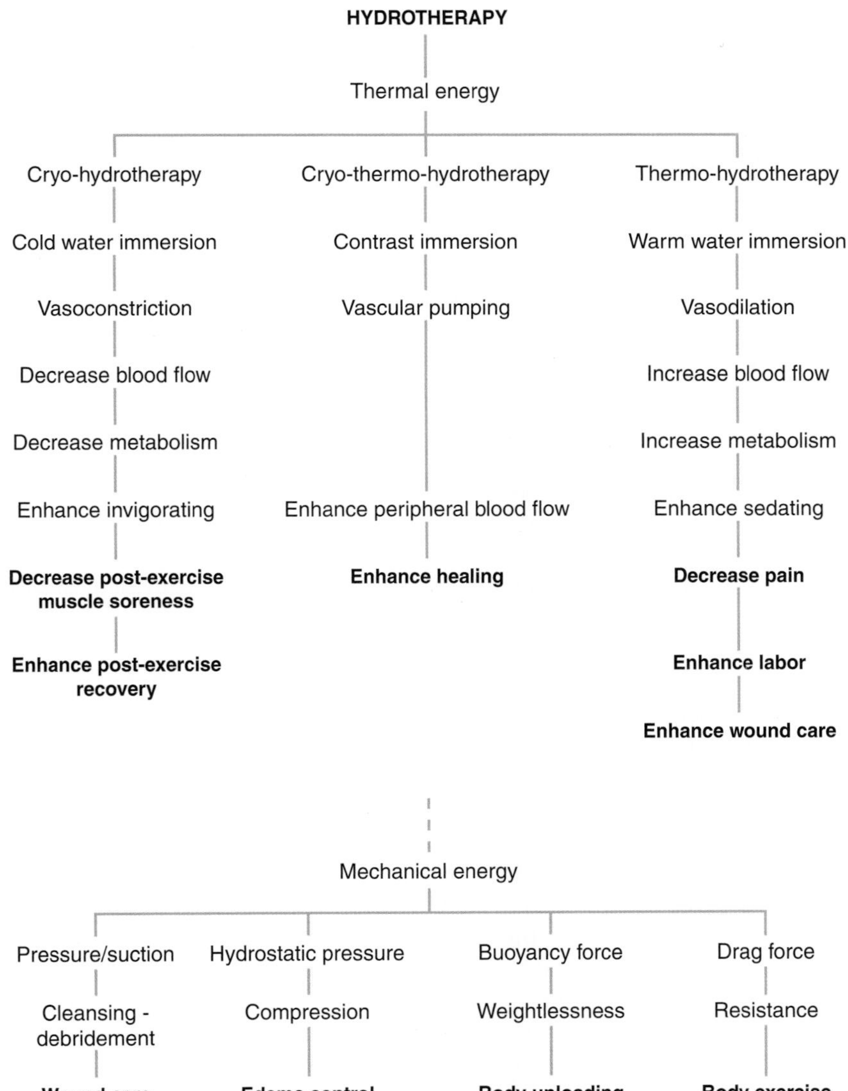

FIGURE 9-6 Proposed physiologic and therapeutic effects of hydrotherapy.

thermotherapy (Chapter 7) and cryotherapy (Chapter 8) agents. This is because lower thermal doses—that is, agent–skin temperature differentials ($T°_{ag-s}$)—are used in hydrotherapy, especially when a significant percentage of the body is immersed in water.

A. THERMAL EFFECTS

1. Cryo-hydrotherapy

Cryo-hydrotherapy is delivered using partial- to full-body immersion in cold water. The resulting effects are vasoconstriction, decreased blood flow, decreased metabolism, and increased invigoration. Together, these effects are presumed to minimize post-exercise muscle soreness and thus enhancing post-exercise recovery.

2. Thermo-hydrotherapy

The delivery of thermo-hydrotherapy is identical to cryo-hydrotherapy, except the body is immersed in warm water. The resulting effects are vasodilation, increased blood flow, increased metabolism, and increased sedation (Fig. 9-6). These effects are presumed to decrease pain, enhance the natural labor experience by reducing an epidural/spinal analgesia requirement during labor, and facilitate wound care. Still and turbulent water in tubs and tanks, when in contact with a wound surface, have a cleansing effect by removing unwanted substances, such as dirt and residual therapeutic cream, which may delay or prevent healing. Turbulent water, created by the use of manual irrigators or electrical turbines, also has a debridement effect on an open wound. *Debridement* is the excision or removal of contused or devitalized tissues (debris) from a wound surface. When infected open wounds are under consideration, nonimmersion irrigator systems should be used for cleansing and debriding (see later discussion).

3. Cryo-Thermo Hydrotherapy

The contrasting effects of cold (cryo) and warm (thermo) water on peripheral blood flow, as shown in Figure 9-6, can be obtained by using contrast immersion (Cochrane, 2004). The first published article on the physiologic effects of contrast immersion appears to be that of Woodmansey et al. (1938), who observed alterations in blood flow through recording surface skin temperatures in healthy subjects versus rheumatic patients after various periods of immersion in cold versus hot water. Because blood vessels dilate in hot water and constrict in cold water, and considering the results of Woodmansey et al. (1938), contrast immersion method was seen by many practitioners as a means of passive vascular exercise similar to the active vascular exercise induced by voluntary contraction. In other words, it was believed that this passive method triggered a peripheral and deep vascular pumping action similar to that documented experimentally during voluntary muscle contractions. It follows that for those patients who have difficulty with voluntary joint movement because of pain or trauma, the use of contrast immersion appears to be an ideal substitute for voluntary contractions to enhance blood flow and decrease residual edema in traumatized soft tissues (Cooper et al., 1979). Is there scientific evidence to suggest that contrast immersion triggers a peripheral and deep vascular pumping effect similar to that induced during voluntary muscle contraction?

a. Passive Contrast Immersion

Results of recent experimental studies involving healthy individuals have raised serious doubts about the deep vascular pumping effect traditionally attributed to contrast immersion (Myrer et al., 1994; Benoit et al., 1996; Myrer et al., 1997; Higgins et al., 1998). Together, the results of these studies indicate that contrast immersion, when applied passively (no movement allowed) on the limbs of healthy individuals, fails to produce any significant intramuscular temperature changes, meaning that this method of water immersion has no significant vasodilation/vasoconstriction effect on the larger and deeper blood vessels. It appears, therefore, that if passive application of contrast immersion is to cause a vascular pumping effect, then this effect is limited to the peripheral blood vessels only.

b. Active Contrast Immersion

Research has shown that vascular, as well as lymphatic, pumping is best achieved by cycles of voluntary muscle contractions and joint motions that we all do on a daily basis. Thus, active, as opposed to passive, contrast immersion, wherein the patient performs short bouts of exercise, may be the best method for obtaining the peripheral and deep vascular pumping effect. In other words, adding an active component (voluntary muscle contractions) to the passive effect of contrast immersion on peripheral blood flow should result in the desired therapeutic vascular and lymphatic therapeutic pumping action.

c. Transition Method

Contrast immersion, because it exposes the body part to cycles of cold and warm water, appears to be one of the best method of transitioning from cryotherapy to thermotherapy, thus facilitating the transition from the early hemostasis/inflammatory stage to the later proliferative maturation stage of soft tissue healing.

4. Burn Wound Cleansing

Infection remains the leading cause of morbidity and mortality from extensive burn injury. There is a consensus in the clinical world that wound cleansing should be an integral step in all wound management, including that used in burn wounds, for which special hydroagents (burn tank and Hubbard tanks) have been developed and used. Is this consensus based on evidence? Interestingly, no study could be found that scientifically compared the outcome of patients who underwent wound cleansing and those who did not (Hayek et al., 2010). In the early 1990s, most burn centers around the world used hydrotherapy for burn wound cleansing. Because numerous reports linked hydrotherapy contamination of water and equipments with the emergence of bacterial outbreaks throughout North America, the traditional body immersion method has been abandoned and replaced by other methods. Today, water irrigation and showering are the preferred methods to treat burn patients (Hayek et al., 2010). When body immersion in a water tank is required, disposable plastic liners should be used to cover the tank to avoid cross-contamination.

B. MECHANICAL EFFECTS

The mechanical effects of hydrotherapy manifest themselves in various ways. First, the water pressure and suction force of irrigators, and turbulence force of turbines, are used for cleansing and debridement, thus enhancing wound care. Second, hydrostatic pressure causes limb compression, thus enhancing control over edema. Third, buoyancy force, through it weightlessness effect, benefits body unloading in cases of difficult and painful weight bearing. Finally, drag forces (surface, profile, and wave) are used to either assist or resist tub- and tank-water–based therapeutic exercises (Al-Qubaeissy et al., 2013).

C. TARGET TEMPERATURE WINDOW

As is the case with the thermotherapy (Chapter 7) and cryotherapy (Chapter 8), scientific evidence suggests that to optimize the clinical effectiveness of hydrotherapy, critical levels of soft tissue heating must be achieved following either cold or warm water immersion. What soft tissue target temperature levels need to be reached to accomplish the above physiologic and therapeutic effects? Figure 9-7 illustrates the therapeutic temperature window of hydrotherapy. It shows that to achieve thermal effects, soft tissues needs to heat up (note upward arrow) to a temperature window ranging from 36° to 40°C (97° to 104°F). If the objective is to cool (note downward arrow) soft tissues, then a temperature window between 27° and 15°C (81° and 59°F) is the target. This therapeutic window is narrower than that of thermotherapy and cryotherapy because water is used, and water—whether hot or cold—is much less tolerable to humans due to its high specific heat and thermal conduction properties.

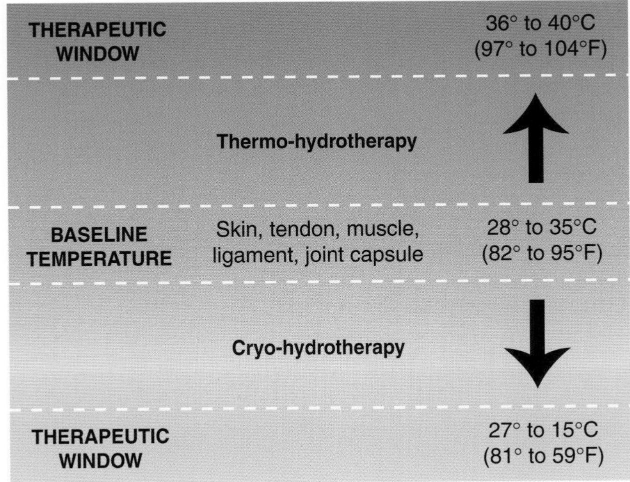

FIGURE 9-7 Therapeutic temperature window of hydrotherapy.

D. RESEARCH-BASED INDICATIONS

The search for evidence behind the use of hydrotherapy, displayed in the Research-Based Indications box, led to the collection of 58 English peer-reviewed human clinical studies. The methodologies, as well as the criteria, used to assess both the strength of evidence and therapeutic effectiveness are described in Chapter 2. As indicated, the strength of evidence is ranked as moderate for delayed-onset muscle soreness/performance recovery, perineal/anal pain, and dermal wound, and as strong for labor pain. Analysis is pending for all other remaining health conditions, because fewer than five studies could be collected. Over all conditions, the strength of evidence behind the use of hydrotherapy is moderate and its therapeutic effectiveness substantiated.

IV. DOSIMETRY

As mentioned in the discussion of thermal agents in Chapters 7 and 8, the practice of evidence-based hydrotherapy also requires that practitioners objectively and quantitatively assess the thermal dose delivered to the tissues, and well as the amount of thermal heating added or extracted to the exposed tissues following the application of these hydroagents. Considering that the rationale for quantitative dosimetry using hydrotherapy is identical to that of thermotherapy and cryotherapy, and to avoid duplication, readers are referred to the material presented on this topic in the Dosimetry section of Chapter 7. In brief, the temperature differential between the hydroagent (ag) and the exposed skin surface (s) is the dose ($T°_{ag\text{-}s}$) delivered to soft tissues. This measurement is easily and rapidly done using a noncontact portable infrared thermometer. The larger the dose, the greater its capacity to either warm or cool soft tissues. The temperature differential between the exposed skin surface before (b) and after (a) treatment ($T°_{b\text{-}a}$) represents the actual skin thermal change caused by the dose. To illustrate how this can be done, let us consider this example. The water temperature inside a Lo-Boy tub is measured at 37°C (99°F), and that of the exposed skin surface at 30°C (86°F), using an infrared portable thermometer. The thermal dose delivered ($T°_{ag\text{-}s}$) thus equals 7°C (13°F), which represents its *potential* heating effect. Immediately after treatment, the exposed

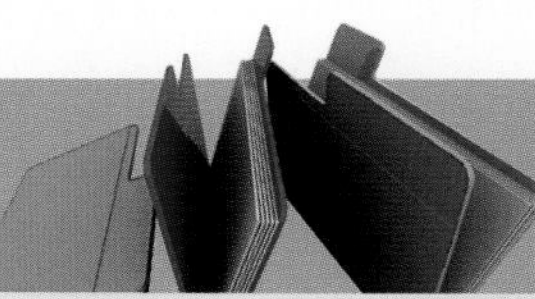

Research-Based Indications

HYDROTHERAPY

Health Condition	Benefit—Yes Rating	Benefit—Yes Reference	Benefit—No Rating	Benefit—No Reference
Delayed-onset muscle soreness/ Performance recovery	I	Kuligowski et al., 1998	I	Howatson et al., 2009
	I	Bailey et al., 2007	II	Sellwood et al., 2007
	I	Yanagisawa et al., 2003	III	King et al., 2009
	I	Vaile et al., 2007	III	Jakeman et al., 2009
	I	Eston et al., 1999	III	Peiffer et al., 2010
	II	Vaile et al., 2008		
	II	Rowsell et al., 2009		
	II	Rowsell et al., 2011		
	II	Montgomery et al., 2008		
	III	Ingram et al., 2009		
	III	Halson et al., 2008		

Strength of evidence: Moderate
Therapeutic effectiveness: Substantiated

Health Condition	Benefit—Yes Rating	Benefit—Yes Reference	Benefit—No Rating	Benefit—No Reference
Labor	I	Rush et al., 1996	I	Eckert et al., 2001
	I	Cammu et al., 1994	I	Schorn et al., 1993
	I	Chaichian et al., 2009		
	I	Da Silva et al., 2009		
	I	Ohlsson et al., 2001		
	I	Woodward et al., 2004		
	II	Eriksson et al., 1997		

Strength of evidence: Strong
Therapeutic effectiveness: Substantiated

Health Condition	Benefit—Yes Rating	Benefit—Yes Reference	Benefit—No Rating	Benefit—No Reference
Perineal/anal pain	I	Dodi et al., 1986	I	Thomas et al., 1993
	II	Ramler et al., 1986	I	Gupta, 2006
	II	Droegemeuller, 1980	II	Gupta, 2007
			II	Pinho et al., 1993

Strength of evidence: Moderate
Therapeutic effectiveness: Conflicting

Health Condition	Benefit—Yes Rating	Benefit—Yes Reference	Benefit—No Rating	Benefit—No Reference
Dermal wound	II	Fruhstorfer et al., 1986	II	Hill, 1989
	II	Juve Meeker, 1998		
	II	Burke et al., 1998		
	III	Gogia et al., 1988		

Strength of evidence: Moderate
Therapeutic effectiveness: Substantiated

Fewer Than 5 Studies

Health Condition	Benefit—Yes Rating	Benefit—Yes Reference	Benefit—No Rating	Benefit—No Reference
Rheumatoid arthritis	II	Ahern et al., 1995	II	Fricke et al., 1952
	II	Hall et al., 1996		
	II	Curkovic et al., 1993		
Osteoarthritis	II	Sylvester, 1990	II	Sterner-Victorin et al., 2004
	II	Green et al., 1993		
	II	Silva et al., 2007		
Multiple sclerosis	II	Boynton et al., 1959	II	Chiara et al., 1988
Ankle sprain	II	Cote et al., 1988		
Clonus	II	Miglietta, 1964		
Soft tissue wounds	II	Abraham et al., 1974		
Postoperative knee pain	II	Barber, 2000		
Traumatic hand injury	II	Hoyrup et al., 1986		
Varicose veins	I	Ernst et al., 1990, 1992		
Colles' fracture			II	Toomey et al., 1986
Bluebottle jellyfish stings	II	Loten et al., 2006		
Exercise-induced hyperthermia	II	Clements et al., 2002		
Hamstring lengthening			II	Burke et al., 2001
Type 2 diabetes			I	Petrofsky et al., 2007

Strength of evidence: Pending
Therapeutic effectiveness: Pending

OVER ALL CONDITIONS
Strength of evidence: Moderate
Therapeutic effectiveness: Substantiated

skin temperature is measured at 34°C (93°F); the *actual* skin heating effect ($T°_{b\text{-}a}$) of this dose was +4°C (+7°F).

A. THERMAL DOSAGE

Three parameters must be considered to set the thermal dose needed: water temperature, body immersion level, and immersion duration.

1. Water Temperature

Water temperature is critical in hydrotherapy because it determines the types of treatment (i.e., cryo- vs. thermo-hydrotherapy) used. The choice of water temperature determines the thermal potential of the hydrotherapeutic application—that is, the greater the temperature differential between the agent and the skin ($T°_{ag\text{-}s}$), whether below (cryo-) or above (thermo-) normal or neutral skin temperature, the more severe the thermal dose received. Water temperature in a *sitz bath* (use in the perineal and genital areas) is usually within the range of 22° to 38°C (72° to 100°F). *Contrast baths* may be used at higher temperature ranging from 10° to 45°C (50° to 113°F). Such high water temperatures can be sustained by patients because the immersion is cyclic, its duration is short (only a few minutes) in each bath, and the body immersion level (see later discussion) is low (only a small percentage of body surface—hands and feet). *Tubs,* which are used for the immersion of the upper or lower extremities (wrists/hands, ankles/feet), may be filled with water at a temperature within the range of 10° to 40°C (50° to 104°F). Finally, water temperatures usually associated with the use of *larger tubs* (Lo- and Hi-Boy), *burn tanks, and Hubbard tanks* fall within the range of 30° to 38°C (86° to 100°F). This narrower temperature range is due to the fact that body immersion levels are the highest with the use of tanks. The larger the percentage of body immersion, the closer the water temperature range should be to the neutral range. Water temperatures outside these ranges increase the risk of the patient's intolerance to treatment, as well as the severity of systemic effects (see later discussion).

2. Body Immersion Level

The level of body immersion, whether partial or full, is also important to dosimetry because it determines if the thermal effects are local (restricted primarily to the treated area) or systemic (spread to the entire body) in nature. There are two levels of immersion from which practitioners can choose—namely, partial- and full-body immersion. *Partial-body immersion* refers to the immersion of one or more body parts. *Full-body immersion,* on the other hand, refers to the immersion of the entire body from the neck down. The larger the dose—that is, temperature differential between water (ag) and the exposed skin ($T°_{ag\text{-}s}$)—and the greater the level or percentage of body immersion in water, the greater the chance to induce systemic thermal reactions, such as increased or decreased heart rate, respiration, and blood pressure, during hydrotherapy.

3. Immersion Duration

Generally speaking, the longer the immersion period or duration, given a similar water temperature, the greater the desired local or systemic effects on the patient. Immersion durations may vary from 10 to 45 minutes, depending on the treated condition and the patient's overall health status.

B. MECHANICAL DOSAGE

Hydrotherapy can induce three mechanical effects on the immersed body part: hydrostatic pressure, buoyancy force, and drag forces. The magnitude of *hydrostatic pressure* (P) is set by the depth at which the affected body part is immersed (see earlier discussion of Pascal's law above and Fig. 9-3). The deeper the immersion, the greater the compressive effect caused by the hydrostatic pressure exerted on the immersed body part. The magnitude of *buoyancy force* (B_f) is determined by the level or percentage of body immersion in water (see Fig. 9-4). For example, a patient standing still and upright in a pool will experience a much greater buoyancy force (effect of weightlessness) if his or her body is immersed fully as opposed to partially. This is explained by Archimedes' principle, which states that the larger the weight of the volume of water displaced by the immersed body, the larger the buoyancy force acting on this body. Finally, the magnitude of each of the three drag forces (surface, profile, and wave) on the immersed body part is influenced by the following elements (see Fig. 9-5). The magnitude of the *surface drag* (S_d) force can be increased by augmenting the roughness of the immersed body part. This can be done by dressing the immersed body part with a shirt or pants. In other words, the smoother the immersed body part (bare skin), the smaller the surface drag force acting on it. The magnitude of the *profile drag* (P_d) force can be increased by (1) augmenting the body part's relative displacement velocity with respect to water and (2) enlarging the body part's surface area that is aligned perpendicular to the flow (Hall, 2006). For example, the patient is asked to move his immersed limb faster to augment the displacement velocity. Floats are attached to the extremities of the immersed moving body part to increase the body surface area. Recall that when either the velocity of movement in water or the surface area of the moving body part is *doubled,* the magnitude of the profile drag force is *quadrupled.* Finally, the magnitude of *wave drag* (W_d) force can be increased by positioning the immersed limb close to the surface of water while causing waves. The closer the immersed body part to the water surface, the greater the wave drag force acting on it. The effects of the elements described earlier on each of the three drag forces will either increase or decrease the total drag force (T_{df}) acting on the immersed and displaced body part during therapy.

C. CLEANSING AND DEBRIDEMENT DOSAGE

There is a consensus in the field of hydrotherapy that tap water should be employed alone, without any other additives. If additive solutions or products are used (e.g., therapeutic soap, antimicrobial, or antibacterial solutions), careful monitoring of the concentrations of such agents is recommended to prevent any cytotoxic reaction. Open wounds, in their inflammatory phase of healing, need debridement to facilitate healing. Wound debridement can be done on land with tweezers and scalpels or water-pressured irrigation systems or under water, also with tweezers, scalpels, and electric turbines. Practitioners should use only certified irrigation systems that are able to deliver water pressure doses within the recommended pressure range (207 to 777 mm Hg or 4 to 15 psi).

V. APPLICATION, CONTRAINDICATIONS, AND RISKS

As is the case for thermotherapy and cryotherapy, to assess and score patients' ability to discriminate between different thermal stimuli prior the first application is capital (see Chapter 7 for details). Very important also is the practitioner's protection against potential contamination from the used water during treatment. The *Application, Contraindications, and Risks* box lists key steps and procedures related to the safe and effective application of hydrotherapy. To facilitate the selection of one agent over the other, comparisons of key considerations are presented in Table 9-2.

APPLICATION, CONTRAINDICATIONS, AND RISKS

Hydrotherapy

IMPORTANT: Because skin thermal damage is always a possibility with the application of hydrotherapy, skin thermal discrimination testing MUST BE CONDUCTED PRIOR to the first application. The description and scoring of this test are documented in Chapter 7. Practitioners using any hydrotherapeutic agents delivered over intact skin and open wounds, whether infected or not, *must always* ensure body protection against the risk of cross-infection or cross-contamination by microorganisms that may be carried in the water or in airborne water droplets by wearing protective gloves, goggles, masks, and waterproof gowns. Cardiopulmonary resuscitation certification for all staff working in hydrotherapy is highly recommended because of the risk associated with electrocution and drowning. The use of clean tap water, without any antimicrobial agent, is recommended. If additives are used, such as antimicrobial or antiseptic agents, their concentration (in parts per million) in water must be carefully monitored and adjusted to prevent cytotoxic reactions that may alter wound healing. Refer to manufacturer recommendations when using therapeutic additive solutions, and never hesitate to ask the opinion of a pharmacist. Regulate hydrotherapy room temperature, ventilation, and humidity. Eliminate any aerosol, mist, or vapor from turbulent water and their additives. A room temperature of 25° to 30°C (77° to 86°F) with a relative humidity of 50% is recommended for most hydrotherapeutic applications. Adequate monitoring of vital signs, including heart rate, blood pressure, ventilation rate, and oral body temperature, should be conducted when systemic reactions are anticipated during or after therapy.

ALL AGENTS

STEP	RATIONALE
1. Check for contraindications.	*Over skin areas where cold/hot sensation discrimination is severely impaired*—skin damage
	Over macerated tissues surrounding a wound—further tissue maceration with prolonged and repeated immersion
	Over a hemorrhagic area—increased bleeding with prolonged and repeated immersion
	In patients presenting with fecal and/or urinary incontinence—auto- and cross-contamination with partial- to full-body immersion
	In patients who are feverish—increased core temperature during prolonged thermo-hydrotherapy immersion
	In patients with multiple sclerosis—increasing fatigue and muscle weakness with thermo-hydrotherapy immersion
	With patients allergic to additive water solutions—inducing unnecessary skin and/or systemic reactions. Carefully monitor the patient's overall response during the first treatment session

STEP	RATIONALE
	With women in the first trimester of pregnancy—fetal teratogenic effects with thermo-hydrotherapeutic agents capable of increasing the basal temperature of a pregnant woman above 39°C (102°F) (Sedgwick Harvey et al., 1981). Healthy, *nonpregnant* women can remain in a thermal tub at 39°C (102°F) for at least 15 minutes and at 41°C (106°F) for at least 10 minutes without risk of reaching a core temperature of 39°C (102°F) or higher (Sedgwick Harvey et al., 1981).
	With patients suffering from severe cardiac and/or respiratory disorders—unduly stressing and overloading the diseased heart–lung system and organs if partial- to full-body immersion is used. Patients will not be able to adapt to the induced systemic effects caused by thermo- and/or cryo-hydrotherapy. There is no justification for refusing hydrotherapy to patients with ankylosing spondylitis who have vital lung capacity less than 1,500 cc (Harrison, 1981).
	In patients who are confused and unreliable—complications during therapy, such as accidental drowning, if full-body immersion is used
2. Consider the risks.	*Thermal skin damage*—Inadequate water temperature (too hot or too cold) can lead to surface skin damage (irritation to burn)
	Macroshock and electrocution—severe tissue burns and possible death by electrocution, for both patients and practitioners, when electrical-line–powered devices and accessories are used because wet skin offers less impedance to current flow. Failure to plug line-powered equipment into ground-fault circuit interrupter (GFCI) receptacles increases this risk.
	Falling—risk of falling in patients and practitioners while walking on slippery floors in hydrotherapy rooms. Wipe floors regularly and install anti-slip mats in strategic areas.
	Fainting and drowning—risk of fainting in patients during full-body immersion in warm to hot water, leading to the risk of drowning. Keep patients alert during treatment, and keep constant visual monitoring of patients during full-body immersion.
	Pathogen transmission and contamination—risk of pathogenic transmission and contamination caused by the proliferation of microbes, such as *Pseudomonas aeruginosa, Staphylococcus aureus,* and *Candida* on the surfaces of hydrotherapy baths, tubs, and tanks, as well as on accessories (McManus et al., 1985; Taddonio et al., 1990; Tredget et al., 1992; Richard et al., 1994; Shandowsky et al., 1994; Hollyoak et al., 1995a,b). These microbes often originate from open wounds, skin surfaces, and fecal flora, and tend to proliferate in warm, moist environments outside the host. Contamination of water, equipment, and accessories can lead to minor skin irritation (folliculitis) and sometimes to local or systemic infection (McGuckin et al., 1981; Berger et al., 1990). Use disposable plastic liners to prevent surface contamination. Apply a regular and rigorous regimen of cleansing, rinsing, and disinfecting procedures after use, and conduct routine culture tests on all equipment and accessories used for therapy.

SITZ BATH

STEP	PROCEDURE
1. Check for contraindications.	See All Agents section.
2. Consider the risks.	See All Agents section.
3. Position and instruct patient.	Ensure comfortable positioning by making sure that the patient is able to reach the floor with the feet while sitting on the basin.
4. Prepare treatment area.	Undress the pelvic and genital areas. Ensure complete privacy during treatment.

STEP	PROCEDURE
5. Prepare the sitz bath.	Place the sitz bath (basin) over the toilet bowl (see Fig. 9-1A). Fill the bath with either warm or cold tap water depending on the condition under treatment. Some sitz baths come with a bag that continuously adds fresh water to the basin. Place the water bag *above* the basin level for gravity drainage. Fill the bag with water that is the same temperature as the basin water. When additional water is added to the bath from a hanging bag, the excess drains through the vents into the toilet bowl below. The vents also allow for overflow of water when the patient first sits in the bath. This type of sitz bath is preferred for those using a continuous flow of water.
6. Determine and measure dose ($T°_{ag\text{-}s}$).	Select the dose that can induce the desired physiologic and therapeutic effects in the targeted tissue. Dose should be high enough to either elevate or lower the targeted tissue temperature within the therapeutic temperature window. Immediately after filling up the basin and bag with water and prior to immersion, measure the dose—that is, the temperature differential between the agent and the skin surface ($T°_{ag\text{-}s}$) over which it is applied.
7. Apply treatment.	Immerse the treated area in the water when sitting in the sitz bath. Soak for 10–15 minutes at a time, and repeat every 4 hours, daily, if needed.
8. Measure skin heating or cooling ($T°_{b\text{-}a}$).	Immediately after immersion, measure the exposed skin temperature and then calculate the differential before and after treatment ($T°_{b\text{-}a}$). Question the patient about the level of coldness that he or she has perceived during treatment.
9. Conduct post-treatment procedures.	Inspect the treated area for any adverse response. Wash and pad dry the treated area.
10. Ensure post-treatment equipment maintenance.	Follow manufacturer recommendations. Empty, wash, and disinfect (if no plastic liner is used) the basin. Empty the water bag. Discard the plastic liner.

CONTRAST BATH

STEP	PROCEDURE
1. Check for contraindications.	See All Agents section.
2. Consider the risks.	See All Agents section.
3. Position and instruct patient.	Ensure comfortable body positioning. Inform patient that he or she should feel vigorous opposite thermal sensations during therapy.
4. Prepare treatment area.	Remove clothing and jewelry. Cleanse the treated extremity by using another plastic container filled with water at room temperature, prior to treatment, to remove skin impurities.
5. Select the contrast bath.	Choose between commercial or custom contrast baths. A custom contrast bath consists of two adjacent and separate plastic water containers. Commercial contrast baths are now available for therapy. Each bath features two adjacent and separate stainless steel water tanks with temperature-controlled switches. Plug the commercial contrast bath into a GFCI receptacle.
6. Prepare the contrast bath.	Fill one container with cold tap water ranging between 10° and 20°C (50° and 68°F). Fill the other container with hot water ranging from 40° to 45°C (104° to 113°F). A disposable plastic liner may be used with a homemade contrast bath to prevent contamination.
7. Determine and measure dose ($T°_{ag\text{-}s}$).	Select the dose that can induce the desired physiologic and therapeutic effects in the targeted tissue. Dose should be high enough to either elevate or lower the targeted tissue temperature within the therapeutic temperature window. Just prior to immersion, measure the dose—that is, the temperature differential between the agent (i.e., the differential between hot and cold water temperature) and the skin surface ($T°_{ag\text{-}s}$) over which it is applied.

STEP	PROCEDURE
8. Apply treatment.	The heat to cold ratio of immersion is measured in minutes (H:C time ratio). The ratios may be kept constant or variable during therapy. An example of a constant H:C time ratio may be 4:2, 4:2, 4:2, and 4:2, meaning immersion in hot water for 4 minutes followed by immersion in cold water for 2 minutes, repeated 4 times, for a total application duration of 24 minutes. An example of a variable H:C time ratio may be 2:3, 1:1.5, and 1:1. There is no evidence to show that a given H:C time ratio is better than the others, that immersion should begin in hot versus cold water, and that constant ratios are better than variable ratios.
9. Conduct post-treatment procedures.	Inspect the exposed treatment area, and record any adverse reaction. Dry the treated segments with towels. Empty, wash, and disinfect (if no plastic liner was used) the contrast bath.
10. Ensure post-treatment equipment maintenance.	For a commercial contrast bath, follow manufacturer recommendations. Immediately report defects or malfunctions to technical maintenance staff.

LO–HI TUBS AND TANKS

STEP	PROCEDURE
1. Check for contraindications.	See All Agents section.
2. Consider the risks.	See All Agents section.
3. Position and instruct patient.	• *For Lo and Hi tubs:* Use a motorized patient-handling system, mounted with a chair (Fig. 9-1F), to move patients to and from the tubs, and to ensure optimal and comfortable body positioning. • *For full-body and Hubbard tanks:* Use a motorized patient-handling system, mounted with a stretcher (Fig. 9-1G), for the same reason as with Lo and Hi tubs. A fixed hydraulic hoist system may also be used to move the patient lying on the stretcher. Inform the patient that he or she should feel a comfortable thermal sensation during therapy.
4. Prepare treatment area.	Partial-body immersion is from the waist level down. Full-body immersion is from the neck down, either in a sitting or lying position in the tank. Ideally, the patient should be completely undressed. If uncomfortable with this situation, the patient may wear loose underwear during water immersion.
5. Prepare the tub or tank.	Fill the tank with warm water (30° to 38°C [86° to 100°F]). To facilitate cleansing and to prevent cross-contamination, cover the tub or tank with a disposable plastic liner.
6. Adjust water turbine.	Adjust the direction and aeration of each turbine. Make sure that the patient's body is not in contact with the turbine ejector.
7. Determine and measure dose ($T°_{ag\text{-}s}$).	Select the dose that can induce the desired physiologic and therapeutic effects in the targeted tissue. Dose should be high enough to elevate the targeted tissue temperature within the therapeutic temperature window. Just prior to immersion, measure the dose—that is, the temperature differential between the agent and the skin surface ($T°_{ag\text{-}s}$) over which it is applied.
8. Apply treatment.	Immerse the body to achieve either partial- or full-body immersion. Apply for 10–30 minutes depending on the condition and the patient's systemic physiologic reactions during immersion. Monitor ventilation, heart rate, and blood pressure in patients susceptible to adverse reactions caused by partial- to full-body immersion in water. Ensure close patient monitoring throughout treatment.
9. Measure skin heating ($T°_{b\text{-}a}$).	Immediately after immersion, measure the exposed skin temperature and then calculate the differential before and after treatment ($T°_{b\text{-}a}$). Question the patient about the level of coldness that he or she has perceived during treatment.

STEP	PROCEDURE
10. Conduct post-treatment procedures.	Remove the patient from the water, and dry the body quickly and thoroughly with towels. Inspect the exposed treatment area, and record any adverse reaction. Wrap or cover the patient immediately to avoid chilling. Drain, rinse, clean, and disinfect (if no plastic liner was used) the tank and turbines.
11. Ensure post-treatment equipment maintenance.	Follow manufacturer recommendations. Immediately report defects or malfunctions to technical maintenance staff.

LAVAGE WITH SUCTION AND IRRIGATION DEVICES

IMPORTANT: These nonimmersion hydrotherapeutic devices are used to cleanse and debride normal and infected wounds. Because they can spray or splash contaminated fluids and soft tissues toward practitioners, wearing the following body protective gears is mandatory: gloves, goggles, mask, waterproof gown, shoe covers, and head covering that include the ears. The patient should also wear a mask and goggles to limit the risk of contamination.

STEP	PROCEDURE
1. Check for contraindications.	See All Agents section.
2. Consider the risks.	See All Agents section.
3. Position and instruct patient.	Ensure comfortable body positioning. Inform the patient that he or she should feel irrigation suction force and pressure over the wounds.
4. Prepare treatment area.	Remove wound dressing to expose the wound.
5. Select and prepare device.	Select between a *manually pressured water irrigator with gravity-assisted drainage* (Fig. 9-2A) or *lavage with a suction device* (Fig. 9-2B). With the latter device, concurrent suction applies a negative pressure to the wound bed during treatment to effectively remove the debris and pathogens. Use sterile normal saline water as the irrigation fluid. Plug electrical devices into GFCI receptacles.
6. Select water pressure.	Pressures ranging between 4 and 15 psi (207 and 777 mm Hg) are recommended. Lower pressures may not adequately debride the wound, whereas higher pressures may cause trauma to the wound bed. Pressures need to be adjusted to the case.
7. Apply treatment.	Most treatments require 15–30 minutes of irrigation. Irrigate until optimal wound cleansing and debriding is achieved.
8. Conduct post-treatment procedures.	Inspect the exposed treatment area, and record any adverse reaction. Reapply wound dressing. Discard handpiece, tubing, coupler, and nozzle.
9. Ensure post-treatment equipment maintenance.	Follow manufacturer recommendations. Immediately report defects or malfunctions to technical maintenance staff.

CASE STUDIES

The following two case studies summarize the concepts, principles, and applications of hydrotherapy discussed in this chapter. Case Study 9-1 addresses the use of cold water immersion for delayed-onset muscle soreness and performance recovery in a young male athlete. Case Study 9-2 is concerned with the application of warm water immersion and irrigation lavage with suction for multiple burn wounds in a middle-aged woman. Each case is structured in line with the concepts of evidence-based practice (EBP), the International Classification of Functioning, Disability, and Health (ICF) disablement model, and SOAP (*s*ubjective, *o*bjective, *a*ssessment, *p*lan) note format (see Chapter 2 for details).

CASE STUDY 9-1: DELAYED-ONSET MUSCLE SORENESS AND PERFORMANCE RECOVERY

EVIDENCE-BASED CLINICAL DECISION MAKING PROTOCOL

1. Formulate the Case History

A 22-year-old elite distance runner is preparing for Olympic qualification. The outdoor trial is soon approaching and hot weather is present. The intensity of training is very high. This athlete is worried about the presence of delayed-onset muscle soreness that could diminish recovery, thus affecting his jumping performance during the trial. Results from past training sessions show severe lower limb muscle soreness, temporary muscular dysfunction, and elevated creatine kinase (CK) activity, all peaking within 48 hours after training. His unique goal is to qualify for and participate in the Olympic Games. He consults for treatments aimed at minimizing muscle damage and soreness, and at enhancing performance recovery following high-intensity training. Previous therapeutics, including nutritional supplements, massage, and stretching, have failed. The practitioner proposes hydrotherapy in the form of post-training bouts of cold water body immersion. The athlete is skeptical about this therapeutic but is willing to try it.

2. Outline the Case Based on the ICF Framework

DELAYED-ONSET MUSCLE SORENESS AND PERFORMANCE RECOVERY		
BODY STRUCTURES AND FUNCTIONS	**ACTIVITIES**	**PARTICIPATION**
Muscle damage, causing delayed muscle soreness and affecting performance recovery	Difficulty with performance recovery	Qualification trial for the Olympics

PERSONAL FACTORS	ENVIRONMENTAL FACTORS
Young healthy man	Elite competitive sports
Elite athlete	Extreme intensity training
Amateur	

3. Outline Therapeutic Goals and Outcome Measurements

GOAL	OUTCOME MEASUREMENT
Decrease perceived soreness	Visual Analogue Scale (VAS; 10 = very, very, sore)
Decrease muscle damage	Serum CK activity
Enhance perceived performance recovery	Rating 0 to 10 (10 = maximum recovery)

4. Justify the Use of Hydrotherapy Based on the EBP Framework

PRACTITIONER'S EXPERIENCE	EVIDENCE SUMMARY	PATIENT'S EXPECTATION
Experienced in hydrotherapy	*Strength:* Moderate	Patient skeptical about benefit
Has used hydrotherapy in similar cases	*Effectiveness:* Substantiated	Just wants to qualify for the Games
Believes that hydrotherapy can be beneficial		

5. Outline Key Intervention Parameters

- **Treatment base:** Private clinic
- **Hydroagent:** *Cold water immersion using Lo-Boy tub.* Inflammation is integral in the etiology of exercise-induced muscle damage. Cryo-hydrotherapy, using partial-body immersion in cold water, appears to be the preferred therapeutic electrophysical agent. There is evidence that cryotherapy (cold water in the present case) can reduce the inflammatory response to injured soft tissues, minimizing secondary tissue damage, and decrease pain. Because delayed-onset muscle soreness is perceived over the entire lower limbs in this jumper, the use of partial-body cold water immersion is preferred over the local application of any other cryoagents because of its circumferential cooling effect. The Lo-Boy tub is preferred over the Hi-Boy tub because full extension of lower limbs is possible during therapy.
- **Application protocol:** Follow the suggested application protocol for tubs in *Application, Contraindications, and Risks* box, and make the necessary adjustments for this case.
- **Patient's positioning:** Sitting on the floor of the tub with extended lower limbs
- **Water immersion level:** From the iliac crest down
- **Water agitation:** Manual. Patient is asked to agitate the cold water with his hands during therapy to avoid the formation of a warmer boundary layer (thermopane), which could diminish therapeutic effectiveness.
- **Application site:** Pelvic area and lower limbs; patient wearing shorts during immersion
- **Water type used:** Tap water
- **Application duration:** 10 minutes
- **Dosage ($T°_{ag-s}$):** 20° ± 2°C (36° ± 2°F). Because the average baseline skin temperature is 30°C (86°F), this dose means that the average water temperature used for each treatment would be kept at approximately 10°C (50°F)—that is, approximately 20°C (36°F) *cooler* than the skin baseline value. To maintain this average temperature differential during the 10-minute treatment, crushed ice was added to the cold water tub.
- **Treatment frequency:** Immediately after each training session
- **Intervention period:** 20 days, or just before the qualification trial
- **Concomitant therapies:** None

6. Report Pre- and Post-Intervention Outcomes

OUTCOME	PRE	POST
Muscle soreness (VAS score)	7/10	2/10
Muscle damage (serum CK)	900 U/L	165 U/L
Perceived performance recovery	4/10	8/10

7. Document Case Intervention Using the SOAP Note Format

S: Elite 22-year-old athletic male Pt presents with delayed-onset muscle soreness following long-jump training, affecting performance recovery.

O: *Test:* Normal thermal discrimination (5/5). *Intervention:* Cold water immersion in Lo-Boy tub; partial-body immersion (sitting with extended leg); manual water agitation to prevent thermopane; dosage ($T°_{ag-s}$): 20° ± 2°C (36°F ± 2°F); treatment schedule: following each training session, application duration of 10 minutes; intervention period lasting 20 days. *Pre–post comparison:* Decrease muscle soreness (VAS 7/10 to 2/10), decrease muscle damage (CK 900 to 165 UL), and increase perceived performance recovery (4/10 to 8/10).

A: No adverse effect. Treatment difficult to tolerate at the beginning but well tolerated thereafter. Pt amazed and very pleased with the results.

P: No further treatment required. Patient discharged the day before the trial.

CASE STUDY 9-2: BURN WOUNDS

EVIDENCE-BASED CLINICAL DECISION MAKING PROTOCOL

1. Formulate the Case History

A 55-year-old woman who was hospitalized for 5 days for multiple burn wounds after a home fire is referred to the burn unit for hydrotherapy in preparation for plastic surgery. The medical diagnosis is multiple first-, second-, and third-degree burn wounds. Physical examination reveals the presence of partially infected large burn wounds over the feet, left leg and thigh, lower abdomen and thorax, and left side of her face. She reports that her wounds are very sensitive and that dry debridement and wound dressing changes, done at the bedside, are extremely painful. She reports increasing pain when she tries to stand or walk and during facial expressions, including eating. Her plastic surgeon is concerned that her wounds may become infected and that healing may be delayed if wound care is inadequate at the bedside. The plastic surgeon's therapeutic objectives are to have all wounds cleaned, and completely debrided, before he proceeds with corrective surgical interventions. The patient spends a large portion of her day lying in bed. Her immediate goals are better pain relief during wound dressing changes and optimal wound preparation for surgery. She is looking forward to hospital discharge and return to her family.

2. Outline Case Based on the ICF Framework

BURN WOUNDS		
BODY STRUCTURES AND FUNCTIONS	**ACTIVITIES**	**PARTICIPATION**
Multiple severe painful burn wounds	Difficulty standing	Unable to take care of her family
	Difficulty walking	Unable to work
	Difficulty with facial expressions	

PERSONAL FACTORS	ENVIRONMENTAL FACTORS
Healthy woman	Home
Mother	Family
	Work

3. Outline Therapeutic Goals and Outcome Measurements

GOAL	OUTCOME MEASUREMENT
Decrease pain during wound cleansing, debridement, and dressing	101-point Numerical Rating Scale (NRS-101)
Achieve complete wound cleansing and debridement	Sussman Wound Healing Tool (SWHT)
Eliminate wound infection	Bacterial count

4. Justify the Use of Hydrotherapy Based on the EBP Framework

PRACTITIONER'S EXPERIENCE	RESEARCH-BASED EVIDENCE	PATIENT'S EXPECTATION
Very experienced in hydrotherapy	*Strength:* Pending	Confident that hydrotherapy will be beneficial
Has used hydrotherapy in similar cases	*Effectiveness:* Pending	Desperate for pain relief using therapeutics other than medication
Confident that hydrotherapy will be beneficial		

5. Outline Key Intervention Parameters

- **Treatment base:** Hospital
- **Hydroagent:** *Warm water immersion using* the *Hubbard tank plus lavage with a suction* unit. The dry or bedside burn wound cleansing, debridement, and dressing is extremely painful and is now becoming unacceptable to the patient. Although there is no evidence to support the use of hydrotherapy for burn wound management, this therapeutic agent is used today in many burn units. Hydrotherapy, through it soothing, moistening, and cleansing effects, is presumed to minimize pain associated with wound management, decrease wound infection, and enhance wound healing. Thermo-hydrotherapy, using full-body immersion in warm water, using the Hubbard tank, appears to be the preferred therapeutic electrophysical agent for all wounds except those present over the face. For those facial wounds, the use of lavage with a suction irrigation unit is preferred because facial immersion is impossible. The use of suction prevents wound debris from falling into the water tank. In the present case, we have a situation where evidence-based practice is justified based on both the practitioner's experience and the patient's expectations, not by the body of scientific evidence behind this practice.
- **Application protocol:** Follow the suggested application protocol for tank and irrigation devices in *Application, Contraindications, and Risks* box, and make the necessary adjustments for this case. Because systemic body reactions are very likely to occur with full-body immersion in the thermo-hydrotherapy mode, vital signs are monitored.
- **Patient's positioning:** Using the motorized patient-handling device, patient lying supine on the stretcher with head supported
- **Water immersion level:** Full-body immersion
- **Water type used:** Tap water with salt. Potable tap water may be as safe and effective as sterile water or normal sterile saline for wound cleansing (Fernandez et al., 2012). The treating dermatologist recommends that salt be added to water to prevent hyponatremia (low concentration of sodium in blood) in this burn patient.
- **Hubbard tank:** Surface covered with a commercial plastic liner to prevent cross-contamination.
- **Application duration:** Approximately 30 minutes, or until wound care is completed
- **Water agitation:** None; cleansing and debriding maneuvers done manually under water
- **Dosage ($T°_{ag\text{-}s}$):** *For body immersion:* 8° ± 2°C (14° ± 2°F) for each application. Because the average baseline skin temperature is 30°C (86°F), this dose means that the average water temperature used for each treatment would be kept at approximately 38°C (100°F)—that is, approximately 8°C (14°F) *warmer* than the skin baseline value. *For facial lavage and suction:* Same temperature dose. Water pressure range from 4 to 15 psi (207 to 777 mm Hg).
- **Treatment frequency:** Daily
- **Intervention period:** 6 days (until ready for surgery)
- **Concomitant therapy:** Hospital wound care

6. Report Pre- and Post-Intervention Outcomes

OUTCOME	PRE	POST
Pain (NRS-101)	90/100	30/100
Wound culture	Infected	No infection
Wound status (WSHT score)	7	3

7. Document Case Intervention Using SOAP Note Format

S: Hospitalized 55-year-old female Pt presents with severely painful multiple burn wounds over several body areas, including the face, following home fire, causing severe pain and affecting general comfort and mobility.

O: *Test:* Thermal discrimination normal (5/5). *Intervention:* Full-body warm water immersion in Hubbard tank plus lavage with suction for wound cleansing and debridement; tap water with salt; dosage: 8° ± 2°C (14° ± 2°F); application duration of approximately 30 minutes; facial wound irrigation using lavage with suction device; daily treatment; intervention period lasting 6 days. *Pre–post comparison:* Decrease pain NRS (90/100 to 30/100), elimination of wound infection, and enhanced wound healing (WSHT 7 to 3).

A: No adverse effect. Treatment very well tolerated. Pt very happy with the outcomes.

P: No further hydrotherapy treatment required. Patient's wounds now ready for dermatologic surgical intervention. Rehabilitation therapy necessary after surgical treatment.

VI. THE BOTTOM LINE

- Hydrotherapy is the use of water's cleansing, thermal and mechanical properties for therapeutic purpose.
- Hydrotherapy can add (thermo), and extract (cryo) heat from soft tissues. It can also induce contrasting thermal effects (thermo/cryo) on peripheral blood circulation.
- Energy is transfer between the hydroagents and soft tissues occur through conduction and convection modes.
- The therapeutic goal with hydrotherapy is to either increase or decrease soft tissues temperature from its baseline to its optimal therapeutic window, which ranges between 36° to 40°C (97° to 104°F) and 15° to 27°C(60° to 80°F)
- The cleansing property of water is used for the management of open wounds.
- The thermal properties of water are used primarily for the management of pain and to enhance wound healing.
- The mechanical properties of water serve primarily for the debridement of wound and for body unloading.
- The conduct of skin thermal discrimination testing is mandatory prior to the first application of hydrotherapy.
- In the context of evidence-based practice, qualitative dosimetry is no longer acceptable has the sole source of dosimetric information. Quantitative dosimetry, based on reliable agent and skin temperature measurements, is required.
- Adopting quantitative dosimetry in day-to-day practice is neither complicated, time consuming and expensive to do.
- Because subcutaneous fat acts as a major thermal barrier between the skin and deeper soft tissues, higher dosages are required with overweight and obese patients.
- All line-powered equipment used for hydrotherapy should be plugged into GFCI receptacles to prevent the occurrence of macroshock.
- The overall research-based indications gathered from human clinical trials shows the strength of evidence behind hydrotherapy to be moderate and its level of therapeutic effectiveness substantiated.

VII. CRITICAL THINKING QUESTIONS

Clarification: What is meant by hydrotherapy and by modes of hydrotherapy?

Assumptions: You assume that clinicians can exert control (i.e., increase or decrease the effects) over many properties of water. How do you justify this assumption?

Reasons and evidence: By what reasoning have you come to the conclusion that the larger the percentage of body immersion in water, the smaller the dose and the greater the possibility of inducing systemic effects?

Viewpoints or perspectives: You are convinced that the buoyancy and drag forces associated with hydrotherapy can play a significant role in some pathologic conditions. What would you say to a colleague who disagrees with you?

Implications and consequences: Knowing that there is moderate evidence to justify the use of hydrotherapy for soft tissue pathology, what might this imply in terms of its current and future use?

About the question: Is it really important to always clean, rinse, and disinfect hydrotherapy equipment and accessories after each use or between each patient? Why do you think I ask this question?

VIII. REFERENCES

Articles

Abraham E, McMaster WC, Krijger M, Waugh TR (1974) Whirlpool therapy for the treatment of soft-tissue wounds complicated by extremity fractures. J Trauma, 14: 222–226

Ahern M, Nicholls E, Simionata E, Clark M, Bond M (1995) Clinical and psychological effects of hydrotherapy in rheumatic diseases. Clin Rehab, 9: 204–212

Atkinson G, Harrison A (1981) Implications of the Health and Safety at Work Act in relation to hydrotherapy departments. Physiotherapy, 67: 263–265

Bailey DM, Erith SJ, Griffin PJ, Dowson A, Brewer DS, Gant N, Williams C (2007) Influence of cold-water immersion on indices of muscle damage following prolonged intermittent shuttle running. J Sports Sci, 25: 1163–1170

Barber FA (2000) A comparison of crushed ice and continuous flow of cold therapy. Am J Knee Surg, 13: 97–101

Benoit TG, Martin DE, Perrin DH (1996) Hot and cold whirlpool treatments of knee joint laxity. J Athl Train, 31: 242–244, 286–287

Berger RS, Seifert MR (1990) Whirlpool folliculitis: A review of its cause, treatment and prevention. Cutis, 45: 97–98

Boynton BL, Garramore PM, Buca JT (1959) Observation of the effect of cold baths for patients with multiple sclerosis. Phys Ther Rev, 39: 297–299

Burke DG, Holt LE, Rasmussen R, MacKinnon NC, Vossen JF, Pelham TW (2001) Effects of hot and cold water immersion and modified proprioceptive neuromuscular facilitation flexibility exercise on hamstring length. J Athl Train, 36: 16–19

Burke DT, Ho CH, Saucier MA, Stewart G (1998) Effects of hydrotherapy on pressure ulcer healing. Am J Phys Med Rehab, 77: 394–398

Cammu H, Clasen K, van Wettere L, Derde MP (1994) To bathe or not to bathe during the first stage of labor. Acta Obstet Gynecol Scand, 73: 468–472

Chaichian S, Akhlaghi A, Rousta F, Safavi M (2009) Experience of water birth delivery in Iran. Arch Iran Med, 12: 468–471

Chiara T, Carlos J, Martin D, Miller R, Nadeau S (1998) Cold effect on oxygen uptake, perceived exertion and spasticity in patients with multiple sclerosis. Arch Phys Med Rehab, 79: 523–528

Clements JM, Casa DJ, Knight JC, McClung JM, Blake AS, Meenen PM, Gilmer AM, Caldwell KA (2002) Ice-water immersion and cold-water immersion provide similar cooling rates in runners with exercise-induced hyperthermia. J Athl Train, 37: 146–150

Cooper DL, Fair J (1979) Contrast baths and pressure treatment for ankle sprains. Physician Sportsmed, 7: 143

Cornwall MW (1994) Effect of temperature on muscle force and rate of muscle force production in men and women. J Orthop Sports Phys Ther, 20: 74–80

Cote DJ, Prentice WE, Hooker D, Shields EW (1988) Comparison of three treatment procedures for minimizing ankle sprain swelling. Phys Ther, 68: 1072–1076

Curkovic B, Vitulic V, Babic-Naglic D, Durrigl T (1993) The influence of heat and cold on the pain threshold in rheumatoid arthritis. Z Rheumatol, 52: 289–291

Da Silva FM, De Olivera SM, Nobre MR (2009) A randomized controlled trial evaluating the effect of immersion bath on labour pain. Midwifery, 25: 286–294

Dodi G, Bogoni F, Infantino A, Pianon P, Mortellaro LM, Lise M (1986) Hot and cold in anal pain. A study of the changes in internal anal sphincter pressure profiles. Dis Colon Rectum, 29: 248–251

Droegemeuller W (1980) Cold sitz baths for relief of perineal pain. Clin Obstet Gynecol, 23: 1039–1043

Eckert K, Turnbull D, MacLenna A (2001) Immersion in water in the first stage of labor: A randomized controlled trial. Birth, 28: 84–93

Eriksson M, Mattson L, Ladfors L (1997) Early or late bath during the first stage of labour: A randomized study of 200 women. Midwifery, 13: 146–148

Ernst E, Saradeth T, Resh KL (1990) A single blind randomized, controlled trial of hydrotherapy for varicose veins. Vasa, 20: 147–152

Ernst E, Saradeth T, Resh KL (1992) Hydrotherapy for varicose veins: A randomized controlled trial. Phlebology, 7: 154–157

Eston R, Peters D (1999) Effects of cold water immersion on the symptoms of exercise-induced muscle damage. J Sports Sci, 17: 231–238

Fricke FJ, Gersten JW. (1952). Effect of contrast baths on the vasomotor response of rheumatoid arthritis patients. Arch Phys Med Rehab, 33: 210–216

Fruhstorfer H, Hermanns M, Latzke L (1986) The effects of thermal stimulation on clinical and experimental itch. Pain, 24: 259–269

Gogia PP, Hurt BS, Zirn TT (1988) Wound management with whirlpool and infrared cold laser treatment. A clinical report. Phys Ther, 68: 1239–1242

Green J, McKenna F, Redfern EJ, Chamberlain MA (1993) Home exercises are as effective as outpatient hydrotherapy for osteoarthritis of the hip. Br J Rheumatol, 32: 812–815

Gupta P (2006) Randomized, controlled study comparing sitz-bath and no-sitz bath treatments in patients with acute anal fissures. ANZ J Surg, 76: 718–721

Gupta PJ (2007) Effects of warm water sitz on symptoms in post-anal sphincterotomy in chronic anal fissure—a randomized and controlled study. World J Surg, 31: 1480–1484

Hall J, Skevington SM, Maddison PJ, Chapman K (1996) A randomized and controlled trial of hydrotherapy in rheumatoid arthritis. Arthritis Care Res, 9: 206–215

Halson SL, Quod MJ, Martin DT, Gardner AS, Ebert TR, Laursen PB (2008) Physiological responses to cold water immersion following cycling in the heat. Int J Sports Physiol Perform, 3: 331–346

Harrison RA (1981) Tolerance of pool therapy by ankylosing spondylitis patients with low vital capacity. Physiotherapy, 67: 296

Hayek S, El Khatib A, Atiyeh B (2010) Burn wound cleansing—a myth or a scientific practice. Ann Burns Fire Disasters, 23: 19–24

Higgins D, Kaminski TW (1998) Contrast therapy does not cause fluctuations in human gastrocnemius intramuscular temperature. J Athl Train, 33: 336–340

Hill PD (1989) Effects of heat and cold on the perineum after episiotomy/laceration. J Obstet Gynecol Neonatal Nurs, 18: 124–129

Hollyoak V, Allison D, Summers J (1995a) Pseudomonas aeruginosa wound infection associated with a nursing home's whirlpool bath. Commun Dis Rep CDR Rev, 23: R100–R102

Hollyoak V, Boyd P, Freeman R (1995b) Whirlpool baths in nursing homes: Use, maintenance and contamination with Pseudomonas aeruginosa. Commun Dis Rep CDR Rev, 23: R102–R104

Howatson G, Goodall S, van Someren KA (2009) The influence of cold water immersion on adaptation following a single bout of damaging exercise. Eur J Appl Physiol, 105: 615–621

Hoyrup G, Kjorvel L (1986) Comparison of whirlpool and wax treatment for hand therapy. Physiotherapy, 38: 79–82

Ingram J, Dawson B, Goodman C, Wallman K, Beilby J (2009) Effect of water immersion methods on post-exercise recovery from simulated team sport exercise. J Sci Med Sports, 12: 417–421

Jakeman JR, Macrae R, Eston R (2009) A single 10-min bout of cold-water immersion therapy after strenuous polymetric exercise has no beneficial effect on recovery from symptoms of exercise-induced muscle damage. Ergonomics, 52: 456–460

Juve Meeker B (1998) Whirlpool therapy on postoperative pain and surgical wound healing: An exploration. Pat Educ Couns, 33: 39–48

Kelly ML, Jarvie GL, Middlebrook JL, McNeer MF, Drabman RS (1984) Decreasing burned children's pain behavior: Impacting the trauma of hydrotherapy. J Appl Behav Anal, 17: 147–158

King M, Duffield R (2009) The effects of recovery interventions on consecutive days of intermittent sprint exercise. J Strength Cond Res, 23: 1795–1802

Kuligowski LA, Lephart SM, Giannantonio FP, Blanc RO (1998) Effect of whirlpool therapy on signs and symptoms of delayed-onset muscle soreness. J Athl Train, 33: 222–228

Loten C, Stokes B, Worsley D, Seymour JE, Jiang S, Isbistergk GK (2006) A randomized controlled trial of hot water (45 degrees C) immersion versus ice packs for pain relief in bluebottle stings. Med J Aust, 184: 329–333

Luedtke-Hoffmann KA, Schader DS (2000) Pulsed lavage in wound cleansing. Phys Ther, 80: 292–300

Magness JL, Garret TR, Erickson DJ (1970) Swelling of the upper extremity during whirlpool baths. Arch Phys Med Rehab, 51: 297–299

McCulloch J, Boyer Boyd A (1992) The effects of whirlpool and the dependent position on lower extremity volume. J Orthop Sports Phys Ther, 16: 169–173

McGuckin M, Thorpe R, Abrutyn E (1981) Hydrotherapy: An outbreak of Pseudomonas aeruginosa wound infections related to Hubbard tank treatments. Arch Phys Med Rehab, 62: 283–285

McManus AT, Mason AD, McManus WF, Pruitt BA (1985) Twenty-five year review of *Pseudomonas aeruginosa* bacteremia in a burn center. Eur J Clin Microbiol, 4: 219–223

Miglietta O (1964) Electromyographic characteristics of clonus and influence of cold. Arch Phys Med Rehab, 45: 508–512

Misasi S, Morin G, Kemler D, Olmstead PS, Pryzgocki K (1995) The effect of toe cap and bias on perceived pain during cold water immersion. J Athl Train, 30: 49–52

Montgomery PG, Pyne DB, Hopkins WG, Dorman JC, Cook K, Minahan CL (2008) The effect of recovery strategies on physical performance and cumulative fatigue in competitive basketball. J Sports Sci, 26: 1135–1145

Myrer JW, Draper DO, Durrant E (1994) Contrast therapy and intramuscular temperature in the human leg. J Athl Train, 29: 318–322

Myrer JW, Measom G, Durrant E, Fellingham GW (1997) Cold and hot-pack contrast therapy: Subcutaneous and intramuscular temperature change. J Athl Train, 32: 238–241

Nimchick PS, Knight KL (1983) Effects of wearing a toe cap or a sock on temperature perceived during ice water immersion. J Athl Train, 18: 144–147

Ohlsson G, Buchhave P, Leandersson U, Nordstrom L, Rydhstrom H, Sjolin I (2001) Warm tub bathing during labor: Maternal and neonatal effects. Acta Obstet Gynecol Scand, 80: 311–314

Peiffer JJ, Abbiss CR, Watson G, Nosaka G, Laursen PB (2010) Effect of cold water immersion on repeated 1-km cycling performance in the heat. J Sci Med Sport, 13: 112–116

Petrofsky J, Lohman E, Lee S, de la Cuesta Z, Labial L, Iouciulescu R, Moseley B, Korson R, Al Malty A (2007) Effects of contrast bath on skin blood flow on the dorsal and plantar foot in people with type 2 diabetes and aged matched controls. Physiother Theory Pract, 23: 189–197

Pinho M, Correa JC, Furtado A, Ramos JR (1993) Do hot baths promote anal sphincter relaxation? Dis Colon Rectum, 36: 273–274

Ramler D, Roberts J (1986) A comparison of cold and warm sitz baths for relief of perineal pain. J Obstet Gynecol Neonatal Nurs, 15: 471–474

Richard P, LeFoch R, Chamoux C, Pannier M, Espaze E, Richet H (1994) Pseudomonas aeruginosa outbreak in a burn unit: Role of antimicrobials in the emergence of multiple resistant strains. J Infect Dis, 170: 377–383

Rowsell GJ, Coutss AJ, Reaburn P, Hill-Haas S (2009) Effects of cold-water immersion on physical performance between successive matches in high-performance junior male soccer players. J Sports Sci, 27: 565–573

Rowsell GJ, Coutss AJ, Reaburn P, Hill-Haas S (2011) Effect of post-match cold-water immersion on subsequent match running performance in junior soccer players during tournament play. J Sports Sci, 29: 1–6

Rush J, Burlock S, Lambert K, Loosley-Millman M, Hutchison B, Enkin M (1996) The effects of whirlpools baths in labor: A randomized controlled trial. Birth, 23: 136–143

Said RA, Hussein MM (1987) Severe hyponatremia in burn patients secondary to hydrotherapy. Burns Incl Therm Inj, 13: 327–329

Schorn NM, McAllister JL, Blanco JD (1993) Water immersion and the effect on labor. J Nurse-Midwifery, 38: 336–342

Sedgwick Harvey MA, McRorie M, Smith DW. (1981). Suggested limits to the use of the hot tub and sauna by pregnant women. Can Med Assoc J, 125: 50–53

Sellwood KL, Brukner P, Williams D, Nicol A, Hinman R (2007) Ice-water immersion and delayed-onset muscle soreness: A randomised controlled trial. Br J Sports Med, 41: 392–397

Shankowsky HA, Cailloux LS, Tredget EE (1994) North American survey of hydrotherapy in modern burn care. J Burn Care Rehab, 15:143–146

Silva LE, Valim V, Passenha AP, Oliveira LM, Myamoto S, Jones A, Natour J (2007) Hydrotherapy versus conventional land-based exercise for the management of patient with osteoarthritis of the knee: A randomized clinical trial. Phys Ther, 88: 12–21

Sterner-Victorin E, Kruse-Smidje C, Jung K (2004) Comparison between electro-acupuncture and hydrotherapy, both in combination with patient education and patient education alone, on the symptomatic treatment of osteoarthritis of the hip. Clin J Pain, 20: 179–185

Sylvester KL (1990) Investigation of the effect of hydrotherapy in the treatment of osteoarthritic hips. Clin Rehab, 4: 223–228

Taddonio TE, Thomson PD, Smith DJ, Prasad JK (1990) A survey of wound monitoring and topical antimicrobial therapy practices in the treatment of burn therapy. J Burn Care Rehab, 11: 423–427

Thomas IL, Erian M, Sarson D, Yan L, White S, Battistutta D (1993) Postpartum hemorrhoids—evaluation of a cooling device (Anorex) for relief of symptoms. Med J Aust, 159: 459–640

Toomey R, Grief-Schwartz R, Piper MC (1986) Clinical evaluation of the effects of whirlpool on patients with Colles' fractures. Physiother Can, 38: 280–284

Tredget EE, Shankowsky HA, Joffe AM, Inkson TI, Volpel K, Paranchych W, Kibsey PC, Alton JD, Burke JF (1992) Epidemiology of infections in Pseudomonas aeruginosa in burn patients: The role of hydrotherapy. Clin Infect Dis, 15: 941–949

Vaile J, Halson S, Gill N, Dawson B (2008) Effects of hydrotherapy on the signs and symptoms of delayed onset muscle soreness. Eur J Appl Physiol, 102: 447–455

Vaile JM, Gill ND, Blazevich AJ (2007) The effect of contrast water therapy on symptoms of delayed onset muscle soreness. J Strength Cond Res, 21: 697–702

Woodmansey A, Collins DH, Ernst MM (1938) Vascular reactions to the contrast bath in health and in rheumatic arthritis. Lancet, 2: 1350–1353

Woodward J, Kelly SM (2004) A pilot study for a randomized controlled trial of waterbirth versus land birth. BJOG, 111: 537–545

Yanagisawa O, Niitsu M, Takahashi H, Goto K, Itai Y (2003) Evaluations of cooling exercised muscle with MR imaging and 31P MR spectroscopy. Med Sci Sports Exerc, 35: 1517–1523

Review Articles

Al-Qubaeissy KY, Fatoye FA, Goodwin PC, Yohannes AM (2013) The effectiveness of hydrotherapy in the management of rheumatoid arthritis: A systematic review. Musculoskeletal Care, 11: 3–18

Cochrane DJ (2004) Alternating hot and cold water immersion for athlete recovery: A review. Phys Ther Sports, 5: 26–32

Fernandez R, Griffiths R (2012) Water for wound cleansing. The Cochrane Library, Issue 2

Jackson R (1990) Waters and spa in the classical world. Med Hist Suppl, 10: 1–13

Chapters of Textbooks

Hall SJ (2006). Human movement in a fluid medium. In: Basic Biomechanics, 5th ed. McGraw-Hill, New York, pp 479–510

Irion JM (1997). Historical overview of aquatic rehabilitation. In: Aquatic Rehabilitation. Ruoti RG, Morris DW, Cole AJ (Eds). Lippincott, Philadelphia, pp 3–14

Sekins KM, Emery AF (1990). Thermal science for physical medicine. In: Therapeutic Heat and Cold, 4th ed. Lehmann JF (Ed). Williams & Wilkins, Baltimore, pp 62–112

Textbooks

Baruch S (1920). An Epitome of Hydrotherapy. WB Saunders, Philadelphia, pp 45–99, 151–198

Kreighbaum E, Barthels KM (1996) Biomechanics: A Qualitative Approach to Studying Human Movement. Allyn and Bacon, Boston, pp 98–99, 104, 414–446, 451–492

PART III

Electromagnetic Agents

Chapter 10

Shortwave Diathermy

Chapter Outline

Learning Objectives

Remembering: List and describe the contraindications, and risks associated with the application of shortwave diathermy therapy.

Understanding: Compare the capacitive and inductive methods of shortwave diathermy delivery.

Applying: Demonstrate how to apply capacitive and inductive applicators over various body areas, using various applicator arrangements.

Analyzing: Explain how the application of shortwave diathermy induces heat in deep soft tissues.

Evaluating: Argue the rationale for using the capacitive method over the inductive method, and vice versa, and discuss the importance of subcutaneous fat tissue overlying the treated tissue.

Creating: Formulate the strength of evidence behind the use of therapeutic shortwave diathermy, and write a recommendation on its overall effectiveness.

I. FOUNDATION

A. DEFINITION

Shortwave diathermy (SWD) is the use of shortwave electromagnetic energy for heating deep soft tissues. The word *shortwave* refers to the shortwave electromagnetic band, or region, of the electromagnetic spectrum, and the word *diathermy* means "through heat" (*dia* = through; *thermy* = heat). The resistance offered by soft tissues to the passage of shortwave electromagnetic energy causes them to heat up.

B. SHORTWAVE DIATHERMY DEVICES

Figure 10-1 shows conventional portable and cabinet-type devices used today to deliver SWD therapy. The portable model is shown with a pair of capacitive flexible pad applicators. The cabinet model is presented with its articulated arms, to which capacitive applicators are attached. A newer type of portable SWD device, the ReBound Therapeutic Warming System, is also shown in the figure. This device is based on technology originally developed by the U.S. Navy deep-sea divers. Electromagnetic energy is applied using garments that envelop the body part (Draper et al., 2013; Hawkes et al., 2013).

C. CAPACITIVE AND INDUCTIVE APPLICATORS

Figure 10-2 shows capacitive and inductive applicators that are used to deliver SWD. They come in different sizes and shapes to accommodate the treated body area. Capacitive plate applicators are made of either rubber or metallic material (see Fig. 10-2A, bottom). Inductive drum applicators, on the other hand, are made of one or more flat spiral copper coils mounted and hidden in a rigid hard plastic casing (see Fig. 10-2A, top). Also shown are the newest inductive garment-type applicators, with their coils embedded in a flexible fabric, also designed in different shapes to accommodate most body segments These garment applicators have the advantage of delivering circumferential heat by wrapping around the body segments.

D. RATIONALE FOR USE

The rationale behind the development and use of SWD therapy lies in the demand for an electrotherapeutic agent capable of deep heating of large surface areas of soft tissues, such as muscles, tendons, ligaments, and joint structures, while minimally heating superficial tissues, such as skin and subcutaneous fat, exposed to the radiating energy. The scope of this chapter relates to the use and application of both continuous shortwave diathermy (CSWD) and pulsed shortwave diathermy (PSWD) therapy using cabinet and portable devices. The survey-based literature on the practice of SWD in the field of physical therapy reveals a relatively high level of ownership combined with a declining level of use (see Shields et al., 2002; Chipchase et al., 2009). The declining use of SWD therapy may be attributed to several concerns, primarily safety. Emission of unwanted stray radiation during therapy, which affects patients, operators, and other personnel in the vicinity of the device, was likely the leading cause of decline in SWD therapy in the latter half of the 20th century.

II. BIOPHYSICAL CHARACTERISTICS

A. ELECTROMAGNETIC SPECTRUM

Electromagnetic radiation is characterized based on frequency, wavelength, and energy per photon. Several

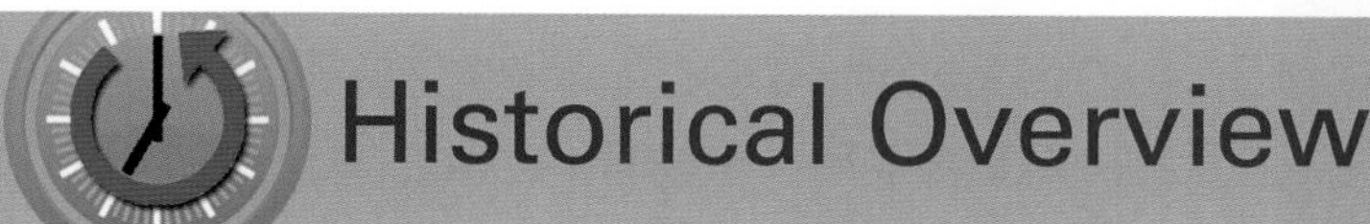

Historical Overview

During the late 1800s, Jacques-Arsène d'Arsonval, a French physician and physiologist, observed that high-frequency electromagnetic currents applied over soft tissues produced perceptible warming without muscle contraction (Kloth et al., 1984; Guy, 1990). This observation led German physician Carl Franz Nagelschmidt to coin the term *diathermy,* meaning "through heating," in 1907. Three generations of SWD devices have been developed and commercialized over the past 80 years. The first generation of diathermy devices, designed in the 1920s, was termed *longwave diathermy* (LWD). The second generation, designed in the early 1940s and termed *shortwave diathermy* (SWD), was built to emit electromagnetic waves within the shortwave region of the electromagnetic spectrum. Frequencies approved by the Federal Communications Commission (FCC) for SWD devices used in clinical practice are 13.56, 27.12, and 40.68 MHz. SWD devices emitting at a frequency of 27.12 MHz are technically easier and less expensive to manufacture; consequently, this is the most commonly found frequency in therapeutic SWD devices manufactured today around the world. During the 1970s, a third model of SWD devices, capable of producing both continuous and pulsed SWD electromagnetic waves, was developed and marketed worldwide. More recently, a portable SWD device, emitting at 13.56 MHz, was introduced on the market. This unit is approved by the U.S. Food and Drug Administration and commercialized as the ReBound System®.

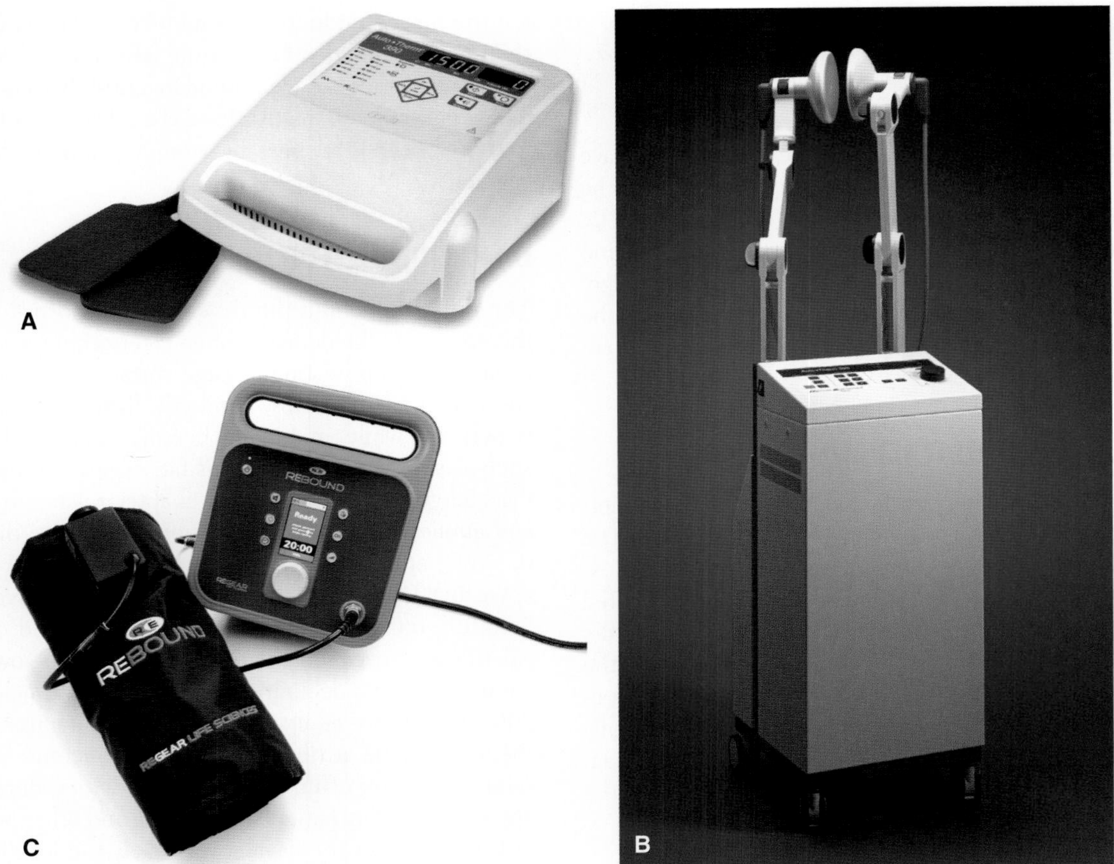

FIGURE 10-1 Conventional portable (**A**), cabinet-type (**B**), and newer (**C**) shortwave diathermy devices. (A, B: Courtesy of Mettler Electronics; C: Courtesy of ReGear Life Sciences Inc.)

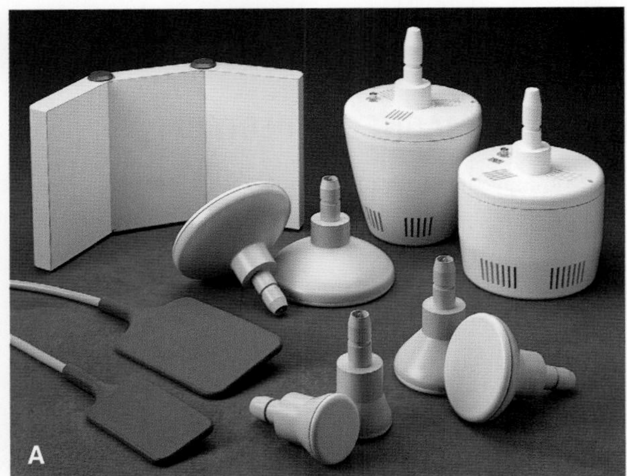

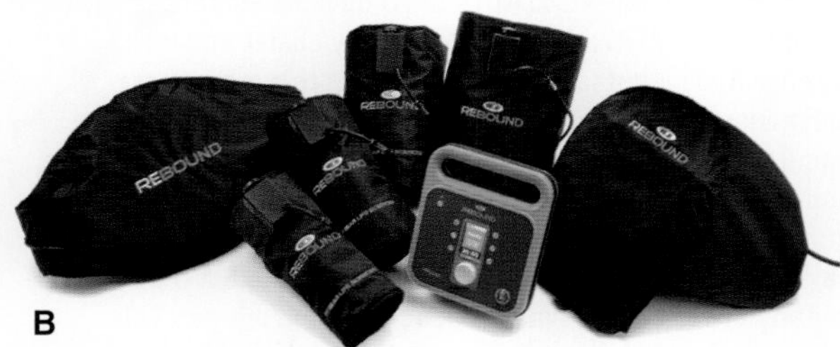

FIGURE 10-2 **A:** Conventional capacitive and inductive plate and drum applicators. **B:** Newer inductive garment applicators. (A: Courtesy of Mettler Electronics; B: Courtesy of ReGear Life Sciences Inc.)

electrophysical agents (EPAs) covered in this textbook, such as SWD, low-level laser therapy (Chapter 11), and ultraviolet therapy (Chapter 12), can be classified based on the electromagnetic spectrum. This spectrum, presented in Table 10-1, shows an inverse relationship between frequency and wavelength, as well as a direct relationship between frequency and energy per photon. It covers electromagnetic radiation from the extremely low frequency to the gamma ray range.

B. ELECTROMAGNETIC WAVE

Figure 10-3 schematizes electromagnetic waves generated from a typical SWD device. An electromagnetic wave is the interaction between an electric and a magnetic field, with each field oriented perpendicular to the other (Low et al., 1994). Electromagnetic waves travel freely in space at a constant velocity equivalent to the speed of light. According to the wave–particle duality found in quantum physics, a photon, defined as the quantum of electromagnetic radiation, may act as either a particle or a wave (see Fig. 10-3).

C. ELECTROMAGNETIC ENERGY

The energy carried by a single photon is measured in unit of electron volt (eV): 1 eV is equal to the amount

TABLE 10-1	**THE ELECTROMAGNETIC SPECTRUM**							
	Nonionizing Radiation					**Ionizing Radiation**		
Parameter	**ELF**	**Radio Wave**	**Microwave**	**Infrared**	**Visible**	**Ultraviolet**	**X-rays**	**Gamma Rays**
Frequency (Hz)	$<3 \times 10^3$	3×10^3 300×10^6	300×10^6 300×10^9	3×10^{12} 4×10^{14}	4×10^{14} 7.5×10^{14}	7.5×10^{14} 3×10^{16}	3×10^{16} 3×10^{19}	$>10^{19}$
Wavelength	>100 km	1 km 1 m	1 m 1 mm	1 mm 750 nm	750 nm 400 nm	400 nm 10 nm	10 nm 0.01 nm	<0.10 pm
Energy per photon	<0.001 eV	< 0.001eV	<0.001eV	.01eV 1.65 eV	1.65 eV 3.1 eV	3.1 eV 124 eV	124 eV 124 KeV	>124 MeV
	Low Long Low			Frequency Wavelength Energy per photon				High Short High
	Use the Online Electromagnetic Spectrum Calculator.							

ELF, extremely low frequency.

of kinetic energy acquired by an electron accelerated by passing through a potential difference of 1 volt (V). The energy of 1 eV is equal to 1.6×10^{-19} joule (J). The main difference between the various types of electromagnetic radiation is the amount of energy (eV value) found in their photons (see Table 10-1). For example, the energy per photon contained in x-rays is much greater than that found in ultraviolet and shortwave rays, respectively.

D. RELATIONSHIP BETWEEN FREQUENCY, WAVELENGTH, AND ENERGY

Table 10-1 shows that the higher the frequency (f) of electromagnetic radiation, the shorter the wavelength (λ) and the higher the energy carried by any given photon (eV). Photons (particles or waves) travel in space at the speed of light (c), which is equal to 300 million meters per second

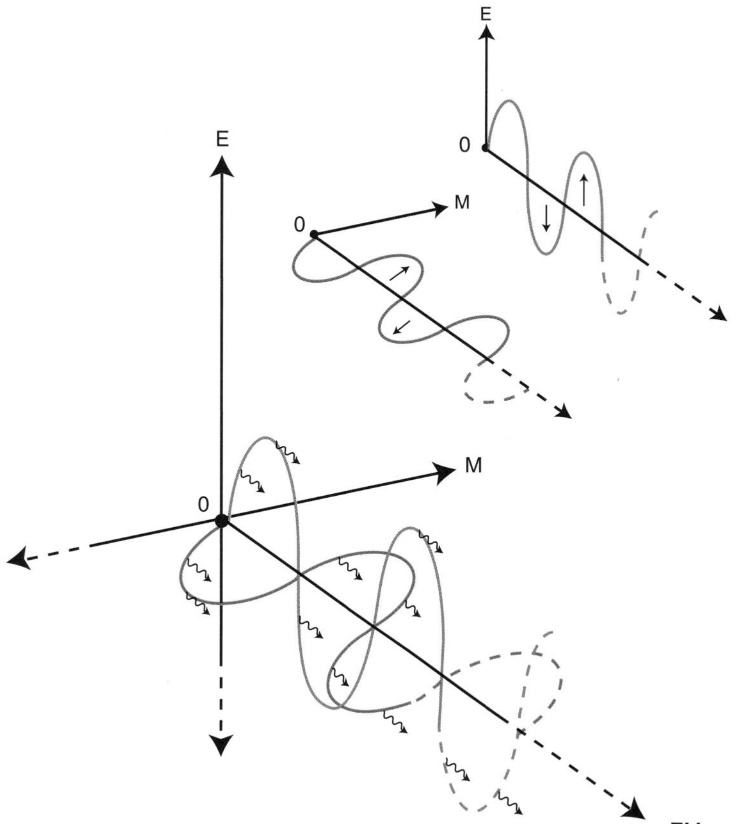

FIGURE 10-3 Schematic representation of electromagnetic (EM) waves generated by a typical SWD device. The electric (E) and magnetic (M) fields are at a right angle (90 degrees) to each other. The variations of amplitude in both fields are sinusoidal and transverse to the direction of travel of the waves. Shown is the wave–photon duality.

(m/s): c = 300 × 10^6 m/s. The wavelength (λ) of a photon is inversely related to its frequency (f) based on this formula: $\lambda = c/f$. The energy (E) carried by a photon, on the other hand, is proportional to its frequency (or inversely proportional to its wavelength) based on the following formula: $E = h \times f$, where h is Planck's constant (h = 4.14 × 10^{15} eV/s). The energy per photon is calculated by multiplying the speed of light and Planck's constant together, and then dividing the product by the wavelength (*Energy per photon* = hc/λ, where hc = 1,241 eV). To facilitate the measurements of frequency, wavelength, and energy per photon related to different types of electromagnetic radiations, readers are invited to use the **Online Dosage Calculator: Electromagnetic Spectrum.**

E. SPECTRUM OF SHORTWAVE DIATHERMY RADIATION

As expected from Table 10-1, and illustrated in Figure 10-4, SWD devices emit energy within the *shortwave* bandwidth of the electromagnetic spectrum, which sits within the radio wave band. Today's commercial therapeutic SWD devices emit at 27.12 MHz and 13.56 MHz, with corresponding wavelengths of 11 and 22 m, respectively ($\lambda = c/f$).

F. IONIZING VERSUS NONIONIZING RADIATION

The types of radiation found in the electromagnetic spectrum are classified as either ionizing or nonionizing radiation based on the amount of energy carried by their photons (see Table 10-1). *Ionization* is the process of removing an electron from its orbit. This process is hazardous for living tissues because it alters cell mitosis, potentially leading to cancerous lesions and cell death.

1. Ionizing Radiation

The Federal Communications Commission (FCC) defines ionization as that with a photon energy greater than 10 eV, of which the energy is equivalent to a vacuum or far ultraviolet wavelength of 124 nm (U.S. Nuclear Regulatory Commission, 2004). As seen in Table 10-1, vacuum ultraviolet, x-rays, and gamma rays are all forms of ionizing radiation than can potentially harm humans. For example, the machines that take x-ray pictures (radiology) produce quantum energy of about 120,000 eV, or 120 KeV per photon. Other radiation machines that are used to treat cancer by destroying cancerous tissues (radiotherapy) are much more powerful, with energies ranging from 2 million to 20 million eV (2 to 20 MeV) per photon.

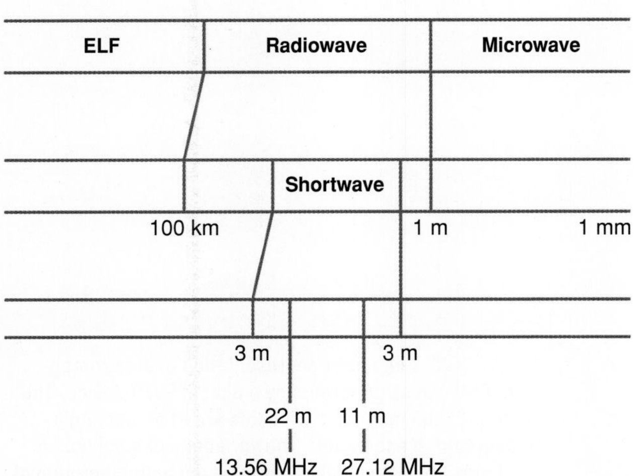

FIGURE 10-4 Shortwave diathermy spectrum of radiation.

2. Nonionizing Radiation

It logically follows from the previous discussion and Table 10-1 that all forms of electromagnetic radiation associated with levels of energy per photon lower than 10 eV, corresponding to wavelengths longer than 124 nm, are nonionizing in nature and thus incapable of causing cellular ionization. Because the energy levels of EPAs covered in this textbook are below the ionizing level, or to the left of vacuum ultraviolet rays, *all* of these therapeutic agents are considered nonionizing or noninvasive in nature.

G. ELECTROMAGNETIC RESONANCE

Electromagnetic resonance is a key biophysical phenomenon associated with SWD therapy. Also known as *tuning*, resonance occurs when the patient circuit (i.e., ions and dipoles in exposed biologic tissues) oscillates at the same frequency as the device circuit (i.e., oscillating current generator), which is either 27.12 or 13.56 MHz. Electromagnetic energy is fully delivered to the tissues only when complete resonance occurs between the two circuits. Resonance occurs automatically in most devices. When it does, a signal, such as a flashing light, appears on the console to inform the operator that full resonance has been achieved. The final power output of the device is always adjusted after resonance is achieved. Resonance between the patient and the device circuit can be lost during a treatment session because of movement at the applicator/skin surface interface. Thus, patients should be instructed to remain still or minimize all body movements to avoid disturbing the applicator arrangement during treatment. It is strongly recommended that the device resonance indicator be checked periodically to ensure that full resonance is maintained through the entire treatment session, which will maximize the flow of electromagnetic radiation in the soft tissues.

H. ENERGY TRANSFER THROUGH RADIATION

SWD uses *radiation* as its mode of energy transfer. Radiation implies the transmission of energy through space. In other words, the electromagnetic energy generated at the applicator's surface travels through an air space before being absorbed by the exposed tissues.

I. INTERACTION BETWEEN RADIATION AND BIOLOGIC TISSUES

When a beam of electromagnetic energy or photons meets biologic tissue, as is the case with SWD, several interactions can disperse the beam. These interactions are transmission, refraction, absorption, reflection, and scattering.

1. Transmission, Refraction, and Absorption

Figure 10-5 illustrates a beam of rays with an incident angle of 0 degrees relative to the normal (N), defined as an imaginary line perpendicular to the surface of the tissue. The beam is transmitted, refracted, and then absorbed by the target tissue. *Transmission* is the process by which a beam of photons passes through the tissues. *Refraction* is the change in direction of a propagating beam of photons when passing through the tissues. *Absorption* is process by which the photonic energy contained in the refracted beam is retained (absorbed) in the radiated tissues.

2. Transmission, Refraction, Absorption, Reflection, and Scattering

Figure 10-6 shows the same beam of rays, this time delivered at a given incident angle relative to the normal (N). A large proportion of its photons are transmitted, absorbed, and refracted within the tissue, whereas the remaining portion is reflected off the tissue surface. *Reflection* is deflection of a beam of radiation from the surface of the radiated tissue. It occurs only when the incident angle is greater than 0 degrees. *Scattering,* on the other hand, is the overall dispersal of a beam of radiation in a range of directions, because of the above physical interactions, due to the collision of photons with the atoms of radiated tissues. It results from the interaction between reflection and refraction.

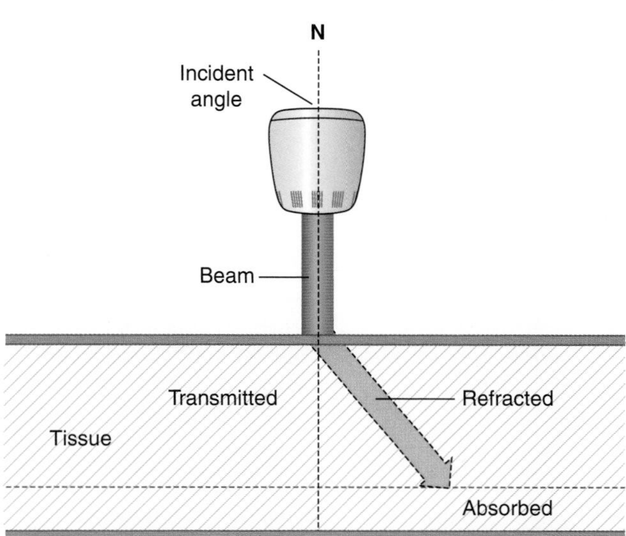

FIGURE 10-5 Geometric interactions between electromagnetic radiation, projected with an incident angle of 0 degrees relative to normal (N), and soft tissues.

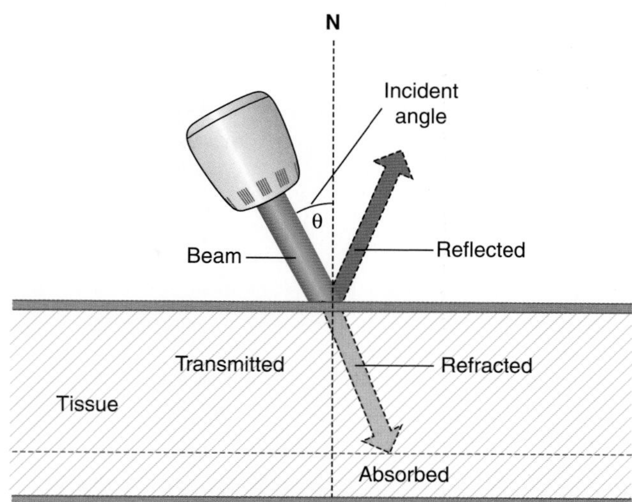

FIGURE 10-6 Geometric interactions between electromagnetic radiation, projected with an incident angle greater than 0 degrees with regard to normal (N), and soft tissues.

J. APPLICATION METHODS

SWD is applied using two methods: capacitive and inductive. The term *capacitive* is drawn from the making of a *capacitor,* meaning two metallic plates (i.e., a pair of rigid or flexible applicators) separated by a dielectric (i.e., the treated body segment). Practically speaking, this corresponds to two capacitive plate electrodes (Fig. 10-2) positioned on either side of the treated body segment. The term *inductive* is derived from the use of an *inductor*—that is, a coil of metal wire housed in the applicator. In practice, this corresponds to inductive drum applicators (Fig. 10-2) positioned over large and flat body areas and to an inductive sleeve (Fig. 10-2) wrapped around a body segment. Table 10-2 presents a comparison between the capacitive and inductive methods with regard to target tissue, fat index, heating depth, and heating pattern.

1. Capacitive Method

When SWD is delivered using the capacitive method, heat will mainly be absorbed and distributed in soft tissues with low electrolyte levels, low water content, or high electrical impedance, such as skin and subcutaneous fat. The greater the thickness of subcutaneous fat in the treated body segment, the more superficial the heat absorption. The use of plate applicators creates a radial heating pattern. The rationale for using SWD rather than other thermal agents is that this agent helps to heat deep soft tissues such as muscles, tendons, ligaments, and joint capsules. Skin can be heated with any thermal agent, and subcutaneous fat is

TABLE 10-2 APPLICATION METHODS

Method	Applicator	Target Tissue	Fat Index	Heating Depth	Heating Pattern
Capacitive	Plate	Articulation Lean body area	Low	Deep	Radial
Inductive	Drum	Muscle Tendon Ligament Joint capsule	Low/high	Deep	Radial
Inductive	Garment	Muscle Tendon Ligament Joint capsule	Low/high	Deep	Circumferential

very rarely a tissue that one wants to heat for therapeutic reasons. Where, then, on the body should the capacitive method be used? This method should be used on articulations with low subcutaneous fat, such as the knee, foot, and shoulder. It can also be used over other body areas such as thighs, arms, and the back if the patient has a low body fat index. The capacitive method should not be used on patients who are overweight or obese.

2. Inductive Method

When SWD is delivered using the inductive method, with either drum- or garment-type applicators, heat will mainly be absorbed and distributed in soft tissues with high electrolyte levels, high water content, or low electrical impedance, such as muscle and the synovial fluid of joint capsules. As shown in Table 10-2, the inductive method should be used if the purpose is to heat the deepest layers of soft tissues, regardless of the thickness of the subcutaneous fat covering them. Using the garment-type applicator, rather than the drum type, has the advantage of creates a circumferential heating pattern.

K. LAWS GOVERNING APPLICATION

Four laws govern the application of SWD. The first two laws stipulate that for SWD to induce thermal effects in soft tissues, a sufficient amount of electromagnetic energy must first be delivered (Arndt-Schultz law) and then absorbed by the targeted tissue (Grotthuss-Draper law). The other two laws stipulate that for optimal results, the applicator surface must be positioned at a distance relatively close to the treated skin surface (inverse square law), and that this same applicator surface must be positioned parallel to the treated skin surface, meaning the beam of radiation applied perpendicular to the treated surface (Lambert's cosine law).

1. Arndt-Schultz Law-Dosage

This law, illustrated in Figure 10-7, states that no physiologic or therapeutic effect (or response) will occur in the target tissues if the amount of radiating energy delivered at the applicator–skin interface (dose) is insufficient to cause adequate energy absorption within the target tissue (response). It further states that small to moderate levels of energy absorption stimulate the therapeutic effects, whereas stronger doses may be toxic and even lethal for the exposed tissues. This law dictates the relationship between dose and response. Practically speaking, this law reminds clinicians of the importance of selecting adequate dosage, knowing that only a percentage of the SWD energy delivered at the applicator–skin interface will be absorbed by the targeted tissues.

2. Grotthuss-Draper Law-Absorption

The Grotthuss-Draper law stipulates that for a radiating energy to have any physiologic or therapeutic effect, or response, the tissues must absorb it. Figure 10-8A shows a beam of rays not absorbed by the soft tissues, thus inducing

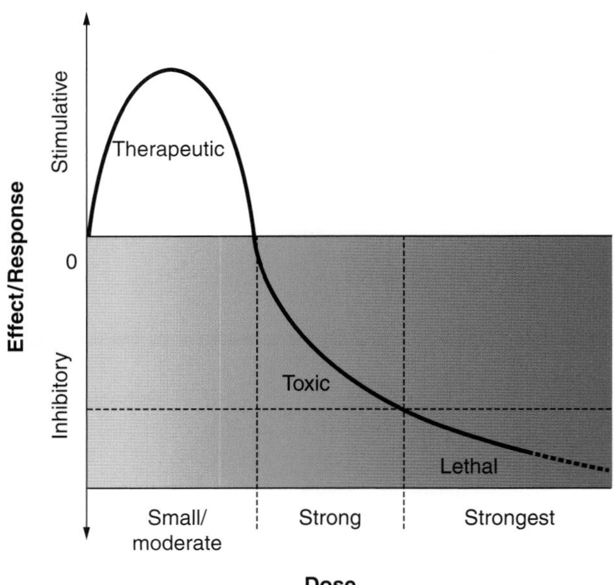

FIGURE 10-7 Arndt-Schultz law.

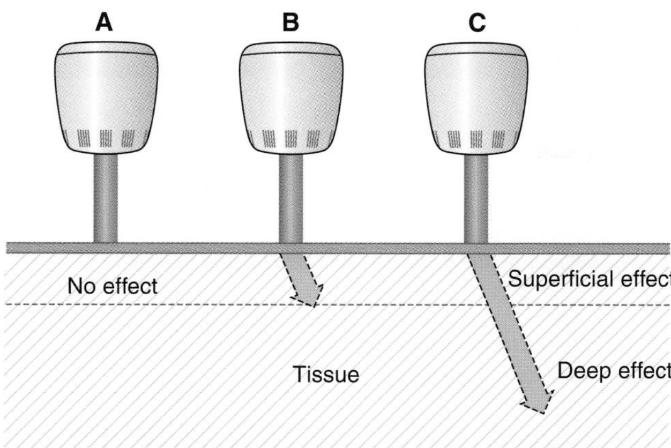

FIGURE 10-8 Grotthuss-Draper law.

no effect. It further states that absorption is inversely related to penetration (or transmission). The greater the absorption of energy by superficial tissues (see Fig. 10-8B), the lesser the penetration (or transmission) of energy in the deeper tissues. Conversely, the lower the absorption in superficial tissues (see Fig. 10-8C), the greater the penetration of energy in the deeper tissues. This law dictates the relationship between radiating energy absorption and effect (or response), and that between energy absorption and penetration (or transmission). Practically speaking, this law relates to the importance of selecting one method of application over the other (i.e., capacitive vs. inductive).

3. Inverse Square Law-Divergence

The inverse square law, illustrated in Figure 10-9, states that the intensity (I) of radiation, or power, observed from a divergent, or noncollimated, radiating source decreases with the square of its distance (D) from the target tissue, as shown in this formula: $I = 1/D^2$. For example, this means that doubling (D2) the original distance between the source and the target tissue (i.e., from D1 to D2) reduces the intensity of energy to one quarter (or 25%) of its original value per surface area radiated ($I = 1/1 = 100\%$; $I = 1/2^2 = 1/4 = 25\%$). In other words, the energy twice as far from the source is spread over four times the original area (A), resulting in one fourth, or 25%, of the intensity per area. Tripling the distance (D3) from the source will further reduce the intensity per area to only one ninth of the original intensity per area. This law dictates the inverse relationship between distance of exposure and energy exposure per surface area in cases of noncollimated radiating sources. A collimated radiating source, such as a laser, does not obey this law (see Chapter 11). Practically speaking, this law relates to the issue of selecting the shortest spacing distance as possible between the applicator and skin surface.

4. Lambert's Cosine Law-Reflection

Lambert's cosine law stipulates that the amount of radiating energy that can be transmitted and absorbed in the tissue is related to the cosine value that the beam's incident

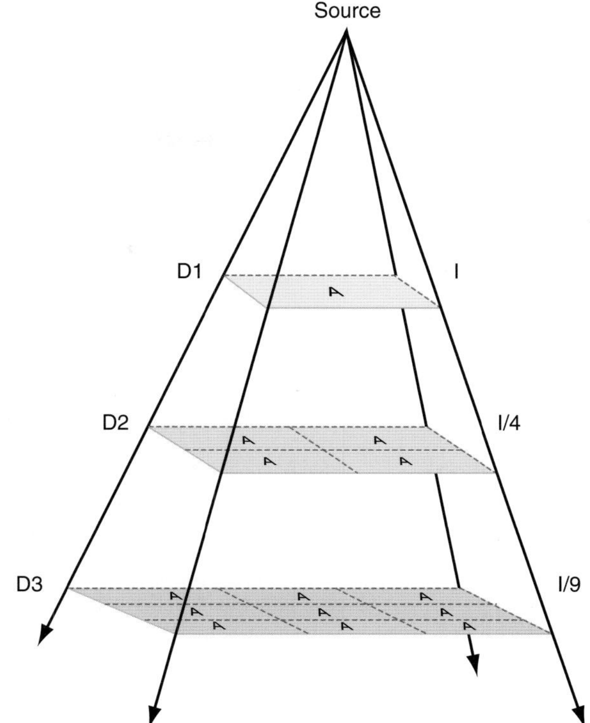

FIGURE 10-9 Inverse square law.

angle makes with the normal (N). In other words, the greater the incident angle relative to normal, the lesser the amount of radiating energy available to the tissues because of wave reflection, as illustrated in Figure 10-10. This law states as follows: Energy available to the tissues = Energy from the source × Cosine of incident angle expressed as a percentage. The examples in this figure show that incident angles of 30 and 60 degrees reduce the amount of energy available to tissues to 86% and 50%, respectively. To obey

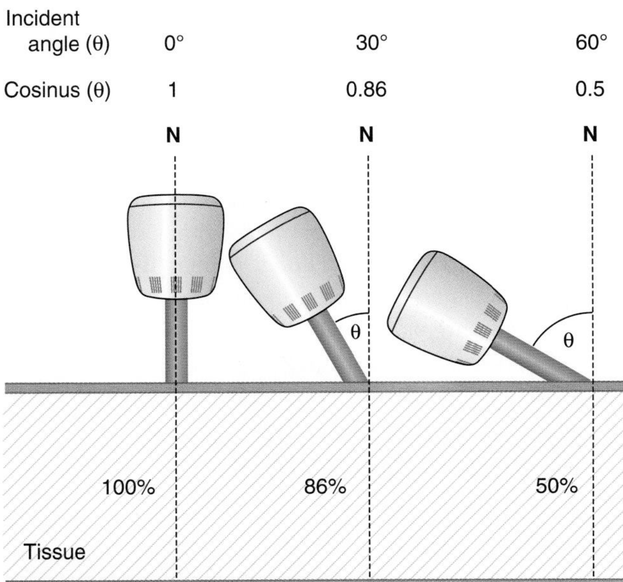

FIGURE 10-10 Lambert's cosine law.

TABLE 10-3	PHYSIOLOGIC EFFECTS OF PULSED SHORTWAVE DIATHERMY ON HEALTHY SUBJECTS
Reference	**Experimental Results**
Draper et al., 1999	PSWD, applied with an average power output of 48 W for 20 minutes, increased gastrocnemius muscle temperature by 3.5°C, 3 cm below the skin surface.
Garrett et al., 2000	PSWD, applied with an average power output of 48 W for 20 minutes, increased triceps surae muscle temperature by 4.5°C, 3 cm below the skin surface.
Peres et al., 2002	PSWD, applied with an average power output of 48 W for 20 minutes before a prolonged static stretch, was more effective in increasing triceps surae elasticity than stretching alone.
Draper et al., 2002	PSWD (unspecified power output) application, combined with short-duration stretching for 15 minutes, was more effective in increasing hamstring elasticity than short-duration stretching alone.
Draper et al., 2004	PSWD, applied with an average power output of 48 W for 20 minutes and combined with low-load and long-duration stretching for 15 minutes, was more effective in increasing hamstring elasticity than low-load, long-duration stretching alone.
Brucker et al., 2005	PSWD, applied with an average power output of 48 W for 20 minutes during stretching, did not improve long-term retention (3 weeks later) of triceps surae muscle elasticity gained.

PSWD, pulsed shortwave diathermy.

this law, practitioners must try to keep the applicator surface as parallel as possible with regard to the treated area. In other words, they must align the beam of radiation as perpendicular to the treated surface as possible.

III. THERAPEUTIC EFFECTS AND INDICATIONS

A. THERMAL VERSUS NONTHERMAL

When soft tissues are exposed to the electromagnetic energy generated by SWD, part of this energy is absorbed, which triggers a cascade of atomic and molecular reactions responsible for the observed physiologic and therapeutic effects. There is general consensus in the literature that SWD induces both thermal and nonthermal effects within soft tissues. A popular view associates the application of PSWD delivered at a low-power output with nonthermal effects in soft tissues. A nonthermal effect is by definition an effect caused by means other than heat. In other words, the term *nonthermal* implies the *absence* of heat. Evidence presented later in our discussion indicates that the nonthermal effect commonly associated with PSWD should be seriously questioned.

B. PULSED SHORTWAVE DIATHERMY AND THERMAL EFFECTS

There is scientific evidence, shown in Table 10-3, to support the claim that PSWD can induce significant soft-tissue heating in healthy subjects (Draper et al., 1999, 2002, 2004; Garrett et al., 2000; Peres et al., 2002; Brucker et al., 2005). Experimental work conducted by two of these authors indicates that PSWD, using an inductive drum applicator applied over a period of 20 minutes and at an average power output as low as 48 watts (W), led to heating human muscles by approximately 4°C at a depth of 3 cm below the skin surface (Draper et al., 1999; Garrett et al., 2000). Four of these authors further demonstrated that the combination of PSWD and stretching, as opposed to stretching alone, could significantly increase joint flexibility because of the heating of the deeper musculotendinous area (Peres et al., 2002; Draper et al., 2002, 2004; Brucker et al., 2005).

C. HYPOTHETICAL NONTHERMAL EFFECTS

No scientific evidence could be found in published English language peer-reviewed studies on humans to support the view that SWD, delivered in its continuous or pulsed mode, induces in situ or in vivo nonthermal effects in soft tissues. Until some evidence is provided, the nonthermal effects associated with PSWD therapy can only be hypothetical. Moreover, the body of scientific evidence presented in Table 10-3 seriously questioned the view, raised by Kloth et al. (1996), that PSWD administered at low power (i.e., less than 38 W) will induce maximum nonthermal and minimal thermal effects. This view should also be considered as hypothetical, considering the fact that PSWD, administered with a mean power output of only 10 W above the threshold value (48 W vs. 38 W) proposed by Kloth et al. (1996), led to an important muscle-heating effect (i.e., an increase of approximately 4°C at a depth of 3 cm below the skin surface). In summary, the current body of scientific evidence indicates that both continuous and pulsed SWD, delivered at an average power output as low as 48 W, are capable of inducing very important thermal effects in human deep soft tissues.

D. CONTINUOUS VERSUS PULSED SHORTWAVE DIATHERMY

There is growing evidence to suggest that over the past two decades, the use of PSWD may have surpassed CSWD as the delivery mode of choice. A possible explanation for this shift may be that the application of PSWD, associated with less stray radiation, is safer for the operator (Tzima et al., 1994). Another likely reason the use of PSWD is on the increase is because a much greater number of clinical studies have been published over the past years showing that low-wattage PSWD can induce a significant deep-heating response in human soft tissues.

E. PROPOSED MECHANISMS BEHIND THERMAL EFFECTS

There is a theoretical consensus in the literature (see Scott, 2002) that the thermal effects induced by the application of SWD, illustrated in Figure 10-11, are primarily caused by two mechanisms: *ionic oscillation* and *dipole rotation*. Soft tissues contain billions of charged particles or ions, such as sodium (Na^+), potassium (K^+), and chloride (Cl^-). When these ions are exposed to the high-frequency oscillating current generated by the device, they are presumed to move to and fro, or oscillate, in response to the oscillating electric (capacitive) and eddy (inductive) current field (Scott, 2002). Soft tissues also contain billions of dipolar, or water, molecules—hydrogen (H^+) and oxygen (O^-). When these dipoles are exposed to this same high-frequency oscillating current, the bipolar molecules are also presumed to rotate in response to the oscillatory current field (Scott, 2002).

F. CONVERSION OF KINETIC ENERGY INTO HEAT

The combined effect of these microscopic oscillatory and rotational movements of particles is the production of *kinetic energy,* which is then converted into *thermal energy* within the exposed tissues (see Fig. 10-11). Kinetic energy is energy that is associated with movement. Thus, the more electromagnetic energy absorbed by a biologic tissue, the greater the ionic oscillatory and dipole rotational movements and, therefore, the greater the heating of deep tissues.

G. THERAPEUTIC EFFECTS

As was the case with the application of other thermal agents (see Chapter 7), the therapeutic goal with SWD is to elevate the temperature of deeper of soft tissues to the desired temperature window, which ranges between 36°C and 45°C (97°F and 113°F). The proposed therapeutic effects of SWD, listed in Figure 10-11, are counterirritation, increase blood flow, increase cell metabolism, increase tissue elasticity and decrease joint viscosity. As a result, SWD is used primarily for the management of pain and wound as well for the management of joint contracture.

H. RESEARCH-BASED INDICATIONS

The search for evidence behind the use of SWD, as displayed in the *Research-Based Indications* box, led to the collection of 56 *English peer-reviewed human clinical* studies. The methodologies, as well as the criteria, used to assess the strength of evidence and therapeutic effectiveness are described in Chapter 2. As indicated, the strength of evidence is ranked as *strong* for osteoarthritis and *moderate* for neck/back pain, ankle pain, and dermal

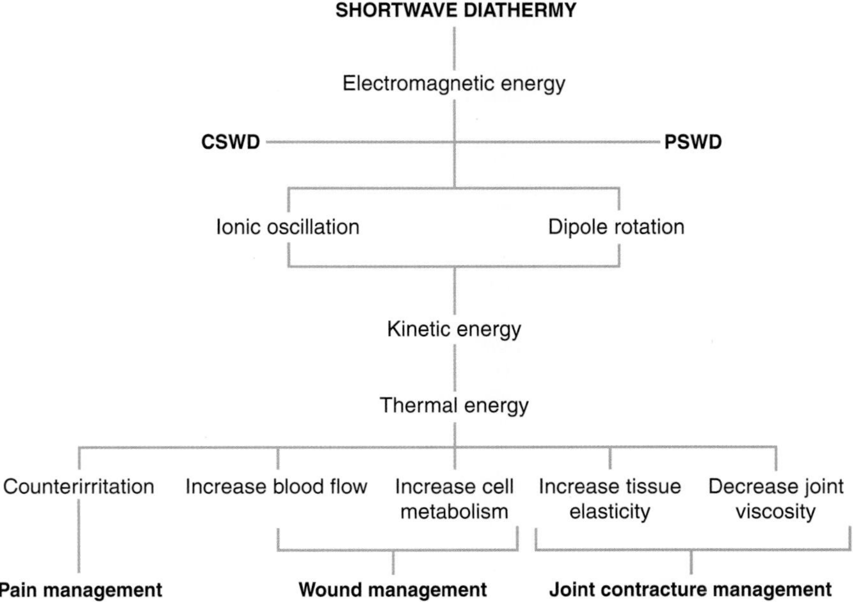

FIGURE 10-11 Proposed physiologic and therapeutic effects of shortwave diathermy.

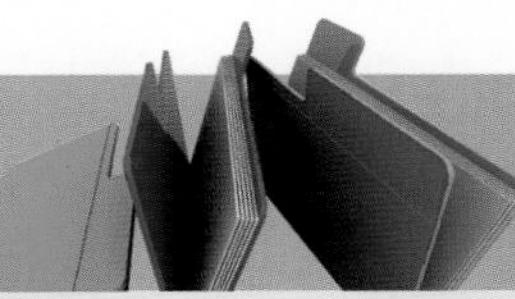

Research-Based Indications

SHORTWAVE DIATHERMY

Health Condition	Benefit—Yes Rating	Benefit—Yes Reference	Benefit—No Rating	Benefit—No Reference
Osteoarthritis	I	Jan et al., 2006	I	Callaghan et al., 2005
	I	Fukuda et al., 2011	I	Klaber-Moffett et al., 1996
	I	Fukuda et al., 2008	I	Clarke et al., 1974
	I	Wright, 1964	I	Svarcova et al., 1988
	II	Chamberlain et al., 1982	I	Moffett et al., 1996
	II	Valtonen et al., 1971	I	Rattanachaiy-anont et al., 2008
	II	Bansil et al., 1975	I	Laufer et al., 2005
	II	Lankhorst et al., 1982	II	Jan et al., 1991
	II	Cetin et al., 2008	II	Akyol et al., 2010
	II	Quirk et al., 1985		

Strength of evidence: Strong
Therapeutic effectiveness: Conflicting

Health Condition	Benefit—Yes Rating	Benefit—Yes Reference	Benefit—No Rating	Benefit—No Reference
Neck/back pain	I	Foley-Nolan et al., 1990	I	Gibson et al., 1985
	I	Foley-Nolan et al., 1992	II	Dziedzic et al., 2005
	I	Lee et al., 2006		
	II	McCray et al., 1984		
	II	Wagstaff et al., 1986		
	II	Ahmed et al., 2009		
	II	Shakoor et al., 2008		

Strength of evidence: Moderate
Therapeutic effectiveness: Substantiated

Health Condition	Benefit—Yes Rating	Benefit—Yes Reference	Benefit—No Rating	Benefit—No Reference
Ankle pain	II	Wilson, 1972	I	Pasila et al., 1978
	II	Wilson, 1974	I	Barker et al., 1985
	II	Pennington et al., 1993	I	McGill, 1988
	III	Seiger et al., 2006		

Strength of evidence: Moderate
Therapeutic effectiveness: Conflicting

Health Condition	Benefit—Yes Rating	Benefit—Yes Reference	Benefit—No Rating	Benefit—No Reference
Dermal wound	I	Comorosan et al., 1993		
	I	Goldin et al., 1981		
	I	Salzberg et al., 1995		
	II	Itoh et al., 1991		
	II	Seaborne et al., 1996		
	II	Cameron, 1964		
	II	Nicolle et al., 1982		

Strength of evidence: Moderate
Therapeutic effectiveness: Substantiated

Fewer Than 5 Studies

Health Condition	Benefit—Yes Rating	Benefit—Yes Reference	Benefit—No Rating	Benefit—No Reference
Postoperative foot pain	I	Kaplan et al., 1968		
	I	Santiesteban et al., 1985		
Neurogenic pain	II	Comorosan et al., 1991		
	II	Allberry et al., 1974		
Temporomandibular pain	I	Gray et al., 1994		
	II	Selby, 1985		
Tendon/ligament lesions	I	Barclay et al., 1983		
	III	Wright, 1973		
Pelvic inflammation	I	Lamina et al., 2011		
	III	Balogun et al., 1988		
Postoperative dental pain	I	Aronofsky, 1971		
Shoulder calcified bursitis	II	Ginsberg, 1961		
Postoperative inguinal pain			I	Reed et al., 1987
Postpartum perineal pain			I	Grant et al., 1989

Strength of evidence: Pending
Therapeutic effectiveness: Pending

ALL CONDITIONS
Strength of evidence: Moderate
Therapeutic effectiveness: Substantiated

wound. Therapeutic effectiveness is *conflicting* for both osteoarthritis and ankle pain, and *substantiated* for both dermal wound and neck/back pain. Analysis is pending for the other remaining health conditions shown in the box because fewer than five studies could be collected. Over all conditions, the strength of evidence behind the use of SWD is determined to be *moderate* and its therapeutic effectiveness *substantiated*.

IV. DOSIMETRY

A. QUALITATIVE VERSUS QUANTITATIVE

Dosimetry associated with SWD therapy may be expressed, as presented in Table 10-4, using two scales: qualitative and quantitative. In the *qualitative scale,* the patient's perception of heat during treatment is ranked according to a four-level dose system (dose I, II, III, or IV). Heat perception is recorded as *none* (dose I), *mild* (dose II), *comfortable* (dose III), or *maximum tolerable* (dose IV). The more heat perceived, the higher the dose number. The *quantitative scale,* on the other hand, describes dosage not in terms of perception, but rather in terms of the amount of electromagnetic energy being delivered to the tissues. In other words, this scale takes into account the actual amount of thermal energy, measured in joules, that the device generates at the applicator–skin interface.

B. KEY PARAMETERS AND FORMULAS

Table 10-4 shows key dosimetric parameters, formulas, and dosimetric examples for both CSWD and PSWD. To facilitate quantitative dosimetry, readers are invited to use the **Online Dosage Calculator: Shortwave Diathermy**. Quantitative dosimetry depends on four key parameters: power, pulse frequency, delivery mode, and application duration. Power (P) is the rate of energy delivered expressed in watts. Peak power (P_p) generated during the continuous mode (CSWD) may be as high as 500 W in many SWD units. If the device is used in its pulsed mode (PSWD), mean power (P_m) is calculated based on peak power, measured in watts; pulse duration (PD), measured in seconds (s); and pulse frequency (F),

TABLE 10-4 SHORTWAVE DIATHERMY DOSIMETRIC SCALE

Qualitative Scale		
Dose	**Description**	
Dose I	No perception of heat	
Dose II	Mild perception of heat	
Dose III	Comfortable perception of heat	
Dose IV	Maximum tolerable perception of heat	
Quantitative Scale		
Parameters*	**CSWD**	**PSWD**
Peak power (P_p)	500 W	500 W
Pulse frequency (F)	N/A	200 Hz
Pulse duration (PD)	N/A	400 μs (0.0004 s)
Application duration (T)	20 min (1,200 s)	20 min (1,200 s)
Mean power (P_m)	N/A	$P_m(W) = P_p(W) \times PD(s) \times F(Hz)$ 40 W = 500 W × 0.0004 s × 200 Hz
Dose (D)	$D(J) = P_p(W) \times T(s)$ 600 kJ	$D(J) = P_m(W) \times T(s)$ 48 kJ
Use the Online Dosage Calculator: Shortwave Diathermy.		

CSWD, continuous shortwave diathermy; PSWD, pulsed shortwave diathermy.
*Case example.

measured in Hz. It is calculated as follows: $P_m = P_p \times PD \times F$. The dose (D), or energy, delivered at the applicator level is expressed in joules (J), and results from the product of power (P), measured in watts, multiplied by the application duration (T), measured in seconds. If CSWD is used, the dose is calculated as follows: $D = P_p \times T$. If PSWD is used, the dose is calculated on the basis of mean power: $D = P_m \times T$.

C. DOSIMETRIC EXAMPLES

Table 10-4 presents examples of those key parameters using both CSWD and PSWD modes of delivery. For the CSWD mode, power is set at 500 W and application duration at 20 minutes or 1,200 s. The dose delivered at the applicator level is 600 kilojoule (kJ): 600,000 J = 500 W × 1,200 s. For the PSWD mode, peak power is set at 500 W, pulse frequency is set at 200 Hz, pulse duration at 400 μs, and application duration at 20 minutes. Mean power equals 40 W (40 W = 500 W × 200 Hz × 0.0004 s). The resulting dose thus equals 48 kJ (48,000 J = 40 W × 1,200 s).

D. ONLINE DOSAGE CALCULATOR: SHORTWAVE DIATHERMY

The qualitative dosimetric scale has the advantage of being very practical and quick: Just ask the patient about his or her perception of heat during therapy and record. Its use, however, requires that the patient show *normal* ability to discriminate thermal sensation, which is not always the case, as well as the ability to be very consistent in his or her appreciation of heat over repeated treatments. Its main disadvantage is that it reveals no information as to the amount of electromagnetic energy being delivered to the tissues during treatment. The qualitative scale, on the other hand, has the advantage of measuring and knowing the amount of energy, or dose, being delivered from one treatment to the next. It has the disadvantage, unfortunately, of being less practical considering the time needed for the practitioner to manually compute the actual dose. The **Online Dosage Calculator: Shortwave Diathermy** can be used to simplify this process. This calculator is designed to lessen the burden associated with recalling those formulas and doing similar hand calculations. Upon entering the dosimetric parameters, the calculator will compute the dose of electromagnetic energy delivered to the tissues. It is important to keep in mind that here is no linear relationship between one scale and the other. For example, a relatively small amount of electromagnetic energy (i.e., 100 kJ) may be perceived by the patient as a comfortable dose (dose III), whereas a greater amount of heat (e.g., 500 kJ) may be perceived by another patient as a mild dose (dose II). Such perception will depend on the patient's ability to discriminate thermal sensation (normal or impaired), the body area exposed, and the methods and types of applicator used. Consequently, this textbook strongly recommends that practitioners use both scales in determining the dose delivered to patients during therapy.

V. APPLICATION, CONTRAINDICATIONS, AND RISKS

Prior to considering the application of SWD, practitioners must first check for contraindications, consider the risks, and then go through key application steps and procedures designed to optimize treatment safety, efficacy, and effectiveness (Shah et al., 2007). To facilitate quantitative dosimetry, readers are invited to use the **Online Dosage Calculator: Shortwave Diathermy.**

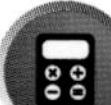

APPLICATION, CONTRAINDICATIONS, AND RISKS

Shortwave Diathermy

IMPORTANT: Because skin thermal damage is always a possibility with the application of shortwave diathermy (SWD), skin thermal discrimination testing MUST BE CONDUCTED PRIOR to the first application. The description and scoring of this test are documented in Table 7-4 of Chapter 7. Illustrated, as examples, are applications of conventional shortwave diathermy with capacitive (Fig. 10-12) and inductive (Fig. 10-13) electrodes, and ReBound diathermy with inductive sleeve electrode (Fig. 10-14).

ALL AGENTS

STEP	RATIONALE
1. Check for contraindications.	*Pregnant operator*—overexposure to the electromagnetic field generated by SWD devices (see later discussion) may be potentially harmful, causing miscarriage and congenital malformations (Martin et al., 1990; Taskinen et al., 1990; Docker et al., 1992; Ouellet-Hellstrom et al., 1993; Lerman et al., 2001). Occasional exposure poses no risk.

STEP	RATIONALE
	Over body areas where sensation to heat is severely impaired—cutaneous burn
	Over patients with electronic implants—electronic interference with the implant caused by the electromagnetic field (Valtonen et al., 1975; Jones, 1976; Medtronic Ltd., 2001; U.S Food and Drug Administration [FDA], 2002; Health and Welfare Canada, 2002)
	Over patients with implanted electrical leads, even if these leads are no longer connected to an implanted device or the device is not turned on—risk of excessive heating in the tissues surrounding the leads (Medtronic Ltd., 2001; FDA, 2002; Health and Welfare Canada, 2002)
	Over surgically implanted metals, such as plates, rods, pins, and nails—tissue burn surrounding the metallic implants (Kloth et al., 1996; Shields et al., 2004). A study on four patients with surgically implanted metals showed that the application of PSWD, with a mean power of 48 W, may be safe (Seiger et al., 2006). This result needs to be replicated on larger populations before surgically implanted metals can be removed from the contraindication list.
	Over metallic objects externally worn by patients and other metallic objects, such as a table or chair, used to deliver the treatment—skin burn if these objects meet the skin, because surface temperatures of metallic objects increase during therapy
	Over cancerous areas—enhanced proliferation of cancer cells
	Over abdominal and pelvic areas of pregnant women—embryonic or fetal congenital malformations if uterine temperature exceeds 39°C (102°F) (Lary et al., 1987; Docker et al., 1992)
	Over abdominal and pelvic areas of women who are actively menstruating—hemorrhagic response
	Over hemorrhagic areas—hemorrhagic response
	Over ischemic areas—tissue necrosis due to the fact that poor peripheral circulation associated with the ischemic disorder may lead to an inadequate thermoregulatory reaction to the thermal effect induced
	Over the testes—infertility due to the increased testicular temperature
	Over the eyes—damage due to increased ocular temperature
	Over epiphyses of growing children—interference with normal bone growth
2. Consider the risks.	*With operator's overexposure* to electromagnetic field during treatment*—risk of miscarriage and higher incidence of congenital malformations in offspring due to stray (unwanted leakage) radiation generated at the applicator and chassis, as well as at the cable level. Current body of evidence indicates that this risk is small (Ouellet-Hellstrom et al., 1993) and not statistically significant (Källen et al., 1982; Logue et al., 1985; Taskinen et al., 1990; Larsen, 1991; Larsen et al., 1991; Guberan et al., 1994).
	Over copper-bearing intrauterine devices—thermal damages to the lining of the uterus (Neilson et al., 1979; Heick et al., 1991)
	With operator's proximity to functioning SWD devices, cables, and applicators—overexposure to stray radiation
	With neighboring patients and personnel wearing implanted electronic devices—exposed to stray radiation causing electronic interference
	In patients who are mentally confused—improper dosimetry

**Overexposure* is defined as an almost daily utilization of SWD devices during which the operator spends a few hours per day working/walking/standing between functioning devices.

CONVENTIONAL SWD DEVICE

STEP	RATIONALE

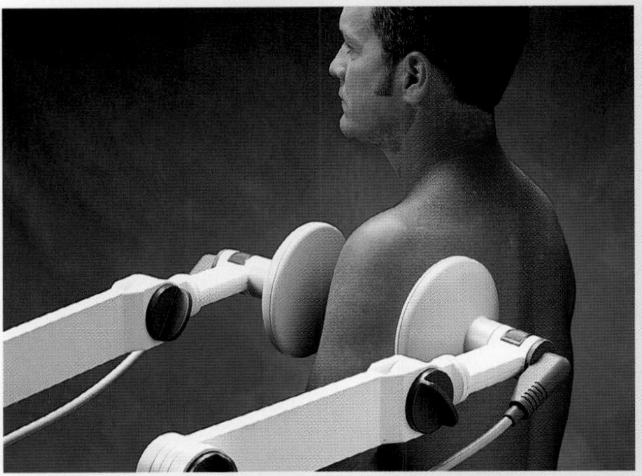

FIGURE 10-12 Application of capacitive electrodes over the shoulder area.

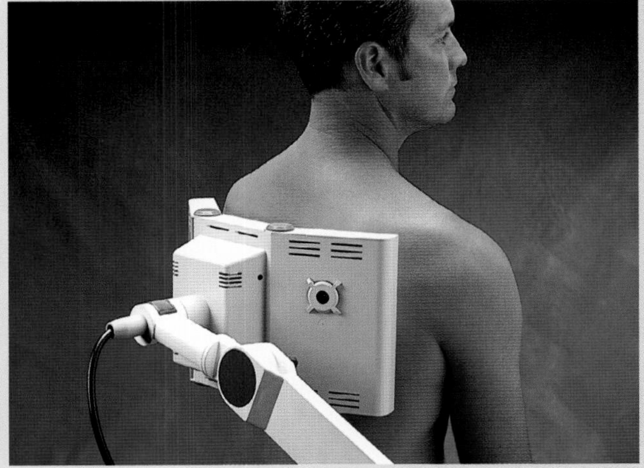

FIGURE 10-13 Application of an inductive drum applicator over the back area.

STEP	RATIONALE
1. **Check for contraindications.**	See All Agents section.
2. **Consider the risks.**	See All Agents section.
3. **Positioned and instruct patient.**	Ensure comfortable body positioning. Instruct the patient to minimize movement of the treated body segment such as to maintained continuous electronic resonance throughout treatment. Further instruct not to touch the device, cables, and applicators and to call for assistance if necessary.
4. **Remove all metallic objects from the treated area.**	Ensure that the radiated body part is free of externally worn metallic objects, such as jewelry and clothing with metal fastenings, and that the treatment material, such as tables and chairs, used for therapy are free of metal.
5. **Prepare treatment area.**	Clean the skin area exposed to the applicator by rubbing it with alcohol, then dry the area with a towel.
6. **Select device type.**	Choose between portable or cabinet SWD devices. Plug line-powered devices into ground-fault circuit interrupter (GFCI) receptacles to prevent the occurrence of macroshocks (see Chapter 5).
7. **Select mode of delivery.**	Choose between CSWD and PSWD. Higher doses are better delivered by using the continuous mode, whereas the pulsed mode is preferable for lower doses.
8. **Select method of application.**	Choose between the capacitive or inductive method: • *Capacitive:* For heating tissues with low water content and high impedance, such as skin and subcutaneous fat • *Inductive:* For heating tissues with high water content and low impedance, such as muscle and synovial fluid The capacitive method is capable of deep tissue heating if applied over patients who are lean (low fat index) because minimal heat absorption will occur in the subcutaneous fat. Conversely, the capacitive method is not recommended for patients who are overweight or obese.
9. **Select applicator.**	• *Capacitive:* Select between rigid or flexible plates. Add a spacer, either a felt pad or a towel, corresponding to a thickness of about 2–3 cm (1 in), between the applicator surface and the exposed skin surface. Spacers are necessary to absorb the sweat during treatment. Sweat bubbles on the skin act as a lens, focusing the beam of radiation and leading to potential skin burn. Adjust spreading distance between the pair of applicators; closer distance creates more superficial heating, whereas farther distance creates deeper heating. Align applicator surface perpendicular to the exposed skin surface to maximize energy transmission.

STEP	RATIONALE
	• *Inductive:* Select between rigid drums, cables, or garments. Add a spacer, such as layers of toweling, corresponding to a thickness of about 2–3 cm (1 in), between the applicator surface and the exposed skin surface. Align drum surface perpendicular to the exposed skin surface to maximize energy transmission. Inductive applicators are most suitable for deep tissue heating regardless of the patient's fat indexes. Recall that the coupling medium is air and that the purpose of spacing materials is to ensure no contact between the applicator and the skin, and to absorb sweating during treatment (toweling). **Avoid contact between the applicator and the exposed skin surface.**
10. Prepare and test device.	Connect applicators to the device. Ensure that the SWD device is located at least 3 m (10 ft) from any other functioning electrophysical agents (EPAs) to minimize cross-electronic interference. Power the device on. Because shortwave radiation is invisible, use the manufacturer's neon check tube and follow testing instructions. If the device is functioning, the neon gas within the tube will glow under the effect of electromagnetic radiation.
 **11. Set dosimetry.**	Use both qualitative and quantitative scales (see Table 10-4 for details). Use the **Online Dosage Calculator: Shortwave Diathermy** to facilitate quantitative dosimetry.
12. Position applicator.	Follow the four laws governing application: Arndt-Shultz (dosage), Gotthuss-Draper (absorption), inverse square (divergence), and Lambert's cosine (reflection).
13. Apply treatment.	Ensure that the device is tuned and remains tuned with the patient during treatment. Ensure adequate monitoring. Inform the patient that the diathermy device will shut down by itself at the end of treatment and that he or she must remain in position until attended by staff. The operator should remain at least 1 m (3 ft) from any functioning SWD devices and 0.5 m (1.5 ft) from their cables and applicators. Minimize operator's body exposure to stray radiation (Stuchly et al., 1982; Health and Welfare Canada, 1983; Martin et al., 1990; Docker et al., 1992; Tzima et al., 1994). Keep neighboring staff and patients at least 5 m (16 ft) from any functioning SWD device.
14. Conduct post-treatment inspection.	Remove applicator. Inspect the treated skin area for any unexpected response. Wash and dry the treated surface area.
15. Ensure post-treatment equipment maintenance.	Follow manufacturer recommendations. Immediately report defects or malfunctions to technical maintenance staff.

See **online video** for more details.

REBOUND SWD DEVICE

STEP	RATIONALE
1. Check for contraindications.	See All Agents section.
2. Consider the risks.	See All Agents section.
3. Position and instruct patient.	Ensure comfortable body positioning. Instruct the patient not to touch the device, cables, and applicators and to call for assistance if necessary.

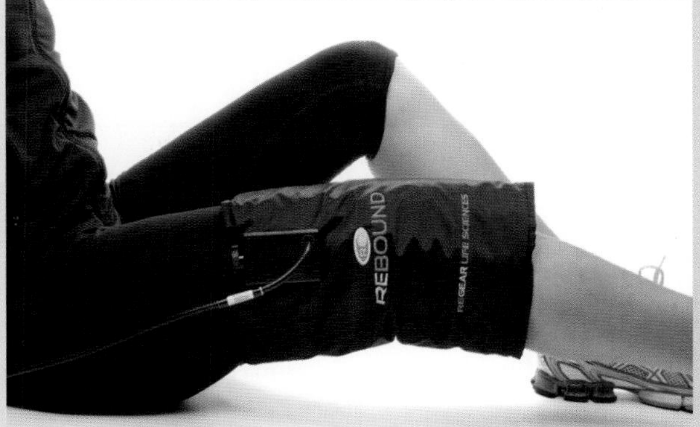

FIGURE 10-14 Application of inductive sleeve wrapped around the knee area.

STEP	RATIONALE
4. Remove all metallic objects from the treated area.	Ensure that the radiated body part is free of externally worn metallic objects, such as jewelry and clothing with metal fastenings, and that the treatment material, such as tables and chairs, used for therapy are free of metal.
5. Prepare treated area.	Clean the skin area exposed to the applicator by rubbing it with alcohol, then dry the area with a towel.
6. Select device.	ReBound garment SWD (see Fig. 10-1C)
7. Choose mode of delivery.	Continuous only
8. Select method of application.	Inductive
9. Select and position garment.	Select the appropriate garment applicator according to the treatment area. Slide the cylindrical garment onto the patient's body part. Allow a spacing of approximately 0.5 cm (1/4 in) between the skin and the garment for optimum effect.
10. Prepare treatment device.	Ensure that the device is located at least 3 m (10 ft) from any other functioning EPAs. Connect garment to device. Place the device on a stable, nonmetal surface in the upright position.
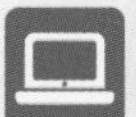 **11. Set dosimetry.**	Ensure that the device is tuned and remains tuned with the patient during the treatment. Use both qualitative and quantitative scales (see Table 10-3 for details). This type of SWD device has a maximum power of 35 W. Use the **Online Dosage Calculator: Shortwave Diathermy** to facilitate quantitative dosimetry.
12. Apply treatment.	Ensure adequate monitoring.
13. Conduct post-treatment inspection.	Remove applicator. Inspect the treated skin area for any unexpected response. Wash and dry the treated surface area.
14. Ensure post-treatment equipment maintenance.	Follow manufacturer recommendations. Immediately report defects or malfunctions to technical maintenance staff. Therapy garments should be cleaned between uses and when they become noticeably dirty. To clean, wipe surface with a damp cloth, antimicrobial wipes, or antimicrobial detergent. To disinfect garments, use a hospital-grade disinfectant. Allow the garments to air-dry.

See **online video** for more details.

CASE STUDIES

Presented are two case studies summarizing the concepts, principles, and applications of SWD discussed in this chapter. Case Study 10-1 addresses its use for the management of an ankle sprain, post-6-week-old cast immobilization, affecting a young athletic man. Case Study 10-2 is concerned with its application for chronic shoulder osteoarthritis affecting a senior sedentary man. Each case is structured in line with the concepts of evidence-based practice (EBP), the International Classification of Functioning, Disability, and Health (ICF) disablement model, and SOAP (*s*ubjective, *o*bjective, *a*ssessment, *p*lan) note format (see Chapter 2 for details).

CASE STUDY 10-1: POST-CAST IMMOBILIZATION ANKLE SPRAIN

EVIDENCE-BASED CLINICAL DECISION MAKING PROTOCOL

1. Formulate the Case History

A 28-year-old man is referred for treatment by his orthopedic surgeon, who has just removed his patient's 6-week-old cast following a baseball-related ankle injury. No surgical intervention was needed, and this severe ankle sprain was treated with cast immobilization. The patient's main complaints are right ankle stiffness and difficulty walking. Physical examination reveals no sign of inflammation, no swelling, a lack of ankle dorsiflexion caused by triceps surae contracture, and ankle joint ankylosis. There is also marked plantarflexor and dorsiflexor muscle atrophy and weakness. The patient has difficulty climbing and descending stairs. He is pain free at rest and when bearing weight on his injured right ankle. His goals are to resume normal activities of daily living (ADLs) and return to play baseball as soon as possible. The treating practitioner, who operates the SWD device, is 5 months pregnant.

2. Outline the Case Based on the ICF Framework

POST-CAST IMMOBILIZATION ANKLE SPRAIN		
BODY STRUCTURES AND FUNCTIONS	**ACTIVITIES**	**PARTICIPATION**
Pain	Difficulty walking	Unable to play baseball
Joint stiffness	Difficulty with stairs	
Calf muscle atrophy	Difficulty with ADLs	
Calf muscle weakness		

PERSONAL FACTORS	ENVIRONMENTAL FACTORS
Young healthy man	Recreational sports
Athletic character	Team play
College educated	Fitness and leisure

3. Outline Therapeutic Goals and Outcome Measurements

GOAL	OUTCOME MEASUREMENT
Decrease pain	Visual Analogue Scale (VAS)
Increase ankle range of motion (ROM)	Goniometry
Increase calf muscle strength	Dynamometer
Improve gait, ability to climb and descend stairs, and accelerate return to normal ADLs and sports activities	Patient-Specific Functional Scale (PSFS)

4. Justify the Use of Shortwave Diathermy Based on the EBP Framework

PRACTITIONER'S EXPERIENCE	RESEARCH-BASED EVIDENCE	PATIENT'S EXPECTATION
Experienced in SWD	*Strength:* Moderate	No opinion on SWD therapy
Has used SWD in previous cases	*Effectiveness:* Conflicting	Just wants to return to full mobility
Hopes that SWD can be beneficial		

5. Outline Key Intervention Parameters

- **Treatment base:** Private clinic
- **Device type:** Cabinet model (27.12 MHz). SWD is used primarily for the management of ankle joint stiffness following prolonged cast immobilization. The goal is to induce deep tissue heating over a large surface area. In this case, the treating practitioner, who operates the SWD device, is 5 months pregnant. Is she at risk? No, because she only occasionally uses SWD in her daily workload. In other words, the use of SWD therapy poses negligible risk to her pregnancy because her work organization shows that she is *not* overexposed to it.
- **Application protocol:** Follow the suggested application protocol presented in *Application, Contraindications, and Risks* box for the conventional SWD device, and make the necessary adjustments for this case.
- **Patient's positioning:** Lying prone
- **Application method:** Inductive
- **Applicator type:** Drum—monode
- **Application site:** Over the triceps surae musculotendinous area
- **Applicator/skin spacing:** 4 layers of towel; 2.5 cm
- **Delivery mode:** PSWD
- **Peak power (P_p):** 200 W
- **Pulse duration (PD):** 0.0004 s
- **Pulse frequency (F):** 800 Hz
- **Application duration (T):** 20 minutes
- **Dose delivered:** 76.8 J, which is equivalent to dose III. **Use the Online Dosage Calculator: Shortwave Diathermy.**
- **Treatment frequency:** Daily; 5 days a week
- **Intervention period:** 10 days
- **Concomitant therapies:** Regimen of ankle flexibility and strengthening exercises

6. Report Pre- and Post-Intervention Outcomes

OUTCOME	PRE	POST
Pain (VAS score)	6/10	1/10
ROM dorsiflexion	–18 degrees	5 degrees
Calf atrophy	–2 cm	–1.5 cm
Calf muscle weakness (deficit)	30%	18%
Functional activities (PSFS score)	4/10	8/10

7. Document Case Intervention Using the SOAP Note Format

S: Young healthy male Pt presents painful post-cast immobilization ankle sprain flexibility and strength deficits leading to difficulty with ADLs and sports activities.

O: *Test:* Normal thermal discrimination test normal (5/5). *Intervention:* SWD (27.12 MHz) applied over the triceps surae area; Pt lying prone; method and applicator: inductive with drum; spacing: 4 layers of toweling; application duration: 20 minutes; dose: 76.8 J (dose III); treatment schedule: daily, 5 days/week, for 10 days. *Pre-Post Comparison:* Significant pain decrease (VAS 6/10 to 1/10), increase ROM dorsiflexion (+23 degrees), reduced muscle atrophy (25%), improved muscle strength (deficit from 30% to 18%), and improved functional activities (PSFS 4/10 to 8/10).

A: No adverse effect. Treatment well tolerated.

P: No further treatment required. Patient discharged. Advise to continue self–ankle muscle strengthening with gradual return to sports activities.

CASE STUDY 10-2: CHRONIC SHOULDER OSTEOARTHRITIS

EVIDENCE-BASED CLINICAL DECISION MAKING PROTOCOL

1. Formulate the Case History

A 77-year-old man who lives in a community aging center is referred with a history of severe osteoarthritis to his right shoulder. This patient is overweight. He complains of chronic shoulder pain and has difficulty mobilizing his right upper limb during ADLs. He spends most of his time sitting, chatting, and watching television. Occasionally, he presents with periods of mental confusion. The patient loves playing darts but can no longer do so. He prefers home therapy. He is well motivated and wants to avoid surgery. He knows a friend who has benefited from SWD therapy for neck pain.

2. Outline the Case Based on the IFC Framework

CHRONIC SHOULDER OSTEOARTHRITIS		
BODY STRUCTURES AND FUNCTIONS	**ACTIVITIES**	**PARTICIPATION**
Pain	Difficulty in mobilizing upper limb	Unable to play darts
Decreased ROM	Unable to mobilize upper limb more than 90 degrees	
Muscle weakness		
Muscle atrophy		

PERSONAL FACTORS	ENVIRONMENTAL FACTORS
Elderly	Social and leisure
Sedentary	Living in a community aging center
Overweight	

3. Outline Therapeutic Goals and Outcome Measurements

GOAL	OUTCOME MEASUREMENT
Decrease pain	101-point Numeric Rating Scale (NRS-101)
Increase shoulder ROM	Goniometry
Increase muscle strength	Dynamometer
Accelerate return to leisure activities	Pain Disability Index (PDI)

4. Justify the Use of Shortwave Diathermy Based on the EBP Framework

PRACTITIONER'S EXPERIENCE	RESEARCH-BASED EVIDENCE	PATIENT'S EXPECTATION
Minimally experienced in SWD	*Strength:* Moderate	Has a friend who received SWD treatment for a similar problem
Has never used SWD in similar cases	*Effectiveness:* Conflicting	Believes that SWD can help him
Wants to see if SWD can be beneficial		

5. Outline Key Intervention Parameters

- **Treatment base:** Private clinic
- **Device type:** Portable ReBound SWD (13.56 MHz). This agent is used primarily for the management of chronic pain and shoulder joint stiffness. The goal is to induce deep tissue heating over a large surface area. In this case, the patient presents with shoulder pain and occasional periods of mental confusion, is overweight, prefers home therapy, and believes that SWD treatment can help his condition. This patient needs to be monitored during treatment to account for his mental confusion. To account for his obesity, and because deep heating is required, the inductive method is selected. Because it is the shoulder joint, circumferential heating is preferred; the shoulder garment applicator is used. Selecting a portable device meets the patient's desire for home therapy.
- **Application protocol:** Follow the suggested application protocol presented for the garment-type SWD system, and make the necessary adjustments for this case.
- **Patient's positioning:** Sitting
- **Application method:** Inductive
- **Application site:** Over shoulder joint
- **Applicator type:** Shoulder garment
- **Applicator/skin spacing:** 0.5 cm (1/4 in)
- **Delivery mode:** CSWD
- **Peak power (P_P):** 30 W
- **Application duration (T):** 30 minutes

- **Dose delivered:** 54 kJ, which is equivalent to dose II. **Use the Online Dosage Calculator: Shortwave Diathermy.**
- **Treatment frequency:** Daily; 5 days a week
- **Intervention period:** 4 weeks
- **Concomitant therapies:** Regimen of shoulder mobilization with flexibility and muscle strengthening exercises

6. Report Pre- and Post-Intervention Outcomes

OUTCOME	PRE	POST
Pain (NRS-101 score)	85	20
ROM elevation	85 degrees	140 degrees
ROM abduction	40 degrees	98 degrees
Muscle strength (deficit)	–42%	–30%
Functional activities (PDI)	3/10	8/10

7. Document Case Intervention Using the SOAP Note Format

S: Elderly Pt who is obese presents with painful R shoulder osteoarthritis causing chronic pain with ROM deficit and muscle weakness, leading to difficulties with ADLs and leisure activities.

O: *Test:* Moderately impaired thermal discrimination test (3/5). *Intervention:* SWD (13.56 MHz) applied over the shoulder joint area; Pt sitting; method and applicator: inductive with shoulder garment; spacing: 0.5 cm (1/4 in); application duration: 30 minutes; dose: 54 kJ (dose III); treatment schedule: daily, 5 days/week, for 4 weeks. *Pre-Post Comparison:* Pain decrease (NRS-101 85 to 20), increase shoulder ROM elevation (+55 degrees) and abduction (+48 degrees), increase muscle strength (+12%), and improved shoulder function (PDI 3/10 to 8/10).

A: Pt needed monitoring during therapy. Treatment well tolerated. Pt very satisfied and happy to avoid surgery.

P: Continue SWD twice a week for an additional 4 weeks or until maximum gains are obtained. Advised to continue mobilizing the shoulder daily, particularly over the 90-degree plane, and encourage to resume favorite leisure activity (darts) as soon and as frequently as possible to maintain R shoulder mobility.

VI. THE BOTTOM LINE

- There is strong scientific evidence to show that both continuous and pulsed SWD can induce significant heating effects on human superficial and deep soft tissues.
- SWD is the delivery of electromagnetic energy, within the shortwave range of the radiowave band.
- Modern SDW devices deliver an electromagnetic energy frequency of 27.12 and 13.56 MHz, respectively.
- SWD is applied to the body using the capacitive and inductive methods.
- Because subcutaneous fat acts as a major thermal barrier between the skin and deeper tissues, the capacitive method is not recommended for patients who are overweight or obese.
- The inductive method is most suited for deep tissue heating regardless of the patient's fat indexes.
- Optimal energy delivery and absorption is achieved when the four laws governing application are applied.
- In the context of EBP, qualitative dosimetry is no longer acceptable has the sole source of dosimetry. Quantitative dosimetry, reflecting the amount of electromagnetic energy delivered at the skin–applicator interface, is required as a complement.
- Using the **Online Dosage Calculator: Shortwave Diathermy** greatly facilitates the adoption of quantitative dosimetry in day-to-day practice by removing the burden of formula memorization and manual calculation.

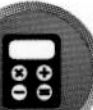

- Thermal sensory discrimination testing is mandatory before initiating SWD therapy.
- The therapeutic goal of SWD is to increase soft-tissue temperature within its therapeutic window, which ranges from 36°C to 45°C (97°F to 113°F).
- The use of SWD poses no risk to the operator's fertility, including pregnancy, as long as overexposure is avoided.
- The overall body of evidence reported in this chapter shows the strength of evidence behind SWD to be *moderate* and its level of therapeutic effectiveness *substantiated*.

VII. CRITICAL THINKING QUESTIONS

Clarification: What is meant by SWD therapy?

Assumptions: You assume that the inductive method may be superior to the capacitive method for inducing heat in deeper soft tissues. How do you justify making that assumption?

Reasons and evidence: What leads you to believe, contrary to common belief in the field, that the application of PSWD at a relatively low dose is capable of inducing significant thermal effect in deeper tissues such as muscle?

Viewpoints or perspectives: How would you respond to a pregnant colleague who says that working regularly with SWD devices poses no risk to her and her unborn child?

Implications and consequences: What are the implications and possible consequences of treating a patient who reports having worn an implantable electronic device a few years ago?

About the question: Is there any scientific evidence in studies on humans that PSWD induces nonthermal effects in soft tissues? Why do you think I ask this question?

VIII. REFERENCES

Articles

Ahmed Ms, Shakoor MA, Khan AA (2009) Evaluation of the effects of shortwave diathermy in patients with chronic low back pain. Bangladesh Med Res Counc Bull, 35: 18–20

Akyol Y, Durmus D, Layli G, Tander B, Bek Y, Canturk F, Tastan Sakarya S (2010) Does short-wave diathermy increase the effectiveness of isokinetic exercise on pain, function, knee muscle strength, quality of life, and depression in patients with knee osteoarthritis? A randomized controlled clinical study. Eur J Phys Rehab Med, 46: 325–336.

Allberry J, Manning FR, Smith EE (1974) Shortwave diathermy for herpes zoster. Physiotherapy, 60: 386

Aronofsky DH (1971) Reduction of dental post-surgical symptoms using nonthermal pulsed high-peak-power electromagnetic energy. Oral Surg, 32: 688–696

Balogun JA, Okonofua FE (1988) Management of chronic pelvic inflammatory disease with shortwave diathermy. A case report. Phys Ther, 68: 1541–1545

Bansil CK, Joshi JB (1975) Effectiveness of shortwave diathermy and ultrasound in the treatment of osteoarthritis of the knee joint. Med J Zambia, 9: 138–139

Barclay V, Collier R, Jones A (1983) Treatment of various hand injuries by pulsed electromagnetic energy (Diapulse). Physiotherapy, 69: 186–188

Barker AT, Barlow PS, Porter J, Smith ME, Clifton S, Andrews L, O'Dowd WJ (1985) A double-blind clinical trial of low-power pulsed shortwave therapy in the treatment of a soft tissue injury. Physiotherapy, 71: 500–504

Brucker JB, Knight KL, Rubley MD, Draper DO (2005) An 18-day stretching regimen, with or without pulsed, shortwave diathermy, and ankle dorsiflexion after 3 weeks. J Athl Train, 40: 276–280

Callaghan MJ, Whittaker PE, Grimes S, Smith L (2005) An evaluation of pulsed shortwave diathermy on knee osteoarthritis using radioleucoscintigraphy: A randomized, double blind, controlled trial. Joint Bone Spine, 72: 150–155

Cameron BM (1964) A three-phase evaluation of pulsed, high frequency, radio short waves (Diapulse) on 646 patients. Am J Orthop, 6: 72–78

Cetin N, Aytar A, Atalay A, Akman MN (2008) Comparing hot pack, shortwave diathermy, ultrasound, and TENS on isokinetic strength, pain, and functional status of women with osteoarthritic knees: A single-blind, randomized, controlled trial. Am J Phys Med Rehabil, 87: 443–451

Chamberlain MA, Care G, Harfied B (1982) Physiotherapy in osteoarthrosis of the knees. A controlled trial of hospital versus home exercises. Int Rehab Med, 4: 101–106

Chipchase LS, Williams MT, Robertson VJ (2009) A national study of the availability and use of electrophysical agents by Australian physiotherapists. Physiother Theory Pract, 25: 279–296

Clarke GR, Willis LA, Stenners L, Nichols PJ (1974) Evaluation of physiotherapy in the treatment of osteoarthrosis of the knee. Rheum Rehab, 13: 190–197

Comorosan S, Pana L, Pop L, Cracium C, Cirlea AM, Paslarv L (1991) The influence of pulsed high peak power electromagnetic energy (Diapulse) treatment on posttraumatic algoneurodystrophies. Rev Roum Physiol, 28: 77–81

Comorosan S, Vasilco R, Arghiropol M, Paslaru L, Jieanu V, Stelea S (1993) The effect of diapulse therapy on the healing of decubitus ulcer. Rom J Physiol, 30: 41–45

Docker M, Bazin S, Dyson M, Kirk DC, Kitchen S, Low J, Simpson G (1992) Guidelines for the safe use of continuous shortwave therapy equipment. Physiotherapy, 78: 755–757

Draper DO, Castro JL, Feland B, Schulties S, Egget D (2004) Shortwave diathermy and prolonged stretching increase hamstring flexibility more than prolonged stretching alone. J Orthop Sports Phys Ther, 34: 13–30

Draper DO, Hawkes AR, Johnson AW, Diede Mt, Rigby JH (2013) Muscle heating with Megapulse II shortwave diathermy and ReBound diathermy. J Athl Train, 48: 477–482

Draper DO, Knight K, Fujiwara T, Castel JC (1999) Temperature change in human muscle during and after pulsed shortwave diathermy. J Orthop Sports Phys Ther, 29: 13–22

Draper DO, Miner L, Knight KL, Ricard MD (2002) The carry-over effects of diathermy and stretching in developing hamstring flexibility. J Athl Train, 37: 37–42

Dziedzic K, Hill J, Lewis MS, Sim J, Daniels J, Hay EM (2005) Effectiveness of manual therapy or pulsed shortwave diathermy in addition to advice and exercise for neck disorders: A pragmatic randomized controlled trial in physical therapy clinics. Arthritis Rheum, 53: 214–222

Foley-Nolan D, Barry C, Coughlan RJ, O'Connor P, Roden D (1990) Pulsed high frequency (27 MHz) electromagnetic therapy for persistent neck pain. A double blind, placebo-controlled study of 20 patients. Orthopedics, 13: 445–451

Foley-Nolan D, Moore K, Codd M, Barry C, O'Connor P, Coughlan RJ (1992) Low energy high frequency pulsed electromagnetic therapy for acute whiplash injuries. Scand J Rehab Med, 24: 51–59

Fukuda TY, Alves da Cunha R, Fukuda VO, Rienzo FA, Cazarini C, Carvalho NAA, Cenrini AA (2011) Pulsed shortwave treatment in women with knee osteoarthritis: A multicenter, randomized placebo-controlled clinical trial. Phys Ther, 91: 1009–1017

Fukuda TY, Ovanessian V, Alves da Cunha R (2008) Pulse short wave effects in pain and function in patients with knee osteoarthritis. J Appl Res, 15: 421–427

Garrett CL, Draper DO, Knight KL, Durrant E (2000) Heat distribution in the lower leg from pulsed short wave diathermy and ultrasound treatments. J Athl Train, 35: 50–55

Gibson T, Grahame R, Harkness J, Woo P, Blagrave P, Hills R (1985) Controlled comparison of shortwave diathermy treatment with osteopathic treatment in non-specific low back pain. Lancet, 1(8440): 1258–1261

Ginsberg AJ (1961) Pulsed shortwave in treatment of bursitis with calcification. Int Rec Med, 174: 71–75

Goldin JH, Broadbent NR, Nancarrow JD, Marshall T (1981) The effects of Diapulse on the healing of wounds: A double blind randomized controlled trial in man. Br J Plast Surg, 34: 267–270

Grant A, Sleep J, McIntosh M, Ashurst H (1989) Ultrasound and pulsed electromagnetic energy treatment for the perineal trauma: A randomized placebo-controlled trial. Br J Obstet Gynaecol, 96: 434–439

Gray RJ, Quayle, AA, Hall CA, Schofield MA (1994) Physiotherapy in the treatment of temporomandibular joint disorders: A comparative study of four treatment methods. Br Dent J, 176: 257–261

Guberan E, Campana A, Faval P, Guberan M, Sweetnam PM, Tuyn JW, Usel M (1994) Gender ratio of offspring and exposure to shortwave radiation among female physiotherapists. Scand J Work Environ Health, 20: 345–348

Hawkes AR, Draper DO, Johnson AW, Diede MT, Rigby JH (2013) Heating capacity of ReBound shortwave diathermy and moist hot packs at superficial depths. J Athl Train, 48: 471–476

Heick A, Esperson T, Pedersen HL, Raahauge J (1991) Is diathermy safe in women with copper-bearing IUDs? Acta Obstet Gynecol Scand, 70: 153–155

Itoh M, Montemayor JS, Matsumoto E, Eason A, Lee MH, Folk FS (1991) Accelerated wound healing of pressure ulcers by pulsed high peak power electromagnetic energy (Diapulse). Decubitus, 4: 24–25

Jan MH, Chai HM, Wang CL, Lin YF, Tsai LY (2006) Effects of repetitive shortwave diathermy for reducing synovitis in patients with knee osteoarthritis: An ultrasonic study. Phys Ther, 86: 236–244

Jan MH, Lai JS (1991) The effect of physiotherapy on osteoarthritic knees of females. J Formos Med Assoc, 90: 1008–1013

Jones SL (1976) Electromagnetic field interference and cardiac pacemakers. Phys Ther, 56: 1013–1018

Källen B, Malmquist G, Moritz U (1982) Delivery outcome among physiotherapists in Sweden. Is nonionizing radiation a fetal hazard? Arch Environ Health, 37: 81–85

Kaplan EG, Weinstock RE (1968) Clinical evaluation of Diapulse as adjunctive therapy following foot surgery. J Am Podiatr Assoc, 58: 218–221

Klaber-Moffett JA, Richardson PH, Frost H, Osborn A (1996) A placebo-controlled double-blind trial to evaluate the effectiveness of pulsed shortwave therapy for osteoarthritic hip and knee pain. Pain, 67: 121–127

Lamina S, Hanif S, Gagarawa YS (2011) Short wave diathermy in the symptomatic management of chronic pelvic inflammatory disease pain: A randomized controlled trial. Physioth Res Int, 16: 50–56

Lankhorst GJ, van de Stadt RJ, van der Korst JK, Hinlopen-Bonrath E, Griffioen FM, de Boer W (1982) Relationship of isometric knee extension torque and functional variables in osteoarthrosis of the knee. Scand J Rehab Med, 14: 7–10

Larsen AI (1991) Congenital malformations and exposure to high-frequency electromagnetic radiation among Danish physiotherapists. Scand J Work Environ Health, 17: 318–323

Larsen AI, Olsen J, Svane O (1991) Gender-specific reproductive outcome and exposure to high-frequency electromagnetic radiation among physiotherapists. Scand J Work Environ Health, 17: 324–329

Lary J, Conover D (1987) Teratogenic effects of radiofrequency radiation. IEEE Eng Med Biol Mag, 6: 42–46

Laufer Y, Zillberman R, Porat R, Nahir AM (2005) Effects of pulsed short-wave diathermy on pain and function of subjects with osteoarthritis of the knee: A placebo-controlled double-blind clinical trial. Clin Rehabil, 19: 255–263

Lee PB, Kim YC, Lim YJ, Lee CJ, Choi SS, Park SH, Lee JG, Lee SC (2006) Efficacy of pulsed electromagnetic therapy for chronic lower back pain: A randomized, double-blind, placebo-controlled study. J Int Med Res, 34: 160–167

Lerman Y, Jacubovich R, Green MS (2001) Pregnancy outcome following exposure to shortwaves among female physiotherapist in Israel. Am J Ind Med, 39: 499–504

Logue JN, Hamburger S, Silverman PM, Chiacchierini RP (1985) Congenital anomalies and paternal occupational exposure to shortwave, microwave, infrared and acoustic radiation. J Occup Med, 27: 451–452

Martin CJ, McCallum HM, Heaton B (1990) An evaluation of radiofrequency exposure from therapeutic diathermy equipment in the light of current recommendations. Clin Phys Physiol Meas, 11: 53–63

McCray RE, Patton NJ (1984) Pain relief at trigger points: A comparison of moist heat and shortwave diathermy. J Orthop Sports Phys Ther, 51: 175–178

McGill SN (1988) The effect of pulsed shortwave therapy on lateral ligament sprain of the ankle. N Z J Physiother, 10: 21–24

Moffett JA, Richardson PH, Frost H, Osborn A (1996) A placebo controlled double blind trial to evaluate the effectiveness of pulsed wave therapy for osteoarthritis hip and knee pain. Pain, 67: 121–127

Neilson NC, Hansen R, Laesen T (1979) Heat induction in copper-bearing IUDs during shortwave diathermy. Acta Obstet Gynecol Scand, 58: 495

Nicolle FV, Bentall RM (1982) The use of radiofrequency pulsed energy in the control of postoperative reaction to blepharoplasty. Aesthetic Plast Surg, 6: 169–171

Ouellet-Hellstrom R, Stewart WF (1993) Miscarriages among female physical therapists who report using radio- and microwave-frequency electromagnetic radiation. Am J Epidemiol, 138: 775–786

Pasila M, Visuri T, Sundholm A (1978) Pulsating shortwave diathermy: Value in the treatment of recent ankle and foot sprains. Arch Phys Med Rehab, 59: 383–386

Pennington GM, Danley DL, Sumko MH, Bucknell A, Nelson JH (1993) Pulsed, non-thermal, high-frequency electromagnetic energy (DIAPULSE) in the treatment of grade I and II ankle sprains. Mil Med, 158: 101–104

Peres SE, Draper DO, Knight KL, Ricard MD (2002) Pulse shortwave diathermy and prolonged long-duration stretching increase dorsiflexion range of motion more than identical stretching without diathermy. J Athl Train, 37: 43–50

Quirk AS, Newman RJ, Newman KJ (1985) An evaluation of interferential therapy, shortwave diathermy and exercise in treatment of osteoarthritis of the knee. Physiotherapy, 71: 55–57

Rattanachaiyanont M, Kuptniratsaikul V (2008) No additional benefit of shortwave diathermy over exercise program for knee osteoarthritis in peri-/post-menopausal women: An equivalence trial. Osteoarthritis Cartilage, 16: 823–828

Reed MW, Bickerstaff DR, Hayne CR, Wyman A, Davies J (1987) Pain relief after inguinal herniorrhaphy. Ineffectiveness of pulsed electromagnetic energy. Br J Clin Pract, 41: 782–784

Salzberg CA, Cooper-Vastola SA, Perez F, Viehbeck MG, Byrne DW (1995) The effects of non-thermal pulsed electromagnetic energy on wound healing of pressure ulcers in spinal-cord-injures patients: A randomized. double-blind study. Ostomy Wound Manage, 41: 42–44

Santiesteban AJ, Grant C (1985) Post-surgical effect of pulsed shortwave therapy. J Am Podiat Med, 75: 306–309

Seaborne D, Quirion-De Girardi C, Rousseau M, Rivest M, Lambert J (1996) The treatment of pressure sores using pulsed electromagnetic energy (PEME). Physiother Can, 48: 131–137

Seiger C, Draper DO (2006) Use of pulsed shortwave diathermy and joint mobilization to increase ankle range of motion in the presence of surgical implanted metal: A case series. J Orthop Sports Phys Ther, 36: 669–677

Selby A (1985) Physiotherapy in the management of temporomandibular joint disorders. Austr Dent J, 30: 273–280

Shah SG, Farrow A (2007) Investigation of practices and procedures in the use of therapeutic diathermy: A study from the physiotherapist's health and safety perspectives. Physioth Res Int, 12: 228–241

Shakoor MA, Rahman MS, Moyeenuzzarman M (2008) Effects of deep heat therapy on the patients with chronic low back pain. Mymensingh Med J, 17: S32–S36

Shields N, Gormley J, O'Hare N (2004) Short-wave diathermy: Current clinical and safety practices. Physioth Res Int, 7: 191–202

Stuchly MA, Repacholi MH, Lecuyer DW, Mann RD (1982) Exposure to the operator and patient during shortwave diathermy treatments. Health Physics, 42: 341–366

Svarcova J, Trnavsky K, Zvarova J (1988) The influence of ultrasound, galvanic currents and shortwave diathermy on pain intensity in patients with osteoarthritis. Scand J Rheumatol Suppl, 67: 83–85

Taskinen H, Kyyronen P, Hemminki K (1990) Effects of ultrasound, shortwave, and physical exertion on pregnancy outcome in physiotherapists. J Epidemiol Community Health, 44: 196–201

Tzima E, Martin CJ (1994) An evaluation of safe practices to restrict exposure to electric and magnetic fields from therapeutic and surgical diathermy equipment. Physiol Meas, 15: 201–206

Valtonen EJ, Alaranta H (1971) Comparative clinical study of the effect of shortwave and longwave diathermy on osteoarthritis of the knee and hip. Scand J Rehab Med, 3: 109–112

Valtonen EJ, Lilius HG, Tiula C (1975) Disturbances in the function of cardiac pacemakers by shortwave and microwave diathermies and pulsed high frequency currents. Ann Clin Gynaecol Fenn, 64: 284–287

Wagstaff P, Wagstaff S, Downey M (1986) A pilot study to compare the efficacy of continuous and pulsed magnetic energy (shortwave diathermy) on the relief of low back pain. Physiotherapy, 72: 563–566

Wilson DH (1972) Treatment of soft tissue injuries by pulsed electrical energy. Br Med J, 2: 269–270

Wilson DH (1974) Comparison of shortwave diathermy and pulsed electromagnetic energy in treatment of soft tissue injuries. Physiotherapy, 60: 309–310

Wright GG (1973) Treatment of soft tissue and ligamentous injuries in professional footballers. Physiotherapy, 59: 385–387

Wright V (1964) Treatment of osteoarthritis of the knees. Ann Rheum Dis, 23: 389–391

Review Articles

Shields N, Gormley J, O'Hare N (2002) Short-wave diathermy: Current clinical and safety practice. Physiother Res Int, 7: 191–2002

Shields N, O'Hare N, Gormley J (2004) Contraindications to shortwave diathermy: Survey of Irish physiotherapists. Physiotherapy, 90: 42–53

Chapters of Textbooks

Guy AW (1990) Biophysics of high-frequency currents and electromagnetic radiation. In: Therapeutic Heat and Cold, 4th ed. Lehmann JF (Ed). Williams & Wilkins, Baltimore, pp 179–236

Kloth LC, Ziskin MC. (1996). Diathermy and pulsed radio frequency radiation. In: Thermal Agents in Rehabilitation, 3rd ed. Michlovitz SL (Ed). FA Davis, Philadelphia, pp 213–254

Low J, Reed A (1994) Waves. In: Physical Principles Explained. Butterworth-Heinemann, London, p 33

Scott S. (2002). Diathermy. In: Electrotherapy Evidence-Based Practice, 11th ed. Kitchen S, Bazin S (Eds). Churchill Livingstone, London, pp 145–165

Monographs

Fact Sheet on Biological Effects of Radiation. Publication date December 2004. The U.S. Nuclear Regulatory Commission (NRC). Retrieved 2010-12-04

Food and Drug Administration (FDA) (2002) Public Health Notification: Diathermy interaction with implanted leads and implanted systems with leads

Health and Welfare Canada (1983) Safety Code 25—Shortwave diathermy guidelines for limited radiofrequency exposure. Publication 83-EHD-98

Health and Welfare Canada (2002) Health Canada is advising Canadians of a dangerous interaction between diathermy therapy and implanted metallic leads

Kloth L, Morrison MA, Ferguson BH (1984) Therapeutic microwave and shortwave diathermy: A review of thermal effectiveness, safe use, and state of the art. U.S. Food and Drug Administration, U.S. Department of Health and Human Services, HHS Publication FDA 85-8237

Medtronic Ltd. (2001) Medtronic Safety Reminder. Contraindication to diathermy for patients implanted with any type of Medtronic neurostimulation system

Internet Resources

http://thePoint.lww.com: Online Electromagnetic Spectrum Calculator

http://thePoint.lww.com: Online Dosage Calculator: Shortwave Diathermy

Chapter 11

Low-Level Laser Therapy

Chapter Outline

Learning Objectives

Remembering: State and describe the fundamental properties of a laser light and the key physical components of a laser device.

Understanding: Distinguish between the process of spontaneous and stimulated emission of photons.

Applying: Demonstrate contact versus noncontact methods as well as gridding, scanning, and stationary application techniques.

Analyzing: Explain how laser energy induces photobiomodulation effects in soft tissues.

Evaluating: Explain the difference between laser and nonlaser light as well as the difference between visible red and infrared laser therapy.

Creating: Formulate the strength of evidence behind the use of low-level laser therapy, and write a recommendation on its overall effectiveness.

I. FOUNDATION

A. DEFINITION

Laser is the acronym for *light amplification by stimulated emission of radiation. Light* is defined as the emission of electromagnetic waves, made of photons, traveling in space. A laser light, in comparison with all other forms of light, such as incandescent (light bulb) and luminescent (fluorescent tube), is monochromatic, collimated, and coherent in nature. The use of lights, or photons, for therapeutic purposes, is known as phototherapy. *Low-level laser therapy,* known under the acronym *LLLT,* is the application of low-power light energy, in the visible red and near-infrared band of the electromagnetic spectrum, for the purpose of photoactivating cellular mechanisms leading to enhanced soft-tissue repair and pain modulation.

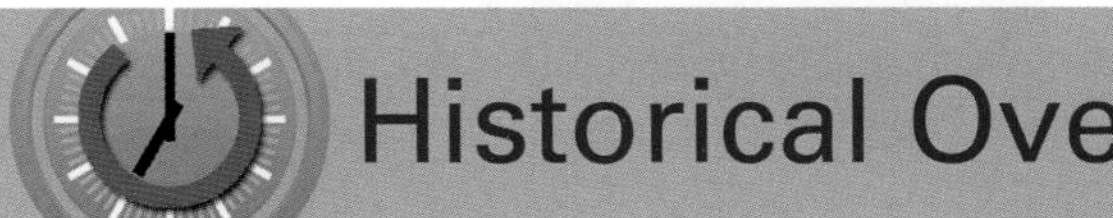

Historical Overview

In 1917, Albert Einstein proposed the theoretical biophysical concept of stimulated (*S*) emission (*E*) of radiation (*R*), which became the central process underlying the production of a la*SER* light. Einstein is thus considered to be the *biophysical father* of all lasers. In 1960, American physicist Theodore Maiman developed and manufactured the first laser, using a solid ruby crystal as the lasing medium (Calderhead, 1988; Baxter, 1994). A year later, another American physicist, Ali Javan, constructed the first HeNe gas laser. The invention of diodes, or semiconductors, in the 1970s led to the development of lower-cost, more powerful lasers than the first HeNe gaseous lasers. Today, the very large majority of lasers used to deliver low-level laser therapy (LLLT) are diode-type lasers made of gallium arsenide (GaAs), and gallium-aluminum-arsenide (GaAlAs) lasing substrates. A few years after the first laser was invented, Hungarian Endre Mester wanted to test whether laser radiation might cause cancer in animals (Mester et al., 1968). He shaved the dorsal hair of mice, divided them in two groups, and exposed one group to a low-power ruby laser. The results were spectacular. Mester showed not only that ruby laser radiation caused no cancer in the skin of the irradiated mice but also that the hair of the treated group of mice grew more quickly than the hair of the untreated group. This was the first demonstration that laser energy can induce photobiostimulation effects on in vivo mammalian soft tissues (Hamlin et al., 2006). Mester is credited with the first human applications of LLLT conducted in patients with various chronic and recalcitrant wounds and ulcers (Mester et al., 1971, 1985, 1989).

B. LASER CLASSIFICATION

Lasers are classified into four major hazard classes (I, II, IIIa/IIIb, and IV) based on the power outputs and exposure time of the devices (Occupational Safety and Health Administration, 2007). Hazard refers to the potential risk of laser to cause biologic damage to the skin and eyes. Class I, II, and IIIa lasers have single-diode power outputs of less than 5 megawatt (mW) and are not used for therapeutic purposes. Class IIIb lasers have power outputs ranging between 5 and 500 mW and are used for therapeutic purposes. These lasers pose eye hazards, such as damage to the retina, if their beams of energy are focused on the human eye. They pose no hazard to the skin. Finally, class IV lasers, which have single-diode power outputs greater than 500 mW, are not used therapeutically, because they pose eye (damage to retina) and skin (cell destruction) hazards if their beams of energy are focused on these biologic tissues.

C. THERAPEUTIC LASERS

Lasers with power outputs less than or equal to 500 mW are labeled as *low-level laser* (LLL) and are used for *therapy* (T), thus the acronym *LLLT.* Lasers with power outputs greater than 500 mW, on the other hand, are labeled as *high-level laser* (HLL) and are used for *surgery* (S). Table 11-1 shows a comparison between class IIIb and

TABLE 11-1 COMPARISON OF LASER TYPES USED IN HEALTH CARE

	LLLT	HLLS
OSHA classification	IIIb	IV
Single diode power	≤500 mW	>500 mW
Use	Therapy	Surgical therapy
Physiologic effect	Photobiomodulation	Photothermal
Therapeutic effect	Enhance cellular function	Cellular destruction

LLLT, low-level laser therapy; HLLS, high-level laser surgery; OSHA, Occupational Safety and Health Administration.

IV lasers used in health care (see Baxter, 1994; Kamami, 1987; Karu, 1998; Schindl et al., 2000; Tuner et al., 2002). The word *therapy* is used in reference to the improved cell function achieved through laser-induced photobiomodulation effects. Class IV lasers, because of their high power level, are used in surgery; this application is known under the acronym *HLLS*. The term *surgery* is used in reference to the cell destruction due to laser-induced photothermal effects. This chapter focuses on the use of low-level laser devices to treat soft-tissue pathologies in the field of physical rehabilitation.

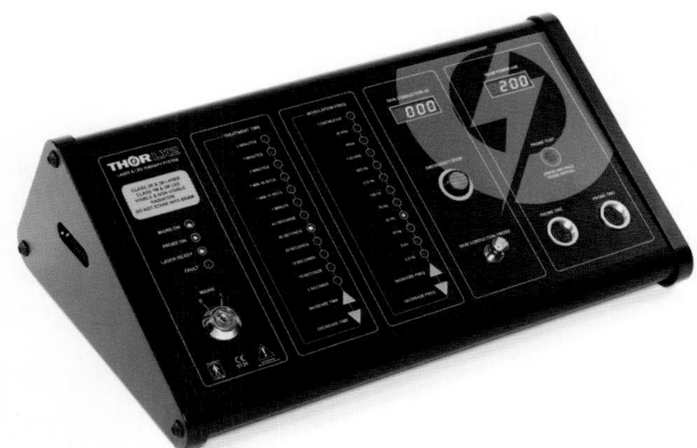

FIGURE 11-1 Typical cabinet diode-type low-level laser therapy device. (Courtesy of THOR Laser, Inc.)

D. LOW-LEVEL LASER DEVICES AND ACCESSORIES

Figure 11-1 illustrates a typical line-powered cabinet-type diode laser used to deliver LLLT. A complete laser device consists of a console (power supply) attached via a cable to the applicator, which contains the diodes. Figure 11-2 shows two common types of applicators or probes used to deliver LLLT. The key difference between the wand (see Fig. 11-2A) and cluster (see Fig. 11-2B) probe is that the former contains only one laser diode (LD), whereas the latter contains a group, or a cluster, of LDs. An array pad applicator, with its diodes positioned in an array as opposed to a cluster fashion, is also used. Practically speaking, wand probes are used to treat smaller areas, whereas cluster probes and array pads are used to treat medium to large treatment surfaces. The use of class IIIb lasers requires *both* the patient and the operator to wear eye protection goggles during therapy (www.osha.gov). Figure 11-2C also shows a typical pair of laser safety goggles. These goggles filter out the wavelength(s) generated by the LLLT device while allowing maximum visible light transmission to the clinician's eye during therapy. For a pair of goggles to be effective, its filter *must* match the photonic wavelength range generated by the laser device being used.

E. RATIONALE FOR USE

The use of LLLT arose from pioneering studies on animals and humans performed in the 1960s and 1970s by the Hungarian Endre Mester, who is regarded by many in the field as the *therapeutic father* of LLLT (Calderhead, 1988; Baxter, 1994, Tuner et al., 2002). More specifically, Mester et al. (1970, 1971, 1985, 1989) claimed that by using a ruby-type laser of low-level power, a therapeutic response rate of approximately 90% was obtained after treating more than 1,000 patients with various chronic and recalcitrant wounds and ulcers. Global recognition of these findings spurred researchers and clinicians to further explore the photobiologic effects induced by LLLT

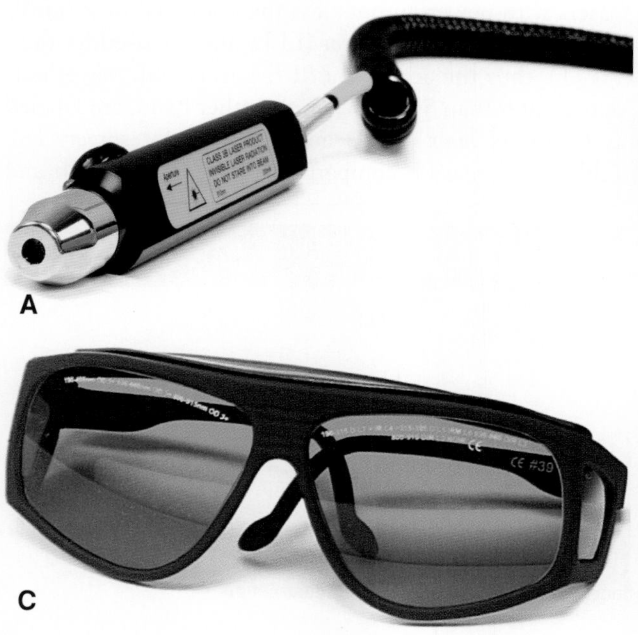

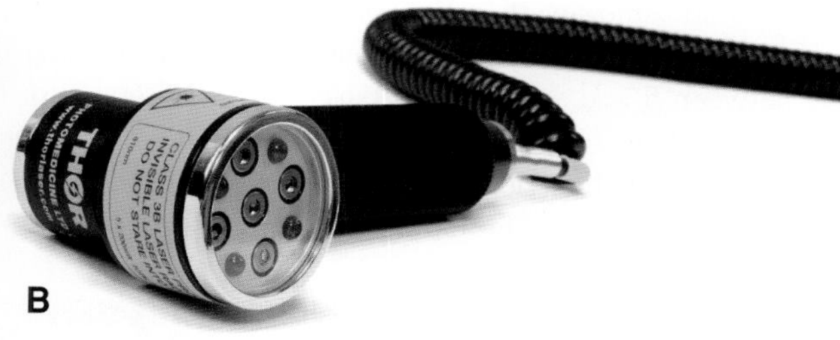

FIGURE 11-2 Typical wand **(A)** and cluster **(B)** applicators used to deliver low-level laser therapy. Each applicator may contain a mix of laser diodes, superluminous diodes, and light-emitting diodes. **C:** Typical laser protective goggles worn by both patient and operator during treatment. (A–C: Courtesy of THOR Laser, Inc.)

in humans. There is clear evidence, based on the body of research, that the use of the gaseous helium–neon (HeNe) laser is now obsolete, with the focus now being on the use of diode-type lasers. This chapter, therefore, focuses on the use of diode-type lasers, emitting within red and infrared lights, for treating soft-tissue pathology. In summary, the rationale for inducing photobiomodulation using LLLT is based on its ability to affect cellular function using a nonthermal, nondestructive source of light energy with no known side effects.

II. BIOPHYSICAL CHARACTERISTICS

A. FUNDAMENTAL ELEMENTS

The biophysics of lasers is a very complex subject (Nolan, 1987; Karu, 1989, 1998; Baxter, 1994; Kamami, 1997; Knappe et al., 2004), and addressing its full complexity is beyond the scope of this chapter. Nonetheless, to understand the basis of laser therapy, one must consider the following three fundamental elements: the properties of light, the physical components of a laser, and the process of laser light emission.

1. Properties of Light

Laser light, as shown in Table 11-2, differs from all other lights based on the following three properties of light: monochromacity, coherence, and collimation (Baxter, 1994; Knappe et al., 2004). *Monochromacity* implies that all photons accounting for the laser light have a single wavelength, and thus a single color. The therapeutic advantage of monochromatic light is that its absorption can be targeted at specific, wavelength-dependent photoacceptor molecules, called *chromophores,* buried within soft tissues. *Coherence* refers to the fact that the photons that make up a laser light travel in phase, in both time (temporal) and space (spatial), with each other. In other words, it means that all photons travel in the same direction at the same time. *Collimation* refers to the ability of a beam of laser light not to diverge, or spread, significantly with distance. The advantage of a collimated beam of light is its ability to be focused precisely on a very small target area. Table 11-2 thus indicates that laser light, generated by an LD, is monochromatic, coherent, and collimated in nature. It also shows that all regular lights (incandescent and fluorescent) are polychrome, incoherent, and noncollimated, with the exception of lights generated by light-emitting diodes (LEDs), and superluminous diodes (SLDs), which are monochomatic and collimated but noncoherent. Lights originating from LEDs and SLDs, therefore, are nonlaser lights (see later discussion).

2. Laser Physical Components

The second element to consider is the three basic physical components of a laser device: active medium, resonance chamber, and power source (Knappe et al., 2004). As shown in Table 11-3 and illustrated in Figure 11-3, LLLT is clinically delivered using gaseous- and diode-type lasers. The first component, the *active medium,* also known as the lasing medium, corresponds to the material used to emit a laser light, for which the laser is named. For example, a laser made of a mixture of two inert gases, such as helium (He) and neon (Ne), is labeled as a HeNe laser (see Fig. 11-3A). Diode lasers, as their name implies, are made of diodes—that is, semiconductors (two slabs of material separated by a junction) made of different chemical lasing elements (see Fig. 11-3B). The three main active media, or organic material, used to construct a diode laser for LLLT are gallium (Ga), aluminum (Al), and arsenide (As). These lasers are thus named *GaAs lasers* and *GaAlAs lasers* (see Table 11-3). The second component of a laser, the *resonance chamber,* is the cavity within the laser device that contains the active medium. In this chamber, the active medium is activated or lased, leading to the production of a beam of laser light. The resonance chamber of a HeNe laser is made of a *sealed glass tube,* housing the active medium (see Fig. 11-3A). This tube is mounted with a fully reflective mirror at one end and a semi-reflective mirror at the other. The beam of laser light is emitted through the semi-reflective mirror. The resonance chamber of a diode laser, on the other hand, corresponds to the *p–n junction gap* between two slabs of semiconductor material sandwiched together (see Table 11-3). This p–n junction gap is commonly referred to as a diode (see Fig. 11-3B). The p–n junction is created by placing a p-type semiconductor material (*p* for positively charged, because it has a deficit of free electrons

TABLE 11-2 PROPERTIES OF LIGHT

Light	Monochromacity	Coherence	Collimation
Laser diode	Monochromatic	Coherent	Collimated
Light-emitting diode Superluminous diode	Monochromatic	Noncoherent	Collimated
Regular	Polychromatic	Noncoherent	Noncollimated

TABLE 11-3 PHYSICAL COMPONENTS OF LOW-LEVEL LASER

Component	Gaseous	Diode
Active medium	Helium–Neon (HeNe)	Gallium arsenide (GaAs) Gallium-aluminum-arsenide (GaAlAs)
Resonance chamber	Sealed glass cylinder	Diode p–n junction gap
Power source	Electrical	Electrical

and therefore contains holes that accept free electrons) in contact with an n-type semiconductor material (*n* for negatively charged, because it has a surplus of electrons). The chamber's parallel reflecting mirrors are obtained by cleaving along the natural planes of the semiconductor materials used to make the diode. The third physical component, the *power source,* is electrical in nature and is common to both gaseous- and diode-type lasers. An electrical current, passing through the resonance chamber, powers the laser, thus stimulating (or lasing) its active medium, which results in the emission of a beam of laser light (see arrows in Fig. 11-3).

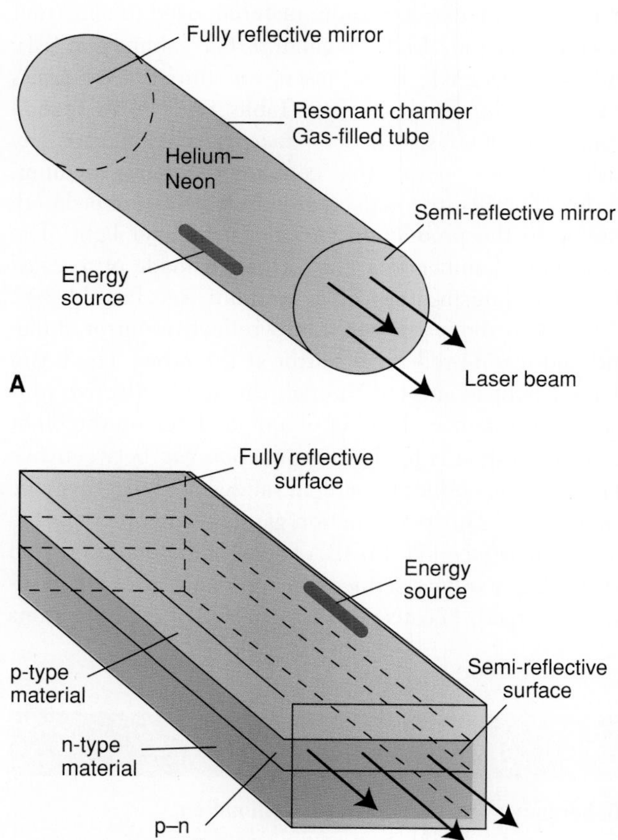

FIGURE 11-3 Schematic physical representation of a helium–neon (**A**) and diode-type (**B**) laser device. The active medium, resonance chamber, and power source are shown for each laser type. The laser beam (shown by *arrows*) for both lasers escapes through the semi-reflective mirror of the resonance chamber.

3. Process of Laser Light Emission

The third and final element that one needs to know in order to understand the nature of laser is the all important *process of light emission,* which results from activation of the active medium, housed in the resonance chamber. The sequential biophysical steps leading to emission of a laser light are described next. These biophysical steps are the same regardless of the laser type. Figure 11-4 illustrates a simple atomic model to help visualize the complex

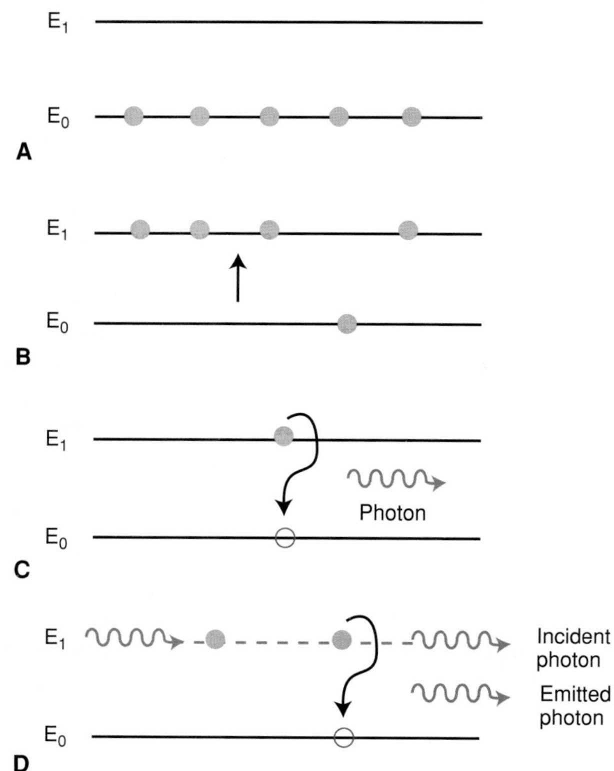

FIGURE 11-4 Schematic sequences of key atomic states and processes leading to emission of a laser beam of light. For simplicity, an active medium population of only five atoms is presented in a system with two energy levels. **A:** Active medium in its resting or ground state. **B:** Pumping of active medium causes the majority of atoms to jump to their metastable energy level, thus causing a population inversion. **C:** Spontaneous emission of a photon traveling parallel to the lateral wall of the resonance chamber. **D:** An incident photon striking an electron in its metastable energy level, thus causing the process of stimulated emission, which corresponds to the release of a newly emitted photon perfectly identical to the incident photon. E_1, metastable energy state; E_0, ground energy state.

fundamental steps needed to create a laser light. This model presupposes the use of an active medium with a population of five atoms, all shown resting (i.e., power Off) at their ground level (see Fig. 11-4A). In reality, any given active medium has a population of millions of molecules and billions of atoms.

a. First Step: Pumping of Active Medium

This step involves the activation, or pumping, of the active medium caused by an electrical current (i.e., power On) passing into the resonance chamber. To pump the active medium is to energize it. It is the process of moving atoms, and therefore their electrons, from their resting ground state (E_0) to their excited state (E_1). This means that in the resonance chamber, there are now a growing number of atoms whose electrons have been excited.

b. Second Step: Population Inversion

This step is achieved when a majority of atoms are in their excited state. Figure 11-4B illustrates this population inversion by showing electrons of four of the five atoms (80%) in their excited state.

c. Third Step: Spontaneous Emission

This step corresponds to the emission of a photon caused by the spontaneous drop of an electron from its excited state to its ground state, as illustrated in Figure 11-4C. As more and more electrons spontaneously drop from their higher energy level, more and more spontaneous photons are emitted in the resonance chamber. All photons not traveling parallel to the wall of the resonance chamber are absorbed by the lining of the wall and cease to exist. These three first steps are common to the production of all light sources.

d. Fourth Step: Stimulated Emission

This fourth step is critical to the creation of a laser light. Remember that the term *laser* stands for *light amplification by stimulated emission of radiation.* This process corresponds to the emission of a photon caused by an incident photon striking an atom's electron into its metastable energy state, which is defined as an excited state that has a long lifetime (i.e., a state that lasts long enough for the incident photon to strike the excited atom before it spontaneously de-excites itself by dropping to its ground state). This striking action, illustrated in Figure 11-4D, causes the electron to drop from its metastable energy level to its resting energy level, releasing a new photon that is identical to the incident photon. Physics has shown that only one spontaneously emitted photon, traveling parallel to the lateral wall of the resonance chamber, is needed to trigger the process of stimulated emission. Both the incident and the newly emitted photons now travel together and in phase with each other in the resonance chamber (see Fig. 11-4D). This process of stimulated emission is self-perpetuating in that these 2 traveling photons will later strike 2 other excited electrons, leading to the emission of 4 photons, and later to 8, 16, 32, 64 photons, and so on.

e. Fifth and Final Step: Amplification

The final step—amplification—is achieved through the back-and-forth movements of incident and newly emitted photons traveling parallel to the lateral wall of the resonance chamber as they are reflected between the parallel reflective and semi-reflective mirrors forming the end walls of the chamber. Physics has shown that the back-and-forth passing of these photons through the active medium dramatically amplifies the process of stimulated emission, triggering a chain reaction as more and more perfectly identical photons fill the resonance chamber (see earlier discussion). The ultimate emission of a beam of laser light through the laser's probe occurs when the amplification process is maximal—that is, when the resonance chamber has reached its maximum capacity to store photons. At this point, and as long as pumping continues (i.e., the laser device is turned On), a percentage of photons escapes the chamber through the semi-reflective mirror to form an almost perfect monochromatic, collimated, and coherent beam of light at the tip of the probe. This beam of laser light is then delivered to soft tissues during LLLT.

B. LOW-LEVEL LASER THERAPY RADIATION SPECTRUM

Photons emitted by LLLT lasers have different wavelengths that are determined by the nature and specific composition of their active medium. Figure 11-5 illustrates the electromagnetic radiation spectrum occupied by LLLT, which spans between the visible red and the infrared band of the electromagnetic spectrum. The *visible band* of the electromagnetic spectrum is between 750 and 400 nm. Visible light is made of six different

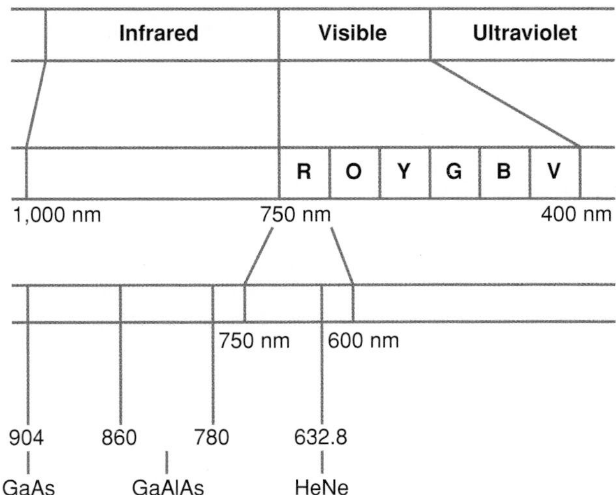

FIGURE 11-5 Low-level laser therapy radiation spectrum. GaAs, gallium arsenide; GaAlAs, gallium-aluminum-arsenide; HeNe, helium–neon. (R, red; O, orange; Y, yellow; G, green; B, blue; V, violet)

lights ranging from violet to red. The *infrared band* is adjacent to the visible band, with wavelengths ranging between 1,000 and 750 nanometers (nm). Infrared light is invisible to the human eye. Low-level laser light is nonionizing in nature because its energy per photon is well below the 10 electron volt (eV) ionizing energy per photon threshold value (see Chapter 10).

C. RED AND INFRARED LASERS

Lasers used to deliver LLLT are commonly referred to as red and infrared lasers. The gaseous HeNe laser emits a light having a specific wavelength of 632.8 nm (10^{-9} m). Its laser light is red and visible to human eyes because it falls within the red band of the visible spectrum (see Fig. 11-5). Within the red band of visible light can be found Mester's original ruby laser, which emitted photons with a wavelength of 694 nm. Diode-type lasers, on the hand, emit lights within the infrared band. Located in Figure 11-5 are the GaAlAs laser, emitting photons within 860 to 780 nm, and the GaAs laser, emitting photons at 904 nm. Infrared light is invisible. Why then do practitioners see a red beam of light at the tip of an infrared laser applicator? What is the purpose of this red light? The red light comes from one or many LEDs embedded in the applicator, which contains one or many LDs. This red visible light has two purposes. First, it serves as a *safety measure* to remind both patient and operator that an invisible therapeutic laser beam is being emitted from the applicator. Second, it serves as a *visual guiding aid* to help in guiding this therapeutic beam of invisible light over the area being treated.

D. DIODE TYPES AND LOW-LEVEL LASER THERAPY LIGHTS

Three types of diodes are found in today's low-level lasers: LDs, SLDs, and LEDs (Fig. 11-6). LDs are the only diodes emitting a *laser light*—that is, a light that is monochromatic, coherent, and collimated. As discussed earlier, SLDs and LEDs emit nonlaser light—that is, a light that is monochromatic and collimated but noncoherent. Depending of the types and proportion of diodes contained in the applicators, modern lasers used to deliver LLLT may deliver laser-only light, or both laser and nonlaser lights to the tissues. Why does the field of laser therapy include nonlaser light? There is evidence to support the view that as soon as the laser light passes through the first millimeters of skin (see Fig. 11-5), its qualities of coherence and collimation are both *lost*. This means that the lights emitted by all three types of diodes should have the same phototherapeutic effects because their lights now share the same property—that of being monochromatic. To make use of nonlaser light in the field of LLLT, one has to postulate that it is the light's wavelength, or monochromacity, that is therapeutically *important,* not its coherence and collimation properties.

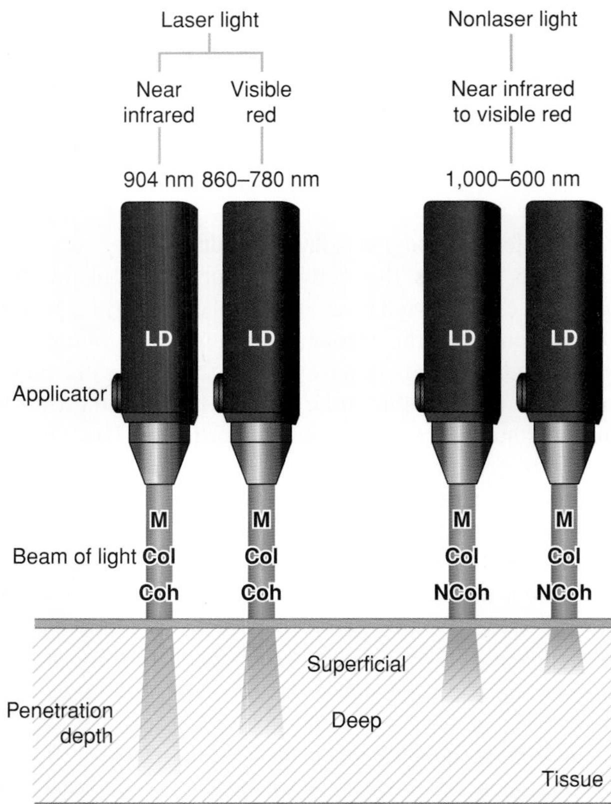

FIGURE 11-6 Laser and nonlaser light properties. LD, laser diode. M, monochromacity; Col, collimation; Coh, coherence.

E. PENETRATION DEPTH

Laser light emitted in the near-infrared band penetrates soft tissue deeper than light emitted in the visible red band (see Fig. 11-6). Why is it so? As shown in Table 11-4, the depth to which a laser beam of light can penetrate soft tissues depends on two factors: absorption and scattering. First, the greater the absorption of photons by superficial tissues, the fewer the number of photons the deeper tissues can absorb. In other words, penetration depth (P) is inversely related to absorption (A), meaning that the greater the absorption superficially, the lesser the penetration depth ($P = 1/A$). Biophysics indicates that visible red laser light is absorbed much more by superficial tissues (skin and blood) than is infrared invisible light (Nussbaum et al., 2003). Second, for any laser light to physiologically and therapeutically affect tissues, it must first be able to penetrate the skin and underlying targeted soft tissue before being absorbed by the wavelength-specific chromophores buried in the layers of this tissue. When a laser beam of light hits soft tissues, a significant portion of its photons is scattered, or deflected, in various directions away from the original direct path to the targeted area. The biophysics of laser indicates that scattering is inversely related to wavelength ($S = 1/\lambda$). It is greatest at short wavelengths and gradually decreases at longer wavelengths (Houza et al., 1993; Nussbaum et al., 2003). This means that photons of red lasers will experience

TABLE 11-4 LOW-LEVEL LASER PENETRATION DEPTH

Parameter	Formula	GaAlAs and GaAs	
Light		Red	Infrared
Wavelength (λ)		600–780 nm	780–904 nm
Absorption (A)		++	+
Scattering (S)	$S = 1/\lambda$	++	+
Penetration (P)	$P = 1/A$	+	++
Penetration (P)	$P = 1/S$	+	++
Penetration depth		~1.0 cm	~5.0 cm

GaAlAs, gallium-aluminum-arsenide; GaAs, gallium arsenide; +, less; ++, more.

more scattering than those of infrared lasers when penetrating soft tissues. Biophysics has also established that penetration depth (P) is inversely related to scattering (S), meaning that penetration depth decreases as scattering increases ($P = 1/S$). As stated earlier, scattering is more pronounced with shorter-wavelength lasers (red) than with longer-wavelength lasers (infrared). Compared to red light lasers, infrared light thus penetrates deeper into soft tissues because it presents less superficial absorption and scattering (see Table 11-4 and Fig. 11-6). Penetration depth value is defined (Low et al., 1990; Baxter, 1994) as the tissue depth, measured in centimeters, at which the laser beam energy is reduced to 37% of its original value (100%). This value is derived from the following formula: *Penetration depth value* = $1/e$, where e is a constant value of 2.718. Penetration depth values for human tissues are approximately less than 1 cm for red light lasers and less than 5 cm for infrared light lasers.

F. APPLICATOR DIODE ARRANGEMENT

The proportion of one type of diode, with each diode having different wavelengths and power, contained in a given applicator, varies from one manufacturer to the next. The wand probe, or single probe, contains one and only one LD. It may also contain one or two SLDs or LDs, if the light emitted by the LD is within the infrared or invisible spectrum. In such a case, the red light emitted by the SLD serves to guide the laser beam and ensure application safety. Cluster probes may contain up to 100 diodes and array pads up to 200 diodes, with both applicators also having different proportions of LDs, SLDs, and LEDs. It is important to keep in mind that the useful life of a laser is predetermined and specified by the manufacturer. This is because the laser's active medium has a finite number of hours, which may vary between 5,000 and 20,000 hours, during which it can be optimally stimulated or lased.

G. LAWS GOVERNING APPLICATION

As is the case with the application of electromagnetic energy using shortwave diathermy therapy (Chapter 10), the application of LLLT is also governed by the same four laws—that is, Arndt-Shultz (dosage), Grotthuss-Draper (absorption), inverse square (divergence), and Lambert's cosine (reflection). These laws are fully described and illustrated in Chapter 10. Note that the inverse square law does not apply to laser light (LD) application because its beam is collimated, thus showing no divergence with distance from the skin.

III. THERAPEUTIC EFFECTS AND INDICATIONS

A. PHOTOBIOMODULATION

The exact physiologic and therapeutic effects of LLLT on human soft tissues are, unfortunately, far from well established or understood. There is a strong consensus in the scientific literature, however, that LLLT induces **photobiomodulation** effects through photochemical interactions between photons and healthy cells within and surrounding the soft-tissue pathology (see Knappe et al., 1994; Reddy, 2004; Hamblin et al., 2006; Lopes-Martin et al., 2007; Bjordal et al., 2010; Chung et al., 2012; Farraresi et al., 2012; Prindeze et al., 2012).

B. PROPOSED THERAPEUTIC EFFECTS

Figure 11-7 illustrates the proposed physiologic and therapeutic effects of LLLT. It shows that the delivery of low-level laser electromagnetic energy within the visible red and near-infrared bands causes chromophore activation, which then triggers *photobiostimulation* effects

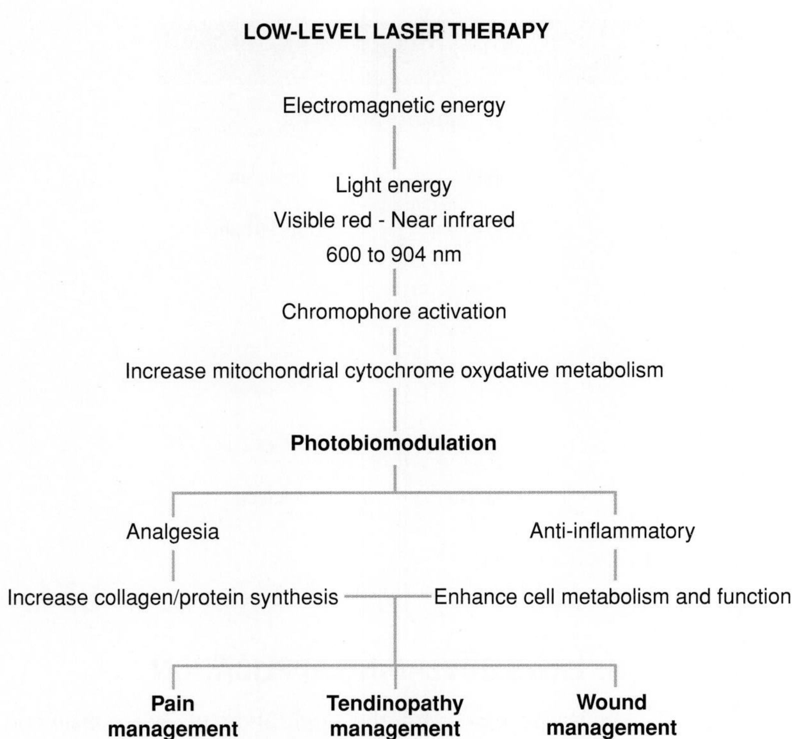

FIGURE 11-7 Proposed physiologic and therapeutic effects of low-level laser therapy.

in soft tissues. A *chromophore,* meaning "color lover" (*chromo* = color; *phore* = lover) is a light-absorbing part of a molecule that gives its color. Melanin (skin darkening), hemoglobin (red blood), and retinal rhodopsin (color vision) are among the best-known chromophores, or pigments, found in human tissues. The photobiologic effects of LLLT at the cellular level are based on the absorption of monochromatic visible (greater than 600 nm) and near-infrared (less than 1 mm) radiation or light by those photoacceptor molecules found in biologic tissues. There is evidence to suggest that LLLT photobiomodulates soft tissues by increasing the oxidative metabolism in mitochondria, which is caused by electronic excitation of components of the respiratory chain (see Smith, 1991 ; Knappe et al., 1994; Chung et al., 2012). The absorption of light energy by those chromophores (i.e., mitochondrial cytochromes) is presumed to trigger the process of photobiomodulation. As shown in Figure 11-7, effects such as analgesia, anti-inflammation, and increased protein and collagen synthesis have been postulated, leading to enhanced cellular metabolism and function promoting soft-tissue healing. The body of research shows that LLLT has been primarily used for the management of wounds, tendinopathies, and pain.

C. RESEARCH-BASED INDICATIONS

The search for evidence behind the use of LLLT, displayed in the *Research-Based Indications* box led to an impressive collection of 157 English peer-reviewed human clinical studies. The methodology, as well as the criteria, used to assess the strength of evidence and therapeutic effectiveness are described in Chapter 2. As indicated, the strength of evidence is ranked as *strong* for all the following conditions: dermal wounds, tendinopathies, myofascial/trigger point pain, rheumatoid arthritis, mixed painful musculoskeletal conditions, osteoarthritis, herpes/postherpetic pain, neck/low back pain, temporomandibular disorders, and carpal tunnel syndrome. Therapeutic effectiveness is *substantiated* for those conditions with the exception of tendinopathies and mixed painful musculoskeletal conditions, where the evidence is found to be *conflicting*. Analysis is *pending* for all other health conditions because fewer than five studies could be collected. Over all conditions, the strength of evidence behind the use of LLLT is found to be *strong* and its therapeutic effectiveness *substantiated.*

IV. DOSIMETRY

A. LASER AND NONLASER LIGHTS

As discussed earlier, there is evidence to show that the monochromacity of both laser (LD) and nonlaser (LED, SLD) lights may be the key property behind the photobiomodulation process attributed to LLLT. This is because both coherence and collimation properties are lost (see Fig. 11-6) as soon as their photons are absorbed by the exposed tissues (Enwemeka, 2006; Jenkins et al., 2011). This explains why today's LLLT lasers may emit laser light only, or a mixture of laser and nonlaser lights, for therapeutic purposes.

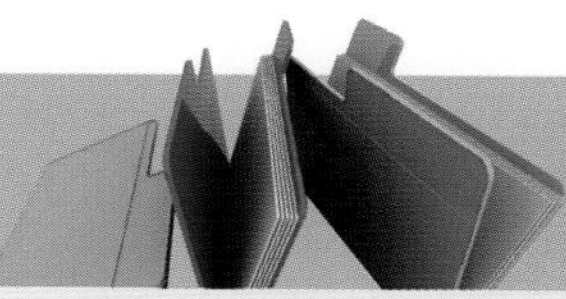

Research-Based Indications

LOW-LEVEL LASER THERAPY

	Benefit—Yes		Benefit—No	
Health Condition	**Rating**	**Reference**	**Rating**	**Reference**
Dermal wound	I	Schindl et al., 1998	I	Kopera et al., 2005
	I	Hopkins et al., 2004	I	Malm et al., 1991
	I	Kymplova et al., 2003	I	Santoianni et al., 1984
	I	Schindl et al., 2002	I	Lundeberg et al., 1991
	I	Gupta et al., 1998	I	Kokol et al., 2005
	I	Iusim et al., 1992	I	Lagan et al., 2002
	II	Robinson et al., 1991	II	Lucas et al., 2000
	II	Bihari et al., 1989	II	Freanek et al., 2002
	II	Sugrue et al., 1990	II	Lucas et al., 2003
	II	Crous et al., 1988	II	Nussbaum et al., 1994
	II	Mester et al., 1971	II	Lagan et al., 2001
	II	Mester et al., 1985		
	II	Schindl, et al., 1999b		
	II	Morita et al., 1993		
	III	Gogia et al., 1988		
	III	Ashford et al., 1999		
	III	Khan, 1984		
	III	Lagan et al., 2000		
	III	Herascu et al., 2005		
	III	Ohshiro et al., 1992		
	III	Schindl et al., 2000		
	III	Schindl et al., 1997		
	III	Schindl et al., 1999		

Strength of evidence: Strong
Therapeutic effectiveness: Substantiated

	Benefit—Yes		Benefit—No	
Health Condition	**Rating**	**Reference**	**Rating**	**Reference**
Tendinopathy	I	Vasseljen et al., 1992	I	Lundeberg et al., 1987
	I	Lam et al., 2007	I	Krashen-innikoff et al., 1994
	I	Simunovic et al., 1998	I	Haker et al., 1990
	I	Lam et al., 2007	I	Papadopoulos et al., 1996
	I	England et al., 1989	I	Haker et al., 1991a
	I	Saunders, 1995	I	Haker et al., 1991b
	I	Bjordal et al., 2006a	I	Basford et al., 2000
	I	Stergioulas et al., 2008	I	Vecchio et al., 1993
	I	Sharma et al., 2002	I	Darre et al., 1994
	II	Terashima et al., 1990	I	Tumilty et al., 2008
	II	Stergioulas, 2007	I	Siebert et al., 1987
	II	Oken et al., 2008	II	Konstantinovic et al., 1997
	II	Palmieri, 1984	II	Oken et al., 2008
	II	Saunders, 2003	II	Vasseljen et al., 1992

Strength of evidence: Strong
Therapeutic effectiveness: Conflicting

	Benefit—Yes		Benefit—No	
Health Condition	**Rating**	**Reference**	**Rating**	**Reference**
Myofascial/trigger point pain	I	Ceccherelli et al., 1989	I	Altan et al., 2005
	I	Ilbuldu et al., 2004	I	Thorsen et al., 1992
	I	Gur et al., 2004	I	Waylonis et al., 1988
	I	Snyder-Mackler et al., 1989	I	Dundar et al., 2007
	I	Olavi et al., 1989	I	Laakso et al., 1997
	I	Simunovic, 1996		
	I	Logdberg-Andersson et al., 1997		
	I	Ceylan et al., 2004		
	II	Hakguder et al., 2003		

Strength of evidence: Strong
Therapeutic effectiveness: Substantiated

	Benefit—Yes		Benefit—No	
Health Condition	**Rating**	**Reference**	**Rating**	**Reference**
Rheumatoid arthritits	I	Palmgren et al., 1989	I	Heussler et al., 1993
	I	Goldman et al., 1980	I	Johannsen et al., 1994
	I	Walker, et al., 1987b	I	Hall et al., 1994
	I	Goats et al., 1996	II	Bliddal et al., 1987
	II	Fulga, 1998		
	II	Fulga et al., 1994		
	II	Longo et al., 1997		
	II	Asada et al., 1989		
	II	Obara et al., 1987		

Strength of evidence: Strong
Therapeutic effectiveness: Substantiated

Health Condition	Benefit—Yes Rating	Benefit—Yes Reference	Benefit—No Rating	Benefit—No Reference
Mixed painful musculoskeletal conditions	I	Walker, 1983	I	De Bie et al., 1998
	I	Atsumi et al., 1987	I	Mulcahy et al., 1995
	I	Emmanoulidis et al., 1986	I	Basford et al., 1998
	II	Shiroto et al., 1989	I	Bingol et al., 2005
	II	Stergioulas, 2004	I	Rogvi-Hansen et al., 1991
	II	Li, 1990		
	II	Gartner et al., 1987		
	II	Tam, 1999		
Strength of evidence: Strong **Therapeutic effectiveness:** Conflicting				
Osteoarthritis	I	Lonauer, 1986	I	Bülow et al., 1994
	I	Willner et al., 1985	I	Basford et al., 1987
	I	Jensen et al., 1987	I	Brosseau et al., 2005
	I	Walker, 1983		
	I	Stelian et al., 1992		
	I	Gur et al., 2003a		
	I	Ozdemir et al., 2001		
	I	Lewith et al., 1981		
	II	Trelles et al., 1991		
Strength of evidence: Strong **Therapeutic effectiveness:** Substantiated				
Herpes/ Postherpetic pain	I	Schindl et al., 1999a		
	I	Moore et al., 1988		
	I	Ohtsuka et al., 1992		
	II	McKibben et al., 1990		
	II	Kemmotsu et al., 1991		
	II	Yaksish, 1993		
	III	Matsumura et al., 1993		
Strength of evidence: Strong **Therapeutic effectiveness:** Substantiated				
Neck/low back pain	I	Basford et al., 1999	II	Klein et al., 1990
	I	Soriano et al., 1998		
	I	Toya et al., 1994		
	I	Chow et al., 2006		
	II	Djavid et al., 2007		
	II	Gur et al., 2003b		
Strength of evidence: Strong **Therapeutic effectiveness:** Substantiated				

Health Condition	Benefit—Yes Rating	Benefit—Yes Reference	Benefit—No Rating	Benefit—No Reference
Temporomandibular disorders	I	Mazzetto et al., 2007	I	Conti, 1997
	I	Kulekcioglu et al., 2003		
	I	Cetiner et al., 2006		
	II	Fikackova et al., 2007		
	II	Nunez et al., 2006		
Strength of evidence: Strong **Therapeutic effectiveness:** Substantiated				
Carpal tunnel syndrome	I	Naeser et al., 2002	I	Irvine et al., 2004
	I	Evcik et al., 2007	II	Ekim et al., 2007
	II	Weintraub, 1997		
Strength of evidence: Strong **Therapeutic effectiveness:** Substantiated				
Fewer Than 5 Studies				
Orofacial/ maxillofacial pain	I	Ong et al., 2001	I	Hansen et al., 1990
	II	Pinheiro et al., 1997		
	II	Pinheiro et al., 1998		
Lymphedema	I	Catari et al., 2003		
	I	Kaviani et al., 2006		
	II	Dirican et al., 2011		
Fibromyalgia	I	Gur et al., 2002		
	II	Matsutani et al., 2007		
Trigeminal pain	I	Eckerdal et al., 1996		
	I	Walker et al., 1987a		
Muscle soreness			I	Craig et al., 1996
			I	Craig et al., 1999
Clonus	I	Walker, 1985		
Postsurgical pain	I	Moore et al., 1992		
Neurogenic pain	I	Kreczi et al., 1986		
Fibrotic lumps	III	Nussbaum, 1999		
Raynaud's phenomenon	I	Hirschl et al., 2004		
Strength of evidence: Pending **Therapeutic effectiveness:** Pending				

ALL CONDITIONS
Strength of evidence: Strong
Therapeutic effectiveness: Substantiated

B. DOSIMETRIC PARAMETERS, FORMULAS, AND UNITS

Correct measurement and reporting of dosimetric parameters still remains a major problem in the field of LLLT (Enwemeka, 2011; Jenkins et al., 2011). For example, there is clear evidence that common measurements, such as power density (mW/cm^2) and energy density (J/cm^2), may only be just two of several parameters that should be documented with each case. To improve the situation, recommendations have been made by the World Association for Laser Therapy (WALT) to help LLLT researchers and clinicians better understand and report all necessary parameters for a repeatable study or treatment (Jenkins et al., 2011; waltza.co.za). Table 11-5 lists key recommended dosimetric parameters, with their formulas and units, that practitioners need to consider and document when delivering LLLT to their patients. These parameters are laser type, wavelength, delivery mode, peak power, mean power, beam irradiation area, power density, irradiation duration per point, energy density, treatment surface area, number of irradiation per treatment session, total number of treatments, dose per point, dose per treatment, and cumulative dose. To further guide the practice of LLLT based on evidence, WALT has published dosage recommendations on its website that were last updated in 2010 (waltza.co.za). These dosage recommendations are summarized in Table 11-6. As shown, the recommendations apply the use of diode-type lasers for the management of tendinopathies and arthritic disorders. The table shows that the minimum dose per point, expressed in joules (J), should be a minimum of 4 J for GaAlAs and a minimum of 1 J for GaAs lasers. It also

TABLE 11-5 KEY LOW-LEVEL LASER THERAPY DOSIMETRIC PARAMETERS*

Parameter	Synonym	Formula	Units
Laser type	*Gaseous:* HeNe *Diode:* GaAlAs; GaAs		
Wavelength (λ)			nm
Delivery mode	Continuous Pulsed		
Peak power (P_p)	Radiant power		mW
Mean power (Pm)		$Pm = P_p \times F \times PD$, where • P_p = peak power in watts • F = frequency in Hertz • PD = pulse duration in seconds	mW
Beam irradiation area (A)	Probe spot size		cm^2
Power density (P_d)	Irradiance	$P_d = P_p/A$ $P_d = P_m/A$	mW/cm^2
Irradiation duration per point (T)			sec
Energy density (E_d)	Fluence	$E_d = P_d \times T$	J/cm^2
Treatment surface area (S)			cm^2
Number of irradiated points per treatment	NbIpTr		
Total number of treatments	ToNbTr		
Dose per point (D_p)	Energy delivered per point	$D_p = P_p \times T$ $D_p = P_m \times T$	J
Dose per treatment (D_t)	Total energy delivered during one treatment session	$D_t = D_p \times$ nb of irradiation points	J
Cumulative dose (D_c)	Total energy delivered over the total number of treatments	$D_c = \Sigma D_t$	J

*Adapted from World Association for Laser Therapy (waltza.co.za).

TABLE 11-6 DOSAGE RECOMMENDATIONS FROM THE WORLD ASSOCIATION FOR LASER THERAPY*

	For Tendinopathies and Arthritic Disorders	
	GaAlAs 780–860 nm	**GaAs 904 nm**
Irradiation duration per point*	20–300 s	30–600 s
Dose per point*	Min 4 J	Min 1 J
Power density per point	Max 100 mW/cm^2	
Treatment frequency	Daily for 2 wk or every other day for 3–4 wk	

GaAlAs, gallium-aluminum-arsenide; GaAs, gallium arsenide.
*Range from ±50% of given values.
From World Association for Laser Therapy (waltza.co.za), revised 2010.

shows that the irradiation duration per point should range between 20 and 600 seconds and that power density per point should be a maximum of 100 mW/cm^2. The dosimetric approach used in the case studies presented in this chapter complies with WALT dosimetric parameters and dosage recommendations.

C. DOSIMETRIC EXAMPLES

Dosage measurement in the field of LLLT, as exemplified earlier, can be complex and often confusing. To help in clarifying and reducing the complexity of the situation, two dosimetric case examples are presented in Table 11-7 and Table 11-8, respectively. In both cases, a diode-type laser is used (GaAlAs). The first example is concerned with the delivery of LLLT in the continuous mode and the second example with the pulsed mode. In each case, parameters related to the application of all three applicators—wand, cluster, and array pad—are shown. To facilitate the understanding of these two examples, let us focus or track the dosimetric parameters and dosage associated with the *cluster probe*.

1. Continuous Mode

The case example presented in Table 11-7 indicates that a cluster probe made of 36 diodes is used for the delivery of continuous LLLT. The cluster probe contains 32 LDs at 880 nm, and 4 LEDs at 660 nm, for a total number of 36 diodes. This GaAlAs laser thus delivers a mix of laser and nonlaser lights to the tissues. The total peak power (P_p) of this cluster probe is 1,400 mW (32 diodes × 40 mW + 4 diodes × 30 mW). The cluster beam's irradiation area (A) has a value of 20 cm^2, and the treatment surface area (S) is measured at 40 cm^2. This means that two irradiations per treatment are necessary in order to cover the full treatment surface area (2 irradiations per treatment = 40 cm^2/20 cm^2). Power density (P_d) is 70 mW/cm^2 (1,400 mW/20 cm^2), of which value is below the 100 mW/cm^2 value recommended by the WALT (see Table 11-5). The application method is stationary with no contact with the exposed skin surface. The practitioner, based on WALT's recommendations (see Table 11-6), wants to deliver a dose per point (D_p) of 7 J. At first sight, it appears that the peak power of this cluster is too high because it can deliver the dose (7 J) in 5 seconds only (7 J = 1,400 mW × 5 s)—much too short an application duration value for effective therapy according to WALT, which recommends that irradiation duration *per point* be between 20 and 300 s (see Table 11-6). Practitioners need to recall that energy, in the present case, is delivered over a much greater surface area (A = 20 cm^2), not over a point, or 1 cm^2, as presented by WALT. If we divide the cluster probe peak power (P_p) by its beam irradiation area (A), we then obtain a power density of 70 mW/cm^2, a value that is below WALT's recommended value of 100 mW/cm^2. Thus, each square centimeter of tissue gets 70 mW, in which case 7 J is achieved at every square, or per point, in 100 seconds (7 J = 70 mW × 100 s). This longer irradiation duration value is now within the WALT guideline (i.e., between 20 and 300 s). As stated earlier, two irradiations per treatment session are needed because the cluster's beam irradiation area (A) is half the treatment surface area (S). This yields a dose per treatment (D_t) equal to 280 J (280 J = 7 J/point × 20 points × 2 applications; 1 point = 1 cm^2). With a total number of eight treatment sessions, the total amount of energy delivered to the tissues, or cumulative dose of light received by the tissues in this case example, is equal to 2,240 J (2,240 J = 280 J × 8).

2. Pulsed Mode

The dosimetric approach for this case example, using pulsed mode, is similar to the one used for continuous mode presented earlier. For the sake of comparison, let us also track the cluster probe values. As shown in Table 11-8, all dosimetric parameters are identical to the previous case with the exception that the laser energy is now pulsed at a frequency (F) of 2,000 Hz, each pulse having 0.0002 s duration (PD). This pulsing yields a mean power (P_m) of 560 mW (560 mW = 1.4 W × 2,000 Hz × 0.0002 s). The

TABLE 11-7 EXAMPLES OF LOW-LEVEL LASER THERAPY DOSIMETRIC MEASUREMENTS FOR CONTINUOUS MODE

	Continuous Mode GaAlAs Laser		
Parameter	**Wand Probe**	**Cluster Probe**	**Array Pad**
Number of diodes	2	36	185
Types of diodes	1 LD 1 LED	32 LD 4 LED	140 LD 30 SLD 15 LED
Wavelength	*LD:* 820 nm *LED:* 600 nm	*LD:* 880 nm *LED:* 660 nm	*LD:* 904 nm *SLD:* 780 nm *LED:* 640 nm
Diode's power	*LD:* 40 mW *LED:* 10 mW	*LD:* 40 mW *LED:* 30 mW	*LD:* 30 mW *SLD:* 50 mW *LED:* 20 mW
Total peak power (P_p)	50 mW	1,400 mW	6,000 mW
Beam irradiation area (A)	0.5 cm^2	20 cm^2	300 cm^2
Treatment surface area (S)	4 cm^2	40 cm^2	260 cm^2
Number of irradiated points per treatment	4	40	300
Power density (P_d)	100 mW/cm^2	70 mW/cm^2	20 mW/cm^2
Energy density (E_d)	6 J/cm^2	7 J/cm^2	8 J/cm^2
Application technique	Stationary with contact	Stationary with no contact	Stationary with contact
Dose per point (D_p)	6 J	7 J	8 J
Irradiation duration (T) per square centimeters or point*	60 s	100 s	400 s
Dose per treatment (D_t)	24 J	280 J	2,400 J
Total number of treatments	6	8	3
Cumulative dose (D_c)	144 J	2,240 J	7,200 J

GaAlAs, gallium-aluminum-arsenide; LD, laser diode; LED, light-emitting diode; SLD, superluminous diode.
***Use the Online Dosage Calculator: Low-Level Laser Therapy.**

mean power density (P_d) value now equals 28 mW/cm^2. This example shows that to deliver the same dose per point (D_p), dose per treatment (D_t), and cumulative dose (D_c) as with the continuous mode, the irradiation duration needs to be longer (from 100 s to 250 s) because of the reduced laser power density resulting from pulsing the beam of energy.

3. Dosage Charting

Current guidelines (waltza.co.za) state that clinical dosage should be expressed, as exemplified earlier, in joules as opposed to joules per square centimeter (J/cm^2), often seen in several electrophysical agent textbooks. WALT suggests that reporting dosage in joules per square centimeter should be confined to studies with small animals and cell cultures, where the treated surface areas are small. When much larger surface areas are treated, as is often the case in humans, the recommendation is to report dosage in joules (Bjordal et al., 2010; waltza.co.za). WALT further recommends documenting, for each clinical case, both the dose per point as well as the cumulative dose of laser energy delivered to the treated soft tissues, as exemplified earlier, also in joules (waltza.co.za). To document LLLT dosage *only* in term of energy density (J/cm^2), or dose per point (J), is incomplete and *can be misleading.* For example, Table 11-9 demonstrates that although energy density or

TABLE 11-8 EXAMPLES OF LOW-LEVEL LASER THERAPY DOSIMETRIC MEASUREMENTS FOR PULSED MODE

	Pulsed Mode GaAlAs Laser		
Parameter	**Wand Probe**	**Cluster Probe**	**Array Probe**
Number of diodes	2	36	185
Types of diodes	1 LD 1 LED	32 LD 4 LED	140 LD 30 SLD 15 LED
Wavelength	*LD:* 820 nm *LED:* 600 nm	*LD:* 880 nm *LED:* 660 nm	*LD:* 904 nm *SLD:* 780 nm *LED:* 640 nm
Diode's power	*LD:* 40 mW *LED:* 10 mW	*LD:* 40 mW *LED:* 30 mW	*LD:* 30 mW *SLD:* 50 mW *LED:* 20 mW
Total peak power (P_p)	50 mW	1,400 mW	6,000 mW
Frequency (F)	3,000 Hz	2,000 Hz	1,000 Hz
Pulse duration (PD)	0.0002s	0.0002 s	0.0005 s
Mean power (P_m)	30 mW	560 mW	3,000 mW
Beam irradiation area (A)	0.5 cm^2	20 cm^2	300 cm^2
Treatment surface area (S)	4 cm^2	40 cm^2	260 cm^2
Number of irradiated points per treatment	4	40	300
Power density (P_d)	60 mW/cm^2	28 mW/cm^2	10 mW/cm^2
Energy density (E_d)	6 J/cm^2	7 J/cm^2	8 J/cm^2
Application technique	Stationary with contact	Stationary with no contact	Stationary with contact
Dose per point (D_p)	6 J	7 J	8 J
Irradiation duration (T) per centimeter or point*	100 s	250 s	800 s
Dose per treatment (D_t)	24 J	280 J	2,400 J
Total number of treatments	6	8	3
Cumulative dose (D_c)	144 J	2,240 J	7,200 J

GaAlAs, gallium-aluminum-arsenide; LD, laser diode; LED, light-emitting diode; SLD, superluminous diode.
***Use the Online Dosage Calculator: Low-Level Laser Therapy.**

dose per point is the same (7 J or 7 J/cm^2) for all four case examples, the dose per treatment and cumulative doses are quite different. This illustrates why it is preferable to document, for each clinical case, all three dosages in joules, because the bottom line is that dosage must represent the amount of light energy (joules) delivered over the entire treated surface area of tissue and not only over 1 cm^2 of it.

D. ONLINE DOSAGE CALCULATOR: LOW-LEVEL LASER THERAPY

As described in Chapter 10 on shortwave diathermy, an **Online Dosage Calculator** is provided with the objective to lessen the burden associated with recalling those formulas and doing similar hand calculations. Upon entering

TABLE 11-9 EXAMPLES OF LOW-LEVEL LASER THERAPY DOSAGE DOCUMENTATION

Applicator	Beam Irradiating Area (A)	Treatment Surface Area (S)	Number of Irradiated Points	Number of Treatment Sessions	Dose per Point or Energy Density	Dose per Treatment	Cumulative Dose
Wand	1 cm^2	1 cm^2	1	10	7 J	7 J	70 J
	1 cm^2	4 cm^2	4	10	7 J	28 J	280 J
Cluster	20 cm^2	40 cm^2	40	10	7 J	280 J	2,800 J
Array pad	300 cm^2	300 cm^2	300	10	7 J	2,100 J	21,000 J

the dosimetric parameters, the calculator will provide the precise irradiation duration required to deliver the desired dose per point, as well as the amount of the dose per treatment and cumulative dose given to each patient during the course of LLLT.

V. APPLICATION, CONTRAINDICATIONS, AND RISKS

Prior to considering the application of LLLT, practitioners must first check for contraindications, consider the risks, and then go through key application steps and procedures designed to optimize treatment safety, efficacy, and effectiveness. Note that the listed contraindications apply to both continuous and pulsed modes. In addition, recall that LLLT can be applied safely over metallic implants and on patients with pacemakers. To facilitate quantitative dosimetry, readers are invited to use the **Online Dosage Calculator: Low-Level Laser Therapy.**

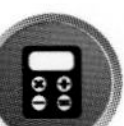

APPLICATION, CONTRAINDICATIONS, AND RISKS

Low-Level Laser Therapy

IMPORTANT: Prior to treatment, test whether the laser device is functioning by applying the applicator over the test photoelectrical cell mounted on the device console. The rationale behind such testing is that infrared lasers generate invisible light, and exposure to the laser beam generates no sensation. *Both patients and practitioners must wear protective glasses or goggles,* which filter the wavelength range emitted by the laser device during therapy. Use a closed room to deliver therapy. Avoid unnecessary exposure to surrounding staff and patients. Shown, as examples, are applications of LLLT using a cluster (Fig. 11-8) and a wand (Fig. 11-9) probe.

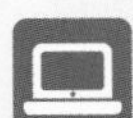

See **online video.**

STEP	RATIONALE AND PROCEDURE
1. Check for contraindications.	*Over the eye*—damage to the retina *Over a malignant lesion*—further enhancement and spread of lesion *Over the abdominal and pelvic area of women who are pregnant*—interference with normal development and growth of the fetus *Over a hemorrhagic area*—exacerbating the condition by laser-induced vasodilation (Baxter, 2002) *Over the thyroid gland*—interfering with normal function of the thyroid gland (Navratil et al., 2002) *In patients with epilepsy*—inducing an epileptic seizure (Navratil et al., 2002) ***Note:*** Metal and plastic implants, as well as pacemakers, are not contraindicated and can be used safely.

STEP	RATIONALE AND PROCEDURE

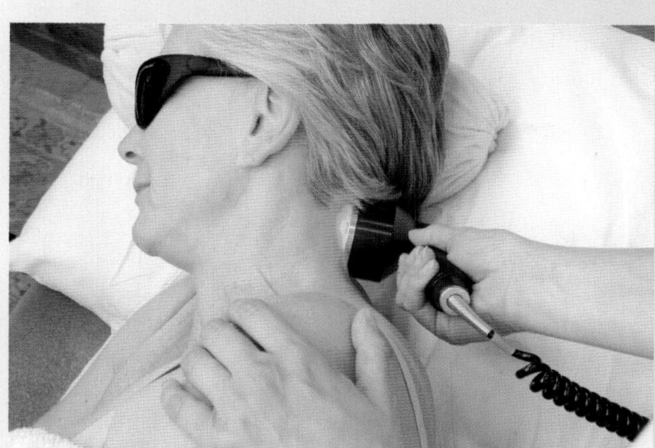

FIGURE 11-8 Application of low-level laser therapy using a cluster probe over the cervical area. (Courtesy of THOR Laser, Inc.)

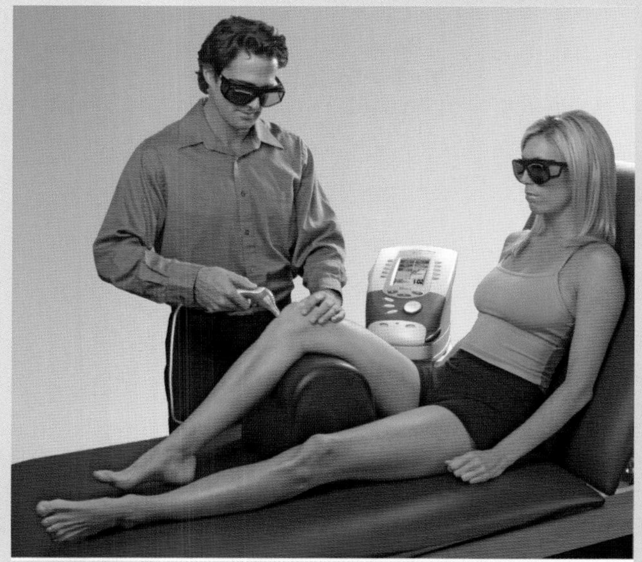

FIGURE 11-9 Application of low-level laser therapy over the knee area with both patient and operator wearing laser protective goggles. (Courtesy of DJO Global.)

STEP	RATIONALE AND PROCEDURE
2. Consider the risks.	*Over an infected area*—risk of stimulating or inhibiting bacterial activity *Over bruised muscle*—risk of enhancing brusing (Gabel, 1995) *Over testicular region*—risk of affecting fertility *Over sympathetic ganglia, vagus nerve, and cardiac region in patients with heart disease*—risk of adverse heart effects (Baxter, 2002) *Over photosensitive skin areas*—risk of adverse reaction. A test dose is recommended before application (Baxter, 2002) *Over bone epiphyseal region of growing children*—risk of affecting bone growth
3. Position and instruct patient.	Ensure comfortable body positioning. Inform the patient that he or she may feel nothing during treatment.
4. Prepare treatment area.	*Normal skin:* Cleanse the exposed skin with rubbing alcohol to remove impurities. Shave excessive hair if necessary. *Wounded skin:* Wash and debride the wound. Wear protective gears like goggles, mask, gown, and gloves to prevent contamination.
5. Estimate location, depth, and surface area of lesion.	Locate the pathologic soft-tissue lesion, estimate its depth (in centimeters) from the skin surface, and measure its surface area (in square centimeters). Information about tissue depth will guide the selection of laser (see later discussion). Measurement of lesion's surface area will guide the selection of applicator's size (see later discussion).
6. Select device type.	Choose between a *cabinet* (in clinic therapy) and a *portable* (bedside or home therapy) type of device. Diode-type lasers have replaced the gaseous type because they are much less expensive to manufacture. Consequently, the remaining elements of this protocol relate *only on the application* of diode-type lasers (GaAlAS and GaAs). Plug line-powered devices into ground-fault circuit interrupter (GFCI) receptacles to prevent macroshock (see Chapter 5).

STEP	RATIONALE
7. Select light range.	Choose between red or infrared, or a mix of both lights. Select laser, superluminous, or light-emitting diodes. • *Red light:* Select diodes emitting within the 600–750 nm range. • *Infrared light:* Select diodes emitting within the 750–1 mm range. The deeper the target tissue, the more infrared light should be used because it is more penetrating.
8. Select applicator type and size.	Choose between the wand, cluster, or array pad applicators. Select the wand probe for small, cluster probe for medium, and array pad for larger treatment areas.
9. Select application technique.	Choose between stationary with contact, stationary with noncontact, gridding, and scanning. • *Stationary with contact:* The applicator makes contact with the skin and is kept in place for the entire irradiating duration or treatment. This method eliminates photonic reflection off the skin surface and minimizes beam divergence because of the probe's close proximity to the treated area. • *Stationary with noncontact:* The applicator makes no contact with the skin and is kept in place for the entire irradiating duration or treatment. The applicator-irradiating surface is maintained at a few millimeters (less than 1 cm) for the skin surface. This method is recommended when patients cannot tolerate the pressure exerted by the applicator on the treated surface. • *Gridding:* This technique, also called *point-by-point,* consists in making a grid by mapping the entire treatment surface area with 1-cm^2 squares to guide the point-by-point application. Each square centimeter corresponds to one point, thus the related term *point-by-point technique.* The grid can be made either visually or with a plastic sheet and a pen. Gridding is used with the wand probe, because its tip or irradiating area is often less than 1 cm^2. • *Scanning:* The entire treatment surface area is scanned (noncontact) using wand- and cluster-type probes. This scanning action may be done by manipulating the wand probe (up-and-down and side-to-side movements). It can also be done automatically by means of robotic displacements of the diodes within the cluster probe positioned over the treatment area.
10. Set dosimetry.	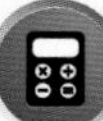 Choose between the *continuous* or *pulsed* mode of delivery. Determine the dose (J) of energy that you want to deliver to the tissues per application. Use Table 11-7 (continuous mode) or Table 11-8 (pulsed mode) as dosimetric templates. Use the dosage recommendations from the WALT as a guideline (see Table 11-6). To facilitate dosimetry, use the **Online Dosage Calculator: Low-Level Laser Therapy.**
11. Position the applicator.	Apply the following two laws governing application (see Chapter 10 for details): • *Lambert's cosine law:* Keep the laser beam as perpendicular as possible to the exposed treated surface area to minimize light reflection. • *Inverse square law:* If noncontact is used, keeps the distance separating the applicator and the exposed skin surface as small as possible, and constant from one application to the next.
12. Put on protective laser goggles.	*Both patients and practitioners must wear protective glasses or goggles,* which filter the wavelength range emitted by the laser device during therapy.
13. Apply treatment.	Ensure adequate monitoring.
14. Conduct post-treatment procedures.	Inspect the exposed treatment area, and record any adverse reaction. Clean and disinfect the applicator faceplate (if contact) to prevent cross-contamination between patients. Ensure optimal device function. True power outputs specified by some manufacturers may be much less than advertised, leading to improper dosimetry (Nussbaum, 1999). Power decreases as the device (diodes) ages, thus requiring routine check and calibration measurements (Jenkins et al., 2011). Lock the laser device, and store the key in a safe place for further use.
15. Ensure post-treatment equipment maintenance.	Follow manufacturer recommendations. Immediately report defects or malfunctions to technical maintenance staff. Keep in mind that lasers are very susceptible to de-calibration over time.

CASE STUDIES

Two case studies follow that summarize the concepts, principles, and applications of LLLT discussed in this chapter. Case Study 11-1 addresses its use for chronic cervical osteoarthritis pain affecting a middle-aged male taxi driver. Case Study 11-2 is concerned with the application of LLLT for an Achilles tendinosis affecting a young male college athlete. Each case is structured in line with the concepts of evidence-based practice (EBP), the International Classification of Functioning, Disability, and Health (ICF) disablement model, and SOAP (*s*ubjective, *o*bjective, *a*ssessment, *p*lan) note format (see Chapter 2 for details).

CASE STUDY 11-1: CERVICAL OSTEOARTHRITIS

EVIDENCE-BASED CLINICAL DECISION MAKING PROTOCOL

1. Formulate the Case History

A 48-year-old male taxi driver, diagnosed with chronic cervical osteoarthritis, consults about his condition. His main complaint is severe neck pain during head movements, particularly when driving his car for relatively long periods without rest. Physical and radiographic examinations suggest that the pain is caused by bilateral osteoarthritic changes affecting facet joints at the C2–C5 level. Physical examination also reveals a loss of 20 degrees of flexion and 10 degrees of extension. There is also a loss of 35 degrees of right head rotation and 25 degrees of left rotation. The patient is looking for an alternative to his current cocktail of analgesic and anti-inflammatory drugs, which in addition to not giving him adequate pain relief is adding to his gastric problems. He fervently wants to reduce the number of pills he is taking. A few months ago, he tried transcutaneous electrical nerve stimulation (TENS) therapy for a period of 6 weeks but received no satisfactory pain relief. He also tried hot pack therapy, but that did not provide lasting pain relief either. Surgery is not indicated. The patient's goals are to reduce his pain level when driving at work for long hours and improve his head mobility.

2. Outline the Case Based on the ICF Framework

CERVICAL OSTEOARTHRITIS		
BODY STRUCTURES AND FUNCTIONS	**ACTIVITIES**	**PARTICIPATION**
Pain	Difficulty rotating his head	Difficulty in driving a car
Joint stiffness		

PERSONAL FACTORS	ENVIRONMENTAL FACTORS
Middle-aged man	Car driving
History of health problems	Stressful job
Low education	

3. Outline Therapeutic Goals and Outcome Measurements

GOAL	OUTCOME MEASUREMENT
Decrease pain	Visual Analogue Scale (VAS)
Reduce drug intake	Pill count in personal diary
Increase cervical range of motion (ROM)	Goniometry
Improve head function	Neck Disability Index (NDI)

4. Justify the Use of Low-Level Laser Therapy Based on the EBP Framework

PRACTITIONER'S EXPERIENCE	RESEARCH-BASED INDICATION	PATIENT'S EXPECTATION
Moderately experienced in LLLT	*Strength:* Strong	No opinion on LLLT
Has never used LLLT in similar cases	*Effectiveness:* Substantiated	Just wants pain relief
Believes that LLLT can be beneficial		

5. Outline Key Intervention Parameters

- **Treatment base:** Private clinic
- **Device type:** Cabinet model (GaAlAs). LLLT is selected because there is evidence to show its effectiveness for chronic pain, and because all previous therapies (medication, TENS, and thermotherapy) have failed to provide adequate relief. Infrared light (904 nm) is used because penetration and absorption by deep tissues in needed. Only one irradiation per treatment is needed because the beam irradiating area fully covers the treatment surface area. Dosage documentation and values complies with WALT recommendations.
- **Application protocol:** Follow the suggested application protocol for LLLT in *Application, Contraindications, and Risks* box, and make the necessary adjustments for this case.
- **Patient's positioning:** Lying prone
- **Application site:** Over the painful posterior neck area
- **Application method:** Stationary with noncontact
- **Applicator type:** Handheld cluster with 36 diodes
- **Diode type and wavelength:** 24 LDs: 904 nm;12 LEDs: 660 nm
- **Delivery mode:** Continuous
- **Peak power*:** 1,200 mW
- **Beam irradiation area:** 20 cm^2
- **Treatment surface area:** 18 cm^2
- **Power density*:** 60 mW/cm^2
- **Dose per point*:** 6 J
- **Application duration*:** 100 s
- **Number of irradiation per treatment:** 1
- **Dose per treatment*:** 120 J
- **Treatment frequency:** Daily; 5 days/week
- **Intervention period:** 2 weeks (15 days)
- **Cumulative dose*:** 1,200 J
- **Concomitant therapies:** Neck manipulation combined with a regimen of ankle flexibility and strengthening exercises

***Use the Online Dosage Calculator: Low-Level Laser Therapy.**

6. Report Pre- and Post-Intervention Outcomes

OUTCOME	PRE	POST
Pain (VAS score)	7/10	2/10
Drug intake (number of pills)	40 pills/week	10 pills/week
Cervical ROM	*Loss:* F 20 degrees; E 10 degrees; RR 35 degrees; LR 25 degrees	*Loss:* F 5 degrees; E 5 degrees; RR 15 degrees; LR 5 degrees
Improve neck function (NDI score)	32/50	12/50

7. Document Case Intervention Using the SOAP Note Format

S: Middle-aged male taxi driver presents with chronic cervical osteoarthritic pain causing difficulty with head mobility, particularly while at work. Previous drug, TENS, and thermotherapy treatments provided mild pain relief and inadequate functional results.

O: *Intervention:* LLLT (GaAlAs; 904 and 660 nm) applied over the posterior neck area; Pt lying prone; method and applicator: stationary with noncontact—cluster probe; dosage: D_p: 6 J; D_t: 120 J; D_c: 1,200 J; treatment schedule: daily, 5 days/week, for 15 days. *Pre–post comparison:* Decrease pain VAS score (7/10 to 2/10), decrease drug intake by 75%, improved cervical range of motion and improved neck function (NDI score 32/50 to 12/50).

A: No adverse effect. Treatment very well tolerated. Pt satisfied with results.

P: No further treatment required. Patient discharged.

CASE STUDY 11-2: ACHILLES TENDINOSIS

EVIDENCE-BASED CLINICAL DECISION MAKING PROTOCOL

1. Formulate the Case History

A 20-year-old college basketball player consults for painful activity- and sports-related symptoms from the right Achilles region. Pain, lasting for 2 months now, is located in the Achilles tendon. There is crepitation and tenderness during palpation. Ankle dorsiflexion is limited to 5 degrees. He has difficulty with jumping and running. He takes over-the-counter analgesic and anti-inflammatory drugs occasionally. Pain and functional limitation persists despite previous treatments, which included cryotherapy and thermotherapy. The playoff season is fast approaching, and he is desperate to get better.

2. Outline the Case Based on the ICF Framework

CERVICAL OSTEOARTHRITIS		
BODY STRUCTURES AND FUNCTIONS	**ACTIVITIES**	**PARTICIPATION**
Pain	Difficulty jumping and running	Difficulty playing competitive basketball
Joint stiffness		

PERSONAL FACTORS	ENVIRONMENTAL FACTORS
Young healthy man	College student
Athletic	Sports scholarship
Competitive	

3. Outline Therapeutic Goals and Outcome Measurements

GOAL	OUTCOME MEASUREMENT
Decrease pain	Visual Analogue Scale (VAS)
Increase ankle dorsiflexion ROM	Goniometry
Improve ankle function	Lower Extremity Functional Scale (LEFS)

4. Justify the Use of Low-Level Laser Therapy Based on the EBP Framework

PRACTITIONER'S EXPERIENCE	RESEARCH-BASED INDICATION	PATIENT'S EXPECTATION
Moderately experienced in LLLT	*Strength:* Strong	Read on the Internet about LLLT
Occasionally has used LLLT in similar cases	*Effectiveness:* Conflicting	Wants full recovery before playoffs
Is curious to see if LLLT can be beneficial		Believes that LLLT may be effective

5. Outline Key Intervention Parameters

- **Treatment base:** Private clinic
- **Device type:** Cabinet model (GaAs). LLLT is selected because there is evidence to show its effectiveness for tendinopathies, and because previous therapies (medication, cryotherapy, and thermotherapy) have failed to provide adequate therapeutic effects. Infrared light is used because penetration and absorption by deep tissues in needed. Four irradiations per treatment are needed to cover or treat the entire treatment surface area. Dosage parameters comply with WALT recommendations.
- **Application protocol:** Follow the suggested application protocol for LLLT in *Application, Contraindications, and Risks* box, and make the necessary adjustments for this case.
- **Patient's positioning:** Lying prone
- **Application site:** Over the painful Achilles tendon area
- **Application method:** Stationary with contact; visual gridding
- **Applicator type:** Handheld wand with 3 diodes
- **Diode type and wavelength:** 1 LD of 820 nm; 2 LDs of 720 nm
- **Delivery mode:** Pulsed
- **Mean power*:** 80 mW
- **Beam irradiation area:** 1 cm^2
- **Treatment surface area:** 4 cm^2
- **Power density*:** 80 mW/cm^2
- **Dose per point*:** 4 J
- **Application duration*:** 50 s
- **Number of irradiations per treatment:** 4
- **Dose per treatment*:** 16 J
- **Treatment frequency:** daily; 5 days/week
- **Intervention period:** 2 weeks
- **Cumulative dose*:** 160 J
- **Concomitant therapies:** A regimen of eccentric exercises combined with static stretching of the triceps surae

***Use the Online Dosage Calculator: Low-Level Laser Therapy.**

6. Report Pre- and Post-Intervention Outcomes

OUTCOME	PRE	POST
Pain (VAS score)	6/10	1/10
Ankle ROM	*Loss:* dorsiflexion 5 degrees	*Loss:* dorsiflexion 0 degrees
Lower limb function (LEFS score)	48/80	64/80

7. Document Case Intervention Using the SOAP Note Format

S: Young athletic Pt presents with right Achilles tendinopathy causing difficulty with regular activities, particularly while playing competitive basketball. Previous drug, cryotherapy, and thermotherapy provided temporary pain relief but limited functional benefit.

O: *Intervention:* LLLT (GaAs; 820 and 720 nm) applied over the Achilles tendon area; Pt lying prone; applicator and application: wand probe, stationary with contact; dosage: D_p: 4 J; D_t: 16 J; D_c: 160 J; treatment schedule: daily, 5 days/week, for 10 days. *Pre–post comparison:* Decrease pain VAS score (6/10 to 1/10), full ankle dorsiflexion, and improved lower limb function (LEFS scores from 4880 to 64/80).

A: No adverse effect. Treatment very well tolerated.

P: No further treatment required. Patient discharged. Asked to better warm up the lower limbs before competitive basketball.

VI. THE BOTTOM LINE

- There is strong scientific evidence to show that LLLT can induce significant photobiologic effects on human superficial and deep soft tissues.
- LLLT is the delivery of electromagnetic energy, within the red visible and near-infrared band of the electromagnetic spectrum, for therapeutic purposes.
- All laser (LD) and nonlaser (LED, SLD) lights are capable of generating therapeutic photobiologic effects on soft tissues.
- LLLT energy is absorbed by chromophores triggering photobiomodulation effects.
- Monochromacity appears to be the key property behind the photobiologic effects of LLLT, because both coherence and collimation are lost as soon as the beam of light enters the skin.
- Near-infrared light is more penetrating than red visible light.
- Optimal energy delivery is achieved when the four laws governing application are applied.

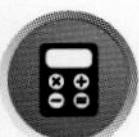

- Using the **Online Dosage Calculator: Low-Level Laser Therapy** removes the burden of hand calculation and promotes the adoption of quantitative dosimetry.
- The dosage recommendations from the WALT provide adequate guidelines for dosimetry.
- Dose per point (D_p), dose per treatment (D_t), and cumulative dose (D_c) should be measured, recorded, and expressed in joules.
- Metal and plastic implants, as well as pacemakers, are not contraindicated in LLLT and can be exposed to light energy safely.
- Until the photobiologic effects associated with pulsed LLLT are better defined, using continuous LLLT remains the gold standard.
- The overall body of evidence reported in this chapter shows the strength of evidence behind LLLT to be *strong* and its level of therapeutic effectiveness *substantiated.*

VII. CRITICAL THINKING QUESTIONS

Clarification: What is meant by low-level laser therapy (LLLT)?

Assumptions: You assume that the therapeutic optical window of LLLT is within the visible red and invisible infrared band of the electromagnetic spectrum. How do you justify making that assumption?

Reasons and evidence: What leads you to believe that monochromacity may be the key property behind the therapeutic effects of LLLT?

Viewpoints or perspectives: How will you respond to a colleague who says that the use of LLLT is well justified today for the treatment of cutaneous wounds and tendinopathies?

Implications and consequences: What are the implications and consequences of (1) using a wand instead of a cluster, or an array pad, applicator, (2) if neither the operator nor the patient wears protective goggles when delivering or receiving LLLT, and (3) if the lasers are not regularly calibrated?

About the question: What is the estimated penetration depth of red and infrared lasers used to deliver LLLT to soft tissues? Why do you think I ask this question?

VIII. REFERENCES

Articles

Altan L, Bibgol U, Aykac M, Yurtkuran M (2005) Investigation of the effect of GaAs laser therapy on cervical myofascial pain syndrome. Rheumatol Int, 25: 23–27

Asada K, Yutani Y, Shimazu A (1989) Diode laser therapy for rheumatoid arthritis. A clinical evaluation of 102 joints treated with low reactive-level laser therapy (LLLT). Laser Ther, 1: 147–151

Ashford R, Lagan K, Brown N, Howell C, Nolan C, Brady D, Walsh M (1999) Low-intensity laser therapy for chronic venous leg ulcers. Nurs Stand, 14: 66–70, 72

Atsumi K, Fijumasa I, Abe Y (1987) Biostimulation effect of low-power energy of diode laser for pain relief. Lasers Surg Med, 7: 77–82

Basford JR, Malanga GA, Krause DA, Harmsen WS (1998) A randomized controlled evaluation of low-intensity laser therapy: Plantar fasciitis. Arch Phys Med Rehabil, 79: 249–254

Basford JR, Sheffield CG, Cieslak KR (2000) Laser therapy: A randomized, controlled trial of the effects of low intensity Nd:Yag laser irradiation on lateral epicondylitis. Arch Phys Med Rehabil, 81: 1504–1510

Basford JR, Sheffield CG, Harmsen WS (1999) Laser therapy: A randomized, controlled trial of the effects of low-intensity Nd:YAG laser irradiation on musculoskeletal back pain. Arch Phys Med Rehabil, 80: 647–652

Basford JR, Sheffield CG, Mair SD, Ilstrup DM (1987) Low-energy helium-neon laser of thumb ostearthritis. Arch Phys Med Rehabil, 68: 794–797

Bihari I, Mester AR (1989) The biostimulative effects of low-level laser therapy of long-standing crural ulcers using helium-neon laser, helium-neon plus infrared lasers, and noncoherent light: Preliminary reports of a randomized double-blind comparative study. Laser Ther, 1: 75–78

Bingol U, Altan L, Yurtkuran M (2005) Low-power laser treatment for shoulder pain. Photomed Laser Surg, 23: 459–464

Bjordal JM, Lopes-Martins RA, Iversen VV (2006a) A randomized placebo controlled trial of low level laser therapy for activated Achilles tendonitis with microdialysis measurement of peritendinous prostaglandin E2 concentration. Br J Sports Med, 40: 76–80

Bliddal H, Hellesen C, Ditlevsen P, Asselberghs J, Lyager L (1987) Soft-laser therapy of rheumatoid arthritis. Scand J Rheumatol, 16: 225–228

Brosseau L, Wells G, Marchand S, Gaboury I, Stokes B, Morin M, Casimiro L, Yonge K, Tugwell P (2005) Randomized controlled trial on lower laser therapy (LLLT) in the treatment of osteoarthritis (OA) on the hand. Lasers Surg Med, 36: 210–219

Bülow PM, Jensen H, Danneskiold-Samsoe B (1994) Low-power Ga-Al-As laser treatment of painful osteoarthritis of the knee. Scand J Rehab Med, 26: 155–159

Catari CJ, Anderson SN, Gannon BJ, Piller NB (2003) Treatment of postmastectomy lymphedema with low-level laser therapy: A double blind, placebo-controlled trial. Cancer, 98: 1114–1122

Ceccherelli F, Altafini L, Lo Castro G, Avila A, Ambrosio F, Giron GP (1989) Diode laser in cervical myofascial pain: A double-blind study versus placebo. Clin J Pain, 5: 301–304

Cetiner S, Kahraman SA, Yucetas S (2006) Evaluation of low-level laser therapy in the treatment of temporomandibular disorders. Photomed Laser Surg, 24: 637–641

Ceylan, Hizmetli S, Silig Y (2004) The effect of infrared laser therapy and medical treatments on pain and serotonin degradation products in patients with myofascial pain syndrome. A controlled trial. Rheumatol Int, 24: 260–263

Chow RT, Barnsley LB, Heller GZ (2006) The effect of 300 mW, 830 nm laser on chronic neck pain: A double-blind, randomized, placebo-controlled study. Pain, 124: 201–210

Conti PC (1997) Low level laser therapy in the treatment of temporomandibular disorders (TMD): A double-blind pilot study. Cranio, 15: 144–199

Craig JA, Barlas P, Baxter GD, Walsh DM, Allen JM (1996) Delayed-onset of muscle soreness: Lack of effect of combined phototherapy/low-intensity laser therapy at low pulse repetition rates. J Clin Laser Med Surg, 14: 375–380

Craig JA, Barron J, Walsh DM, Baxter GD (1999) Lack of effect of combined low-intensity laser therapy/phototherapy (CLILT) on delayed onset muscle soreness in humans. Lasers Surg Med, 24: 223–230

Crous LC, Malherbe CP (1988) Laser and ultraviolet light irradiation in the treatment of chronic ulcers. S Afr J Physiother, 44: 73–77

Darre EM, Klokker M, Lund P, Rasmussen JD, Hansen K, Vedtoffe PE (1994) Laser therapy of Achilles tendonitis. Ugeskr Laeger, 156: 6680–6683

De Bie RA, de Vet HC, Lenssen TF, van den Wildenberg FA, Kootstra G, Knispschild PG (1998) Low-level laser therapy in ankle sprains. A randomized clinical trial. Arch Phys Med Rehabil, 79: 1415–1420

Dirican A, Andacoglu O, Johnson R, McGuire K, Mager L, Soran A (2011) The short-term effects of low-level laser therapy in the management of breast-cancer related lymphedema. Support Care Cancer, 19: 685–690

Djavid GE, Mehrdad R, Ghasemi M, Hasan-Zedeh H, Sotoodeh-Manesh A, Pouryaghoub G (2007) In chronic low-back pain, low-level laser therapy combined with exercise is more beneficial than exercise alone in the long term: A randomized trial. Aust J Physiother, 53: 155–160

Dundar U, Evcik D, Samli F, Pusak H, Kacuncu V (2007) The effects of gallium arsenide laser therapy in the management of cervical myofascial pain syndrome: A double blind, placebo-controlled study. Clin Rheumatol, 26: 930–934

Eckerdal A, Bastian HL (1996) Can low reactive–level laser therapy be used in the treatment of neurogenic facial pain? A double-blind, placebo-controlled investigation of patients with trigeminal neuralgia. Laser Ther, 8: 247–252

Ekim A, Armagan O, Tascioglu F, Oner C, Colak M (2007) Effect of low-level laser therapy in rheumatoid patients with carpal tunnel syndrome. Swiss Med Wkly, 137: 347–352

Emmanoulidis O, Diamantopoulos C (1986) CW IR low-power laser application significantly accelerates chronic pain rehabilitation of professional athletes. A double-blind study. Lasers Surg Med, 6: 173–178

England S, Farrell AJ, Coppock JS, Struthers G, Bacon PA (1989) Low-power laser therapy of shoulder tendonitis. Scand J Rheumatol, 18: 427–431

Enwemeka CS (2011) The relevance of accurate comprehension of treatment parameters in photobiomodulation. Photomed Laser Surg, 29: 783–784

Evcik D, Kavuncu V, Cakir T, Subasi V, Yaman M (2007) Laser therapy in the treatment of carpal tunnel syndrome: A randomized controlled trial. Photomed Laser Surg, 25: 34–39

Fikackova H, Dostalova T, Navratil L, Klaschka J (2007) Effectiveness of low-level laser therapy in temporomandibular joint disorders: A placebo-controlled study. Photomed Laser Surg, 25: 297–303

Freanek A, Krol P, Kucharzewski M (2002) Does low output laser stimulation enhance the healing of crural ulceration? Some critical remarks. Med Eng Phys, 24: 607–615

Fulga C (1998) Anti-inflammatory effect of laser therapy in rheumatoid arthritis. Rom J Intern Med, 36: 273–279

Fulga C, Fulga IC, Prodescu M (1994) Clinical study of the effect of laser therapy in rheumatic degenerative diseases. Rom J Intern Med, 32: 227–233

Gabel P (1995) Does laser enhance bruising in acute sporting injuries? Aust J Physiother, 41: 273–275

Gartner CH, Becker M, Dusoir T (1987) Pain control in spondyloarthritis with infrared laser. Lasers Surg Med, 7: 79–81

Goats GC, Flett E, Hunter JA, Stirling A (1996) Low-intensity laser and phototherapy for rheumatoid arthritis. Physiotherapy, 82: 311–320

Gogia PP, Hurt BS, Zirn TT (1988) Wound management with whirlpool and infrared cold laser treatment. Phys Ther, 68: 1239–1242

Goldman JA, Chiapella J, Casey H, Bass N, Graham J, McClatchey W, Dronavalli RV, Brown R, Bennet WJ, Miller SB, Wilson CH, Pearson B, Haun C, Persinski L, Huey H, Muckerheide M (1980) Laser therapy in rheumatoid arthritis. Laser Surg Ther, 1: 93–101

Gupta AK, Filimenko N, Salansky N, Sauder DN (1998) The use of low energy photon therapy (LEPT) in venous leg ulcers: A double-blind, placebo-controlled study. Dermatol Surg, 24: 1383–1386

Gur A, Cosut A, Sarac AJ, Cevik R, Nas K, Uyar A (2003a) Efficacy of different therapy regimes of low-power laser in painful osteoarthritis of the knee: A double-blind and randomized-controlled trial. Lasers Surg Med, 33: 330–338

Gur A, Karakoc M, Cevik R, Nas K, Sarac AJ, Karakoc M (2003b) Efficacy of low power laser therapy and exercise on pain and functions in chronic low back pain. Lasers Surg Med, 32: 233–238

Gur A, Kakaroc M, Nas K, Cevik R, Sarac J, Ataoglu S (2002) Effects of low power laser and low dose amitriptyline therapy on clinical symptoms and quality of life in fibromyalgia: A single-blind, placebo-controlled trial. Rheumatol Int, 22: 188–193

Gur A, Sarac AJ, Cevik R, Altindag O, Sarac S (2004) Efficacy of 904 nm gallium arsenide low level laser therapy in the management of chronic myofascial pain in the neck: A double-blind and randomized-controlled trial. Lasers Surg Med, 35: 229–235

Haker EH, Lunderberg T (1990) Laser treatment applied to acupuncture points in lateral humeral epicondylalgia. A double-blind study. Pain, 43: 243–247

Haker EH, Lundeberg TC (1991a) Lateral epicondylalgia: Report of noneffective midlaser treatment. Arch Phys Med Rehabil, 72: 984–988

Haker EH, Lundeberg TC (1991b) Is low energy laser treatment effective in lateral epicondylalgia? J Pain Symptom Manage, 6: 241–246

Hakguder A, Birtane M, Gurcan S, Kokino S, Turan FN (2003) Efficacy of low level laser therapy in myofascial pain syndrome: An algometric and thermographic evaluation. Lasers Surg Med: 33: 339–343

Hall J, Clarke AK, Elvins DM, Ring EF (1994) Low-level laser therapy is ineffective in the management of rheumatoid arthritic finger joints. Br J Rheumatol, 33: 142–147

Hansen HJ, Thoroe U (1990) Low-power laser biostimulation of chronic oro-facial pain. A double-blind, placebo-controlled cross-over study in 40 patients. Pain, 43: 169–179

Herascu N, Velciu B, Calin M, Savastru D, Talianu C (2005) Low-level laser therapy (LLLT) efficacy in post-operative wounds. Photomed Laser Surg, 23: 70–73

Heussler JK, Hinchey G, Margiotta E, Quinn R, Butler P, Martin J, Sturgess AD (1993) A double-blind, randomized trial of low-power laser treatment in rheumatoid arthritis. Ann Rheum Dis, 52: 703–706

Hirschl M, Katsenschlager R, Francesconi C, Kundi M (2004) Low level laser therapy in primary Raynaud's phenomenon—results of a placebo controlled, double blind intervention study. J Rheumatol, 31: 2408–2412

Hopkins JT, McLoda TA, Seegmiller JG, Baxter GD (2004) Low-level laser therapy facilitates superficial wound healing in humans: A triple-blind, sham-controlled study. J Athl Train, 39: 223–229

Houza G, Gerenemus R, Dover J, Arndt K (1993) Lasers in dermatology. Arch Dermatol, 129: 1026–1035

Ilbuldu E, Cakmak A, Disci R, Aydin R (2004) Comparison of laser, dry needling, and placebo laser treatments in myofascial pain syndrome. Photomed Laser Surg, 22: 306–311

Irvine J, Chong SL, Amirjani N, Chan KM (2004) Double-blind randomized controlled trial of low-level laser therapy in carpal tunnel syndrome. Muscle Nerve, 30: 182–187

Iusim M, Kimchy J. Pillar T (1992) Evaluation of the degree of effectiveness of Biobeam low level narrow band light on the treatment of skin ulcers and delayed postoperative wound healing. Orthopedics, 15: 1023–1026

Jenkins PA, Carroll JD (2011) How to report low-level laser therapy (LLLT)/photomedicine dose and beam parameters in clinical and laboratory studies. Photomed Laser Surg, 29: 785–787

Jensen H, Herreby M, Kjer J (1987) Infrared laser-effect in painful arthrosis of the knee? Ugeskr Laeger, 149: 3104–3106

Johannsen F, Hauschild B, Remvig L, Johnsen V, Petersen M, Bieler T (1994) Low-energy laser therapy in rheumatoid arthritis. Scand J Rheumatol, 23: 145–147

Kaviani A, Fateh M, Nooraie RY, Alinagi-Zadeh MR, Ataie-Fashtami L (2006) Low-level laser therapy in management of postmastectomy lymphedema. Lasers Med Sci, 21: 90–94

Kemmotsu O, Sato K, Furumido H, Harada K, Takigawa C, Kaseno S, Yokota S, Hanaoka Y, Yamamura T (1991) Efficacy of low reactive–level laser therapy for pain attenuation of postherpetic neuralgia. Laser Ther, 3: 71–76

Khan J (1984) Case reports: Open wound management with the HeNe (632.8 nm) cold laser. J Orthop Sports Phys Ther, 6: 203–204

Klein RG, Eek BC (1990) Low-energy laser treatment and exercise for chronic low back pain: Double-blind controlled trial. Arch Phys Med Rehabil, 71: 34–37

Knappe V, Frank F, Rohde E (2004) Principles of lasers and biophotonic effects. Photomed Laser Surg, 22: 411–417

Kokol R, Berger C, Haas J, Kopera D (2005) Venous leg ulcers: No improvement of wound healing with 685-nm low level laser therapy. Randomized, placebo-controlled, double blind study. Hautarzt, 56: 570–575

Konstantinovic L, Antonic M, Badareski Z (1997) Combined low-power laser therapy and local infiltration of corticosteroids in the treatment of radial humeral epicondylitis. Vojnosanit Pregl, 54: 489–463

Kopera D, Kokol R, Berger C, Haas J (2005) Does the use of low-level laser influence wound healing in chronic venous leg ulcers? J Wound, 14: 391–394

Krasheninnikoff M, Ellitsgaard N, Rogvi-Hansen B, Zeuthen A, Harder K, Larsen R, Gaardbo H (1994) No effect of low-power laser in lateral epicondylitis. Scand J Rheumatol, 23: 260–263

Kreczi T, Klinger D (1986) A comparison of laser acupuncture versus placebo in radicular and pseudoradicular pain syndromes as recorded by subjective responses of patients. Acupunct Electrother Res, 11: 207–216

Kulekcioglu S, Sivrioglu K, Ozcan O, Parlak M (2003) Effectiveness of low-level laser therapy in temporomandibular disorders. Scan J Rheumatol, 32: 114–118

Kymplova J, Navratil L, Knizek J (2003) Contribution of phototherapy to the treatment of episiotomies. J Clin Laser Med Surg, 21: 35–39

Laakso E, Richardson C, Cranond T (1997) Pain scores and side effects in response to low level laser therapy (LLLT) for myofascial trigger points. Laser Ther, 9: 67–72

Lagan KM, Clements BA, McDonough S, Baxter GD (2001) Low intensity laser therapy (830nm) in the management of minor postsurgical wounds: A controlled clinical study. Lasers Surg Med, 28: 27–32

Lagan KM, McDonough SM, Clements BA, Baxter GD (2000) A case report of low intensity laser therapy (LILT) in the management of venous ulceration: Potential effects of wound debridement upon efficacy. J Clin Laser Med Surg, 18: 15–22

Lagan KM, McKenna T, Witherow A, Johns J, McDonough SM, Baxter GD (2002) Low-intensity laser therapy/combined phototherapy in the management of chronic venous ulceration: A placebo-controlled study. J Clin Laser Med Surg, 20: 109–116

Lam KL, Cheing GL (2007) Effects of 904-nm low-level laser therapy in the management of lateral epicondylitis: A randomized controlled trial. Photomed Laser Surg, 25: 65–71

Lewith GT, Machin D (1981) A randomized trial to evaluate the effects of infrared stimulation on local trigger points, versus placebo, on the pain caused by cervical osteoarthritis. Acupunct Electrother Res, 6: 277–284

Li XH (1990) Laser in the department of traumatology: With a report of 60 cases of soft tissue injury. Laser Ther, 2: 119–122

Logdberg-Andersson M, Mutzell S, Hazel A (1997) Low level laser therapy of tendinitis and myofascial pain: A randomized double-blind controlled study. Laser Ther, 9: 79–86

Lonauer G (1986) Controlled double-blind study on the efficacy of HeNe laser beams versus HeNe infrared laser beams in the therapy of activated osteoarthritis of finger joints. Lasers Surg Med, 6: 172–175

Longo L, Simunovic Z, Postiglione M, Postiglione M (1997) Laser therapy for fibromyositic rheumatisms. J Clin Laser Med Surg, 15: 217–220

Lucas C, Coenen CH, De Haan RJ (2000) The effect of low level laser therapy on stage III decubitus ulcers: A prospective, randomized single-blind, multicenter pilot study. Lasers Med Sci, 15: 94–100

Lucas C, van Gemet MJ, de Haan RJ (2003) Efficacy of low-level laser therapy in the management of stage III decubitus ulcers: A prospective, observer-blinded multicentre randomised clinical trial. Lasers Med Sci, 18: 72–77

Lundeberg T, Haker E, Thomas M (1987) Effect of laser versus placebo in tennis elbow. Scand J Rehab Med, 19: 135–138

Lundeberg T, Malm M (1991) Low-power HeNe laser treatment of venous leg ulcers. Ann Plastic Surg, 27: 537–539

Malm M, Lundeberg T (1991) Effect of low power gallium arsenide laser on healing of venous ulcers. Scand J Plast Reconstr Surg Hand Surg, 25: 249–251

Matsumura C, Ishikawa F, Imai M, Kemmotsu O (1993) Useful effect of application of helium-neon LLLT on an early stage of case of herpes zoster: A case report. Laser Ther, 5: 43–46

Matsutani LA, Marques AP, Ferreira EA, Assumpcao A, Lage LV, Casarotto RA, Pereira CA (2007) Effectiveness of muscle stretching exercises with and without laser therapy at tender points for patients with fibromyalgia. Clin Exp Rheumatol, 25: 410–415

Mazzetto MO, Carasco TG, Bidinelo EF, de Andrade Pizzo RC, Mazetto RG (2007) Low intensity laser application in temporomandibular disorders: A phase I double-blind study. Cranio, 25: 186–192

McKibben LS, Downie R (1990) Treatment of postherpetic pain using a 904 nm low-energy infrared laser. Laser Ther, 2: 20–25

Mester E, Korenyi-Both A, Spiry T, Tisza S (1970) The effect of laser irradiation on the regeneration of muscle fibres (preliminary report). Z Exp Chirurg, 8: 258–262

Mester E, Mester A (1989) Wound healing. Laser Ther, 1: 7–15

Mester E, Mester AF, Mester A (1985) The biomedical effect of laser application. Lasers Surg Med, 5: 31–39

Mester E, Spiry T, Szende B, Tota JG (1971) Effect of laser rays on wound healing. Am J Surg, 122: 532–535

Mester E, Szende B, Gartner P (1968) The effect of laser beams on the growth of hair in mice. Radiobiol Radiother, 9: 621–626

Moore KC, Hira N, Broome IJ, Cruikshank JA (1992) The effect of infrared diode laser irradiation on the duration and severity of postoperative pain. A double-blind trial. Laser Ther, 4: 145–150

Moore KC, Hira N, Kumar PS, Jayakumar CS, Oshiro T (1988) A double-blind crossover trial of low-level laser therapy in the treatment of post herpetic neuralgia. Laser Ther, 1: 7–9

Morita H, Kohno J, Hori M, Kitano Y (1993) Clinical application of low reactive–level laser therapy (LLLT) for atopic dermatitis. Keio J Med, 42: 174–176

Mulcahy D, McCormack D, McElwain J, Wagstaff S, Conroy C (1995) Low-level laser therapy: A prospective double-blind trial of its use in an orthopedic population. Injury, 26: 315–317

Naeser MA, Han KA, Lieberman BE, Branco KF (2002) Carpal tunnel syndrome pain treated with low-level laser and microamperes transcutaneous electric nerve stimulation: A controlled study. Arch Phys Med Rehabil, 83: 978–988

Navratil L, Kymplova J (2002) Contraindications in non-invasive laser therapy: Truth and fiction. J Clin Laser Med Surg, 20: 341–343

Nolan LJ (1987) Laser physics and safety. Clin Podiatr Med Surg, 4: 777–786

Nunez SC, Garces AS, Suzuki SS, Ribeiro MS (2006) Management of mouth opening in patients with temporomandibular disorders through low-level laser therapy and transcutaneous electrical nerve stimulation. Photomed Laser Surg, 24: 45–49

Nussbaum EL (1999) Low-intensity laser therapy for benign fibrotic lumps in the breast following reduction mammaplasty. Phys Ther, 79: 691–698

Nussbaum EL, Biemann I, Mustard B (1994) Comparison of ultrasound/ultraviolet-C and laser for treatment of pressure ulcers in patients with spinal cord injury. Phys Ther, 74: 812–823

Nussbaum EL, Van Zuylen J, Baxter GD (1999) Specification of treatment dosage in laser therapy: Unreliable equipment and radiant power determination as confounding factors. Physiother Can, 51: 159–167

Obara J, Yanase M, Motomura (1987) The pain relief of low-energy laser irradiation on rheumatoid arthritis. Pain Clinic, 8: 18–22

Ohshiro T, Maeda T (1992) Application of 830-nm diode laser LLLT as successful adjunctive therapy of hypertrophic scars and keloids. Laser Ther, 4: 155–168

Ohtsuka H, Kemnotsu O, Doazaki S, Imai I (1992) Low reactive–level laser therapy near the stellate ganglion for postherpetic facial neuralgia. Masui, 91: 1809–1813

Oken O, Kahraman Y, Ayhan F, Canpolat S, Yorgancioglu ZR, Oken OF (2008) The short-term efficacy of laser, brace, and ultrasound treatment in lateral epicondylitis: A prospective, randomized, controlled trial. J Hand Ther, 21: 63–67

Olavi A, Pekka R, Pertti K (1989) Effects of the infrared laser therapy at treated and non-treated trigger points. Acupunct Electrother Res, 14: 9–14

Ong KS, Ho VC (2001) Pain reduction by low-level laser therapy: A double-blind, controlled, randomized study in bilaterally symmetrical oral surgery. Am J Pain Manage, 11: 12–16

Ozdemir F, Birtane M, Kokino S (2001) The clinical efficacy of low-power laser therapy on pain and function in cervical osteoarthritis. Clin Rheumatol, 20: 181–184

Palmgren N, Jensen GF, Kaa K, Windelin M, Colov HC (1989) Low-power laser therapy in rheumatoid arthritis. Laser Med Sci, 4: 193–196

Palmieri B (1984) Stratified double blind crossover study on tennis elbow in young amateur athletes using infrared laser therapy. Med Laser Report, 1–7

Papadopoulos ES, Smith RW, Cawley MI, Mani R (1996) Low-level laser therapy does not aid the management of tennis elbow. Clin Rehab, 10: 9–11

Pinheiro AL, Cavalcanti ET, Pinheiro TI, Alves MJ, Manzi CT (1997) Low-level laser therapy in the management of disorders of the maxillofacial region. J Clin Laser Med Surg, 15: 181–183

Pinheiro AL, Calvalcanti ET, Pinheiro TI, Alves MJ, Miranda ER, De Quevedo AS, Manzi CT, Vieira AL, Rolim AB (1998) Low-level laser therapy is an important tool to treat disorders of the maxillofacial region. J Clin Laser Med Surg, 16: 223–226

Robinson B, Walters J (1991) The use of low laser therapy in diabetic and other ulcerations. J Br Pod Med, 46: 10–14

Rogvi-Hansen B, Ellitsgaard N, Funch M, Dall-Jensen M, Prieske J (1991) Low-level laser treatment of chondromalacia patellae. Int Orthop, 15: 359–361

Santoianni P, Monfrecola G, Martellota D, Ayala F (1984) Inadequate effect of helium-neon laser on venous leg ulcers. Photodermatology, 1: 245–249

Saunders L (1995) The efficacy of low-level laser therapy in supraspinatus tendinitis. Clin Rehab, 9: 126–134

Saunders L (2003) Laser versus ultrasound in the treatment of supraspinatus tendinosis: Randomized controlled trial. Physiotherapy, 89: 365–373

Schindl A, Heinze G, Schindl M, Pernerstorfer-Schon H, Schindl L (2002) Systemic effects of low-intensity laser irradiation on skin microcirculation in patients with diabetic microangiopathy. Microvasc Res, 64: 240–246

Schindl A, Neumann R (1999a) Low-intensity laser therapy is an effective treatment for recurrent herpes simplex infection. Results from a randomized, double-blind, placebo-controlled trial. J Invest Med, 113: 221–223

Schindl A, Schindl M, Pernerstorfer-Schon H, Kerschan K, Knobler R, Schindl L (1999b) Diabetic neuropathic foot ulcer: Successful treatment by low-intensity laser therapy. Dermatology, 198: 314–316

Schindl A, Schindl M, Pernerstorfer-Schon H, Mossbacher U, Schindl L (2000) Low-intensity laser irradiation in the treatment of recalcitrant radiation ulcers in patients with breast cancer—long-term results of three cases. Photodermatol Photoimmunol Photomed, 16: 34–37

Schindl A, Schindl M, Schindl L (1997) Successful treatment of persistent radiation ulcer by low-power laser therapy. J Am Acad Dermatol, 37: 646–648

Schindl A, Schindl M, Schon H, Knobler R, Havelec L, Schindl L (1998) Low-intensity laser irradiation improves skin circulation in patients with diabetic microangiopathy. Diabetes Care, 21: 580–584

Schindl M, Kerschan K, Schindl A, Schon H, Heinzl H, Schindl L (1999) Induction of complete wound healing in recalcitrant ulcers by low-intensity laser irradiation depends on ulcer cause and size. Photodermatol Photoimmunol Photomed, 15: 18–21

Sharma R, Thukral A, Kumar S, Bhargarva SK (2002) Effect of low level lasers in de Quervains tenosynovitis: Prospective study with ultrasonographic assessment. Physiotherapy, 88: 730–734

Shiroto C, Ono K, Onshiro T (1989) Retrospective study of diode laser therapy for pain attenuation in 3635 patients: Detailed analysis by questionnaire. Laser Ther, 1: 41–48

Siebert W, Seichert N, Seibert B, Wirth CJ (1987) What is the efficacy of "soft" and "mild" lasers in therapy of tendinopathies? A double-blind study. Arch Orthop Trauma Surg, 106: 358–363

Simunovic Z (1996) Low-level laser therapy with trigger points technique: A clinical study of 243 patients. J Clin Laser Med Surg, 14: 163–167

Simunovic Z, Trobonjaca T, Trobonjaca Z (1998) Treatment of medial and lateral epicondylitis—tennis and golfer's elbow—with low-level laser therapy: A multicenter double-blind, placebo-controlled clinical study on 324 patients. J Clin Laser Med Surg, 16: 145–151

Smith KC (1991) The photobiological basis of low-level laser radiation therapy. Laser Ther, 3: 19–24

Snyder-Mackler L, Barry AJ, Perdins AI, Soucek MD (1989) Effects of helium-neon laser irradiation on skin resistance and pain in patients with trigger points in the neck or back. Phys Ther, 69: 336–341

Soriano S, Rios R (1998) Gallium arsenide laser treatment of chronic low back pain: A prospective, randomized and double blind study. Laser Ther, 10: 175–180

Stelian J, Gil I, Habot B (1992) Improvement of pain and disability in elderly patients with degenerative osteoarthritis of the knee treated with narrow band light therapy. J Am Geriatr Soc, 40: 23–26

Stergioulas A (2004) Low-level laser treatment can reduce edema in second degree ankle sprains. J Clin Laser Med Surg, 22: 125–128

Stergioulas A (2007) Effects of low-level laser and plyometric exercises in the treatment of lateral epicondylitis. Photomed Laser Surg, 25: 205–213

Stergioulas A, Stergioulas M, Aarskog R, Lopes-Martins RA, Bjordal JM (2008) Effects of low level laser therapy and eccentric exercises in the treatment of recreational athletes with chronic Achilles tendinopathy. Am J Sports Med, 36: 881–887

Sugrue ME, Carolan J, Leen EJ, Feeley TM, Moore DJ, Shanik GD (1990) The use of infrared laser therapy in the treatment of venous ulceration. Ann Vasc Surg, 4: 179–181

Tam G (1999) Low-power laser therapy and analgesic action. J Clin Laser Med Surg, 17: 29–33

Terashima H, Okajima K, Motegi M (1990) Low laser level irradiation for lateral humeral epicondylitis and De Quervain's disease. Laser Ther, 2: 27–32

Thorsen H, Gam AN, Svensson BH, Jess M, Jensen MK, Piculell I, Schack LK, Skjott K (1992) Low-level laser therapy for myofascial pain in the neck and shoulder girdle. A double-blind, cross-over study. Scand J Rheumatol, 21: 139–141

Toya S, Motegi M, Inomata K, Ohshiro T, Maeda T (1994) Report on a computer randomized double blind clinical trial to determine the effectiveness of the GaAlAs (830 nm) diode laser for attenuation in selected pain groups. Laser Ther, 6: 143–148

Trelles MA, Rigau J, Sala P (1991) Infrared diode laser in low reactive–level laser therapy (LLCLT) for knee osteoarthritis. Laser Ther, 3: 198–153

Tumilty S, Munn J, Abbott JH, McDonough S, Hurley DA, Baxter JD (2008) Laser therapy in the treatment of Achilles tendinopathy. A pilot study. Photomed Laser Surg, 26: 25–30

Vasseljen O, Hoeg N, Kjelstad B, Johnsson A, Larsen S (1992) Low-level laser versus placebo in the treatment of tennis elbow. Scand J Rehab Med, 24: 37–42

Vecchio P, Cave M, King V, Adebajo AO, Smith M, Hazleman BL (1993) A double-blind study of the effectiveness of low-level laser treatment of rotator cuff tendonitis. Br J Rheumatol, 32: 740–742

Walker J (1983) Relief from chronic pain by low-power laser irradiation. Neurosci Lett, 43: 339–344

Walker JB (1985) Temporary suppression of clonus in humans by brief photostimulation. Brain Res, 340: 109–113

Walker JB, Akhanjee LK, Cooney MM (1987a) Laser therapy for pain of trigeminal neuralgia. Clin J Pain, 3: 183–187

Walker JB, Akhanjee LK, Cooney MM, Goldstein J, Tamayoshi S, Segal-Gidan F (1987b) Laser therapy for pain of rheumatoid arthritis. Clin J Pain, 3: 54–59

Waylonis GW, Wilke S, O'Toole D, Waylonis DA, Waylonis DB (1988) Chronic myofascial pain: Management by low-output helium-neon laser therapy. Arch Phys Med Rehabil, 69: 1017–1120

Weintraub MI (1997) Noninvasive laser neurolysis in carpal tunnel syndrome. Muscle Nerve, 20: 1029–1031

Willner R, Abeles M, Myerson G (1985) Low-power infrared laser biostimulation of chronic osteoarthritis in hand. Laser Surg Med, 5: 149–150

Yaksish I (1993) Low-energy laser therapy for treatment of post-herpetic neuralgia. Ann Acad Med Singapore, 22 (Suppl 3): 441–442

Review Articles

Bjordal JM, Lopes-Martins RA, Joensen J, Iverson VV (2010). The anti-inflammatory mechanism of low level laser and its relevance for clinical use in physiotherapy. Phys Ther Rev, 15: 286–293

Chung H, Dai T, Sharma SK, Huang YY, Carroll JD, Hamblin MR (2012) The nuts and bolts of low-level laser (light) therapy. Ann Biomed Eng, 40: 516–533

Farraresi C, Hamblin MR, Parizotto NA (2012) Low-level laser (light) therapy (LLLT) on muscle tissue: Performance, fatigue and repair benefit by the power of light. Photonics Lasers Med, 1: 267–286

Hamblin MR, Demidova TN (2006) Mechanisms of low level light therapy. Proc of SPIE, 6140: 1–12

Lopes-Martins R, Penna SC, Joensen J, Iversen VV, Bjordal JM (2007) Low level laser therapy (LLLT) in inflammatory and rheumatic diseases: A review of therapeutic mechanisms. Cur Rheumatol Rev, 3: 147–154

Prindeze NJ, Moffatt LT, Shupp JW (2012) Mechanisms of action for light therapy: A review of molecular interactions. Exp Biol Med, 237: 1241–1248

Reddy GK (2004) Photobiological basis and clinical role of low-intensity lasers in biology and medicine. J Clin Laser Med Surg, 22: 141–150

Schindl A, Schindl M, Pernerstorfer-Schon H, Schindl L (2000) Low-intensity laser therapy: A review. J Invest Med, 48: 312–326

Textbooks

Baxter GD (1994) Therapeutic Lasers: Theory and Practice. Churchill Livingstone, New York

Kamami YV (1997) Le laser en pratique medicale. Masson, Paris

Karu T (1998) The Science of Low-Power Laser Therapy. Gordon & Breach Science, Amsterdam

Tuner J, Hode L (2002) Laser Therapy: Clinical Practice and Scientific Background. Prima Books, Grangesberg

Miscellaneous

Enwemeka CS (2006) The place of coherence in light induced tissue repair and pain function. Photomed Laser Surg, 24: 457

Occupational Safety and Health Administration (OSHA)—U.S. Department of Labor (2007)

U.S. Food and Drug Administration (FDA)—Department of Health & Human Services (2002) Section 510K n.k0101175 Notification of Premarket Approval, February 6, 2002

Internet Resources

waltza.co.za: World Association for Laser Therapy

www.naalt.org: North American Association for Light Therapy

http://thePoint.lww.com: Online Dosage Calculator: Low-Level Laser Therapy

Suggested Review Articles

Al-Shenqiti AM, Oldham JA (2009) The use of low intensity laser therapy in the treatment of myofascial trigger points. An updated critical review. Phys Ther Rev, 14: 115–123

Bjordal JM (2007) On "is low-level laser therapy effective . . ." Phys Ther, 87: 224–226

Bjordal JM, Bogen B, Lopes-Martin RA, Klovning A (2005) Can Cochrane reviews in controversial areas be biased? A sensitive analysis based on the protocol of a systematic Cochrane review on low-level laser therapy in osteoarthritis. Photomed Laser Surg, 23: 453–458

Bjordal JM, Couppé C, Chow RT, Tuner J, Ljunggren EA (2003) A systematic review of low level laser therapy with location-specific doses for pain from chronic joint disorders. Aust J Physiother, 49: 107–116

Bjordal J, Couppé C, Ljunggren A (2001) Low-level laser therapy for tendinopathy. Evidence of a dose-response pattern. Phys Ther Rev, 6: 91–99

Bjordal JM, Johnson MI, Iversen VV, Aimbire FR (2006b) Low level laser therapy (LLLT) in acute pain: A systematic review of possible mechanisms of action and clinical effects in randomized placebo-controlled trials. Photomed Laser Surg, 24: 158–168

Bjordal JM, Johnson MI, Lopes-Martins RA, Bogen B, Chow R, Ljunggren AE (2007) Short-term efficacy of physical interventions in osteoarthritic knee pain. A systematic review and meta-analysis of randomized placebo-controlled trials. BMC Musculoskelet Disord, 22: 8–51

Bjordal JM, Lopes-Martins RA, Joensen J, Couppe C, Ljunggren AE, Stergioulas A, Johnson MI (2008) A systematic review with procedural assessments and meta-analysis of low level laser therapy in lateral elbow tendinopathy (tennis elbow). BMC Musculoskelet Disord, 9: 75–89

Brosseau L, Welch V, Wells G, Tugwell P, de Bie R, Gam A, Harman K, Shea B, Morin M (2000) Low-level laser therapy for osteoarthritis and rheumatoid arthritis: A meta-analysis. J Rheumatol, 27: 1961–1969

Chang WD, Wu JH, Yang WJ, Jiang JA (2010) Therapeutic effects of low-level laser on lateral epicondylitis from different interventions of Chinese-Western medicine: Systematic review. Photomed Laser Surg, 28: 327–336

Chow RT (2009) Efficacy of low-level laser therapy in the management of neck pain: A systematic review and meta-analysis of randomized placebo or active-treatment controlled trials. Lancet, 374: 1897–1908

Enwemeka CS (1988) Laser biostimulation of healing wounds: Specific effects and mechanisms of action. J Orthop Sports Phys Ther, 9: 333–338

Enwemeka CS, Parker JC, Dowdy DS, Harkness EE, Sanford LE, Woodruff LD (2004) The efficacy of low-power laser in tissue repair and pain control: A meta-analysis study. Photomed Laser Surg, 22: 323–329

Hashmi JT, Huang YY, Sjarma SK, Kurup DB, de Taboada L, Carroll JD, Hamblin MR (2010) Effects of pulsing in low-level light therapy. Lasers Surg Med, 42: 450–466

Hawkins D, Houreld N, Abrahamse H (2005) Low level laser therapy (LLLT) as an effective therapeutic modality for delayed wound healing. Ann N Y Acad Sci, 1056: 486–493

Joensen J, Demmink JH, Johnson MI, Iversen VV, Lopes-Martins RA, Bjordal JM (2011) The thermal effects of therapeutic lasers with 810 and 904 nm wavelengths on human skin. Photomed Laser Surg, 29: 145–153

Lucas C, Stanborough RW, Freeman CL (2000) Efficacy of low level laser therapy on wound healing in human subjects: A systematic review. Lasers Med Sci, 15: 83–94

Maher S (2006) Is low-level laser therapy effective in the management of lateral epicondylitis? Phys Ther, 86: 1161–1167

Naeser MA (2006) Photobiomodulation of pain in carpal tunnel syndrome: Review of seven laser therapy studies. Photomed Laser Surg, 24: 101–110

Nussbaum EL, Baxter GD, Lilge L (2003) A review of laser technology and light-tissue interactions as a background to therapeutic applications of low intensity lasers and other light sources. Phys Ther Rev, 8: 31–44

Nussbaum EL, Burke S, Johnstone L, Lahiffe G, Robitaille E, Yoshida K (2007a) Use of electrophysical agents: Findings and implications of a survey of practice in Metro Toronto. Physiother Can, 59: 118–131

Nussbaum EL, Van Zuylen J, Jing F (2007b) Transmission of light through human skin folds during phototherapy: Effects of physical characteristics, irradiation wavelength, and skin-diode coupling. Physiother Can, 59: 194–207

Peplow PV, Chung TY, Baxter GD (2010) Application of low level laser technologies for pain relief and wound healing: Overview of scientific bases. Phys Ther Rev, 15: 253–285

Pereira da Silva J, Alves da Silva M, Figueiredo Almeida AP, Lombardi I, Matos AP (2010) Laser therapy in the tissue repair process: A literature review. Photomed Laser Surg, 28: 17–21

Posten W, Wrone DA, Dover JS, Arndt KA, Silapunt S, Alam M (2005) Low-level laser therapy for wound healing: Mechanism and efficacy. Dermatol Surg, 31: 334–340

Smith KC (2005) Laser (and LED) therapy is phototherapy. Photomed Laser Surg, 23: 78–80

Sobanko JF, Alster TS (2008) Efficacy of low-level laser therapy for chronic cutaneous ulceration in humans: A review and discussion. Dermatol Surg, 34: 991–1000

Stasinopoulos DI, Johnson MI (2005) Effectiveness of low-level laser therapy for lateral elbow tendinopathy. Photomed Laser Surg, 23: 425–430

Tumilty S, Munn J, McDonough S, Hurley DE, Basford JR, Baxter GD (2010) Low level laser treatment of tendinopathy: A systematic review with meta-analysis. Photomed Laser Surg, 28: 3–16

Woodruff LD, Bounkeo JM, Brabbon WM, Dawes KD, Barham CD, Waddell DA, Enwemeka CS (2004) The efficacy of laser therapy in wound repair: A meta-analysis of the literature. Photomed Laser Surg, 22: 241–247

World Association for Laser Therapy (2006) Consensus agreement on the design and conduct of clinical studies with low-level laser therapy and light therapy for musculoskeletal pain and disorders. Consensus Agreement Paper. Photomed Laser Surg, 24: 761–762

Chapter 12

Ultraviolet

Chapter Outline

Learning Objectives

Remembering: State and describe the major side effects of ultraviolet (UV) therapy for the management of dermatoses.

Understanding: Distinguish between UVA, UVB, and UVC therapy.

Applying: Show the steps required to determine the initial dose using the minimum erythemal dose and the skin phototype method.

Analyzing: Explain the proposed physiologic and therapeutic effects of UVB and UVC therapy.

Evaluating: Formulate the dosimetric parameters that phototherapists need to consider and calculate to deliver safe and effective UV therapy.

Creating: Discuss the role of narrowband UVB, relative to broadband UVB and UVA, in the management of dermatoses.

I. FOUNDATION

A. DEFINITION

Sunlight is the greatest source of ultraviolet (UV) radiation on earth. **Ultraviolet light** is defined as electromagnetic radiation with wavelength shorter than that of visible light (thus invisible) but longer than x-rays. UV radiation, as illustrated in Figure 12-1, covers a small portion of the electromagnetic spectrum, spanning a wavelength region ranging from 400 to 10 nanometers (nm = 10^{-9} m). *Ultraviolet therapy* is thus defined as the use of artificial UV light or photons for therapeutic purposes. It is commonly referred to in the literature as *phototherapy.* The main application of UV therapy is for the management of dermatoses. Because the biologic effects caused by UV radiation vary enormously within wavelengths, the therapeutic UV spectrum is further subdivided into different subtypes (see Fig. 12-1). Following in order from longest to shortest wavelengths are UVA (400 to 320 nm), UVB (320 to 290 nm), and UVC (290 to 100 nm). Vacuum UV, not used for therapeutic purposes, occupies almost all of the shortest half of the UV spectrum (200 to 10 nm). The UVA subtype is further subdivided into psoralen UVA (PUVA; 400 to 320 nm) and UVA1 (400 to 340 nm). The UVB subtype is subdivided into broadband UVB (BBUVB; 320 to 290 nm) and narrowband UVB (NBUVB; 313 to 309 nm) UVB. Finally, UVC (290 to 200 nm) occupies the band between BBUVB and vacuum UV.

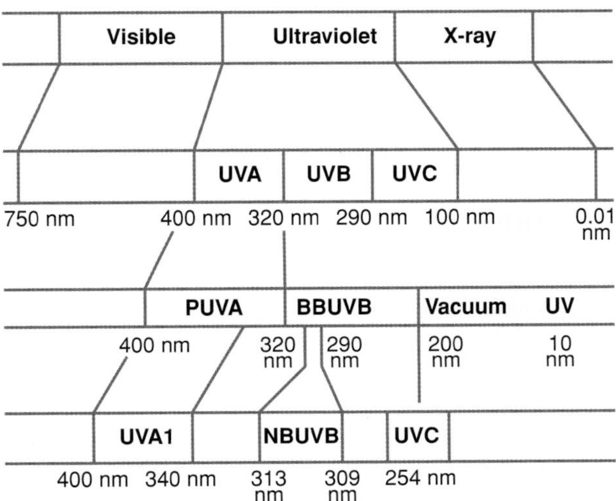

FIGURE 12-1 Ultraviolet spectrum of radiation.

B. UVA THERAPY

Ultraviolet A (UVA) is therapeutically delivered using two modes: PUVA and UVA1 (British Photodermatology Group, 1994; Halpern et al. 2000; Dawe, 2003). PUVA requires the use of a natural photosensitizing agent, *psoralen,* to enhance the patient's erythemal response, which would be weak if exposed to UVA light alone. Psoralen may be administered orally (oral PUVA) or topically, either with a psoralen cream rubbed over the treated skin area (cream PUVA) or by means of a psoralen bath, in which the treated body part is immersed before irradiation (bath PUVA). UVA1 therapy is easier or more practical to use because no sensitizing agent is required (Dawe, 2003; Tuchinda et al., 2006). Research has shown that PUVA penetrates deep into the skin, reaching the hypodermis, and induces a *photochemical* effect resulting from the interaction between psoralen and UVA light. UVA1 therapy, on the other hand, induces a *phototherapy* effect on the skin because no photosensitizing agent is

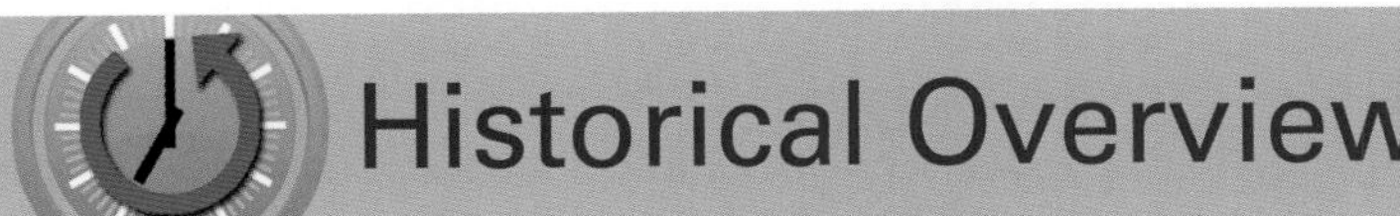

The use of sunlight to treat skin disease, also known as *heliotherapy,* dates back to 1400 BC, when Hindus used plant extracts on the skin followed by sun exposure to treat patients with vitiligo (Rajpara et al., 2010). Phototherapy utilizing artificial light sources emerged in the late 1890s, when Danish physician Niels Finsen was awarded the 1903 Nobel Prize for Medicine for his successful treatment of lupus vulgaris by using a carbon-arc UV lamp (Diffey et al., 2002; Roelandts, 2002; Dogra et al., 2004). Over the past decades, significant technical developments led to the creation of various sources of artificial UV radiation, moving from Finsen's original carbon-arc–type lamp to today's mercury-arc lamps and fluorescent tubes (Diffey et al., 2002; Dogra et al., 2004). In 1974, Parrish and colleagues reported the useful role of UVA radiation in combination with oral psoralen in the treatment of psoriasis; this application led to what is known as PUVA therapy (Parrish et al., 1974). A few years later, Wiskemann and colleagues introduced BBUVB therapy for the treatment of psoriasis and uremic pruritus (Dogra et al., 2004). In the late 1980s, Van Weelden et al. (1988) and Green et al. (1988) introduced NBUVB, also known as TL-01 UVB therapy, for the treatment of psoriasis. A few years earlier, Larko et al. (1979) first introduced successful home phototherapy for psoriasis by using BBUVB on patients who lived too far away to access a clinic. NBUVB therapy came about after Philips Lighting, of the Netherlands, developed and manufactured the new TL-01 fluorescent tube capable of delivering UVB light in the narrower (N) band (range of 313 to 309 nm, with a peak at 311 nm) of the broad (B) band (320 to 290 nm) of UV light. With such a tube, the shorter and more damaging UV wavelengths are absent during radiation, thus minimizing the skin's carcinogenic risk. In today's literature and in this textbook, NBUVB and TL-01 UVB therapy are used interchangeably.

used (British Photodermatology Group, 1994; Halpern et al., 2000; Dawe, 2003; Tuchinda et al., 2006).

C. UVB THERAPY

Ultraviolet B (UVB) is also therapeutically delivered via two modes: broadband and narrowband UVB (Bilsland et al., 1997; Bandow et al., 2004; Dogra et al., 2004; Ibbotson et al., 2004; Gambichler et al., 2005). No sensitizing agent is required to deliver UVB therapy. NBUVB is a subset of BBUVB, as shown in Figure 12-1. NBUVB is delivered within a much narrower band (313 to 309 nm), with its peak emission at 311 nm. This mode is also known as TL-01 UVB in the UV phototherapy literature. Research has shown that UVB, within either its broadband or narrowband, penetrates the dermis and induces a *phototherapy* effect on the skin tissue (Bilsland et al., 1997; Bandow et al., 2004; Dogra et al., 2004; Ibbotson et al., 2004; Gambichler et al., 2005).

D. UVC THERAPY

Ultraviolet C (UVC), and especially the light emitted at 254 nm (see Fig. 12-1), has been shown to penetrate the epidermis and to deactivate or kill, both in vitro and in vivo, normal and antibiotic-resistant strains of bacteria and other families of germs. UVC thus has a *photogermicidal* effect on dermatoses (Conner-Kerr et al., 1998, 2007; Sullivan et al., 1999; Thai et al., 2002, 2005).

E. DECLINING UVA, BBUVB, AND UVC THERAPY

The practice of phototherapy using UVA and UVB has evolved over the past two decades, but that of UVC has remained rather stagnant, marginal, and sporadic. There is a clear trend in the current literature indicating that the practice of UVA (PUVA and UVA1) therapy is gradually declining in favor of UVB therapy. Because of its high carcinogenic risk, combined with its increased skin phototoxicity with repeated treatments, it is recommended that PUVA therapy should be kept only for dermatoses that do not respond to other treatments (Halpern et al., 2000). The practice of BBUVB therapy is also slowly declining because of its higher carcinogenic risk in favor of NBUVB therapy, which is today recognized as the first line of treatment for many of the most frequent dermatoses affecting humans (Bandow et al., 2004; Dogra et al., 2004; Ibbotson et al., 2004; Gambichler et al., 2005). Finally, the body of scientific evidence related to the practice of UVC therapy, in contrast to UVA and UVB therapy, is very limited, suggesting sporadic and declining clinical usage.

F. TODAY'S INCREASING USE OF NBUVB

The practice of NBUVB therapy (313- to 309-nm band, with its peak spectra at 311 nm) is rapidly gaining in popularity today among dermatologists, phototherapists, and patients around the world. NBUVB has several key advantages over PUVA and BBUVB, such as similar to higher therapeutic efficacy, greater patient preference, minimal side effects, faster clearance, reduced erythemogenic effect, and reduced carcinogenic risk (Parrish et al., 1981; Fisher et al., 1984; Van Weelden et al., 1988; Lee et al., 2005; Dogra et al., 2010; Nolan et al., 2010; Rajpara et al., 2010). The growing popularity or use of NBUVB therapy is also supported by the fact that it is a safe, effective, and well-tolerated treatment for most dermatoses, not only in adults but also in children (Tan et al., 2010).

G. SCOPE OF CHAPTER

The scope of this chapter is on the use of UVB light therapy. As mentioned previously, there is consensus today is that PUVA therapy, with its severe side effects and high carcinogenic risk, should be restricted to the most severe dermatoses—those recalcitrant to topical and systemic therapies as well as to all the other forms of UV therapy. As for the use of UVC therapy, this chapter will show that its clinical usage is marginal, if not obsolete, with only three human peer-reviewed studies published since its introduction on the clinical scene.

H. ULTRAVIOLET DEVICES

There is a strong evidence to suggest that the practice of ultraviolet therapy is slowly shifting from outpatient therapy (clinical setting) to home therapy because the latter can be as safe, effective and cost-effective as outpatient phototherapy (see Nolan et al., 2010; Rajpara et al., 2010). Figure 12-2 illustrates typical devices used today to deliver UV therapy to large, small, and spotty body areas. These devices are mounted with single to multiple UV lamps, or tubes, capable of emitting artificial UV light within the UVA, UVB, or UVC spectrum.

I. ULTRAVIOLET ACCESSORIES

Because UV radiation is harmful to the eyes, protective UV goggles, similar to those shown in Figure 12-3A, must be worn *at all times* by both patients and practitioners during UV radiation. Other accessories, such as commercial cardboard punctured with holes and skin phototesting templates (see Fig. 12-3B), are used to establish the patient's starting dose based on the minimum erythermal dose (MED) approach (see the Dosimetry section).

J. RATIONALE FOR USE

Many thousands of individuals are affected over the course of their lives by a wide variety of skin pathologies or dermatoses, such as psoriasis, acne vulgaris, atopic dermatitis (eczema), and vitiligo, to name only a few. These skin disorders are traditionally treated by general practitioners and dermatologists by using an array of oral anti-inflammatory/antibiotic drugs and topical creams. Over the past decades, however, UV therapy has gained popularity as an alternative treatment for several dermatoses. Therapy has evolved

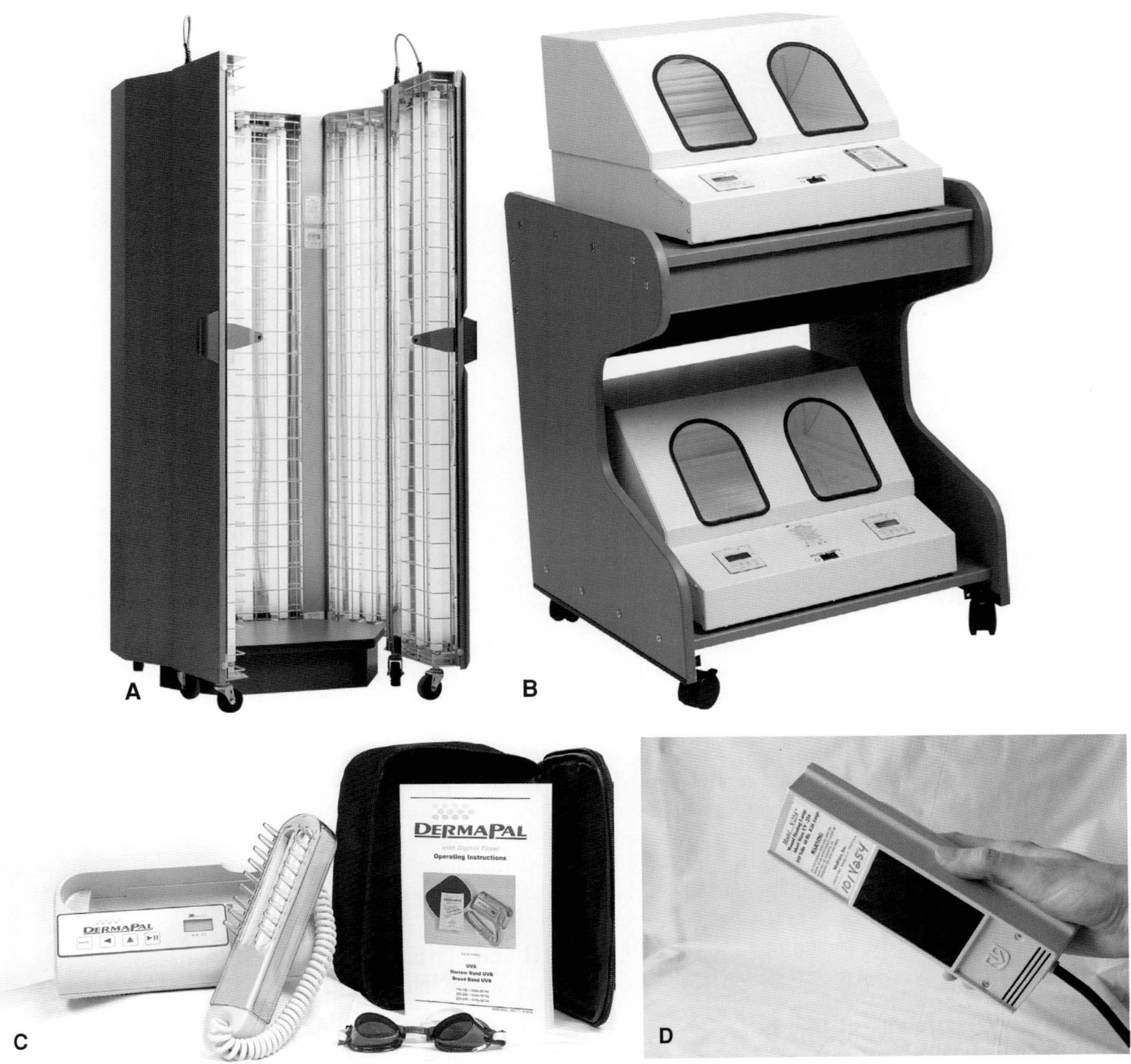

FIGURE 12-2 Home ultraviolet B devices: whole-body cubicle (**A**); hands/feet cabinet (**B**); handheld wand (**C**); ultraviolet C lamp (**D**). (A–C: Courtesy of Daavlin; D: Courtesy of Medfaxx.)

over the years from the use of PUVA to BBUVB, and from BBUVB to NBUVB therapy. Today, UV therapy is recognized, as this chapter will demonstrate, as an important alternative therapy to conventional topical creams and oral drugs, providing significant clearance of multiple dermatoses for periods lasting weeks to months.

II. BIOPHYSICAL CHARACTERISTICS

A. ULTRAVIOLET LIGHT GENERATORS

Therapeutic artificial UV light comes from two types of light-emitting generators: mercury-arc lamps and fluorescent tubes. *Mercury-arc lamps* are made of a small quantity of mercury gas sealed into a UV quartz transmitting tube. After an electrical arc passes into the tube, the mercury atoms are excited, being heated up (the incandescence process) at a very high temperature (approximately 8,000°C [14,432°F]), and emit photons, primarily in the UVB spectrum (Davis, 2002). During radiation, the pressure inside the quartz tube is high, and the tube is hot. The hot tube must be cooled and this is done by means of a circulating air or water jacket. These lamps require a warm-up period before peak emission is achieved and a cool-down period after being turned off before they can be used again (Davis, 2002). *Fluorescent tubes* consist of a small quantity of mercury vapor sealed in a UV transmitting tube, mounted with an electrical filament and coated with phosphors. After an electrical current passes through the filament and into the tube, the mercury atoms are excited and produce low-pressure photons in the full UV range (see Diffey et al., 2002). These tubes, sold in

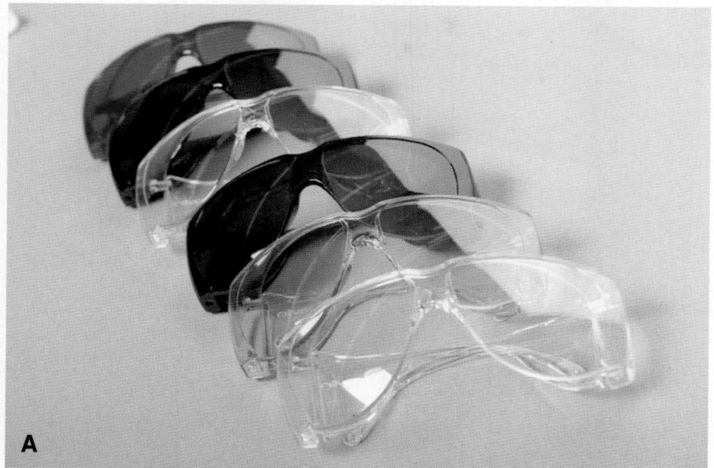

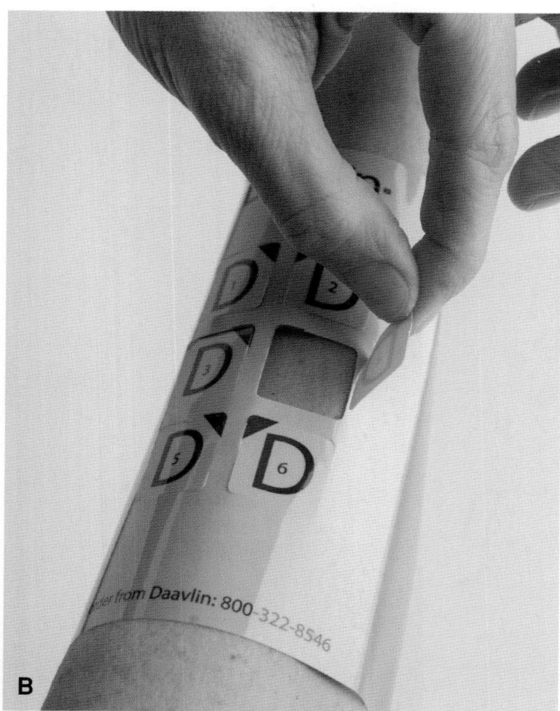

FIGURE 12-3 Ultraviolet protective goggles (**A**) and skin phototesting templates (**B**). These commercial panels are made of UV-opaque fabrics and are completely washable. Each piece has several apertures or exposure ports that can be covered and uncovered during testing. Homemade templates or panels can also be used. (A, B: Courtesy of Daavlin.)

different sizes and lengths, are gradually replacing mercury-arc gas lamps in modern UV devices. Today, practitioners can choose from several types of fluorescent tubes with varying UV spectral emissions to deliver UV therapy. All UV tubes have a lifetime ranging between 5,000 and 10,000 hours (Diffey et al., 2002). Regular maintenance and prompt replacement of burnt-out lamps and tubes is mandatory to ensure optimal irradiation and precise dosimetry.

B. SPONTANEOUS EMISSION OF ULTRAVIOLET LIGHT

The process of UV light emission is based on the concept of *spontaneous emission* of photons, resulting from the sudden and spontaneous drop of electrons from their activated state to their resting state. This important biophysical process is discussed at length in Chapter 11, which deals with the emission of laser light. To avoid duplication, readers are invited to consult Chapter 11 for full details of this concept and other biophysical processes leading to spontaneous emission of photons.

III. THERAPEUTIC EFFECTS AND INDICATIONS

A. PHOTOTHERAPY

Research has demonstrated, as illustrated in Figure 12-4, that photons of lights within the UVA and UVB regions of the UV spectrum can induce *photochemical* and *photobiologic* effects on the skin, with those within the UVC region inducing a *photogermicidal* effect (British Photodermatology Group, 1994; Halpern et al., 2000; Dawe, 2003; Weichenthal et al., 2005; Tuchinda et al., 2006).

B. ERYTHEMAL RESPONSE AND CARCINOGENIC RISK

The practice of UVA and UVB therapy relies on the capacity of each region of the electromagnetic spectrum to induce a skin erythemal response following exposure. *Erythema* is defined as skin redness due to dilation of the superficial blood vessels. There is evidence to show that the induced erythemal response is strong in both PUVA and BBUVB therapy, moderate in NBUVB therapy, and absent in UVC therapy (Bilsland et al., 1997; Cameron et al., 2002a). It is scientifically established that prolonged or repeated skin exposure to either solar or artificial UV radiation may cause skin cancer (for a review, see Saladi et al., 2005). Unfortunately for patients, many dermatoses, such as psoriasis and eczema, require numerous treatment exposures before the condition will clear up, and lifetime UV treatment may be required because of the recurrent nature of these dermatoses. There is strong evidence to suggest that UVA therapy, particularly PUVA and BBUVB, have a much higher carcinogenic risk than NBUVB therapy, because their erythemal response is much stronger than that of NBUVB (see Stern et al. 1994; Lee et al., 2005; Man et al., 2005; Saladi et al., 2005).

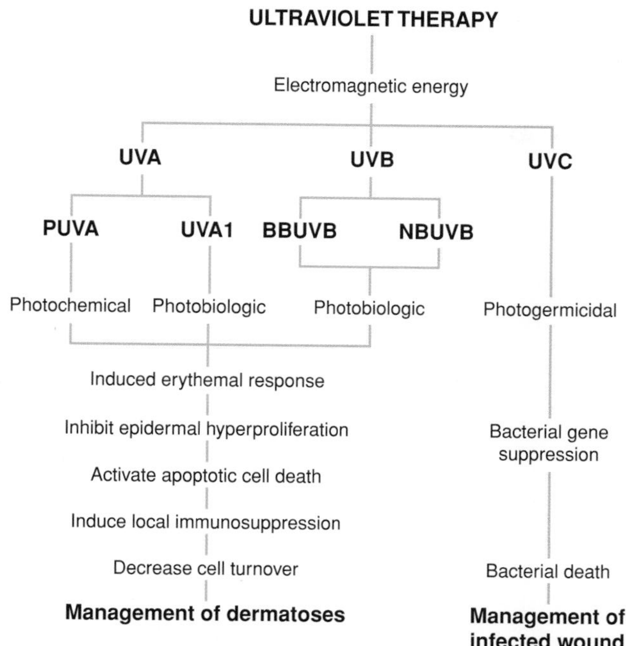

FIGURE 12-4 Proposed physiologic and therapeutic effects of ultraviolet therapy.

C. PROPOSED MECHANISMS BEHIND PHOTOTHERAPY

The exact mechanisms behind the therapeutic effects of UV light remain obscure (Weichenthal et al., 2005; Weisberg et al., 2006). There is evidence, however, to support some of its proposed mechanisms of action, which are illustrated in Figure 12-4. UVA and UVB lights induce a skin erythemal response that in turn triggers a cascade of physiologic effects, such as inhibiting epidermal hyperproliferation, activating apoptotic cell death, and inducing local immunosuppression. Together, these physiologic effects decrease cellular turnover over time (for details, see Weichenthal et al., 2005 Weisberg et al., 2006; Menter et al., 2010; York et al., 2010). UVC light, on the hand, is believed to suppress bacterial gene activation, resulting in bacterial death (Conner-Kerr et al., 1998, 2007; Sullivan et al., 1999; Cohill et al., 2008). Both UVA and UVB lights are indicated for the management of most dermatoses, whereas UVC light is used only for the management of infected wounds.

D. RESEARCH-BASED INDICATIONS

The search for evidence behind the use of ultraviolet B and C therapy, displayed in the *Research-Based Indications* box, led to the collection of 78 English peer-reviewed human clinical studies. The methodologies and criteria used to assess the strength of evidence and therapeutic effectiveness are described in Chapter 2. As indicated in the box, the strength of evidence behind UVB is ranked as *strong* for psoriasis, atopic dermatitis, vitiligo, and mycosis fungoides. Therapeutic effectiveness is *substantiated* for all of these dermatoses. Analysis is *pending* for all the other health conditions related to UVB and UVC because fewer than five studies could be collected. Over all conditions treated with UVB, the strength of evidence is found to be *moderate* and its therapeutic effectiveness *substantiated.*

IV. DOSIMETRY

A. KEY PARAMETERS, FORMULAS, AND UNITS

Table 12-1 shows key parameters, with formulas and units, related to the dosimetry of UV therapy. The irradiance (I), or power density, is measured by means of a UV sensor mounted on the device and is expressed in mW/cm^2. The irradiance of a given UV device is thus determined by its total number of lamps or tubes. Each tube has its own irradiance. The greater the number of tubes within a device, the greater that device's total irradiance. The exposure duration (T) is the time, measured in seconds, during which the skin is exposed to UV light. It varies in relation to the treatment dose used and the device's irradiance.

TABLE 12-1 ULTRAVIOLET THERAPY DOSIMETRIC PARAMETERS, FORMULAS, AND UNITS

Parameter	Synonym	Formula	Unit
Irradiance (I)	Intensity or power density	Read from a UV sensor	mW/cm^2
Exposure duration (T)	Treatment time		sec
Dose per treatment (D_t)	Amount of energy delivered to the skin during a single treatment	$D_t = I \times T$	mJ/cm^2
Cumulative dose (D_c)	Summation of all doses per treatment within a treatment period or over a lifetime	$D_c = \Sigma D_t$	J/cm^2

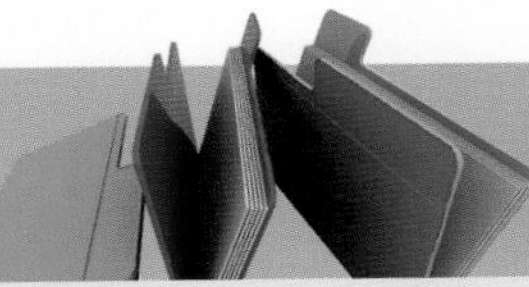

Research-Based Indications

ULTRAVIOLET

Health Condition	Benefit—Yes		Benefit—No	
	Rating	Reference	Rating	Reference
Ultraviolet B				
Psoriasis	I	Boztepe et al., 2006		
	I	Cameron et al., 2002a		
	II	Kirke et al., 2007		
	II	Dawe et al., 2003		
	II	Dawe et al., 1998		
	II	Gokdemir et al., 2005		
	II	Picot et al., 1992		
	II	Kollner et al., 2005		
	II	Van Weelden et al., 1988		
	II	Lim et al., 2006		
	II	Leenutaphong et al., 2000		
	II	Yones et al., 2006		
	II	Van Weelden et al., 1990		
	II	Parrish et al., 1981		
	II	Fisher et al., 1984		
	II	Hofer et al., 1998		
	II	Coven et al., 1997		
	II	Green et al., 1988		
	II	Karvonen et al., 1989		
	II	Larko, 1989		
	II	Tanew et al., 1999		
	II	Storbeck et al., 1993		
	II	Gordon et al., 1999		
	II	Ortel et al., 1993		
	II	Stern et al., 1986		
	II	Yones et al., 2005		
	II	Jury et al., 2006		
	II	Sezer et al., 2007a		
	II	Aydogan et al., 2006		
	III	Wainwright et al., 1998		
	III	Kaur et al., 2006		

Strength of evidence: Strong
Therapeutic effectiveness: Substantiated

Health Condition	Benefit—Yes		Benefit—No	
	Rating	Reference	Rating	Reference
Atopic dermatitis	II	Clayton et al., 2006		
	II	Valkova et al., 2004		
	II	Hjerppe et al., 2001		
	II	Grundmann-Kollmann et al., 1999		
	II	George et al., 1993		
	II	Reynolds et al., 2001		
	II	Der-Petrossian et al., 2000		
	II	Legat et al., 2003		
	II	Jekler, 1992		
	II	Sjovall et al., 1987		
	II	Sezer et al., 2007b		

Strength of evidence: Strong
Therapeutic effectiveness: Substantiated

Health Condition	Rating	Reference	Rating	Reference
Vitiligo	II	Yones et al., 2007		
	II	Bhatnagar et al., 2007		
	II	Westerhof et al., 1997		
	II	Parsad et al., 2006		
	II	Njoo et al., 2000		
	II	Kanwar et al., 2005		
	II	Scherschun et al., 2001		
	II	Tjioe et al., 2002		
	II	Don et al., 2006		
	II	Hamzavi et al., 2004		
	II	Yashar et al., 2003		
	II	Natta et al., 2003		

Strength of evidence: Strong
Therapeutic effectiveness: Substantiated

Health Condition	Rating	Reference	Rating	Reference
Mycosis fungoides	II	Ahmad et al., 2007		
	II	Brazzelli et al., 2007		
	II	Hofer et al., 1999		
	II	Clark et al., 2000		
	II	Gokdemir et al., 2006		
	II	Gathers et al., 2002		
	II	Diederen et al., 2003		

Strength of evidence: Strong
Therapeutic effectiveness: Substantiated

Health Condition	Benefit—Yes Rating	Benefit—Yes Reference	Benefit—No Rating	Benefit—No Reference
Fewer Than 5 Studies				
Lichen planus	II	Taneja et al., 2002		
	II	Saricaoglu et al., 2003		
	II	Wackernagel et al., 2007		
Pruritus	II	Seckin et al., 2007		
	II	Baldo et al., 1996		
	II	Baldo et al., 2002		
Chronic urticaria	II	Berroeta et al., 2004		
Seborrheic dermatitis	II	Pirkhammer et al., 2000		
Nodular prurigo	II	Tamagawa-Mineoka et al., 2007		
Polymorphic eruption	II	Bilsland et al., 1993		

Health Condition	Benefit—Yes Rating	Benefit—Yes Reference	Benefit—No Rating	Benefit—No Reference
Localized scleroderma	I	Kreuter et al., 2006		
Pressure ulcers	I	Wills et al., 1983		
Psoriasis with HIV	III	Fotiades et al., 1995		
Mix of dermatoses	III	Tay et al., 1996		
Strength of evidence: Pending				
Therapeutic effectiveness: Pending				
Ultraviolet C				
Fewer Than 5 Studies				
Infected wounds	II	Taylor, 1972		
	II	Thai et al., 2005		
	III	Thai et al., 2002		
Strength of evidence: Pending				
Therapeutic effectiveness: Pending				
ALL CONDITIONS				
Strength of evidence: Moderate				
Therapeutic effectiveness: Substantiated				

B. DOSE PER TREATMENT

The dose per treatment (D_t), measured in mJ/cm^2, is determined by the device's irradiance (I) multiplied by the application time (T), as shown in Table 12-1 (Taylor et al., 2002; Van der Leun et al., 2005). For example, a dose per treatment of 450 mJ/cm^2 will be delivered to a patient's skin if the phototherapist exposes a UV device with an irradiance of 3 mW/cm^2 for 150 s (450 mJ/cm^2 = 3 mW/cm^2 × 150 s). Dosage is in keeping with the *reciprocity law,* also known as the Bunsen-Roscoe law, which refers to the inverse relationship between irradiance and exposure time. This means that a similar dose (D) can result from decreasing application duration (T) or increasing irradiance (I), or vice versa (Van der Leun et al., 2005). For example, a dose of 400 mJ/cm^2 may be obtained as follows: 400 mJ/cm^2 = 2 mW/cm^2 × 200 s or 4 mW/cm^2 × 100 s. In other words, the dose is similar if the irradiance is halved and the exposure time doubled, or if the irradiance is doubled while the exposure time is halved.

C. CUMULATIVE DOSE

Because several UV treatments are needed for the management and maintenance of most dermatoses, and repeated exposure to UV lights over weeks, months, and years presents a greater carcinogenic risk for the skin, it is essential that the cumulative dose (D_c) received by the patient be calculated and recorded in the patient's file (Taylor et al., 2002; Ibbotson et al., 2004). The cumulative dose is calculated by adding up each dose per treatment that the patient has received during the course of his or her treatment period, which may last weeks or months (see Table 12-1). The greater the cumulative dose per treatment period and the larger the number of treatment periods over time, the greater the risk of developing a skin cancer. Therefore, the ultimate goal of any practitioner is to achieve optimal treatment outcomes with the smallest cumulative dose possible. To facilitate dosimetry, readers are invited to use the **Online Dosage Calculator: Ultraviolet**.

D. DETERMINATION OF INITIAL UVB DOSE

The determination of the initial or starting dose is crucial in the field of UV phototherapy because of the patient's carcinogenic risk as discussed previously. Research on UV therapy has clearly established that too low of a starting dose will not induce a therapeutic benefit, whereas too high of a starting dose may induce serious side effects such as skin burning and pain, brought on by a strong skin erythemal response to too much UV energy (Lee et al., 2005; Weichenthal et al., 2005). This important initial dose determination is done by using one of the following two methods: the minimum erythemal dose (MED) method or Fitzpatrick's skin phototype method (Bilsland et al., 1997; Halpern et al., 2000; Taylor et al., 2002; Ibbotson et al., 2004; Menter et al., 2010; Nolan et al., 2010). In general, MED-based phototherapy protocols are thought to be safer than skin-type–based protocols, but most practitioners today *prefer* the latter because it is much more convenient to use (Menter et al., 2010; Rajpara et al., 2010). To illustrate why the Fitzpatrick skin phototype method is gaining in popularity over the MED method, both methods are described and exemplified next.

1. Minimum Erythemal Dose Testing Method

Exposure of human skin to UVB light induces an erythemal response, which can vary among people. Erythema is skin redness caused by vascular dilation. This induced skin redness may be mediated by prostaglandin release from the epidermis, or by the DNA-damaging effect of UV radiation (Diffey et al., 2002). It is critical that a *minimal dose causing erythema* (MED) be determined, because development of UVB-induced erythema will limit the UV dose that can be given at each treatment. As stated earlier, the ultimate therapeutic goal is to deliver an effective dose of UV light to the skin lesion while minimizing the erythemal effect on the surrounding healthy skin cells. MED is defined as the lowest, or *minimal,* dose of UV radiation that will produce a barely detectable erythema 24 hours after exposure (Taylor et al., 2002). MED is synonymous to an E-1, or first-degree erythemal dose (Conner-Kerr et al., 2007).

Minimum Erythemal Dose Determination

Figure 12-5 illustrates how, using an example, practitioners can determine the MED for their patients. Phototesting is done, in this example, on the skin over the lower back of a patient. Testing can also be done over the buttock, abdomen, or anterior forearm areas. The testing UVB lamp's surface is positioned perpendicular to the lower back skin surface, in keeping with Lambert's cosine law. The lamp is positioned at a fixed distance of 30 cm (12 inches) from the skin surface, according to the inverse square law. This lamp emits light in the NBUVB range and has an irradiance value fixed at 3 mW/cm^2. As shown in Figure 12-5, a homemade UV-opaque flexible plastic rectangular template with five apertures (circles) is used. Only the bare skin areas exposed in each of these apertures is submitted to UV light, with the surrounding skin covered by a towel. Commercial MED testing templates may also be used. After the lamp has reached its full power, the following aperture uncovering sequence is initiated. To begin, all of the apertures are covered, except for the first one. The UV lamp is on and the timer is activated (time 0). The aperture *uncovering time* sequence is 160, 80, 40, 20, and 20 seconds. This means that after the first 160 seconds, the second aperture is uncovered and irradiated for 80 seconds. Then, the third aperture is uncovered and exposed for 40 seconds. The fourth is then uncovered and exposed for 20 seconds. Then, the fifth aperture is uncovered and irradiated for 20 seconds. According to this uncovering sequence, the *exposure time* of the skin surface within the first aperture is 320 seconds (160 + 80 + 40 + 20 + 20), with the following skin surfaces irradiated for 160 seconds (second), 80 seconds (third), 40 seconds (fourth), and 20 seconds (fifth). The corresponding *testing dose* delivered, from the first to the fifth aperture, is 960 (3 mW/cm^2 × 320 s), 480, 240, 120, and 60 mJ/cm^2, respectively. At 24 hours after testing, the practitioner visually determines that the dose given to the aperture showing just perceptible erythema (*MED*), with no erythema visible on the adjacent lower dose apertures, is seen, as illustrated in Figure 12-5, in the fourth aperture and corresponds to an MED value of 240 mJ/cm^2.

2. Fitzpatrick's Skin Phototype Testing Method

It is a common observation that human skin, depending on its color, responds differently to the sun's UV rays. Table 12-2 shows an exemplified determination of skin phototype using Fitzpatrick's skin phototype method. Fitzpatrick's classification of human skin phototypes is based on the interaction between skin color and burning or tanning reaction to the sun (Fitzpatrick, 1988). This classification includes six skin types and shows that whiter skins (types I and II) are more likely to display a burning, or erythemogenic reaction, to UV radiation than are browner (types III, IV, and V) and blacker (type VI) skins. In the present example, the patient presents a light brown skin color. Asked about his tanning and sunburning history, he replies than he tends to burn moderately and tan gradually. Based on this information, the practitioner then determines that this patient has a type III skin phototype. What is the MED value, or initial dose, corresponding to a type III skin phototype? Based on the practice guideline developed by the American Academy of Dermatology (discussed next), the answer is 30 mJ/cm^2 for BBUVB and 260 mJ/cm^2 for NBUVB (Menter et al., 2010).

E. UVB DOSING AND SCHEDULING RECOMMENDATIONS

To facilitate the practice of UVB therapy, practitioners may use the following dosage and scheduling

EXEMPLIFIED DETERMINATION OF MINIMUM ERYTHEMAL DOSE (MED)

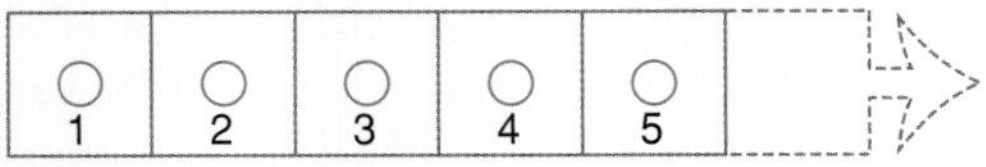

Template with apertures	1	2	3	4	5
Uncovering time (s)	160	80	40	20	20
Exposure time (s)	320	160	80	40	20
Testing dose (mJ/cm2)	960	480	240	120	60
MED (mJ/cm2)				240	

FIGURE 12-5 Exemplified determination of minimum erythemal dose (MED).

TABLE 12-2 EXEMPLIFIED DETERMINATION* OF SKIN PHOTOTYPE

Fitzpatrick's Skin Phototype	Skin Color	Tanning and Sunburn History
Type I	Lighter white	Burns easily; never tans
Type II	Darker white	Burn easily; tans minimally
Type III	Light brown	Burns moderately; tans gradually
Type IV	Moderate brown	Burns minimally; tans well
Type V	Dark brown	Burns rarely; tans profusely
Type VI	Black	Never burns; insensitive to tanning

**Determination:* The patient has a type III skin phototype. This determination is based on the patient's skin color and on his full verbal tanning and sunburn history.

guidelines developed by the American Academy of Dermatology (Menter et al., 2010). UV initial dose, incremental dosage, and scheduling, for both BBUVB and NBUVB, based on the MED method is presented in Table 12-3, whereas that based on Fitzpatrick's skin phototype is shown in Table 12-4. Because the skin photoadapts to repeated UV light exposures, the initial or starting dose must be constantly increased during the entire course of therapy to induce a therapeutic erythemal response with each treatment (Davis, 2002; Diffey et al., 2002).

1. Dosage and Scheduling Based on Minimum Erythemal Dose

As shown in Table 12-3, the initial dose, which corresponds to 50% of MED value, is similar for both BB- and NBUVB therapy. In keeping with the example developed earlier (see Fig. 12-5), this means that the initial dose should be 120 mJ/cm^2 (240 mJ/cm^2 × 50%). The table shows that the dose increment percentages from one treatment period to the next are different for BBUVB and NBUVB. As for the treatment frequency, it is similar for both BB- and NBUVB therapy (see Table 12-3).

2. Dosage and Scheduling Based on Skin Phototype

The American Academy of Dermatology recommends lower initial dosages for BBUVB (approximately five times lower) than for NBUVB because of the former higher skin erythemal effect (Menter et al., 2010). As expected, initial doses for both BB- and NBUVB increase with skin color darkness (I to VI). As mentioned earlier and in keeping with the example discussed previously (see Table 12-2), the initial dose for a patient presenting a type III skin phototype is 30 mJ/cm^2 for BBUVB and 260 mJ/cm^2 for NBUVB; increment values vary between skin types and UV bands. Note that these recommendations are primarily for the treatment of psoriasis and psoriatic arthritis disorders, which represent a large percentage of all dermatoses treated with UV phototherapy. It is the practitioner's responsibility to make the necessary adjustments to these guidelines based on

TABLE 12-3 RECOMMENDED* ULTRAVIOLET DOSING AND SCHEDULING BASED ON MINIMUM EFFECTIVE DOSE

Dosage	BBUVB	NBUVB
Initial dose	50% of MED	50% of MED
Treatments 2–10	Increase by 25% of initial MED	Increase by 10% of initial MED
Treatments 11–20	Increase by 10% of initial MED	Increase by 10% of initial MED
Treatments ≥21	As prescribed by dermatologist	As prescribed by dermatologist
Treatment frequency	3–5 treatments per week	

BBUVB, broadband ultraviolet B; NBUVB, narrowband ultraviolet B; MED, minimum effective dose.
*Adapted from Menter et al., 2010, and Zanolli et al., 2004.

TABLE 12-4 RECOMMENDED* ULTRAVIOLET DOSING AND SCHEDULING BASED ON SKIN PHOTOTYPE

	BBUVB		NBUVB	
Skin Phototype	**Initial Dose (mJ/cm^2)**	**Increment After Each Treatment (mJ/cm^2)**	**Initial Dose (mJ/cm^2)**	**Increment After Each Treatment (mJ/cm^2)**
I	20	5	130	15
II	25	10	220	25
III	30	15	260	40
IV	40	20	330	45
V	50	25	350	60
VI	60	30	400	65
Treatment frequency	3–5 treatments per week			

BBUVB, broadband ultraviolet B; NBUVB, narrowband ultraviolet B.
*Adapted from Menter et al., 2010, and Zanolli et al., 2004.

the types of dermatoses for which they plan to use UVB phototherapy.

F. PHOTOTESTING CONVENIENCE

Which of the two methods—MED versus skin phototype—is more clinically convenient? A simple comparison clearly demonstrates why the skin phototype method is gaining in popularity among practitioners. The MED method is clearly less convenient—that is, more difficult and time consuming to execute. One major difficulty is the precision required to gradually expose the apertures at specific times, which requires good hand–eye coordination (i.e., precise timing, using a chronograph, combined with precise manual uncovering). The skin-type method, on the other hand, is very practical, fast, and convenient for both practitioners and patients, requiring only a single visit that may last no longer than 10 minutes. Readers need to recall that the focus of this chapter, as stated earlier, is on the practice of UVB and UVC therapy, not UVA therapy. The description of phototesting protocols used to determine the minimum phototoxic dose (MPD) before oral or topical (e.g., cream, bath) administration of PUVA are thus beyond the scope of this chapter. Readers interested in such protocols may refer to the review articles by Halpern et al. (2000) and Dawe (2003) for details.

G. ONLINE DOSAGE CALCULATOR: ULTRAVIOLET

As is the case in the previous chapters on shortwave diathermy and low-level laser therapy, an **Online Dosage Calculator** is provided with the objective to lessen the burden associated with recalling formulas and doing hand calculations. Upon entering the dosimetric parameters, the calculator will provide the precise dose per treatment and cumulative dose given to patients.

V. APPLICATION, CONTRAINDICATIONS, AND RISKS

Prior to considering the application of UV therapy, practitioners must first check for contraindications, consider the risks, and then go through key application steps and procedures designed to optimize treatment safety, efficacy, and effectiveness. Important elements of this protocol involve the determination of the initial dose, using the MED or skin phototype method, and the selection of the applicator and method of application. To facilitate quantitative dosimetry, readers are invited to use the **Online Dosage Calculator: Ultraviolet**. UV phototherapy delivered in a clinical setting (hospital or therapeutic UV centers) is common. Repeated journeys to these clinical centers for treatments, however, can be time consuming and expensive for many patients, considering that a given UV treatment session lasts only a few minutes. An alternative is for these patients to treat themselves at home using UV devices found in hospitals. Home-based therapy, therefore, is suitable only if found to be as safe and effective as hospital-based therapy. Today's consensus on this subject is that home-based UV therapy should be used with caution and restricted to those patients with overwhelming difficulties in visiting hospitals (Sarkany et al., 1999; Cameron et al., 2002b; Langan et al., 2004; Koek et al., 2006; Yelverton et al., 2006). Moreover, there is strong opinion that home-based UV phototherapy is a suboptimal treatment with greater attendant risks than phototherapy delivered in a

hospital environment (Sarkany et al., 1999). There can be no doubt that the safe use of UV therapy is directly related to the carcinogenic risk associated with it (Lee et al., 2005; Man et al., 2005). Dermatologists and phototherapists must be fully aware of this responsibility when prescribing unsupervised home-based UV phototherapy. Before authorizing home-based UV therapy, the treating phototherapist must ensure that the patient receives appropriate guidelines, training, and follow-up (Cameron et al., 2002b; Haykai et al., 2006).

APPLICATION, CONTRAINDICATIONS, AND RISKS

Ultraviolet

IMPORTANT: Prior to treatment, the patient's maximum erythemal dose (MED), or skin phototype, MUST be determined. Steps and procedures related to MED determination are illustrated and described in Figure 12-5. Those for skin phototype determination are presented in Table 12-2. **The wearing of ultraviolet (UV) protective goggles, by both practitioner and patient during therapy, is mandatory.** Shown, as examples, are applications of ultraviolet therapy using a handheld wand (Fig. 12-6) and a hand cabinet (Fig. 12-7).

See **online video** for more details.

STEP	RATIONALE AND PROCEDURE

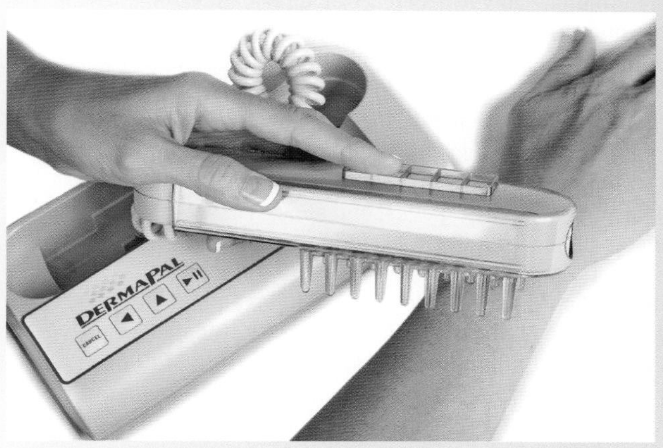

FIGURE 12-6 Application of ultraviolet therapy for a forearm spotty area using a handheld wand applicator. (Courtesy of Daavlin).

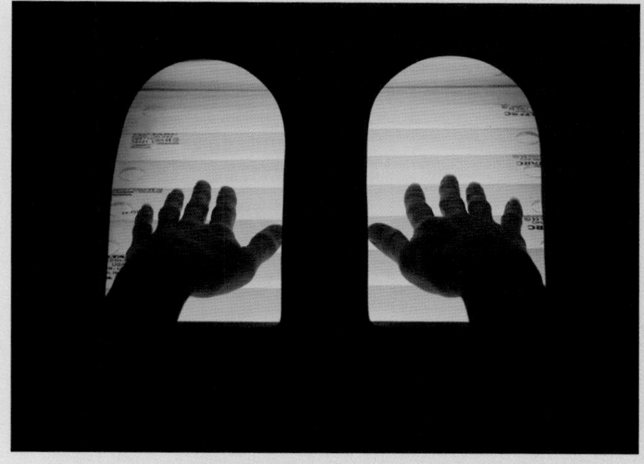

FIGURE 12-7 Application of ultraviolet for the hand area using a commercial hand cabinet. (Courtesy of Daavlin).

1. Check for contraindications.

Over the eye—temporary damage to the conjunctiva (photoconjunctivitis), or to the cornea (photokeratitis), causing ocular pain, eye watering, and blurred vision

Over a malignant skin lesion—further enhancing and spreading the lesion

History of melanoma—further enhancing and spreading the lesion

Lupus erythematosus, porphyrias, pellagra, sarcoidosis, herpes simplex—exacerbation of these pathologies (Cameron et al., 2003; Weisberg et al., 2006; Rajpara et al., 2010)

Active pulmonary tuberculosis—exacerbation of infection

Significant kidney, cardiac, and liver diseases—decreased tolerance of UV radiation

Hyperthyroidism, diabetes mellitus—severe itching from interaction of UV light with thyroid medication and insulin

Acute eczema or dermatitis—re-exacerbation of these conditions

STEP	RATIONALE AND PROCEDURE
2. Consider the risks.	*Over areas recently exposed to other radiation therapies*—risk of skin carcinoma (Cameron et al., 2003; Weisberg et al., 2006) *With patients who are photosensitive (acquired or drug related)*—risk of increased sensitivity to UV radiation (Weisberg et al., 2006) *With patients who are feverish*—risk of elevating core temperature (Weisberg et al., 2006) *With patients having a large cumulative dose*—risk of late adverse effect such as photoaging, wrinkling, and photocarcinogenesis *Discuss the risk of UV therapy-induced skin cancer with each patient prior to therapy and obtain written consent*—protection against this risk in case of litigation; record the consent in writing and file it (Ibbotson et al., 2004). *With women who are pregnant or lactating and children*—although UVB therapy is considered safe (Menter et al., 2010; Rajpara et al., 2010; Tan et al., 2010; Pavlovsky et al., 2011), caution is advised.
3. Position and instruct patient.	Ensure comfortable body positioning. Instruct the patient to minimize movement of the treated body segment such as to ensure optimal irradiation. Further instruct not to touch the UV tubes, to stay at least 30 cm (12 in) from UV tubes, and to call for assistance if necessary.
4. Prepare trearment area.	Remove jewelry and clothing. Most dermatoses involve several lesional plaques on the skin affecting a certain percentage of the body. Before each application, cleanse the treated areas with water to remove all impurities, including any therapeutic cream or emollient. Theoretically speaking, only the lesions should be treated. Unfortunately, this is rarely entirely possible, considering the locations and extent of these lesional plaques in relation to normal skin. Normal skin areas in between, or surrounding, the plaques should be protected from UV radiation by means of UV-protective creams and materials such as goggles, face shields, or other UV-blocking clothing such as shorts, gloves, and socks. Always shield the genital (to prevent tumor) as well as the nipple (to prevent blistering) areas.
5. Select device type.	Select the most appropriate UV device according to the location of the plaques affecting the body. For example, a whole-body cubicle (see Fig. 12-2A) may be selected if a large proportion of the body is affected. Conversely, a handheld UV wand (see Fig. 12-2C) may be used if the lesions are spread over a smaller area of the body. Make use of devices with key-locked ON–OFF switches and built-in controlled prescription timers to optimize treatment safety (Nolan et al., 2010).
6. Select mode of delivery.	Choose between BBUVB and NBUVB. When possible, select NBUVB over BBUVB because of its lower carcinogenic risk.
7. Power up the device.	Plug line-powered devices into ground-fault circuit interrupter (GFCI) receptacles to prevent the occurrence of macroshocks (see Chapter 5). Follow the manufacturer's instructions about how to power up the UV device and about the time needed (warm-up time) before optimal operation.
8. Set dosimetry and scheduling.	• *If based on MED value:* Follow the recommendations presented in Table 12-3. • *If based on skin phototype:* Follow the recommendations presented Table 12-4. • Note that most modern UVB devices are equipped with dosimeter control centers. The dose per treatment (D_t) is entered as prescribed. A special UV sensor measures the irradiance (I), or intensity, of light, and adjust the irradiation duration (T) to compensate for any irradiance variation due to aging of the tubes, thus keeping the dose per treatment constant during treatment ($D_t = I \times T$). One-touch operation allows the patient to conveniently begin, pause, or resume his or her treatment. A removable safety key prevents unauthorized use, which is particularly important for home treatment, where children may be present. Use the **Online Dosage Calculator: Ultraviolet** to facilitate dosimetry .

STEP	RATIONALE AND PROCEDURE
9. Position the applicator.	Apply the following two laws governing application (see Chapter 10 for details): • *Lambert's cosine law:* For every treatment, keep the UV lamp's irradiating surface area *perpendicular* to the skin surface being treated. • *Inverse square law:* For every treatment, keep the distance separating the UV lamp's surface from the treated skin surfaces the same.
10. Put on UV protective goggles.	Both patient and practitioners *must* wear UV-protective goggles during skin phototesting and therapy. If the facial area is free of lesions and a whole-body device is be used, a UV face shield, instead of simple goggles, should be used to protect the patient's facial area.
11. Apply treatment.	Ensure adequate monitoring. Continue treatment until complete clearance or until no further improvement to optimize treatment plan (Nolan et al., 2010)
12. Conduct post-treatment inspection.	Inspect the treated skin area for any unexpected response.
13. Ensure regular follow-up.	Because UV energy is cumulative, it is extremely important to monitor the cumulative dose received by the patient over time. Regular follow-up is mandatory.
14. Ensure post-treatment equipment maintenance.	Follow manufacturer recommendations (Taylor et al., 2002). Immediately report any defects or malfunctions to technical maintenance staff. Precise and quantitative dosimetry is mandatory with UV therapy because the carcinogenic risk increases relative to the cumulative dose the patient will receive over his or her lifetime. Conduct regular maintenance and calibration to optimize dosimetry and treatment efficacy. Change in irradiance can occur as lamp output declines with age. Pairs of internal cabin detectors may be used to automatically adjust treatment time to keep the dose constant (Amatiello et al., 2006). The alternative is to replace lamps as they burn out or otherwise fail.

CASE STUDIES

Presented are two case studies that summarize the concepts, principles, and applications of UV therapy discussed in this chapter. Case Study 12-1 addresses the use of NBUVB for psoriasis affecting a young athletic man. Case Study 12-2 is concerned with the application of NBUVB for hand eczema (atopic dermatitis) affecting a young mother. Each case is structured in line with the concepts of evidence-based practice (EBP), the International Classification of Functioning, Disability, and Health (ICF) disablement model; and SOAP (*s*ubjective, *o*bjective, *a*ssessment, *p*lan) note format (see Chapter 2 for details).

CASE STUDY 12-1: PSORIASIS

EVIDENCE-BASED CLINICAL DECISION MAKING PROTOCOL

1. Formulate the Case History

A 32-year-old active man, diagnosed 4 years ago with severe psoriasis causing multiple lesions on various body segments, is referred by his treating dermatologist for UVB therapy. Psoriasis is a noncontagious, common, chronic, and incurable disease that occurs when faulty signals in the immune system causes skin cells to regenerate too quickly. This man has no history of skin cancer. His skin phenotype is II (darker white skin, burns easily, tans minimally). His past treatments have included oral drugs, topical creams, and five regimens (or therapeutic periods) of oral PUVA. Because of the significant side effects associated with his previous PUVA therapy sessions (nausea, skin phototoxicity), and the growing awareness of his carcinogenic risk, the patient declined further PUVA treatment and asked his dermatologist for an alternative, less carcinogenic form of UV therapy. His main complaints are pain and restricted elbow, knee, and trunk movements caused by the lesional plaques. He also complains of difficulty with some activities of daily living (ADLs) and with his favorite sport activity—cycling. His goal is to achieve a reasonable, enduring resolution of his plaques, enough to reduce his pain and increase his overall ability to perform most of his ADLs and cycling activities. The patient presently suffers from Achilles tendinitis, for which he takes the anti-inflammatory and photosensitizing drug Celebrex. He prefers receiving treatment in the UV center. If UVB treatment is effective, he may consider home-based therapy.

2. Outline the Case Based on the ICF Framework

PSORIASIS		
BODY STRUCTURES AND FUNCTIONS	**ACTIVITIES**	**PARTICIPATION**
Pain	Limited bilateral elbow and knee range of motion	Difficulty with cycling
Multiple skin lesional plaques	Limited trunk range of motion	Difficulty with ADLs

PERSONAL FACTORS	ENVIRONMENTAL FACTORS
Young man	Recreational sports
Athletic character	Team play
College educated	Fitness and leisure

3. Outline Therapeutic Goals and Outcome Measurements

GOAL	OUTCOME MEASUREMENT
Decrease pain	Visual Analogue Scale (VAS)
Decrease plaque severity	Psoriasis Area Severity Index (PASI)
Increase articulation range of motion	Goniometry
Facilitate ADLs and cycling	Patient-Specific Functional Scale (PSFS)

4. Justify the Use of UVB Therapy Based on the EBP Framework

PRACTITIONER'S EXPERIENCE	RESEARCH-BASED INDICATIONS	PATIENT'S EXPECTATION
Experienced in UVB	*Strength:* Strong	Looking forward to receive less carcinogenic-type UV therapy
Has used UVB in similar cases	*Effectiveness:* Substantiated	Hope for good results
Is convinced that UVB will be beneficial		

5. Outline Key Intervention Parameters

- **Treatment base:** UV treatment center
- **Device type:** Whole-body cubicle (see Fig. 12-2A), mounted with 48 fluorescent TL-01 tubes emitting NBUVB light. The narrowband is selected over the broadband because its peak spectral irradiation (313 to 309 nm) is well within the action spectrum of psoriasis. NBUVB is also selected because it eliminates the nontherapeutic, strong erythemogenic response caused by the shorter band (310 to 290 nm) of BBUVB rays. NBUVB is further justified because it presents no side

effects and a lower carcinogenic risk when compared to BBUVB. Because of the broad coverage of his lesions, the patient is treated using a whole-body cubicle device. During therapy, the patient's intact skin areas and key organs are protected with a face shield (for facial protection), shorts (for genital protection), gloves, and socks. The repeated erythemal effect of UV light is expected to clear most of the plaques. The use of UVB presents a risk for the patient, because he is currently using an anti-inflammatory and photosensitizing drug, Celebrex, for his acute Achilles tendinitis. Caution is advised.

- **Application protocol:** Follow the suggested application protocol for UVB presented in *Application, Contraindications, and Risks* box, and make the necessary adjustments for this case.
- **Patient's positioning:** Standing
- **Application site:** Over skin lesions
- **UV protection:** Over eyes (goggle), nipple, and genital (clothing) areas
- **Application method:** Stationary with noncontact; body kept at approximately 30 cm (12 in) from tubes
- **Dosimetry:** Based on the skin phototype method
- **Patient's skin phototype:** Type III (see Table 12-2)
- **Initial dose:** 260 mJ/cm^2, which corresponds to phototype III using NBUVB (see Table 12-4)
- **Increment after each treatment:** 40 mJ/cm^2 (see Table 12-4)
- **Treatment frequency:** 3 per week
- **Total number of treatments:** 24
- **Intervention period:** 8 weeks
- **Cumulative dose*:** 14.4 J/cm^2
- **Concomitant therapy:** Daily meticulous skin care

***Use the Online Dosage Calculator: Ultraviolet.**

6. Report Pre- and Post-Intervention Outcomes

OUTCOME	PRE	POST
Pain (VAS score)	4/10	1/10
Plaque lesion status (PASI score)	4/7	1/7
Functional activities (PSFS score)	7/10	9/10

7. Document Case Intervention Using the SOAP Note Format

S: Middle-aged active Pt, diagnosed with severe psoriasis, presents with multiple skin lesions distributed over several body areas, causing pain and difficulty with ADLs and sports activities. Concerned with increasing risk of skin cancer, PT wants to move away from PUVA.

O: *Test:* Skin phototype: III. *Intervention:* NBUVB applied over skin lesions; Pt standing; whole-body UV cubicle; stationary without contact; initial dose: 260 mJ/cm^2; dose increment after each treatment: 40 mJ/cm^2; treatment schedule: 3 per week for 8 weeks. *Pre–post comparison:* Decrease pain (4/10 to 1/10), improve skin lesion status (decrease PASI score from 4/7 to 1/7), and improve functionality (increase PSFS score from 7/10 to 9/10).

A: No adverse effect, despite Pt taking photosensitizing drug. Treatment well tolerated. PT very pleased with results.

P: Considering the unfortunate recurrent nature of psoriasis, Pt considers renting or purchasing UV device for home therapy conducted under the supervision of his dermatologist.

CASE STUDY 12-2: CHRONIC HAND ECZEMA

EVIDENCE-BASED CLINICAL DECISION MAKING PROTOCOL

1. Formulate the Case History

A 28-year-old Caucasian woman and mother to two young children is referred to phototherapy for moderate chronic bilateral hand eczema (atopic dermatitis) that is irresponsive to conventional drug and cream therapies. She is now 5 months pregnant. Her main complaints are itching, skin dryness, and pain. She has also major difficulty with practically all ADLs. Physical examination reveals, on both hands, moderate to severe signs of pruritus, exudation, and excoriation. She still copes well with her disease, which has been present for the past 5 years, but is desperate for pain relief and improved hand function. She read on the Internet that UV therapy might be beneficial. Her preference is for home therapy because of her young children.

2. Outline the Case Based on the ICF Framework

CHRONIC HAND ECZEMA		
BODY STRUCTURES AND FUNCTIONS	**ACTIVITIES**	**PARTICIPATION**
Pain	Difficulty with handling	Difficulty with ADLs
Multiple skin lesions		

PERSONAL FACTORS	ENVIRONMENTAL FACTORS
Young healthy woman	Housewife
Mother of young children	Child care

3. Outline Therapeutic Goals and Outcome Measurements

GOAL	OUTCOME MEASUREMENT
Decrease signs and symptoms related to skin lesions	Atopic Dermatitis Quickscore (ADQ)
Improve hand function	Manual Ability Measure (MAM-16)

4. Justify the Use of UVB Therapy Based on the EBP Framework

PRACTITIONER'S EXPERIENCE	RESEARCH-BASED INDICATIONS	PATIENT'S EXPECTATION
Moderate experience in UVB	*Strength:* Strong	Read on the Internet about UV therapy
Has never used UVB in similar cases	*Effectiveness:* Substantiated	Wants home therapy
Believes that UVB can be beneficial		

5. Outline Key Intervention Parameters

- **Treatment base:** Home; patient rents the UV device for a month.
- **Device type:** Hand cabinet (see Fig. 12-2B) mounted with 30 fluorescent TL-01 tubes emitting NBUVB light
- **Risk and precaution:** Pregnancy is not a contraindication to UVB therapy. The narrowband is selected over the broadband because its peak spectral irradiation (313 to 309 nm) is well within the action spectrum of psoriasis. NBUVB is also selected because it eliminates the non-therapeutic strong erythemogenic response caused by the shorter band (310 to 290 nm) of BBUVB rays. NBUVB is further justified because it presents no side effects and has a lower carcinogenic risk when compared to BBUVB.
- **Application protocol:** Follow the suggested application protocol presented for UVB in *Application, Contraindications, and Risks* box, and make the necessary adjustments for this case.
- **Patient's positioning:** Sitting with both hands resting in the cabinet
- **Application site:** Over hands
- **UV protection:** Over eyes (goggles)
- **Application method:** Stationary with noncontact
- **Dosimetry:** Based on the MED method (see Fig. 12-5)
- **MED value:** 400 mJ/cm^2
- **Initial dose:** 200 mJ/cm^2 or 5% of MED (see Table 12-3)
- **Treatment scheduling:** According to recommendation for NBUVB presented in Table 12-3
- **Treatment frequency:** 5 per week
- **Total number of treatments:** 20
- **Intervention period:** 4 weeks
- **Cumulative dose*:** 5.9 J/cm^2
- **Concomitant therapy:** Daily meticulous skin care

***Use the Online Dosage Calculator: Ultraviolet.**

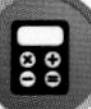

6. Report Pre- and Post-Intervention Outcomes

OUTCOME	PRE	POST
Skin lesion status—ADQ score	48/70	15/70
Hand function—MAM score	48/64	15/64

7. Document Case Intervention Using the SOAP Note Format

S: A 28-year-old pregnant woman, mother of 2 young children, presents with moderate chronic bilateral hand eczema (atopic dermatitis) that is irresponsive to conventional drug and cream therapies.

O: *Test:* MED determination over forearm; 400 mJ/cm^2. *Intervention:* NBUVB applied over both hands; Pt sitting; UV hand cabinet; stationary without contact; initial dose: 20 mJ/cm^2; treatment schedule daily, 5 per week for 4 weeks. *Pre–post comparison:* Improve skin lesions (ADQ 48/70 to 15/70) and improved hand function (MAM 48/64 to 15/64).

A: No adverse effect. Treatment very well tolerated. PT very pleased with results.

P: Considering the unfortunate recurrent nature of atopic dermatitis, Pt will purchase UV device for home therapy conducted under the supervision of her dermatologist.

VI. THE BOTTOM LINE

- There is strong scientific evidence to show that UVB therapy can induce significant therapeutic effects (clearance of lesions) on human dermatoses. The use of UVC for infected wounds is pending. The use of UVA (PUVA and UVA1) is beyond the scope of this chapter.
- UV therapy is the delivery of electromagnetic energy within the visible and x-ray band of the electromagnetic spectrum for therapeutic purposes.
- The use of NBUVB is increasing because of its therapeutic effectiveness and lower risk of inducing skin cancer over the years.
- UV therapy poses an important risk of developing skin cancer over the years.
- Skin phototesting is mandatory prior to using UV therapy.
- The initial UV dose is determined by using the MED or the skin phototype method.
- The skin phototype method is much more convenient, practical, and easy to use than the MED method.
- The dosage and treatment scheduling recommendations from the American Academy of Dermatology provide helpful and easy guidance to dosimetry.
- Each dose per treatment (mJ/cm^2) and cumulative dose (J/cm^2) should be documented in the patient's file.
- Using the **Online Dosage Calculator: Ultraviolet** removes the burden of hand calculation and promotes the adoption of quantitative dosimetry.
- The overall body of evidence reported in this chapter shows the strength of evidence behind BBUVB and NBUVB to be *moderate* and its level of therapeutic effectiveness *substantiated*.

VII. CRITICAL THINKING QUESTIONS

Clarification: What is meant by ultraviolet (UV) therapy?

Assumptions: You have assumed that the carcinogenic risk associated with NBUVB is lower than that associated with BBUVB. How do you justify making that assumption?

Reasons and evidence: Why do you believe that the use of NBUVB is as effective as and less carcinogenic than PUVA and BBUVB for most dermatoses?

Viewpoints or perspectives: How will you respond to a colleague who says that skin phototesting is optional prior to using UV therapy?

Implications and consequences: What are the implications and consequences of operating a UV device without considering the reciprocity law, Lambert's cosine law, and the inverse square law?

About the question: Why is it so important to do phototesting before UV therapy and monitor cumulative doses over the patient's lifetime? Why do you think I ask this question?

VIII. REFERENCES

Articles

Ahmad K, Rogers S, McNicholas PD, Collins P (2007) Narrowband UVB and PUVA in the treatment of mycosis fungoides: A retrospective study. Acta Derm Venereol, 87: 413–417

Aydogan K, Karadogan SK, Tunali S, Adim SBG, Ozcelik T (2006) Narrowband UVB phototherapy for small plaque parapsoriasis. J Eur Acad Dermatol Venereol, 20: 573–577

Baldo A, Sammarco E, Monfrecola M (1996) UVB phototherapy for pruritus in polycythaemia vera. J Dermatol Treat, 7: 245–246

Baldo A, Sammarco E, Plaitano R, Martinelli V, Monfrecola A (2002) Narrow (TL-01) ultraviolet B phototherapy for pruritus polycythaemia vera. J Dermatol, 147: 979–981

Berroeta I, Clark C, Ibbotson SH, Ferguson J, Dawe RS (2004) Narrowband (TL-01) ultraviolet B phototherapy for chronic urticaria. Clin Exp Dermatol, 29: 97–99

Bhatnagar A, Kanwar AJ, Parsad D, De D (2007) Comparison of systemic PUVA and NB-UVB in the treatment of vitiligo: An open prospective study. J Eur Acad Dermatol Venereol, 21: 638–642

Bilsland D, George SA, Gibbs NK (1993) A comparison of narrow band phototherapy (TL-01) and phototherapy (PUVA) in the management of polymorphic light eruption. Br J Dermatol, 129: 708–712

Boztepe G, Karaduman A, Sahin S, Hayran M, Koleman F (2006) The effect of maintenance narrow-band ultraviolet B therapy on the duration of remission of psoriasis: A prospective randomized clinical trial. In J Dermatol, 45: 245–250

Brazzelli V, Antoninetti M, Palazzini S, Prestinari F, Berroni G (2007) Narrow-band ultraviolet therapy in early-stage mycosis fungoides: A study on 20 patients. Photodermatol Photoimmunol Photomed, 23: 229–233

Cameron H, Dawe RS, Yule S, Murphy J, Ibbotson SH, Ferguson J (2002a) A randomized observer-blinded trial of twice vs. three times weekly narrowband ultraviolet B phototherapy for chronic plaque psoriasis. Br J Dermatol, 147: 973–978

Cameron H, Yule S, Moseley H, Dawe RS, Ferguson J (2002b) Taking treatment to the patient: Development of a home TL-01 ultraviolet B phototherapy service. Br J Dermatol, 147: 957–965

Clark C, Dawe RS, Evans AT, Lowe G, Ferguson J (2000) Narrowband TL-01 phototherapy for patch-stage mycosis fungoides. Arch Dermatol, 136: 748–752

Clayton TH, Clark SM, Turner D, Goulden V (2006) The treatment of severe atopic dermatitis in children with narrowband ultraviolet B phototherapy. Clin Exp Dermatol, 32: 28–33

Conner-Kerr TA, Sullivan PK, Gaillard J, Franklin ME, Jones RM (1998) The effect of ultraviolet radiation on antibiotic-resistant bacteria in vitro. Ostomy Wound Manage, 44: 50–56

Coven TR, Burack LH, Gilleaudead R, Keogh M, Ozawa M, Krueger JG (1997) Narrow-band UV-B produces superior clinical and histopathological resolution of moderate-to-severe psoriasis in patients compared with broadband UV-B. Arch Dermatol, 133: 1514–1522

Dawe RS, Cameron H, Yule S, Man I, Wainwright NJ, Ibbotson SH, Ferguson J (2003) A randomized controlled trial of narrowband ultraviolet B vs. bath-psoralen plus ultraviolet A photochemotherapy for psoriasis. Br J Dermatol, 148: 1194–1204

Dawe RS, Wainwright NJ, Cameron H, Ferguson J (1998) Narrow-band (TL-01) ultraviolet B phototherapy for chronic plaque psoriasis: Three times or five times weekly treatment? Br J Dermatol, 139: 833–839

Der-Petrossian M, Seeber A, Honigsmann H, Tanew A (2000) Half-side comparison study on the efficacy of 8-methoxysporalen bath-PUVA versus narrow-band ultraviolet B phototherapy in patients with severe chronic atopic dermatitis. Br J Dermatol, 142: 39–43

Diederen PV, Van Weelden H, Sanders CJ, Toonstra J (2003) Narrow-band UVB and psoralen-UVA in the treatment of early-stage mycosis fungoides. A retrospective study. J Am Acad Dermatol, 48: 215–219

Don P, Iuga A, Dacko A, Hardick K (2006) Treatment of vitiligo with broadband ultraviolet B and vitamins. Int J Dermatol, 45: 63–65

Fisher T, Alsins J, Berne B (1984) Ultraviolet action spectrum and evaluation of ultraviolet lamps for psoriasis healing. Int J Dermatol, 23: 633–637

Fitzpatrick TB (1988) The validity and practicality of sun-reactive skin types I through VI. Arch Dermatol, 124: 869–871

Fotiades J, Lim HW, Jiang SB, Soter NA, Sanchez M, Moy J (1995) Efficacy of ultraviolet B phototherapy for psoriasis in patients infected with human immunodeficiency virus. Photodermatol Photoimmunol Photomed, 11: 107–115

Gathers RC, Scherschun L, Malick F, Fivenson DP, Lim HW (2002) Narrowband UVB phototherapy for early-stage mycosis fungoides. J Am Acad Dermatol, 47: 191–197

George SA, Bilsland DJ, Johnson BE, Ferfuson J (1993) Narrowband (TL-01) UVB air-conditioned phototherapy for chronic severe adult atopic dermatitis. Br J Dermatol, 128: 49–56

Gokdemir G, Barutcuoglu B, Sakiz D, Koslu A (2006) Narrowband UVB phototherapy for early-stage mycosis fungoides: Evaluation of clinical and histopathological changes. J Eur Acad Dermatol Venereol, 20: 804–809

Gokdemir G, Kivanc-Altunay I, Koslu A (2005) Narrow-band ultraviolet B phototherapy in patients with psoriasis: For which types of psoriasis is it more effective? J Dermatol, 32: 436–441

Gordon PM, Diffey BL, Matthews JN, Farr PM (1999) A randomized comparison of narrow-band TL-01 phototherapy and PUVA photochemotherapy for psoriasis. J Am Acad Dermatol, 41: 728–732

Green C, Ferguson J, Lakshmipathi T, Johnson BE (1988) 311 nm UVB phototherapy—an effective treatment for psoriasis. Br J Dermatol, 119: 691–696

Grundmann-Kollmann M, Behrens S, Podda M, Peter RU, Kaufmann R, Kerscher M (1999) Phototherapy for atopic eczema with narrowband UVB. J Am Dermatol, 40: 995–997

Hamzavi I, Jain H, McLean D, Shapiro J, Zeng H, Lui H (2004) Parametric modeling of narrowband UV-B phototherapy for vitiligo using a novel quantitative tool: The vitiligo area scoring index. Arch Dermatol, 140: 677–683

Haykai KA, DesGroseilliers JP (2006) Are narrow-band ultraviolet home units a viable option for continuous or maintenance therapy of photoresponsive diseases? J Cutan Med Surg, 10: 234–240

Hjerppe M, Hasan T, Saksala I, Reunala T (2001) Narrow-band UVB treatment in atopic dermatitis. Acta Derm Venereol, 81: 439–440

Hofer A, Cerroni L, Kerl H, Wolf P (1999) Narrowband (311 nm) UV-B therapy for small plaque parasporiasis and early-stage mucosis fungoides. Arch Dermatol, 135: 1377–1380

Hofer A, Fink-Puches R, Kerl H, Wolf P (1998) Comparison of phototherapy with near vs. far erythemogenic doses of narrow-band ultraviolet B in patients with psoriasis. Br J Dermatol, 138: 96–100

Jekler J (1992) Phototherapy of atopic dermatitis with ultraviolet radiation. Acta Dermatol Venereol, 72: 1–37

Jury CS, McHenry P, Burden AD, Lever R, Bilsland D (2006) Narrowband ultraviolet B (NBUVB) phototherapy in children. Clin Exp Dermatol, 31: 196–199

Kanwar AJ, Dogra S, Parsad D, Kumar B (2005) Narrow-band UVB for the treatment of vitiligo: An emerging effective and well-tolerated therapy. Int J Dermatol, 44: 57–60

Karvonen J, Kokkonen EL, Ruotsalainen E (1989) 311 nm UVB lamps in the treatment of psoriasis with the Ingram regimen. Acta Derm Venereal, 69: 82–85

Kaur M, Oliver B, Hu J, Feldman SR (2006) Nonlaser UVB-targeted phototherapy treatment of psoriasis. Cutis, 78: 200–203

Kirke SM, Lowder S, Lloyd JJ, Diffey BL, Matthews JN, Farr PM (2007) A randomized comparison of selective broadband UVB and narrowband UVB in the treatment of psoriasis. J Invest Dermatol, 127: 1641–1646

Kollner K, Wimmershoff MB, Hintz C, Landthaler M, Hohenleutner U (2005) Comparison of the 308-nm excimer laser and a 308-nm excimer lamp with 311-nm narrow-band ultraviolet B in the treatment of psoriasis. Br J Dermatol, 152: 750–754

Kreuter A, Hyun J, Stiker M, Sommer A, Altmeyer P, Gambichler T (2006) A randomized controlled study of low-dose UVA1, medium dose UVA1, and narrowband UVB phototherapy in the treatment of localized scleroderma. J Am Acad Dermatol, 54: 440–447

Langan SM, Heerey A, Barry M, Barnes L (2004) Cost analysis of narrow-band UVB phototherapy in psoriasis. J Am Acad Dermatol, 50: 623–626

Larko O (1979) Home solarium treatment for psoriasis. Br J Dermatol, 101: 13–16

Larko O (1989) Treatment of psoriasis with a new UVB-lamp. Acta Dermatol Venereol, 69: 357–359

Leenutaphong V, Nimkulrat P, Sudtim S (2000) Comparison of phototherapy two times and four times a week with low doses of narrow-band ultraviolet B in Asian patients with psoriasis. Photodermatol Photoimmunol Photomed, 16: 202–206

Legat FJ, Hofer A, Brabek E, Quehenberger F, Kerl H, Wolf P (2003) Narrowband UV-B vs medium-dose UV-A1 phototherapy in chronic atopic dermatitis. Arch Dermatol, 139: 223–224

Lim C, Brown P (2006) Quality of life in psoriasis improves after standardized administration of narrowband UVB phototherapy. Australas J Dermatol, 47: 37–40

Man I, Crombie OK, Dawe RS, Ibbotson SH, Ferguson J (2005) The photocarcinogenic risk of narrowband UVB (TL-01) phototherapy: Early follow-up data. Br J Dermatol, 152: 755–757

Natta R, Somsak T, Wisuttida T, Laor L (2003) Narrowband ultraviolet B radiation therapy for recalcitrant vitiligo in Asians. J Am Acad Dermatol, 49: 473–476

Njoo MD, Bos JD, Westerhof W (2000) Treatment of generalized vitiligo in children with narrow-band (TL-01) UVB radiation therapy. J Am Acad Dermatol, 42: 245–253

Ortel B, Perl S, Kinaciyan T, Calzavara-Pinton PG, Honigsmann H (1993) Comparison of narrow-band (331 nm) UVB and broad band UVA after oral or bath-water 8-methoxypsoralen in the treatment of psoriasis. J Am Acad Dermatol, 29: 736–740

Parrish JA, Fitzpatrick TB, Tanenbaum L, Pathak MA (1974) Photochemotherapy of psoriasis with oral methoxsalen and long-wave ultraviolet light. N Engl J Med, 291: 1207–1211

Parrish JA, Jaenicke KF (1981) Action spectrum for phototherapy of psoriasis. J Invest Dermatol, 76: 359–362

Parsad D, Kanwar AJ, Kumar B (2006) Psoralen-ultraviolet A vs. narrow-band ultraviolet B phototherapy for the treatment of vertiligo. J Eur Acad Dermatol Venereol, 20: 175–177

Pavlovky M, Baum S, Shpiro D, Pavlovky L, Pavlovky F (2011) Narrowband UVB: Is it effective and safe for paediatric psoriasis and atopic dermatitis. Eur Acad Dermatol Venereol, 25: 727–729

Picot E, Meunier I, Picot-Debeze MC (1992) Treatment of psoriasis with a 311-nm UVB lamp. Br J Dermatol, 127: 509–512
Pirkhammer D, Seeber A, Honigsmann H, Tanew A (2000) Narrowband ultraviolet B (TL-01) phototherapy is an effective and safe treatment for patients with seborrhoeic dermatitis. Br J Dermatol, 143: 964–968
Reynolds NJ, Franklin V, Gray JC, Diffey BL, Farr PM (2001) Narrow-band ultraviolet B and broad-band ultraviolet A phototherapy in adult atopic eczema: A randomized controlled trial. Lancet, 357: 2012–2016
Saricaoglu H, Karadogan SK, Baskan EB, Tunali S (2003) Narrowband UVB therapy in the treatment of lichen planus. Photodermatol Photoimmunol Photomed, 19: 265–267
Scherschun L, Kim JJ, Lim HW (2001) Narrow-band ultraviolet B is a useful and well-tolerated treatment for vitiligo. J Am Acad Dermatol, 44: 999–1003
Seckin D, Demircay Z, Akin O (2007) Generalized pruritus treated with narrowband UVB. Int J Dermatol, 46: 367–370
Sezer E, Erbil AH, Kurumlu Z, Tastan HB, Etikan I (2007a) Comparison of the efficacy of local narrowband ultraviolet B (NB-UVB) phototherapy versus psoralen plus ultraviolet A (PUVA) paint for palmoplantar psoriasis. J Dermatol, 34: 435–440
Sezer E, Etikan I (2007b) Local narrowband UVB phototherapy vs. local PUVA in the treatment of chronic hand eczema. Photodermatol Photoimmunol Photomed, 23: 10–14
Sjovall P, Christensen O (1987) Local and systemic effect of UV-B irradiation in patients with chronic hand eczema. Acta Dermatol Venereol, 67: 538–541
Stern RS, Armstrong RB, Anderson TF, Bickers DR, Lowe NJ, Harber L, Voorhees J, Parrish J (1986) Effect of continued ultraviolet B phototherapy on the duration of remission of psoriasis: A randomized study. J Am Acad Dermatol, 15: 546–556
Storbeck K, Holzle F, Schurer N, Lehmann P, Plewig G (1993) Narrow-band UVB (311 nm) versus conventional broad-band UVB with and without dithranol in phototherapy for psoriasis. Br J Dermatol, 28: 227–231
Sullivan PK, Conner-Kerr TA, Smith ST (1999) The effects of UVC irradiation on group A streptococcus in vitro. Ostomy Wound Manage, 45: 50–54, 56–58
Tamagawa-Mineoka R, Katoh N, Ueda E, Kishimoto S (2007) Narrow-band ultraviolet B phototherapy in patients with recalcitrant nodular prurigo. J Dermatol, 34: 691–695
Tan E, Lim D, Rademaker M (2010) Narrowband UVB phototherapy in children: A New Zealand experience. Australasian J Dermatol, 51: 268–273
Taneja A, Taylor CR (2002) Narrow-band UVB for lichen planus treatment. Int J Dermatol, 41: 282–283
Tanew A, Radakovic-Fijan S, Schemper M, Honigsmann H (1999) Paired comparison study on narrow-band (TL-01) UVB phototherapy versus photochemotherapy (PUVA) in the treatment of chronic plaque type psoriasis. Arch Dermatol, 135: 519–524
Tay YK, Morelli JG, Weston WL (1996) Experience with UVB phototherapy in children. Pediatr Dermatol, 13: 406–409
Taylor R (1972) Clinical study of ultraviolet in various skin conditions. Phys Ther, 52: 279–282
Thai TP, Houghton PE, Campbell KE, Woodbury MG (2002) Ultraviolet light C in the treatment of chronic wounds with MRSA: A case study. Ostomy Wound Manage, 48: 52–60
Thai TP, Keast DH, Campbell KE, Woodbury G, Houghton PE (2005) Effect of ultraviolet light C on bacterial colonization in chronic wounds. Ostomy Wound Manage, 51: 32–45
Tjioe M, Gerritsen MJ, Juhlin L, Van Der Kerkof PC (2002) Treatment of vitiligo vulgaris with narrow band UVB (311 nm) for one year and the effect of addition of folic acid and vitamin B12. Acta Derm Venereol, 82: 369–372
Valkova S, Velkova A (2004) UVA/UVB phototherapy for atopic dermatitis revisited. J Dermatolog Treat, 15: 239–244
Van Weelden H, De la Faille B, Young E, Van der Leun JC (1988) A new development in UVB phototherapy of psoriasis. Br J Dermatol, 119: 11–19
Van Weelden H, De la Faille B, Young E, Van der Leun JC (1990) Comparison of narrowband UV-B phototherapy and PUVA photochemotherapy (PUVA) in the treatment of psoriasis. Acta Derm Venereol, 70: 212–215
Wackernagel A, Legat FJ, Hofer A, Quehenberger F, Kerl H, Wolf P (2007) Psoralen plus UVA vs. UVB-311 nm for the treatment of lichen planus. Photodermatol Photoimmunol Photomed, 23: 15–19
Wainwright NJ, Dawe RS, Ferguson J (1998) Narrowband ultraviolet B (TL-01) phototherapy for psoriasis: Which incremental regimen? Br J Dermatol, 39: 410–414
Weichenthal M, Schwarz T (2005) Phototherapy: How does UV work? Photodermatol Photoimmunol Photomed, 21: 260–266
Westerhof W, Nieuweboer-Krobotova L (1997) Treatment of vitiligo with UV-B radiation vs topical psoralen plus UV-A. Arch Dermatol, 133: 1525–1528
Wills EE, Anderson TW, Beatie LB, Scott A (1983) A randomized placebo controlled trial of ultraviolet in the treatment of superficial pressure sores. J Am Geriatr Soc, 31: 131–133
Yashar SS, Gielcayk R, Scherschum L, Lim HW (2003) Narrow-band ultraviolet B treatment for vitiligo, pruritis, and inflammatory dermatoses. Photodermatol Photoimmunol Photomed, 19: 164–168
Yelverton CB, Kulkarni AS, Balkrishnan R, Feldman SR (2006) Home ultraviolet B phototherapy: A cost-effective option for severe psoriasis. Manage Care Interface, 19: 33–36, 39
Yones SS, Palmer RA, Garibaldinos TT, Hawk JK (2006) Randomized double-blind trial of the treatment of chronic plaque psoriasis: Efficacy of psoralen-UV-A therapy vs. narrowband UV-B therapy. Arch Dermatol, 142: 836–842
Yones SS, Palmer RA, Garibaldinos TT, Hawk JK (2007) Randomized double-blind trial of treatment of vitiligo. Efficacy of psoralen-UV-A therapy vs narrowband-UV-B therapy. Arch Dermatol, 143: 578–584
Yones SS, Palmer RA, Kuno Y, Hawk JL (2005) Audit of the use of psoralen photochemotherapy (PUVA) and narrowband UVB phototherapy in the treatment of psoriasis. J Dermatolog Treat, 16: 108–112

Review Articles

Amatiello H, Martin CJ (2006) Ultraviolet phototherapy: Review and options for cabin dosimetry and operation. Phys Med Biol, 51: 299–309
Bandow GD, Koo JY (2004) Narrow-band ultraviolet B radiation: A review of the current literature. Int J Dermatol, 43: 555–561
Bilsland D, Dawe R, Diffey BL, Farr P, Ferguson J, George S, Gibbs NK, Green C, McGregor J, Van Weelden H, Wainwright NJ, Young AR (1997) An appraisal of narrowband (TL-01) UVB phototherapy. British Photodermatology Group Workshop Report (April 1996). Br J Dermatol, 137: 327–330
British Photodermatology Group (1994) Guidelines for PUVA. Br J Dermatol, 130: 246–255
Cohill TP, Sagripanti JL (2008) Overview of the inactivation by 254 nm ultraviolet radiation of bacteria with particular relevance to biodefense. Photochem Photobiol, 84: 1084–1090
Dawe RS (2003) Ultraviolet A1 phototherapy. Br J Dermatol, 148: 626–637
Dogra S, De D (2010) Narrowband ultraviolet B in the treatment of psoriasis: The journey so far! Ind J Dermatol Venerol Lepro, 76: 652–661
Dogra S, Kanwar AJ (2004) Narrow band UVB phototherapy in dermatology. Indian J Dermatol Venereal Leprol, 70: 205–209
Gambichler T, Breuckmann F, Booms S, Altmeyer P, Kreuter A (2005) Narrowband UVB phototherapy in skin conditions beyond psoriasis. J Am Acad Dermatol, 52: 660–670
Halpern SM, Anstey AV, Dawe RS, Diffey BL, Farr PM, Ferguson J, Hawk JL, Ibbotson S, McGregor JM, Murphy GM, Thomas SE, Rhodes LE (2000) Guidelines for topical PUVA: A report of a workshop of the British Photodermatology Group. Br J Dermatol, 142: 22–31
Ibbotson SH, Bilsland D, Cox NH, Dawe RS, Diffey B, Edwards C, Farr PM, Ferguson J, Hart G, Hawk J, Loyd J, Martin C, Moseley H, McKenna K, Rhodes LE, Taylor DK (2004) An update and guidance on narrowband ultraviolet B phototherapy: A British Photodermatology Group Workshop Report. Br J Dermatol, 151: 283–297
Koek MB, Buskens E, Bruijnzeel-Koomen CA, Sigurdsson V (2006) Home ultraviolet B phototherapy for psoriasis: Discrepancy between literature, guidelines, general opinion and actual use. Results of a literature review, a web search, and a questionnaire among dermatologists. Br J Dermatol, 154: 701–711

Lee E, Koo J, Berger T (2005) UVB phototherapy and skin cancer risk: A review of the literature. Int J Dermatol, 44: 355–360

Menter A, Korman NJ, Elmets CA, Feldman SR, Gelfand JM, Gordon KB, Gottlieb A, Koo JY, Lebwohl M, Lim HW, van Voorhees AS, Beutner KR, Bhushan R (2010) Guidelines of care for the management of psoriasis and psoriatic arthritis. J Am Acad Dermatol, 62:114–135

Nolan BV, Yentzer BA, Feldman SR (2010) A review of home phototherapy for psoriasis. Dermatol Online J, 16 (2): 1–14

Rajpara AN, O'Neil JL, Nolan BV, Yentzer BA, Feldman SR (2010) Review of home phototherapy. Dermatol Online J, 16 (12): 1–23

Roelandts R (2002) The history of phototherapy: Something new under the sun? J Am Acad Dermatol, 46: 926–930

Saladi RN, Persaud AN (2005) The causes of skin cancer: A comprehensive review. Drugs Today (Barc), 41: 37–53

Sarkany RP, Anstey A, Diffey BL, Jobling R, Langmack K, McGregor JM, Moseley H, Murphy GM, Rhodes LE, Norris PG (1999). Home phototherapy: Report on a workshop of the British Photodermatology Group. December 1996. Br J Dermatol, 140: 195–199

Stern RS, Laird N (1994) The carcinogenic risk of treatments for severe psoriasis. Photochemotherapy Follow-up Study. Cancer, 73: 2759–2764

Taylor DK, Anstey AV, Coleman AJ, Diffey BL, Farr PM, Ferguson J, Ibbotson S, Langmack K, Lloyd JJ, McCann P, Martin CJ, Menage H, Murphy G, Pye SD, Rhodes LE, Rogers S (2002) Guidelines for dosimetry and calibration in ultraviolet radiation therapy: A report of a British Phototherapy Group Workshop. Br J Dermatol, 146: 755–763

Tuchinda C, Kerr HA, Taylor CR, Jacobe H, Bergamo BM, Elmets C, Rivard J, Lim HW (2006) UVA1 phototherapy for cutaneous diseases: An experience of 92 cases in the United States. Photodermatol Photoimmmunol Photomed, 22: 247–253

Van der Leun JC, Forbes PD (2005) Ultraviolet tanning equipment: Six questions. Photodermatol Photoimmunol Photomed, 21: 254–259

York NR, Jacobe HJ (2010) UVA1 phototherapy: A review of mechanism and therapeutic application. Int J Dermatol, 49: 623–630

Chapters of Textbooks

Conner-Kerr T, Albaugh KW, Woodruff LD, Cameron M, Bill A (2007) Phototherapy in wound management. In: Wound Care: A Collaborative Practice Manual for Health Care Professionals, 3rd ed. Sussman C, Bates-Jensen B (Eds). Lippincott Williams & Wilkins, Baltimore, pp 591–611

Davis JM (2002) Ultraviolet therapy. In: Therapeutic Modalities for Physical Therapists, 2nd ed. Prentice WE (Ed). McGraw-Hill, New York, pp 343–357

Diffey B, Farr P (2002) Ultraviolet therapy. In: Electrotherapy Evidence-Based Practice, 11th ed. Kitchen S (Ed). Churchill Livingstone, London, pp 191–207

Weisberg J, Balogun JA (2006) Ultraviolet radiation. In: Integrating Physical Agents in Rehabilitation, 2nd ed. Hecox B, Mehreteab TA, Weisberg J, Sanko J (Eds). Pearson Prentice Hall, Upper Saddle River, New Jersey, pp 429–446

Textbooks

Zanolli MD, Feldman SR (2004) Phototherapy Treatment Protocols for Psoriasis and Other Phototherapy-Responsive Dermatoses, 2nd ed. Informa-Healthcare, New York

Internet Resources

www.aad.org: American Academy of Dermatology

http://thePoint.lww.com: Online Dosage Calculator: Ultraviolet

PART IV

Electrical Agents

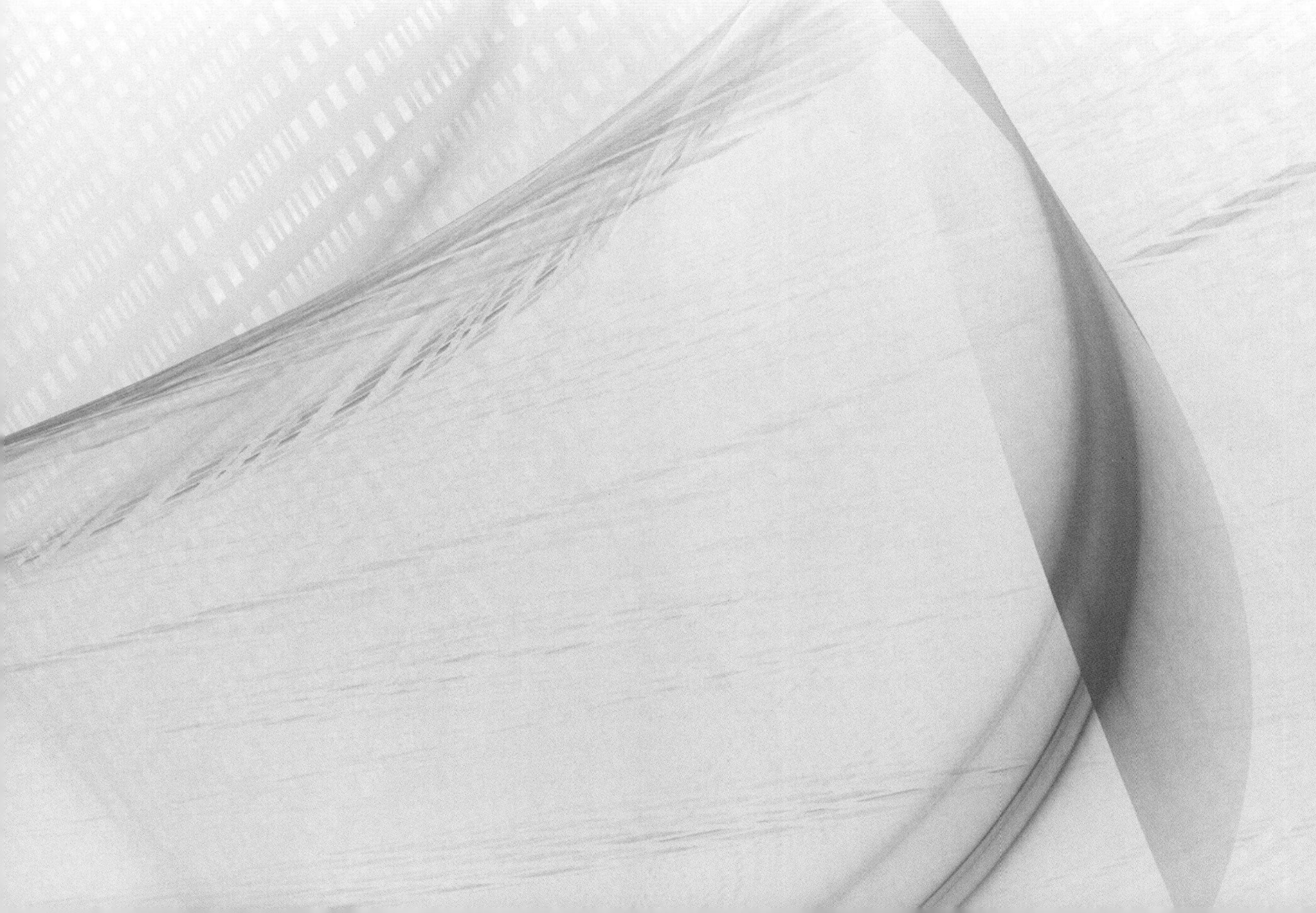

Chapter 13

Neuromuscular Electrical Stimulation

Chapter Outline

Learning Objectives

Remembering: Describe the biophysical characteristics associated with biphasic pulse, Russian, and interferential currents.

Understanding: Distinguish between electrically evoked versus volitional muscle contraction.

Applying: Demonstrate the four electrode configurations (monopolar, bipolar, quadripolar, multipolar) and the three stimulation modes (synchronous, reciprocal, overlap).

Analyzing: Explain how the current modulation underlying Russian current differs from the current modulation used to generate interferential current.

Evaluating: Formulate the dosimetric parameters that practitioners need to consider and calculate to deliver safe and effective neuromuscular electrical stimulation.

Creating: Discuss the evidence behind the therapeutic use of neuromuscular electrical stimulation.

I. FOUNDATION

A. DEFINITION

1. Neuromuscular Nerve Stimulation

The practice of NMES rests on the use of pulsed electrical currents applied to skeletal muscles with the objective to elicit contraction caused by the electrical depolarization of intramuscular nerve branches. Electrical stimuli are delivered using surface electrodes that are positioned over muscle bellies. The main purpose of NMES is to preserve and recover muscle function in patients and to improve muscle strength in healthy individuals (Bax et al., 2005; Gondin et al., 2011 Hortobagyi et al., 2011; Kim et al., 2010; Filipovic et al., 2011, 2012).

2. Functional Electrical Stimulation

The application of NMES for enhancing the control of movement and posture falls under the field of *functional electrical stimulation* (FES). More specifically, this therapeutic field focuses on the enhancement of impaired motor functions, such as hand grasping, locomotion, and respiration, using complex transcutaneous and percutaneous electrical muscle stimulation systems. The main purpose of FES is to enable motor function by replacing, or assisting, a patient's voluntary ability to execute or control the impaired functions. A subgroup of FES is the application of electrical current for *denervated* skeletal muscles, known as EMS, which stands for *electrical muscle stimulation* (APTA, 2001; Selkowitz, 2010). Coverage of FES, including EMS, is beyond the scope of this chapter because it usually requires complex and specially designed therapeutic equipment available for research purposes but not commonly available on the market for regular clinical applications (for an overview, see Glinsky et al., 2007; Roche et al., 2009; Selkowitz, 2010).

B. ELECTRICAL CURRENTS

The body of evidence presented in this chapter indicates that three types of electrical currents are commonly used to deliver clinical NMES. Practitioners can choose between **biphasic pulsed, Russian,** and **interferential** currents. When examining the force-generating capability of these electrical currents, similarities among electrical parameters must be considered before making any statement as to which current waveform is better than the other for muscle strengthening (Bellew et al., 2012). The biophysical characteristic of each of these currents is presented in the Biophysical Characteristics section.

C. ELECTRICAL STIMULATORS

NMES is delivered by using a variety of cabinet and portable electrical stimulators. Figure 13-1A illustrates a cabinet-type, multi-current, line-powered stimulator capable of generating Russian, interferential, and pulsed biphasic currents. The stimulator may be placed on top of a plain table or on a movable cart, as shown; the cart integrates with the stimulator in addition to providing storage bins and mobility. Also shown are two portable, battery-powered stimulators capable of generating Russian and interferential currents (see Fig. 13-1B,C). There is evidence to suggest that battery-powered stimulators are as effective as line-powered stimulators in producing current amplitudes necessary to generate the training muscle force outputs required for therapy (Laufer et al., 2001; Lyons et al., 2005). Additionally illustrated are a cabinet, line-powered interferential stimulator with a vacuum unit, which allows the use of stimulating suction-type electrodes (see Fig. 13-1D and later discussion), as well as the newer, all-in-one, garment-type electrical stimulator that is designed specifically for the treatment of the quadriceps muscle (see Fig. 13-1E).

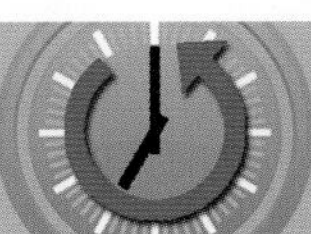

Historical Overview

The foundation of neuromuscular electrical stimulation (NMES) rests on Italian Luigi Galvani's work on frogs, conducted in the 1790s, showing that electrical current (static electricity) can evoke muscle contraction. A few years later, the discovery of electromagnetic induction by British Michael Farady led to the development of modern electrical stimulators. Then came the work of French Duchenne de Boulogne, in the 1800s, on human muscle showing that faradic current (pulsed current) applied with moistened surface electrodes can evoke muscle contraction. In 1950, Austrian Hans Nemec patented a concept that led to the creation of the first interferential current (IFC) therapy device (Nemec, 1959; Hooke, 1998). IFC therapy was first introduced in Europe during the 1960s and then in Australia, Canada, and the United States in the 1980s. The mid-1970s saw the introduction of Russian current, by Russian scientist Yakov Kots. His work opened the door to the use of NMES for enhancing muscle strength to healthy nonathletic and athletic individuals who want to increase their muscle strength without submitting themselves to traditional regimens of voluntary muscle training (Delitto, 2002; Ward et al., 2002). In response to scientific and public interests for this newly discovered current, commercial production of Russian current stimulators began in Canada and the United States in the 1980s.

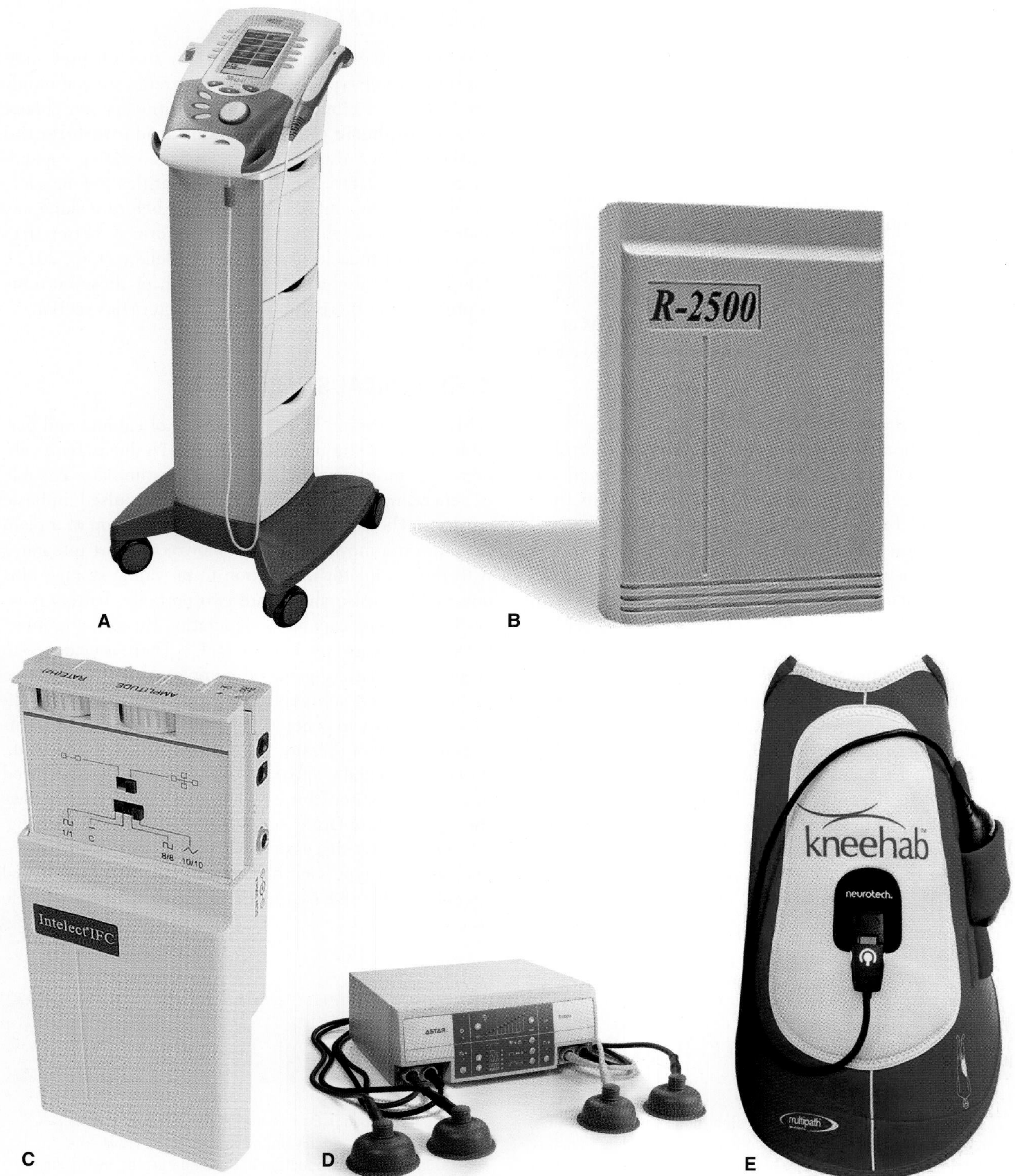

FIGURE 13-1 **A:** Cabinet-type, line-powered, multi-current stimulator mounted on cart, capable of generating Russian, interferential, and pulsed biphasic currents. Portable, battery-powered Russian (**B**) and interferential (**C**) stimulators. **D:** Cabinet-type, line-powered, interferential with vacuum unit, to which is attached a pair of suction electrodes. **E:** Newer, one size fits all, battery-powered, garment-based electrical stimulator designed specifically for the quadriceps muscle. (A–C: Courtesy of DJO Global; D: Courtesy of Astar; E: Courtesy of Neurotech Bio-Medical Research Ltd.)

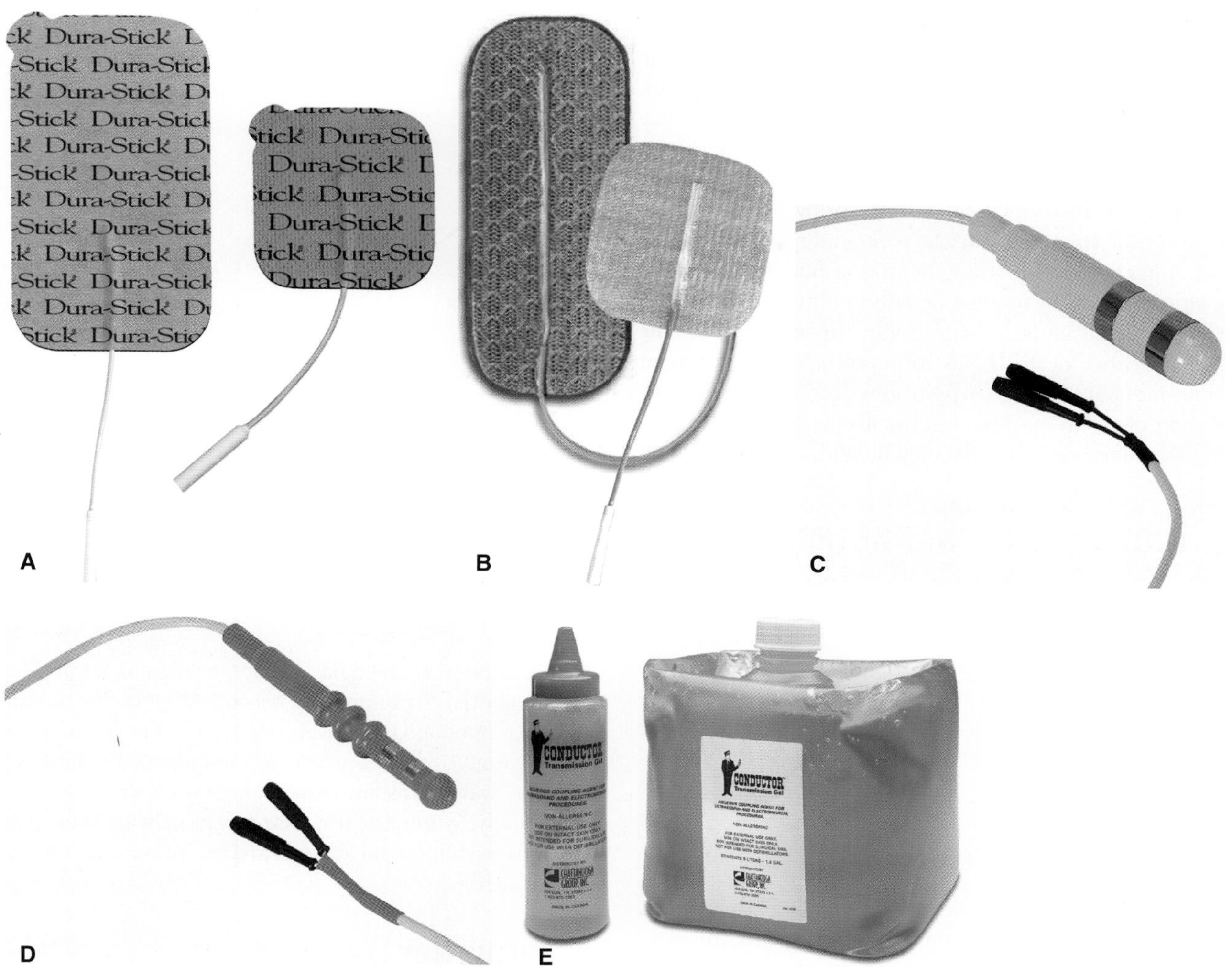

FIGURE 13-2 Surface rubber carbon-impregnated electrodes (**A**) and pliable stainless steel knit fabric electrodes (**B**). Reusable intravaginal (**C**) and intrarectal electrodes (**D**). Electroconductive gel (**E**). (A, B, and E: Courtesy of DJO Global; C, D Courtesy of Enraf-Nonius.)

D. ELECTRODES AND COUPLING MEDIUM

NMES is applied by using a variety of reusable and disposable electrodes connected to the stimulator using various cables. Figure 13-2 shows common surface plate electrodes made of carbon rubber material (A) or pliable stainless steel knit fabrics (B). These electrodes may be applied over flat body areas, with the exception of the pelvic area, where attachment may be a problem. When the purpose is to deliver NMES to the pelvic floor muscles for conditions such as urinary incontinence, special stimulating electrodes may be required. One option is to use intravaginal and intrarectal electrodes (Fig. 13-2C,D, respectively). If patients are not comfortable with the invasive nature of these electrodes, practitioners may select suction cup electrodes as a second option. These electrodes, connected to a vacuum interferential unit (see Fig. 13-1D), can be quickly and easily attached without adhesive tape or straps, and adapt comfortably to the contours of the pelvic area, thus ensuring optimal contact between the electrode and the skin. For NMES of the quadriceps muscle, practitioners may select a "one size fits all" garment electrode with stimulator unit (see Fig. 13-1E) as an alternative to traditional surface plate electrodes. To optimize electrical conduction at the electrode–tissue interface, electrodes must be covered with a thin layer of electroconductive gel (Fig. 13-2E). Both intravaginal and intrarectal electrodes must also be covered with a sterile lubricant prior to use.

E. RATIONALE FOR USE

Common goals in the field of physical rehabilitation are to preserve, recover, and enhance muscle function in patients following disease and trauma, and in healthy individuals for recreational purpose. There is unquestionable evidence in the scientific literature to show that the best method practitioners can use to enhance muscle function (i.e., strengthening) is to submit individuals to bouts of muscle maximum voluntary contractions (MVCs), done under isometric, isotonic, or isokinetic conditions. Which muscle-strengthening method should clinicians use with patients who are unable to perform volitional exercise at adequate intensity and duration to gain benefits, because of related factors such as physical deconditioning, pain, severe muscle atrophy, or lack of motivation? The use of NMES provides practitioners with an *alternative* muscle-strengthening method that *mimics* volitional training methods. By using NMES alone, or by superimposing it on top of voluntary muscle contractions, practitioners can enhance muscle strengthening in both patients and healthy subjects by improving motor unit (MU) activation while inducing muscle hypertrophy. In other words, the main objective of NMES is to improve MU recruitment while inducing muscle hypertrophy through serial bouts of short duration maximal electrically evoked muscle contractions done against resistance or load.

II. BIOPHYSICAL CHARACTERISTICS

As mentioned earlier, the delivery of NMES rests on using three different electrical currents, namely biphasic pulsed, Russian, and interferential currents. To describe electrical current in terms of waveform and frequency is common in the field of NMES. Let us consider these two important concepts before addressing the biophysical characteristics of these three electrical currents.

A. CURRENT WAVEFORM

Waveform is the geometric configuration of a current, which is described based on its phase, symmetry, electrical balance, and shape. First, a current waveform may be monophasic or biphasic in nature. The word *phase* describes an electrical event that begins when the current departs from the isoelectric line and ends when it returns to the baseline (APTA, 2001). A *monophasic* current waveform is made of only one phase that moves in only one direction (+ or – polarity) from the zero baseline to return to it after a finite time (Fig. 13-3). A *biphasic* current waveform, on the other hand, is made of two phases: moving in one direction and then in the opposite direction from the zero baseline, then returning to that baseline after a finite time. Second, a biphasic current waveform may be symmetrical or asymmetrical. It is *symmetrical* when its positive phase is geometrically identical to its negative phase and *asymmetrical* when its two phases are geometrically different (Fig. 13-4). Third, a biphasic waveform may also be balanced or unbalanced. The waveform is *balanced* when there are equal electrical charges in each phase (see *A* in Fig. 13-4). Such a balanced waveform is often referred to as having "zero net charge" or "zero net DC," because the amount of positive charges minus the amount of negative charges equals zero (APTA, 2001). The waveform is said to be *unbalanced* when there are unequal electrical charges in each phase—that is, when there is a net accumulation of charges within the waveform (see *B* in Fig. 13-4). Fourth, biphasic waveforms may have various shapes such as rectangular, square, triangular, sinusoidal, or exponential. To summarize based on the mentioned terminology, monophasic waveforms are neither symmetrical nor asymmetrical, but are always unbalanced. Moreover, biphasic waveforms are either symmetrical or asymmetrical. Finally, symmetrical waveforms are always balanced, whereas asymmetrical waveforms are either balanced or unbalanced.

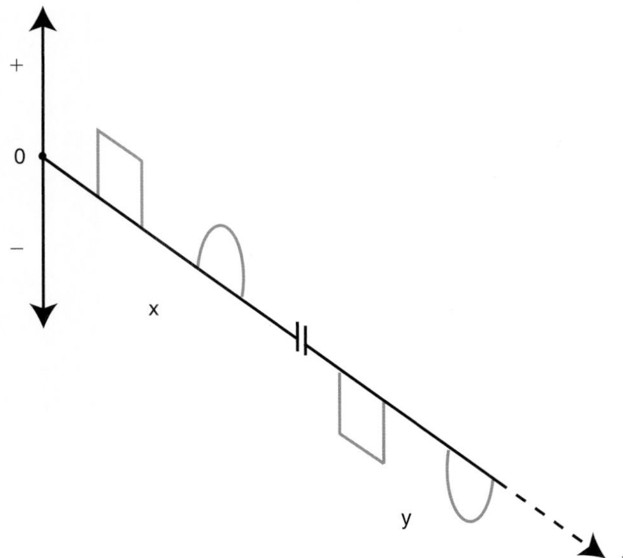

FIGURE 13-3 Monophasic waveforms with either positive (*x*) or negative (*y*) polarity.

B. FREQUENCY

As discussed next, electrical currents used for NMES may be delivered in pulses, bursts, and beats. A *pulse* is a single momentary and sudden fluctuation of current. Pulses may have various shapes; when it has a sinusoidal shape, it is

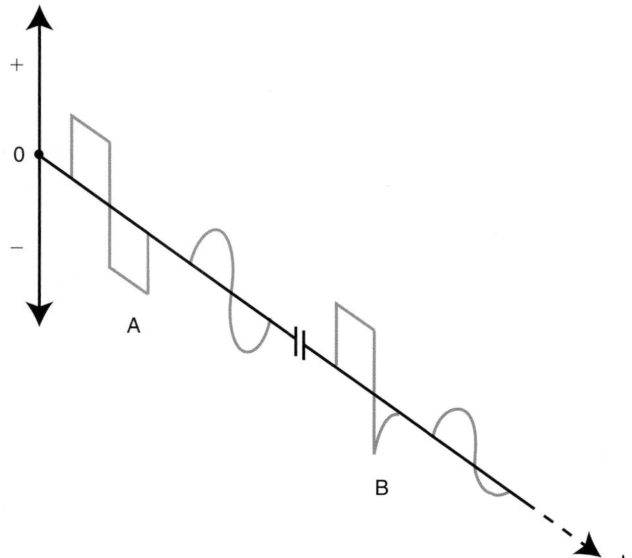

FIGURE 13-4 Biphasic symmetrical (*A*) and asymmetrical (*B*) waveforms.

called a *cycle.* A *burst,* as well as a *beat,* is a group of two or more successive pulses or cycles separated by a time interval during which no electrical activity occurs (APTA, 2001). *Duration,* whether it is pulse duration (PD), cycle duration (CD), burst duration (BuD), or beat duration (BeD), is the time elapsed between the beginning of the first phase and the end of the last phase. The time elapsed between each corresponds to interpulse duration (IPD), intercycle duration (ICD), interburst duration (IBuD), and interbeat duration (IBeD), respectively. *Frequency* (f) is defined as the number of times per second that a pulse, cycle, burst, or beat will repeat itself. It is calculated using the formula $f = 1/P$, where P, the period, is equal to the summation of either PD and IPD, CD and ICD, BuD and IBD, and BeD and IBeD, respectively.

C. BIPHASIC PULSED CURRENT

The use of biphasic pulsed currents is very common in the field of NMES. Figure 13-5 illustrates a typical biphasic pulsed waveform. This particular current waveform may be described as biphasic, asymmetrical, and unbalanced, with a rectangular positive phase and exponential negative phase. Shown is the delivery of successive pulses (Fig. 13-5A) and successive bursts of pulses (Fig. 13-5B), with each burst containing five pulses (see later discussion for details).

D. RUSSIAN CURRENT

The term *Russian current* stems from the work conducted in the field of NMES by Russian physiologist Yakov Kots (1971, 1977). Figure 13-6 illustrates the biophysical characteristics associated with this current. There is a consensus in the literature (Alon, 1999) that the *original* Russian current stems from the time modulation of a continuous alternating sine-wave current (AC), having a carrier frequency of 2,500 cycles per second (cps) or Hertz (Hz), in the form of bursts of electrical cycles. The technical term for Russian current is *burst-modulated sinusoidal alternating current.* As shown in the figure, the continuous sine-wave current underlying Russian current is modulated into bursts of cycles, with each burst containing several cycles. Each burst (Bu) has a fixed duration (BuD) of 10 milliseconds (ms) and a fixed interburst duration (IBuD) of 10 ms. Knowing that $f = 1/P$, where P is equal to the summation of BuD and IBuD, the result is a pulsed AC with a fixed-burst frequency of 50 bursts per second [bups] [$f = 1/(\text{BuD} + \text{IBuD}]$; 50 bups = 1/(10 ms + 10 ms). The inset in Figure 13-6 shows this single typical burst of current, lasting 10 ms and made of 25 continuous biphasic symmetrical sinusoidal cycles. With a carrier frequency of 2,500 cps, the duration of each sine-wave cycle within a burst, of which the duration is equivalent to the period (P), is 400 μs ($P = 1/f$; 400 μs = 1/2,500 cps), with each half-cycle having a duration of 200 μs. In other words, the cycle

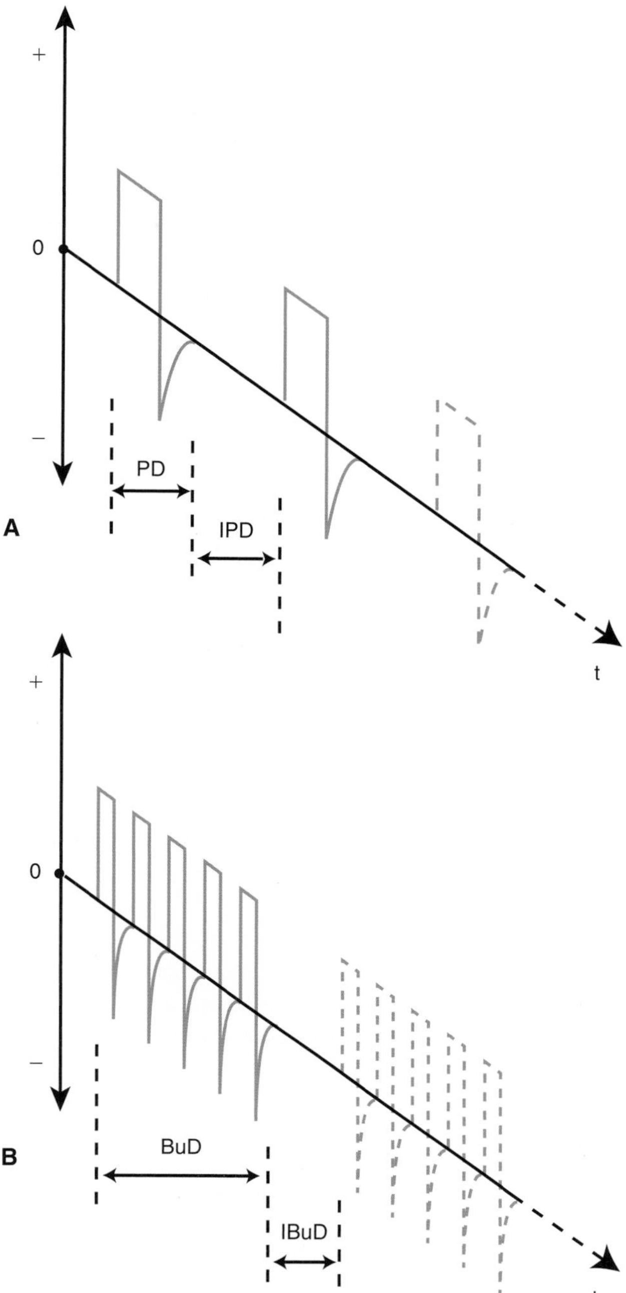

FIGURE 13-5 Typical biphasic pulsed current used for neuromuscular electrical stimulation. Pulse modulation (**A**) and burst modulation (**B**) are shown. PD, pulse duration; IPD, interpulse duration; BuD, burst duration; IBuD, interburst duration.

duration (CD) and the phase duration (PhD) of this cycle equate to 400 μs and 200 μs, respectively.

E. INTERFERENTIAL CURRENT

Interferential current, designated under the acronym IFC, is defined and described as a low-frequency, amplitude-modulated electrical current that results from the *interference* (hence, the word *interferential*) caused by crossing two or more medium-frequency alternating sine-wave

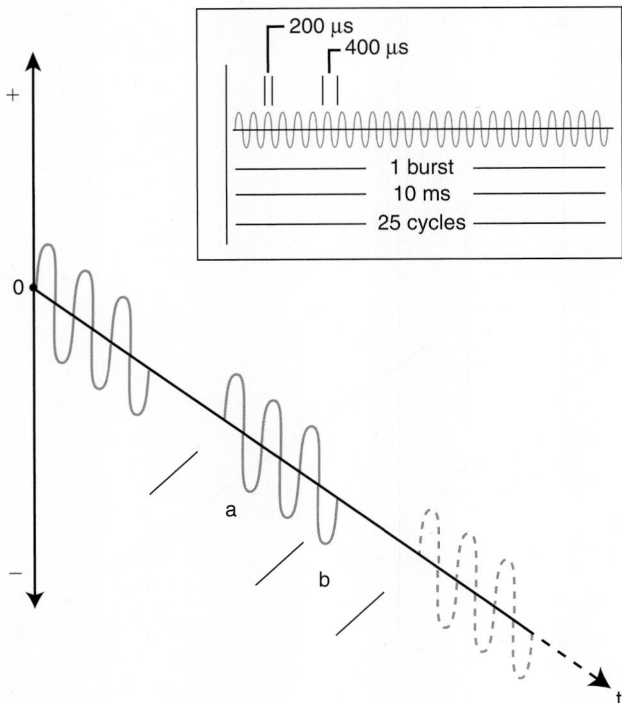

FIGURE 13-6 Original Russian current, with its sine-wave carrier frequency of 2,500 cps delivered in bursts of 10 ms (*a*) followed by 10-ms interburst duration (*b*), leading to a burst frequency of 50 bups (not drawn to scale). The inset shows the 25 cycles contained in each 10-ms burst, with each half-cycle and cycle in the burst lasting 200 and 400 μs, respectively.

currents with different carrier frequencies (Alon, 1999). The carrier frequency of these medium alternating sine-wave currents ranges between 3,000 and 5,000 cps. The technical term for IFC is *beat amplitude-modulated sinusoidal alternating current.*

1. Interference and Beat

The biophysical concept underlying the creation of an IFC is the *interference* caused by superimposing two (and sometimes three; see later discussion) medium-frequency sinusoidal currents generated by independent oscillatory circuits incorporated into the interferential devices (Alon, 1999; Lambert et al., 1993). The terms *low frequency* and *medium frequency* refer to a traditional and arbitrary classification stipulating that current output frequencies of less than 1,000 cps be designated as low-frequency currents, whereas those oscillating between 1,001 and 10,000 cps be classified as medium-frequency currents (Alon, 1999). Medium-frequency sinusoidal currents used today to generate IFC have a carrier frequency ranging from 3,000 to 5,000 cps. Figure 13-7 is the making of an IFC. For example, the first (C_1) and second (C_2) circuits have a carrier frequency (f_c) of 3,000 and 3,050 cps or Hz, respectively. By electronically allowing C_1 to interfere with C_2, and vice versa, a beat amplitude-modulated IFC is created. The beat frequency resulting from the interference of these two AC currents is calculated as the *absolute* frequency difference between the two circuits: *Beats per second (beps)* = $f_{C1} - f_{C2}$. In this example, the interferential beat frequency is equal to 50 beps (50 beps = 3,000 cps − 3,050 cps). The term *beat* (be) is borrowed from the acoustic literature to designate the characteristic "beat of sound" that can be heard when two acoustic waves of different frequencies interfere with each other (Hooke, 1998). The carrier frequencies of each AC circuit are programmable to deliver low amplitude-modulated beat frequency in the range of 1 to 200 beps.

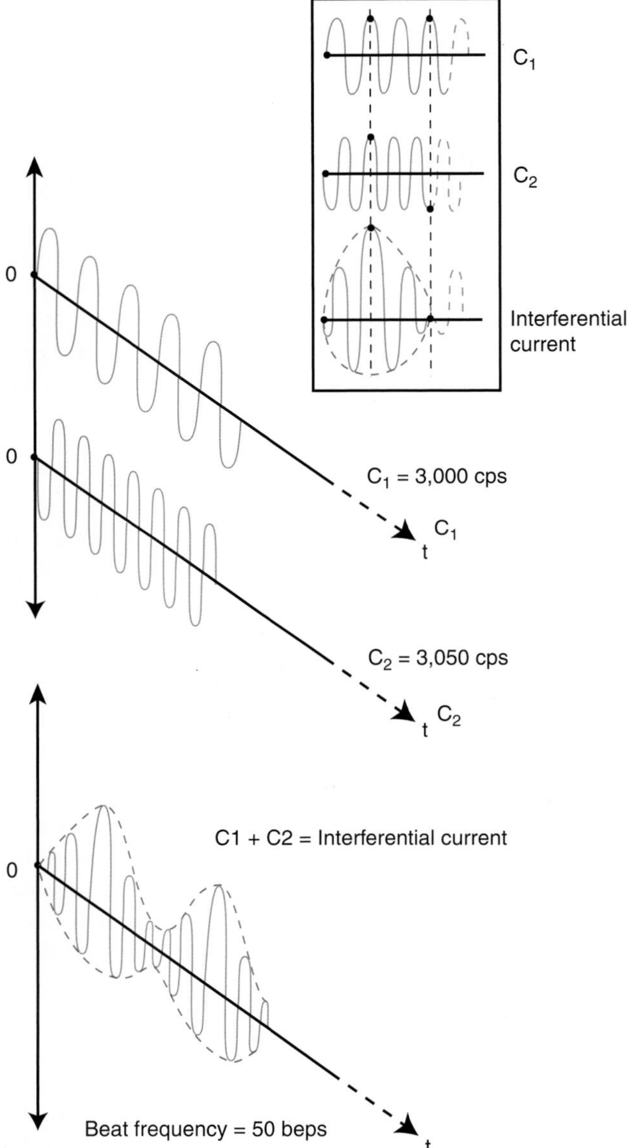

FIGURE 13-7 Bipolar, or premodulated, interferential current resulting from the interference, within the stimulator circuitry, of two medium-frequency sinusoidal currents with different frequencies leading to a beat frequency of 50 beps. Shown in the inset is the characteristic rhythmic rise and fall in the current amplitude (thus, the term *amplitude modulation*) resulting from mixing the two medium-frequency currents, creating an oval-shaped interferential current field.

2. Delivery Modes

There are four basic modes to delivery IFC to soft tissues: bipolar or premodulated, quadripolar or true interferential, quadripolar with automatic vector scan, and stereodynamic modes. Each mode has its unique biophysical characteristics, as shown next.

a. Bipolar or Premodulated Mode

This first mode is illustrated in Figure 13-7. The term *bipolar* means that this mode is delivered using two (bi) electrodes applied over the target muscle (see later discussion). The word *premodulated* means that electronic interference or modulation between the two medium-frequency sine-wave currents occurs within the electronic circuitry of the device, as opposed to within the soft tissues or muscles, as is the case with the other three modes (see later discussion). In other words, the resulting IFC is modulated before (thus, the word *pre*) being delivered to soft tissues. As shown in the figure, each bipolar or premodulated beat has an oval shape composed of several sinusoidal cycles of varying amplitudes.

b. Quadripolar or True Interferential Mode

This second mode is illustrated in Figure 13-8. It is called *quadripolar* because it is applied using four (thus, the word *quadri*) electrodes, each pair of electrodes connected to its respective circuit or channel of stimulation. This mode is also called *true interferential* because current interference occurs within the soft tissues, as opposed to the within the electronic circuitry, as was the case with the premodulated mode described earlier. The figure shows the electronic interference caused by crossing, using two pairs of electrodes or four electrodes (see circles) placed over the target muscle, one medium-frequency sinusoidal current set at 3,000 cps (C1) with another medium-frequency sinusoidal current set at 3,050 cps (C2). The interferences occurring between these two medium-frequency sine-wave currents lead to the formation of a low-frequency (50 beps) beat amplitude-modulated current. When the two medium-frequency sine-wave currents intersect at 90 degrees to each other, the maximum resultant amplitude of the IFC field is halfway between these two lines of current (in this case, at 45 degrees from each circuit). The resulting current field associated with this IFC mode is pictured as having a four-leaf clover shape.

c. Quadripolar with Automatic Vector Scan Mode

As with the previous mode, this third mode is also generated using two unmodulated medium-frequency sine-wave currents delivered using four electrodes. It differs from the true or quadripolar mode, as illustrated in Figure 13-9, by allowing current amplitude in one circuit to slowly vary between 50% and 100% of the maximum set value, with the current amplitude of the second circuit set automatically at a fixed value (e.g., 75% of its maximum amplitude). The automatic and periodic current amplitude variation in one circuit relative to the other creates an electronic phenomenon described as *vector scan*. As shown, the four-leaf clover–shaped current field, observed using the true or quadripolar mode, automatically rotates back and forth between the two lines of current, thus scanning the

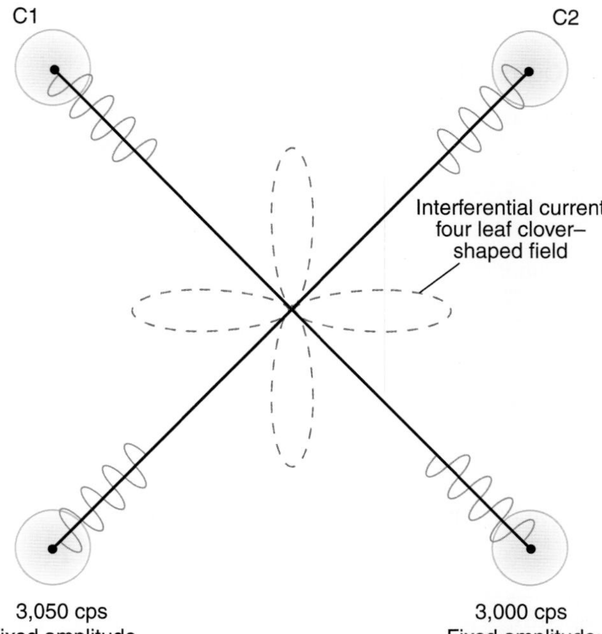

FIGURE 13-8 Quadripolar, or true, mode resulting from the interference, at the level of the targeted tissue, of two medium-frequency sinusoidal currents with different frequencies. The resulting interferential current field is pictured as having a four-leaf clover shape.

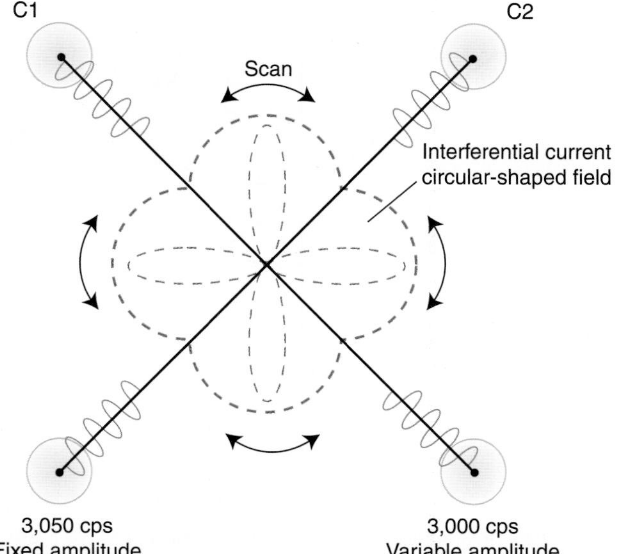

FIGURE 13-9 Quadripolar with automatic vector scan mode is identical to the quadripolar or true interferential current (IFC) except that the four-leaf clover–shaped field is now automatically rotating or scanning back and forth (see *arrows*). This vector scanning produces an enlarged field of IFC with the characteristic circular shape.

treatment surface within this area. This scanning action results in an enlarged treatment area due to the enlarged field of IFC. The purpose of using this mode over the quadripolar or true IFC mode is, therefore, to *enlarge* the stimulating treatment area. In the present example, because the carrier frequency of each circuit remains the same as with the two previous methods (3,000 and 3,050 cps), the beat frequency remains the same at 50 beps. The characteristic four-leaf clover–shaped current field seen in the true or quadripolar or true IFC mode is now pictured as having a more circular shape.

d. Stereodynamic Mode

This last delivery mode is much less common than the three already described and requires the use of a special type of IFC stimulator. This mode, illustrated in Figure 13-10, is created by adding a third (C3) medium-frequency sinusoidal current to interfere with the other two circuits. The resulting IFC mode is called *stereodynamic* because of the three-dimensional (3D) effect achieved within the targeted muscle tissues, as these three sinusoidal currents interfere with each other within the muscle. Because this mode requires simultaneous use of three circuits, six electrodes (or three pairs) are required for application. Two pairs of Y-shaped electrodes, each made of three poles, are commonly used to apply this delivery mode. The stereodynamic mode allows the effective IFC field, or stimulated area, to be enlarged three dimensionally, contrary to the quadripolar mode with automatic vector scan, which allows enlargement of the treatment field only two dimensionally. The IFC field pattern caused by mixing three medium-frequency circuits is pictured to have a six-petal flower shape.

3. Distinguishing Between IFC Modes

The four IFC delivery modes, with their respective numbers of output circuits and electrode requirements, are illustrated in Figure 13-11. The following distinguishing characteristics can be observed. First, only in the bipolar mode is the IFC premodulated. Second, only the quadripolar with vector scan mode offers a dynamic (i.e., rotating or scanning) interferential field; the other three modes offer a static field only. Third, only the stereodynamic mode offers a 3D interferential field. Readers should not confuse the terms *bipolar* and *quadripolar delivery modes* of IFC with the terms *bipolar and quadripolar electrode configurations* commonly used to apply NMES (see Application, Contraindications, and Risks).

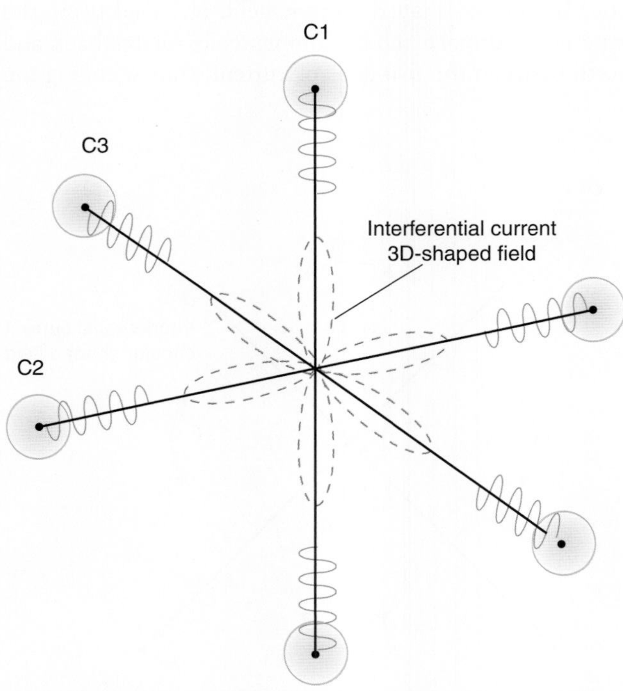

FIGURE 13-10 Stereodynamic mode refers to the interference, at the level of the targeted tissue, of three medium-frequency sinusoidal currents, leading to the characteristic three-dimentional (3D), six-petal flower–shaped field of interferential current. This method requires the use of six electrodes, which are presented as a pair of star- or Y-shaped electrodes. Each star or Y electrode has three poles or three electrodes, and each pair is connected to its respective channel.

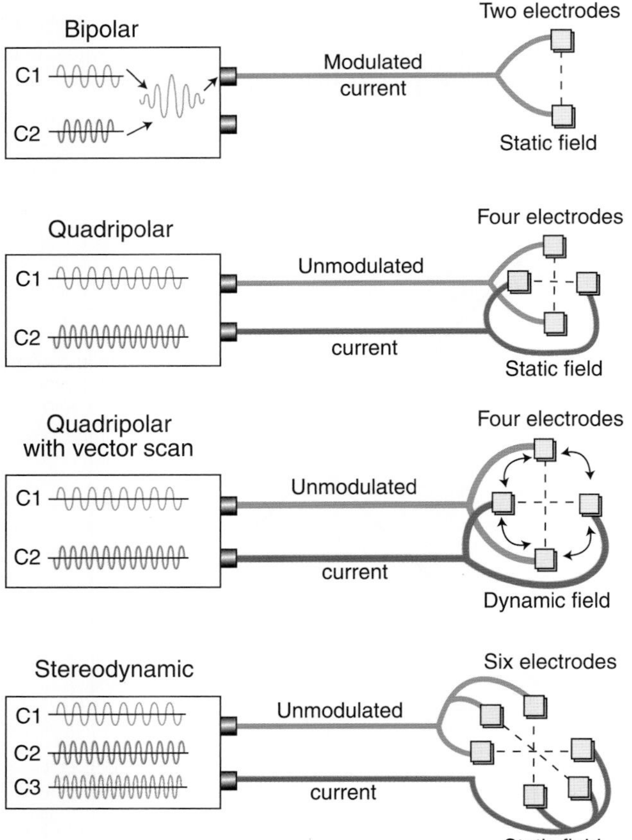

FIGURE 13-11 Interferential current delivery modes with electrode configurations.

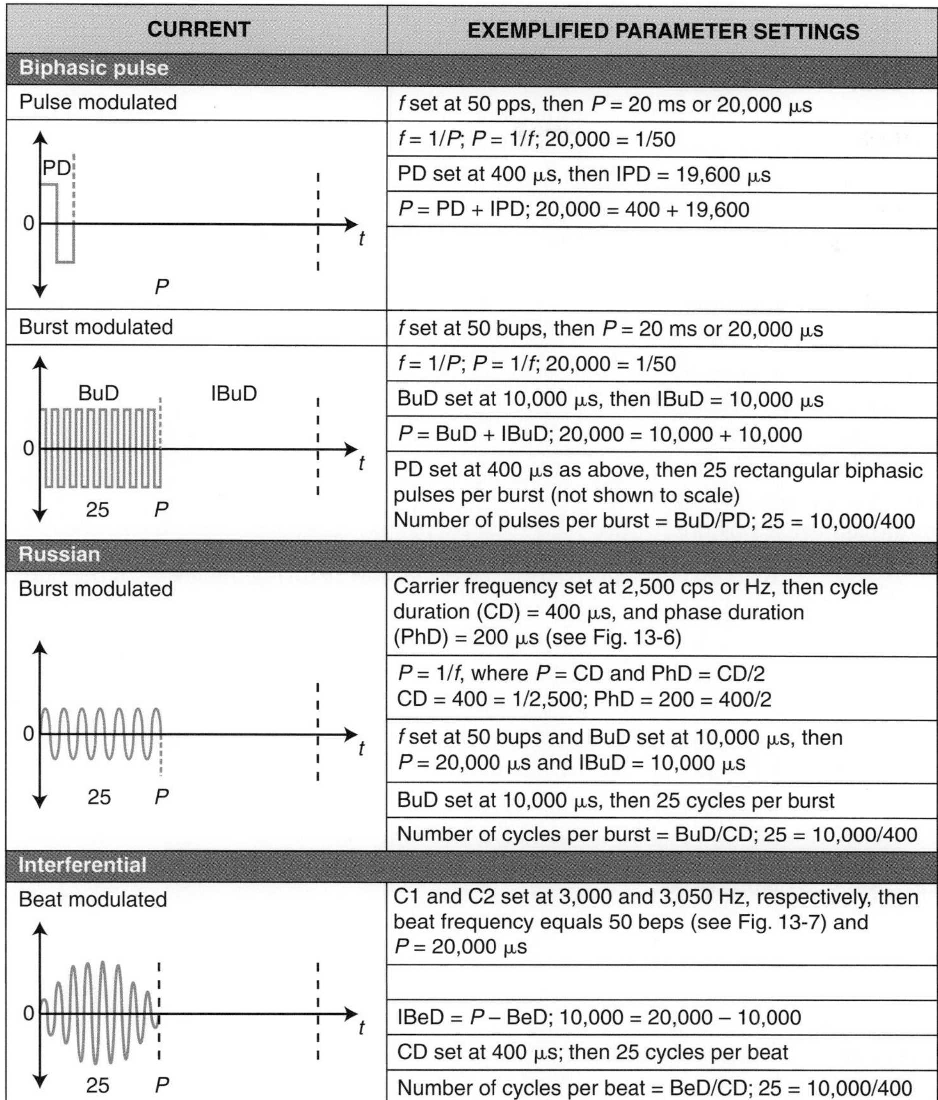

CURRENT	EXEMPLIFIED PARAMETER SETTINGS
Biphasic pulse	
Pulse modulated	*f* set at 50 pps, then *P* = 20 ms or 20,000 µs
	f = 1/*P*; *P* = 1/*f*; 20,000 = 1/50
	PD set at 400 µs, then IPD = 19,600 µs
	P = PD + IPD; 20,000 = 400 + 19,600
Burst modulated	*f* set at 50 bups, then *P* = 20 ms or 20,000 µs
	f = 1/*P*; *P* = 1/*f*; 20,000 = 1/50
	BuD set at 10,000 µs, then IBuD = 10,000 µs
	P = BuD + IBuD; 20,000 = 10,000 + 10,000
	PD set at 400 µs as above, then 25 rectangular biphasic pulses per burst (not shown to scale) Number of pulses per burst = BuD/PD; 25 = 10,000/400
Russian	
Burst modulated	Carrier frequency set at 2,500 cps or Hz, then cycle duration (CD) = 400 µs, and phase duration (PhD) = 200 µs (see Fig. 13-6)
	P = 1/*f*, where *P* = CD and PhD = CD/2 CD = 400 = 1/2,500; PhD = 200 = 400/2
	f set at 50 bups and BuD set at 10,000 µs, then *P* = 20,000 µs and IBuD = 10,000 µs
	BuD set at 10,000 µs, then 25 cycles per burst
	Number of cycles per burst = BuD/CD; 25 = 10,000/400
Interferential	
Beat modulated	C1 and C2 set at 3,000 and 3,050 Hz, respectively, then beat frequency equals 50 beps (see Fig. 13-7) and *P* = 20,000 µs
	IBeD = *P* – BeD; 10,000 = 20,000 – 10,000
	CD set at 400 µs; then 25 cycles per beat
	Number of cycles per beat = BeD/CD; 25 = 10,000/400

FIGURE 13-12 Current parameters and waveform modulation.

F. COMPARATIVE BIOPHYSICAL CHARACTERISTICS

To distinguish between biphasic pulsed, Russian, and interferential currents based on biophysical parameters such as waveform, frequency, pulse duration, interpulse duration, and period can be confusing. To appreciate the similarities and differences between these three currents, Figure 13-12 illustrates and exemplifies the characteristics of each current.

1. Biphasic Pulsed Current

Biphasic pulsed current can be *pulse modulated* or *burst modulated.* In the example for *pulse modulation,* pulse frequency (f) and pulse duration (PD) are set at 50 pulses per second (pps) or Hz and 400 µs, respectively. The current waveform is biphasic, symmetrical, balanced, and square. These settings yield a period (P) and interpulse duration (IPD) of 20,000 µs and 19,600 µs, respectively. In the example for *burst modulation,* burst frequency (bups) and burst duration (BuD) are set at 50 bups and 10,000 µs, respectively. With these settings, the period (P) remains the same at 20,000 µs, and the interburst duration (IBuD) now equates 10,000 µs. Keeping PD at 400 µs, each burst is composed of 25 rectangular biphasic pulses.

2. Russian Current

In the example presented for Russian current, the carrier frequency is set at 2,500 cps or Hz, which yields a cycle duration (CD) and phase duration (PhD) of 400 and 200 µs, respectively. Burst frequency is set at 50 bups, and burst duration (BuD) is equal to 10,000 µs. The interburst duration (IBuD) equals 10,000 µs, and each burst is composed of 25 cycles.

3. Interferential Current

In the example shown in Figure 13-12, beat frequency and beat duration (BeD) are set at 50 beps and 10,000 µs, respectively. Cycle duration (CD) thus equates 400 µs, and each beat is made of 25 cycles.

4. Overall Similarities and Differences

Figure 13-12 reveals great similarities between biphasic pulsed burst modulation, Russian burst modulation, and inferential beat modulation. Waveforms differ only in shape (square for biphasic pulsed current vs. sinusoidal for Russian and interferential currents) and current amplitude (constant for Russian current and modulated for IFC). Practically speaking, these three electrical current will deliver similar amount of electrical energy per second to the target muscle. Theoretically speaking, this means that selecting one burst-modulated current over another should makes no significant difference when comes the time to depolarize motor nerves, which will induce muscle contraction. If there were some significant differences between the capacities of these three currents to evoked muscle contraction, these should be attributed to other factors such as the ability to tolerate the discomfort or pain caused by the passage of electrical current (see later discussion).

III. THERAPEUTIC EFFECTS AND INDICATIONS

Figure 13-13 shows the proposed physiologic and therapeutic effects associated with the application of NMES. The main therapeutic effect, using all three currents, is to increase muscle strength in both patients and healthy individuals. Secondary therapeutic effects associated with the application of IFC are for pain modulation and bowel dysfunction (see later discussion).

A. MUSCLE STRENGTHENING

1. Evoked Motor Nerve Depolarization

Research has long established that nerves are excitable structures and that the passage of pulsed currents can excite or depolarize them (Robinson, 2008), thus triggering MU activation leading to evoked tetanic muscle contraction (see later discussion). Let us first consider the process of electrical nerve depolarization. Nerve fibers at rest are polarized, with the inside of their membranes being negatively charged. To *depolarize* a nerve means to reverse this polarized state, causing the inside of the nerve membrane to become positively charged. This reversal of potential across the nerve semi-permeable membrane leads to the formation of an action potential, or nerve impulse. Illustrated in Figure 13-14, and summarized next, are key physiologic events related to the process of electrically induced nerve depolarization.

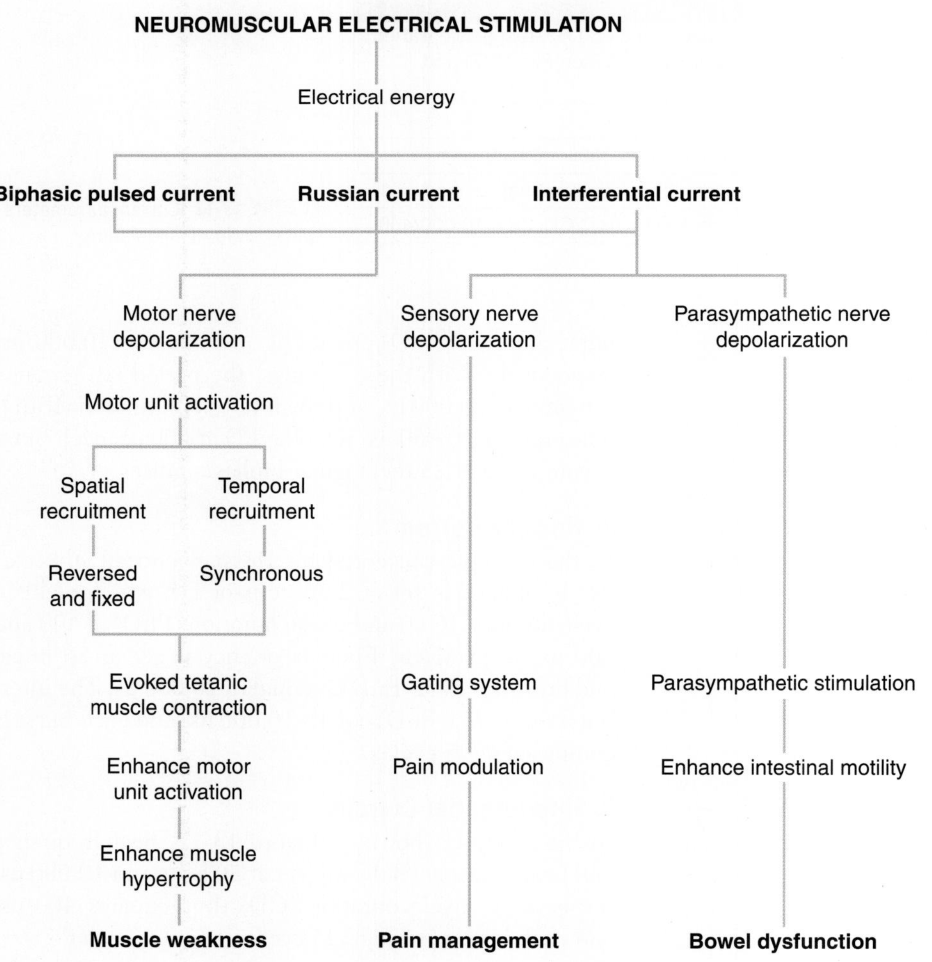

FIGURE 13-13 Proposed physiologic and therapeutic effects associated with neuromuscular electrical stimulation. *Note:* Please see text with regard to abbreviations used in the figure.

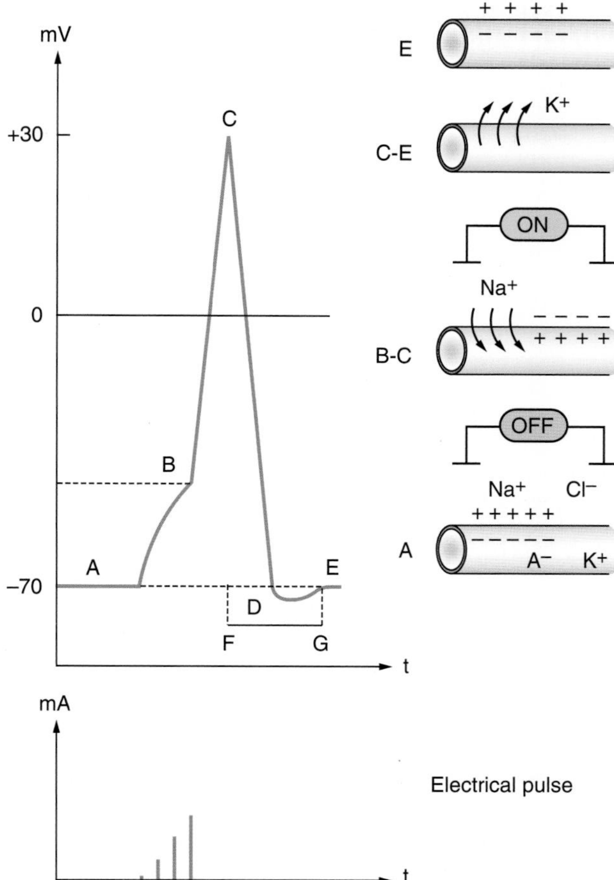

FIGURE 13-14 Electrically induced nerve depolarization. Schematized are key physiologic events leading to the production of an action potential or nerve impulse.

a. Resting Membrane Potential

At rest (stimulator OFF), excitable nerve membranes are readily permeable to potassium (K^+) ions, slightly permeable to sodium (Na^+) and chloride (Cl^-) ions, and impermeable to a number of large negatively (–) charged proteins and phosphates named *anions* (A^-). Research has shown that the flow, or gating, of Na^+ and K^+ ions in and out of the membrane is regulated by voltage-sensitive channels (Robinson, 2008; see later discussion). Because anions are trapped within the intracellular space, the inside of the nerve membrane remains negatively charged. A resting membrane potential (RMP) is thus established and measured, in humans, at approximately −70 mV.

b. Electrical Stimulation Threshold

What will happen to the nerve RMP if a pulsed electrical current of gradually increasing amplitudes is applied, as is the case with NMES? As illustrated in Figure 13-14, the gradual increase of current amplitude will decrease the RMP, passing from approximately −70 to −30 mV (A to B). When the nerve membrane potential finally reaches a critical voltage level (B), a cascade of events (B to E) triggers the process of nerve depolarization (B to C), which leads to the formation of an action potential or nerve impulse (B to E). This critical voltage level corresponds to the nerve membrane *threshold* of activation (B).

c. Depolarization

The process of depolarization (B to C) is caused by the rapid and massive opening of voltage-gated Na^+ channels, resulting in the reversal of potential inside the nerve membrane. In other words, the massive influx of positively charged sodium ions makes the inside of the nerve membrane more positive. This depolarization phase coincides with the beginning of the action potential (B to C).

d. Repolarization or Hyperpolarization

After being depolarized, the nerve membrane quickly repolarizes itself (C to D). This process begins with the complete closure of the voltage-gated Na^+ channels (C) and manifests itself by the rapid and massive opening of the voltage-gated potassium (K^+) channels. In other words, the massive efflux of positively charged potassium ions makes the inside of the nerve membranes more negative, until its RMP is once again restored (from C to D). During this repolarization phase, the nerve membrane is slightly hyperpolarized (D to E) for a very short period of time because the potassium channels stay open a bit too long in the process. The RMP is then quickly restored by the Na^+–K^+ ATPase pumps (E). The process of *depolarization–repolarization* is self-perpetuating, triggering a chain reaction of action potential along the nerve fiber. The influx of Na^+ depolarizes the axon and the outflow of K^+ repolarizes it (see Fig. 13-14).

e. Action Potential/Nerve Impulse Propagation

The passage of a pulse current through a nerve membrane results in the creation of an action potential (B to D), also called *nerve impulse.* Such nerve impulses propagate, or travel, along the nerves carrying neural information from organs to the central nervous system (CNS) or from the CNS to the organs. When the threshold for stimulation (B) is reached, an action potential of a fixed size will always be generated. In other words, there is no big- or small-amplitude action potential—all action potentials, for a given nerve, are of the same size. We have, therefore, two possibilities—either the nerve threshold for depolarization is not achieved (no action potential generated—*none*) or the threshold is achieved (full action potential generated—*all*). This all-or-none situation underlies the *all-or-none principle.* Thus, there is no such thing as a fraction of action potential generated—the potential is either full or none. This also means that increasing the electrical pulse amplitude (subthreshold to supramaximal levels) will not induce larger-size action potentials.

f. Nerve Refractory Period

Nerve fibers require a certain period to recover before they can be depolarized again. There is a short period of time, named the *refractory period* and illustrated in Figure 13-14 (F to G), during which the nerve fiber will

TABLE 13-1 VOLITIONAL VERSUS ELECTRICALLY EVOKED MUSCLE CONTRACTION

Contraction	Volitional	Electrically Evoked
Motor command	Upper motoneurons	Electrical stimulator
Spatial recruitment	Dispersed Smaller to larger MUs	Restricted Larger to smaller MUs
Temporal recruitment	Asynchronous	Synchronous
Onset of muscle fatigue	Slow	Rapid
Muscle force development	Optimal	Suboptimal
Muscle-strengthening mechanisms	*Neurotrophic* *Neural:* Enhanced MU recruitment *Trophic:* Enhanced muscle hypertrophy	

MUs, motor units.

be refractory to the delivery (incapable of being depolarized) of another subthreshold electrical pulse. Within this refractory period, which lasts less than 1 ms, there is an *absolute* period, during which it is impossible to depolarize the nerve, and a *relative* period, during which an action potential can be generated if one applies an electrical pulse having a greater amplitude. The refractory period limits the pulse frequency that practitioners can choose to depolarize peripheral nerve fibers.

2. Evoked Motor Unit Activation

There are fundamental differences, as shown in Table 13-1, between the neurophysiologic mechanisms at work during volitional versus electrically evoked muscle contraction. Skeletal muscle contraction, whether voluntary or electrically evoked, results from the activation, or recruitment, of motor units (MUs).

a. Spatial Recruitment

The term *spatial recruitment* refers to the number and order of MUs recruited during the process of muscle contraction. *Number* refers to the amount, or percentage, of MUs activated within a given muscle or muscle group. *Order* relates to the sequence of activation based on the size of each MU. A muscle may contain hundreds to thousands of MUs depending of its size and function. Research has established that a skeletal muscle is made of a mosaic of three types of MUs. The first type is the slow-twitch (S) unit made of slow-twitch oxidative (SO) fibers, which are very resistant to fatigue. The second type is the fast-twitch/fatigue-resistant (FR) unit made of fast-twitch, oxidative-glycolytic (FOG) muscle fibers. The third type relates to the fast-twitch/fatigable (FF) units made of fast-twitch glycolytic (FG) muscle fibers. FG and FOG muscle units contract faster and generate more force than SO units. In some textbooks, SO units are classified as type I units, whereas FF and FR units are classified as type IIB and type IIA units, respectively.

b. Temporal Recruitment

The term *temporal recruitment* refers to the rate of discharge, or frequency, with which MUs are recruited during the process of muscle contraction. Temporal recruitment is also referred to, in the literature, as rate coding.

c. Motor Unit Recruitment During Volitional Muscle Contraction

During a voluntary effort, the command for muscle contraction originates in the upper motoneurons (volition), which is then transmitted down to the spinal motoneurons. The number of MUs activated is proportional to the magnitude of the voluntary command, and MU activation is dispersed within the muscle. MUs are spatially recruited according to their size—that is, from the smaller (SO) to the larger (FG, FR) units. This is known as the size principle of MU activation (Henneman et al., 1965). Temporal recruitment is asynchronous, or random, meaning that a given MU may be activated several times per second, whereas another MU may be activated only a few times per second, or not at all, during a particular volitional muscle contraction.

d. Motor Unit Recruitment During Electrically Evoked Muscle Contraction

During an electrically evoked muscle contraction, the command for muscle contraction is given by the electrical stimulator, which is programmed to deliver electrical pulses of given amplitudes and frequencies, resulting in motor nerve depolarization. In such a case, the entire motoneuron pool (upper and lower) is bypassed, meaning that muscle contraction results from the local depolarization of motor nerves buried in the muscle. In contrast to the volitional process described earlier, spatial recruitment is restricted to the units that are closer to the electrodes and occurs in the reversed size order—that is, from the larger (FF, FG) to the smaller (SO) units (Delitto et al., 1990; Sinacore et al., 1990; Trimble et al., 1991). This order reversal is explained by the fact that the large-diameter motor axons of FF and FR units are more easily excited by imposed electrical current than are the small-diameter axons of the SO units (Maffiuletti et al., 2011). Also demonstrated is the fact that temporal recruitment is *synchronous*—that is, at a fixed frequency, which corresponds to the frequency setting on the electrical stimulator. In summary, electrical current passes through soft tissues and depolarizes motor nerve fibers, causing nerve impulses to reach neuromuscular junctions initiating muscle contractions. Spatial MU recruitment occurs in a reverse size order (from the larger to the smaller units), and temporal recruitment is synchronous (fixed frequency) in nature.

e. Physiologic Impact of Restricted and Reverse Order Spatial Motor Unit Recruitment

The fact that spatial MU recruitment is restricted and occurs in a reversed order during NMES implies that the same large fatigable MUs—that is, those FOG and FF units closest to the surface electrodes—are repeatedly activated by the same amount of electrical current that, over time, will hasten the onset of muscle fatigue (Maffiuletti et al., 2011). It is well established in the literature that muscle fatigue represents a major limitation to the use of NMES. What can the practitioner do to minimize muscle fatigue during NMES? From one therapeutic session to the next, the practitioner can (1) vary current amplitude, (2) modify electrode configuration and/or electrode placement, and (3) modify muscle length.

f. Physiologic Impact of Synchronous Temporal Recruitment

The temporal synchronous recruitment associated with NMES implies that these same more superficial and large MUs are firing at the same frequency during electrical stimulation. It is well established that SO units have a much lower tetanic fusion frequency (20 to 30 Hz) than FG and FF units (50 to 70 Hz) because their twitch contraction times are longer. This means that setting the stimulator's frequency at 40 Hz, for example, will be optimal for the temporal recruitment of SO units but less than optimal for the larger units. This will result in a suboptimal evoked muscle contraction because the greater force generating fast units (FOG and FF) will fire at their suboptimal frequency. One way to minimize this synchronous effect is to vary the current frequency from one therapeutic session to the next.

3. Evoked Muscle Contraction

The repeated delivery of pulses, bursts, or beats of current cause repeated motor nerve depolarization, triggering a series of muscle twitches that will combine to form an evoked smooth fused tetanic muscle contraction similar to that of maximal voluntary contraction. Neuromuscular research has shown that full tetanic muscle contraction of human skeletal muscles occurs at a fusion frequency of about 50 Hz (i.e., 50 pps; 50 bups; 50 beps). Some muscles may fuse at a higher frequency (i.e., 60 to 80 Hz) if their MU content is primarily made of FF and FR units, and some at lower frequency (i.e., 30 to 40 Hz) if their MU content is primarily made of SO MUs.

4. Claims Behind Interferential and Russian Currents

Several important claims have been made over the past decades with regard to the physiologic effects of these two electrical currents on soft tissues. Let us review these claims and look at the evidence behind them.

a. Interferential Current

Hans Nemec (1959) made remarkable claims related to his newly discovered IFC. He *first* claimed that crossing and superimposing two medium-frequency alternating sine-wave currents of different frequencies will cause the two currents to *interfere* with each other, producing an interferential or low-frequency beat amplitude-modulated current. His *second* claim was that IFC generated by crossing sine-wave currents with medium carrier frequencies (i.e., between 3,000 and 5,000 Hz) will *decrease skin impedance,* leading to deeper tissue stimulation with less current amplitude, thus making it more comfortable than the other currents.

i. Interferential Effect: Supported

There is biophysical evidence to support Nemec's claim that superimposing two medium-frequency alternating sine-wave currents, each with different medium frequency, will interfere with each other causing output interference, resulting in a newly formed amplitude-modulated frequency, or beat, IFC (see Fig. 13-8).

ii. Decreased Skin Impedance: Supported

There is also biophysical evidence to support the claim that the application of IFC, resulting from the interaction of medium-frequency sinusoidal alternating current (2,000 to 5,000 Hz) can decrease skin impedance because it lowers its capacitive reactance component. To assess this claim, brief considerations must be given to the concepts of impedance and capacitive reactance. Biophysicists see biologic tissues, such as the skin, as being made of a mix of resistors (R), capacitors (C), and inductors (L). *Impedance,* designated by the letter Z and measured in ohms (Ω), is defined as the total opposition offered by these three sources, namely, resistance (R), capacitive reactance (X_C), and inductive reactance (X_L), to the passage of an electrical current. The equation denoting capacitive reactance is as follows: $X_C = 1/2\pi fC$, where $\pi = 3.14$, f = current frequency, and

C = skin capacitance, measured in farads. This formula thus indicates that the higher the current carrier frequency, as is the case with IFC (2,000 to 5,000 Hz), the lower the capacitive reactance, thus the lower the skin impedance.

iii. Decreased Skin Impedance: Misleading

To claim that interferential current is the *only* current capable of decreasing skin impedance is misleading. As discussed earlier, impedance is inversely related to frequency ($Z = 1/f$), and frequency is inversely related to the period ($f = 1/T$). By substitution, it turns out that impedance (Z) is *proportional* to the period (*P*). Stated differently, the shorter the period, the lower the skin impedance. In pulsed currents, the period equals pulse duration plus interpulse duration. On the basis of $T = 1/f$, the period (T) of present IFC (2,000 to 5,000 Hz) will range between 500 and 200 μs. Theoretically speaking, it follows than any pulsed current (such as biphasic pulsed and Russian) having a period (T) ranging between 200 and 500 μs is also capable of reducing skin impedance. In summary, IFC does not reduce skin impedance and does not penetrate deeper than other pulsed currents having similar frequency or period.

b. Russian Current

Kots made three revolutionary claims, never before heard in the field of NMES, when he introduced the Russian current to the clinical and research communities (Kots, 1971, 1977; Belanger 1992; Ward et al., 2002). His *first* claim was that his Russian current, unlike all the other known neuromuscular stimulating currents, is *painless,* causing no sensory discomfort during maximal evoked muscle tetanic contraction. Because it is painless, Kots postulated that higher current amplitude can be delivered to soft tissues so that the deeper motor nerve fibers, which are associated with those larger high-force, fast-twitch MUs (FF, FR), can be depolarized, thus increasing the magnitude of the electrically evoked tetanic contraction. Kots's *second* claim was that his Russian current, delivered at a higher current amplitude (because it is painless) than all the other stimulating currents, could generate up to *30% more force* than that generated during the course of an MVC. He postulated that during a maximal voluntary effort, a percentage of those large FF MUs (FG muscle fibers) are not recruited. There is a substantial body of scientific evidence to support this postulate (Belanger et al., 1981; Rutherford et al., 1986; Dowling et al., 1994; Behm et al., 1996). Kots further theorized that applying his painless and deeply penetrating current would compensate for this lack of voluntary MU activation by activating, or depolarizing, those inactive large MUs, thus generating more muscle force. Kots's *third* and last claim was that a few weeks of muscle training using his Russian current can produce *lasting muscle strength gains* in healthy people.

i. Painless Current: Refuted

There is very strong evidence to refute the painless nature of Russian current (Curwin et al., 1980; Laughman et al., 1983; Owens et al., 1983; Currier et al., 1984; Boutelle et al., 1985; Selkowitz, 1985; Delitto et al., 1986a,b; Kubiak et al., 1987; Ferguson et al., 1989; Grimby et al., 1989; Snyder-Mackler et al., 1989; Brooks et al., 1990; Underwood et al., 1990; Franklin et al., 1991; Laufer et al., 2001; Delitto et al., 1992; Hartsell et al., 1992; Rooney et al., 1992). In fact, all subjects enrolled in the mentioned studies reported various levels of sensory discomfort and pain when subjected to Russian current stimulation. No studies could be found to support this claim.

ii. Greater Force: Refuted

Only one study (Selkowitz, 1985) supports Kots's claim that Russian current can evoke greater muscular force than that generated following a maximal voluntary effort. All of the following studies refute this claim (Owens et al., 1983; Noel et al., 1987; Snyder-Mackler et al., 1989; Laufer et al., 2001; Hartsell et al., 1992).

iii. Lasting Force Gains: Supported

There is evidence to support Kots's claim that that the gains of muscle force following Russian current are lasting, as is the case with voluntary muscle training (Currier et al., 1983Laughman et al., 1983; Selkowitz, 1985; Kubiak et al., 1987; Soo et al., 1988). Only one study refutes this claim (St-Pierre et al., 1986).

5. Muscle-Strengthening Mechanisms

Research has shown that repeated muscle contractions, whether voluntarily or electrically evoked, done against resistive external loads induces neurotrophic muscle adaptation (Maffiuletti, 2010; Gondin et al., 2011; Hortobagyi et al., 2011). In strenuous strength-training regimens using biphasic pulsed, Russian, or interferential currents, skeletal muscles get larger and stronger from the hypertrophy, or enlargement, of their muscle fibers, not from the addition of new muscle fibers (hyperplasia). In other words, muscle strengthening following NMES results from the interaction between a *neural* (improved MU recruitment and firing) and a *trophic* (hypertrophy) mechanism (Table 13-2). The patient's or subject's ability to improve MU activation and to enlarge muscle fibers through voluntary or electrically evoked training will determine the extent of muscle strengthening achieved.

6. Quadriceps Versus Pelvic Floor Muscle Strengthening

The evidence from the scientific literature shows that the use of biphasic pulsed and Russian currents has been primarily for the strengthening of lower muscles, primarily the quadriceps muscle, whereas that of IFC has been almost exclusively reserved for pelvic floor muscles

TABLE 13-2 RECOMMENDED DOSIMETRIC PARAMETERS FOR MUSCLE STRENGTHENING

Parameter	Biphasic Pulsed Current	Russian Current	Interferential Current
Carrier frequency	NA	2,000–5,000 Hz	
Pulse duration	100–600 μs	NA	
Burst/beat duration	5–10 ms		
Pulse/burst/beat frequency	30–60 Hz		
Current amplitude*	As high as tolerable—high enough to evoke muscle force equivalent to 40%–70% of maximum voluntary contraction (% MVC)		
ON time**	5–10 s		
OFF time**	5–50 s		
Ramp up time	0.5–2 s		
Ramp down time	0.5–2 s		
Treatment frequency	3 training sessions per week for 4–6 wk		
Acclimatization period	To optimize the application of NMES, subjects and patients need to accommodate to the delivery of electrical current. Training intensities (current amplitude and number of training sessions) should be increased step by step.		

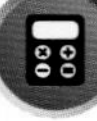

Use the Online Dosage Calculator: Neuromuscular Electrical Stimulation.

NA, not applicable; MVC, maximum voluntary contraction; NMES, neuromuscular electrical stimulation.
*Can be expressed in milliamperes or as percentage of MVC. Usually expressed as peak amplitude (A_{pk}) for biphasic current. Usually expressed as root mean square (rms) amplitude (A_{rms}) for Russian and interferential current. $A_{rms} = 0.707 \times A_{pk}$; $A_{pk} = 1.414 \times A_{rms}$.
**ON time includes ramp up and down times, plus plateau time. Setting the ON time and OFF time automatically sets off the ON:OFF time ratio and duty cycle.

(Oh-oka, 2010; see Research-Based Indications box). Why is this so? The fact that most clinical studies using NMES have focused on the quadriceps muscle, as opposed to other muscle groups, is due to the influence of Kots's work, which focused on this muscle group. It can also be attributed to the fact that knee injuries are very common and that quadriceps strengthening is key to optimal rehabilitation in such cases. That IFC is used primarily for pelvic floor muscle weakness, mostly for cases of incontinence is explained by the fact that these muscles are located deeper in the pelvis and thus require a more penetrating current field for effective NMES. The delivery of IFC, using the quadripolar mode, provides such a penetrating current field that can be focused on these muscles. Moreover, using vacuum IFC with suction electrodes greatly facilitates electrode attachment in this particular body area (perineum). Another option for pelvic floor muscle stimulation is to use any currents with either intravaginal or intrarectal electrodes (see Application, Contraindications, and Risks box for details).

B. INTESTINAL MOTILITY

Aside for muscle weakness, there is limited evidence to suggest that IFC may effective for the treatment of bowel dysfunctions (see Research-Based Indications box). In 1987, Emmerson and colleagues reported diarrhea as a side effect of using IFC for urinary incontinence caused by overactive bladder (Emmerson, 1987). This observation led some clinicians and researchers to theorize that if IFC can induce diarrhea, this electrical current may be beneficial for the treatment of bowel dysfunction such as slow transit constipation (see Chase et al., 2005). They postulated that the deeply penetrating IFC is likely to stimulated vagal sympathetic and parasympathetic outflow to the intestine, thus facilitating bowel movement by increasing intestinal motility leading to defecation (see Fig. 13-13). To provoke this physiologic effect, the electrode configuration is such that current interference occurs, or is focused, at the intestinal level (see Application, Contraindications, and Risks box).

C. PAIN MODULATION

Survey research has demonstrated that IFC is often used clinically for the management of pain (see Beatti et al., 2010; Fuentes et al., 2010). It is postulated that sensory and motor nerve depolarization resulting from the passage of IFC could modulate pain, as is the case for transcutaneous electrical nerve stimulation (see Chapter 14), through various mechanisms, including the gate and opiate systems (see Fig. 13-13). Listed in the Research-Based Indications are human studies, on the effectiveness of IFC on pain.

1. Experimental Pain

Experimental or induced pain significantly differs from clinical or real pain because the former is lacking the all-important affective (cognitive and emotional) component of pain. Caution is advised, therefore, before inferring the effectiveness of IFC based on experimental pain findings. The body of evidence on the effectiveness of IFC for human experimental pain is conflicting, with approximately half of the studies showing no benefit (Stephenson et al., 1995; Johnson et al., 1997, 2003b; Johnson et al., 1999; Minder et al., 2002; Cheing et al., 2003; Johnson et al., 2003a,c; Stephenson et al., 2003; McManus et al., 2006; Shanahan et al., 2006; Fuentes et al., 2010; Fuentes et al., 2011). No clear conclusion, therefore, can be drawn on the effectiveness of IFC on experimental pain (see Beatti et al., 2010).

2. Clinical Pain

Conversely, there is substantial evidence to support the use of IFC for the management of human clinical pain (see Research-Based Indications box). Fuentes and colleagues' (2010) recent meta-analysis on this subject suggests that IFC, when applied concomitantly with other therapeutic interventions, is more effective than when applied alone.

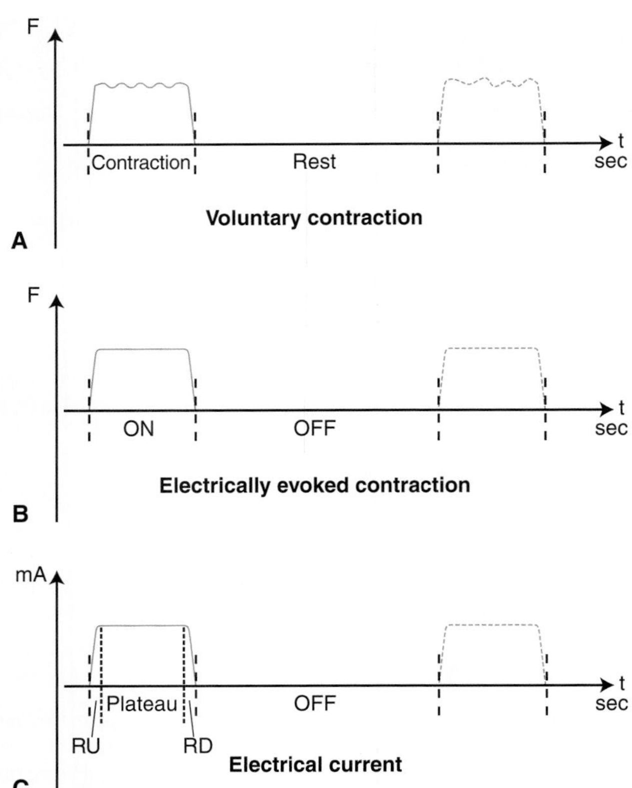

FIGURE 13-15 Interrelationship between maximum voluntary contraction (**A**), maximum electrically evoked contraction (**B**), and current amplitude (**C**). Time modulation of electrical current allows the evoked muscle contraction to mimic voluntary contraction. ON time includes ramp up (RU) and ramp down (RD) times, as well as plateau time.

D. RESEARCH-BASED INDICATIONS

The search for evidence behind the use of NMES, displayed in the *Research-Based Indications* box, led to the collection of 102 English peer-reviewed human clinical studies. The methodologies and criteria used to assess the strength of evidence and therapeutic effectiveness are described in Chapter 2. As indicated, the strength of evidence behind NMES is ranked as *moderate* for quadriceps muscle weakness in both healthy individuals and patients. There is also *moderate* evidence, primarily using IFC, for pelvic floor muscle strengthening, bowel dysfunction, and pain. Over all conditions treated using NMES, the strength of evidence is found to be *moderate* and its therapeutic effectiveness *substantiated.*

IV. DOSIMETRY

The main application of NMES is for muscle strengthening in patients suffering from disuse atrophy and in healthy individuals wanting to improve their muscle strength. The objective is to program the stimulator such as to generate an evoked muscle contraction, which resembles, or mimics, as closely as possible that generated during volitional effort. Figure 13-15 illustrates this concept. During voluntary muscle strengthening (see Fig. 13-15A), patients perform a bout or series of muscle contractions, often under isometric condition, lasting a few seconds (3 to 6 s), with each contraction interrupted by a rest period equivalent to a multiple of contraction time (one to eight times longer). A voluntary muscle contraction is a smooth contraction characterized by a short gradual rise and fall of force at the beginning and end of contraction, respectively. For an electrically evoked muscle contraction to mimic such a smooth contraction (see Fig. 13-15B), several parameters need to be set on the electrical stimulator (see Fig. 13-15C). Let us consider each of them.

A. ELECTRICAL PARAMETERS

Practitioners, using any given type of electrical stimulator for NMES, need to set various electrical parameters prior to therapy. Those key parameters are illustrated and exemplified in Figure 13-12 and listed in Table 13-2. Common settings are carrier frequency (for Russian and interferential currents), pulse duration (for biphasic pulse current), pulse/burst/beat duration, pulse/burst/beat frequency, and current amplitude.

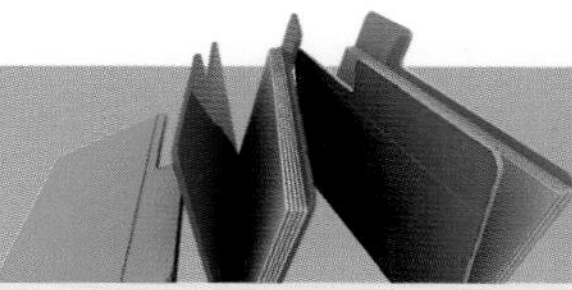

Research-Based Indications

NEUROMUSCULAR ELECTRICAL STIMULATION

	Benefit—Yes		Benefit—No	
Health Condition	**Rating**	**Reference**	**Rating**	**Reference**
Muscle weakness in healthy untrained and trained individuals	I	Laughman et al., 1983		
	I	Parker et al., 2003		
	I	Bircan et al., 2002		
	I	Gondin et al., 1995		
	I	Herrero et al., 2010a		
	I	Herrero et al., 2010b		
	I	Owens et al., 1983		
	I	Boutelle et al., 1985		
	I	Kubiak et al., 1987		
	I	Fahey et al., 1985		
	II	Caggiano et al., 1994		
	II	Halback et al., 1980		
	II	Hartsell, 1986		
	II	Lai et al., 1988		
	II	Nobbs et al., 1986		
	II	Eriksson et al., 1981		
	II	Cabric et al., 1987		
	II	Romero et al., 1982		
	II	Currier et al., 1983		
	II	St-Pierre et al., 1986		
	II	Fahey et al., 1985		
	II	McMiken et al., 1983		
	II	Parker et al., 2005		
	II	Laufer et al., 2001		
	II	Hortobagyi et al., 1992		
	II	Pfeifer et al., 1997		
	II	Selkowitz, 1985		
	II	Soo et al., 1988		
	II	Underwood et al., 1990		
	II	Ruther et al., 1995		
	III	Delitto et al., 1989		

Strength of evidence: Moderate
Therapeutic effectiveness: Substantiated

	Benefit—Yes		Benefit—No	
Health Condition	**Rating**	**Reference**	**Rating**	**Reference**
Muscle weakness following postoperative knee reconstruction	I	Jarit et al., 2003	II	Sisk et al., 1987
	II	Lieber et al., 1996		
	II	Wigerstad-Lossing et al., 1988	II	Paternostro-Sluga et al., 1999
	II	Fitzgerald et al., 2003		
	II	Delitto et al, 1988b		
	II	Feil et al., 2011		
	II	Anderson et al., 1989		
	II	Draper et al., 1991		
	II	Snyder-Mackler et al., 1995		
	II	Snyder-Mackler et al., 1994		
	II	Snyder-Mackler et al., 1991		
	II	Williams et al., 1986		
	II	Curwin et al., 1980		
	II	Avramidis et al., 2003		
	II	Martin et al., 1991		
	III	Petterson et al., 2006		
	III	Stevens et al., 2004		
	III	Lewek et al., 2001		
	III	Mintken et al., 2007		
	III	Delitto et al., 1988a		
	III	Eriksson et al., 1979		

Strength of evidence: Moderate
Therapeutic effectiveness: Substantiated

Health Condition	Rating	Reference	Rating	Reference
Pelvic floor muscle weakness following incontinence	I	Laycock et al., 1993	III	Sylvester et al., 1987
	I	Kajbafzadeh et al., 2009		
	I	Vahtera et al., 1997		
	II	Oh-oka, 2008		
	II	Dougall, 1985		
	II	McQuire, 1975		

Health Condition	Benefit—Yes Rating	Benefit—Yes Reference	Benefit—No Rating	Benefit—No Reference
	II	Demirturk et al., 2008		
	II	Switzer et al., 1988		
	II	Laycock et al., 1988		
	II	Dumoulin et al., 1995a		
	II	Dumoulin et al., 1995b		
	II	Olah et al., 1990		
	II	Wilson et al., 1987		
	II	Turkan et al., 2005		
	II	Van Poppel et al., 1985		
	III	Henella et al., 1987		
Strength of evidence: Moderate **Therapeutic effectiveness:** Substantiated				
Bowel dysfunction	I	Clarke et al., 2009a		
	I	Clarke et al., 2009b		
	I	Koklu et al., 2010		
	I	Kajbafzadeh et al., 2011		
	III	Chase et al., 2005		
Strength of evidence: Strong **Therapeutic effectiveness:** Substantiated				
Painful conditions	I	Gundog et al., 2011	I	Man et al., 2007
	I	Adedoyin et al., 2002	I	Van der Heijden et al., 1999
	I	Hurley et al., 2001	I	Taylor et al., 1987
			II	Gaines et al., 2004
	I	Defrin et al., 2005	II	Quirk et al., 1985
	I	Cheing et al., 2008	II	Werners et al., 1999
	I	Zambito et al., 2007		
	I	Zambito et al., 2006		
	II	Shafshak et al., 1991		
	II	Callaghan et al., 2001		
	II	Hurley et al., 2001		
	II	Ni Chiosig et al., 1994		
	II	Burch et al., 2008		
	II	Philipp et al., 2000		
	II	Tugay et al., 2007		
	III	Walker et al., 2006		
	III	Nitz et al., 1987		
Strength of evidence: Strong **Therapeutic effectiveness:** Substantiated				
Fewer Than 5 Studies				
Muscle weakness following chronic heart failure	I	Nuhr et al., 2004		
	I	Quittan et al., 2001		
	II	Dobsak et al., 2006		
	II	Harris et al., 2003		
Strength of evidence: Pending **Therapeutic effectiveness:** Pending				
ALL CONDITIONS **Strength of evidence:** Moderate **Therapeutic effectiveness:** Substantiated				

1. Pulse/Burst/Beat Frequency

Why is the concept of frequency very important in the field of NMES? Because the physiologic correlate of *frequency* is *temporal MU activation.* In other words, to set the pulse/burst/beat frequency is to set the frequency at which all the activated MUs will fire during the evoked muscle contraction. As shown in Figure 13-13, pulsed biphasic current may be delivered as pulses (pulse frequency) or bursts of pulses (burst frequency), Russian current as bursts of sinusoidal cycles (burst frequency), and IFC as beats of sinusoidal cycles (beps). Setting the frequency between 30 and 60 pps/bups/beps is necessary to obtain optimal temporal MU activation during the fused tetanic muscle contraction, because research has established that the mean fusion frequency for skeletal muscles is approximately 50 pps/bups/beps.

2. Current Amplitude

Why is setting current amplitude so critical in the field of NMES? Because the physiologic correlate of *current amplitude* is *spatial MU activation.* The higher the current amplitude used, the greater the number of motor units activated, and the larger the evoked muscle contraction output of force. A common procedure to set current amplitude is as follows. First, measure the force generated by the target muscle group during an MVC under isometric conditions (100% MVC). Second, increase current amplitude as high as tolerable or high enough to obtain an evoked muscle contraction force equivalent to 40% to 70% of that obtained under a maximal voluntary effort (MVC). Subsequently, express the level of each electrically evoked contraction as a percentage of the MVC force (% MVC). This important parameter provides an indication of the intensity of the NMES training (see Selkowitz, 1985; Stevens et al., 2004; Maffiuletti, 2010). The higher the current amplitude, the higher the effectiveness of NMES for muscle strengthening in both healthy individuals and patients (see Maffiuletti, 2010).

3. Constant Current Stimulator

Stimulators used for NMES are *constant current–type* (CC-type) stimulators, meaning that a set current amplitude (say, 80 mA read on the digital meter) remains constant (hence, the term *constant current*) during treatment, regardless of changes in tissue impedance over time. According to Ohm's law, defined by the formula $V = R \times I$ or $V = Z \times A$ (see below), to maintain current amplitude (I or A) constant during treatment, voltage (V) needs to be automatically adjusted to account for the fluctuation of soft-tissue impedance (R or Z) over time. Ohm's law can thus be rewritten as follows: $V = Z \times A$, where the letter *R* (resistance) is replaced by the letter Z (impedance), and where the letter *I* (intensity) is substituted for the letter *A* (amplitude). The main advantage of CC-type stimulators is that they deliver predictable levels of electrical stimulation, making therapy more predictable and comfortable for the patient (no surge of current).

B. ON:OFF TIME RATIO

Now that the electrical parameters mentioned earlier are set. Which other parameters need to be set? As shown in Figure 13-15C, practitioners need to set the ON and OFF times. The *ON time* is the time, measured in seconds, during which electrical current is delivered to the target muscle. Its duration corresponds to the duration of the volitional muscle contraction. Conversely, the *OFF time* is the time, also measured in seconds, during which there is no current flowing in the target muscle. Its duration corresponds to the duration of the rest period between two successive contractions. The relationship between ON time and OFF time is commonly expressed as a ratio. For example, setting a 5-second ON time and a 30-second OFF time would produce a ON:OFF time ratio of 10s:30s. Such a ratio means that the resting time between two successive evoked contractions is three times longer than that of contraction time (1:3). The term *ON:OFF time ratio* is not synonymous with *duty cycle*, as discussed later.

C. RAMP UP AND DOWN TIMES

As shown in Figure 13-15A, the time course of a volitional contraction begin with a gradual upward ramping, from the beginning to the plateau phase of contraction, followed by a similar smooth downward ramping at the end of contraction. This physiologic ramping effect is part of the full muscle contraction time or ON time. To mimic this ramping volitional effect during NMES (see Fig. 13-15B), practitioners need to adjust the stimulator's ramp up and down times accordingly. Note that the ON time *includes* the ramp up and down times, as well as the time during which the contraction is maintained relatively constant (plateau time). Setting ramp up and down times within the ON time *mimic* as closely as possible the gradual build up and relaxation phases seen at the beginning and the end of a voluntary muscle contraction, as shown in Figure 13-15C. Ramp up and down times are usually set between 0.5 and 2 seconds to prevent the sudden, or jerky, rise and fall of evoked muscle contractions, thus making its time course as smooth as possible (see Table 13-2).

D. DUTY CYCLE

Setting the ON:OFF time ratio automatically sets up the duty cycle, which is defined as the ratio of ON time to the combined ON and OFF times, expressed as a percentage, using the following formula: Duty cycle = [ON/(ON + OFF)] × 100. For example, an ON:OFF time ratio of 10s:50s sets up a duty cycle of 16.7% (16.7% = [10 s/(10 s + 50 s)] × 100). A duty cycle of 16.7% means that muscle contraction occurs during an amount of time (10 s) that is 16.7% of the elapsed time (60 s; 10 s + 50 s) between two successive electrically evoked muscle contractions. To document or chart only the duty cycle value *without* the corresponding ON:OFF time ratio is misleading because ON:OFF time ratios of 5 s:20 s and 10 s:40 s, for example, would yield exactly the same 20% duty cycle value but different ON and OFF times. Both the duty cycle and its corresponding ON:OFF time ratio must therefore be charted in the patient's file. To recap, an ON:OFF time ratio of 10s:50s means that the resting time between two successive evoked contractions is five times that of contraction time. The corresponding 16.7% duty cycle, on the other hand, implies that muscle contraction occurred during 16.7% of the time during two successive evoked contractions.

E. ONLINE DOSAGE CALCULATOR: NEUROMUSCULAR ELECTRICAL STIMULATION

As presented earlier, to set up the multiple dosimetric parameters related to the application of NMES requires the use of several formulas and implies multiple calculations. To facilitate dosimetry, this textbook offers the **Online Dosage Calculator: Neuromuscular Electrical Stimulation**. Log on, select the type of current, enter parameters, and let the calculator do the work for you!

V. APPLICATION, CONTRAINDICATIONS, AND RISKS

Prior to considering the application of NMES, practitioners must first check for contraindications, consider the risks, and then go through key application steps and procedures designed to optimize treatment safety, efficacy, and effectiveness. As discussed next, several important elements need to be taken into consideration to achieve optimal application.

A. SKIN PREPARATION

Adequate skin preparation prior to NMES is critical because in order to depolarize motor nerve fibers, electrical current must first flow through the skin. The skin provides the greatest opposition, resistance, or impedance to current flow because the epidermis contains very little fluid. Dry skin offers a much greater opposition than wet skin. Dry skin resistance may be in the mega ohm range (MΩ), whereas wet skin may in the kilo ohm range (KΩ). Cleansing the skin surface areas over which stimulation electrodes are placed with rubbing alcohol, or with a mixture of water and soap, will remove impurities (i.e., dirt, dry cells, and sebum) and significantly decrease skin resistance, thus facilitating current flow to the target muscles. Never apply stimulation electrodes without first cleansing the skin surface.

B. ELECTRODES AND CABLES

The delivery of electrical energy to the neuromuscular apparatus is done by using a variety of surface electrodes. *Electrodes* are the means by which the electron flow from the stimulator is converted to an ionic current flow in soft tissues. A minimum of two electrodes are required to direct the stimulator current to the target tissues, thus completing the electrical circuit. The most commonly used electrodes are made of flexible and reusable carbonized rubber and mesh flexible materials. They come in various shapes and sizes. Electrical connection is made between the stimulator output jacks and the stimulation electrodes using via lead wires or cables. *Bipolar cables* are used to connect pairs of electrodes to the stimulator output channels. Multiple electrodes can be connected to a single channel using *bifurcated cables*. The rationale for using bifurcated cables—that is, to connect more than two electrodes per channel—is to enlarge the stimulation area per channel. As was the case for the skin (see earlier discussion), electrodes and cables also offer opposition of resistance to current flow. Over time and repeated use, electrode material deteriorates and causes electrode resistance to increase, thus making electrical stimulation less effective. It is recommend to *discard* reusable stimulation electrodes after 6 months of use. Repeated use can also damage cables, causing a break in electrical continuity. Periodic checks of electrode resistance and cable electrical continuity, using a basic multimeter device, is strongly recommended to ensure optimal electrical stimulation.

C. ELECTRODE COUPLING

For a stimulation electrode to function properly, it must be coupled to the skin both electrically and mechanically. Electrical coupling is achieved by the application of an electrolytic gel between the electrode and the skin surface. In the past, water-soaked gauzes, sponges, or pads were used. Today, improved water-soluble electroconductive gels are commonly used. To ensure optimal electroconduction at the electrode–skin interface, all electrodes must be mechanically attached to the skin. Most surface electrodes are mechanically attached to the skin using regular hypoallergic tape, or pre-cut adhesive patches. Good skin surface attachment is necessary to ensure that the entire electrode stimulating surface area is in contact with the skin surface to avoid unintentional variations of current density in one region of the skin during the application.

D. ELECTRODE CURRENT DENSITY

Current density (CD) is the ratio of maximum current amplitude (A) to electrode stimulating surface area (S), expressed in milliamperes per square centimeter (mA/cm^2) and calculated as follows: $CD = A/S$. Research shows that the higher the current density under the electrode, the more discomfort or pain the patient feels beneath that electrode. Because current density under a given electrode often dictates whether the application is more or less comfortable, using larger sizes electrodes is recommended, especially when the current amplitude used to evoke muscle contraction is relatively high. Note that using larger stimulating electrodes may have the disadvantage of stimulating undesired muscles or muscle groups located in the immediate vicinity of the targeted muscle area. Note that a small electrode will focus the current over a small area, whereas a larger electrode will disperse it over a larger area.

E. ELECTRODE SPACING

Spacing between pairs of electrodes influences current dispersion within the tissues, which in turn affects the current's penetration depth. Generally speaking, the wider the spacing between electrodes, the more dispersed the current and the deeper the current penetration into the tissue. In contrast, the closer the spacing between electrodes, the less dispersed the current and the more superficial the stimulating effect.

F. ELECTRODE CONFIGURATION

Four electrode configurations are routinely used in the field of NMES: monopolar, bipolar, quadripolar, and multipolar. These configurations, each illustrated in Figure 13-16, are based on clinical situations in which one stimulator, with

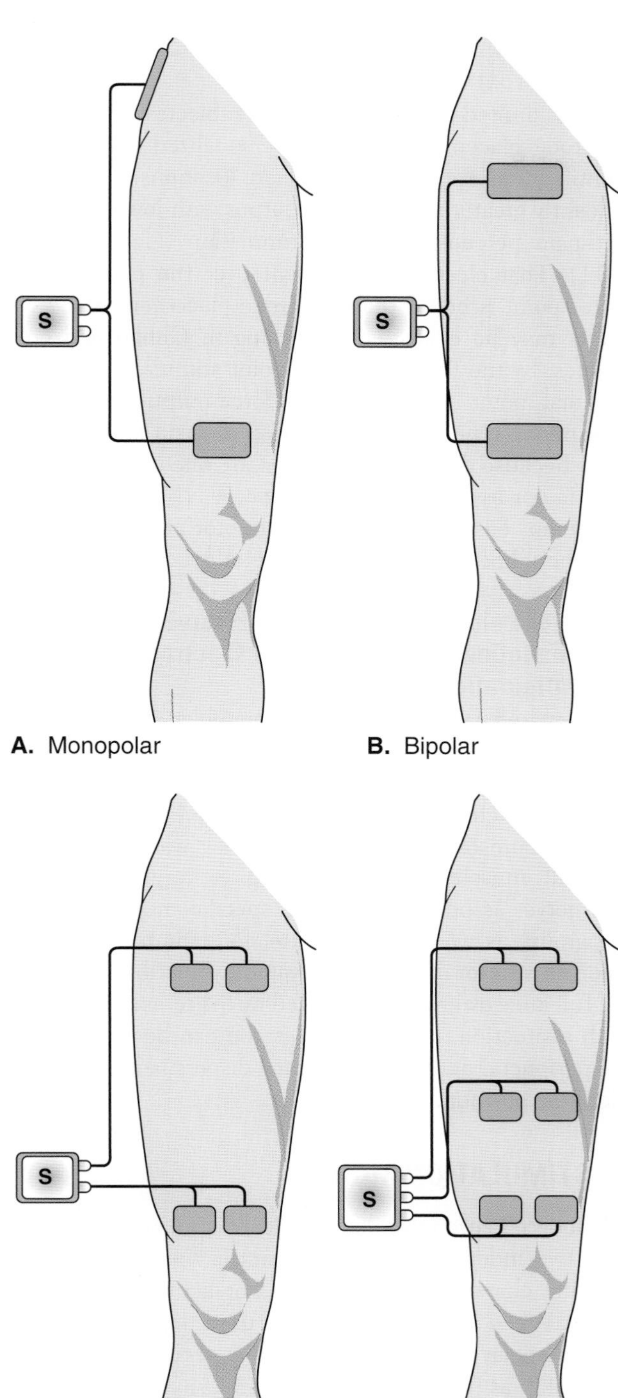

FIGURE 13-16 Monopolar (**A**), bipolar (**B**), quadripolar (**C**), and multipolar (**D**) electrode configurations.

two or three output channels, is used. Recall that each electrode has a pole; hence, the term *polar.*

1. Monopolar

One (mono-) electrode is placed *over* the targeted muscle contractile area with the other positioned at some distance away from the targeted muscle or muscle group. In the example illustrated in Figure 13-16A, one electrode is placed over the targeted quadriceps area with the other positioned away from the targeted area, over the upper lateral hip area.

2. Bipolar

Two (bi-) electrodes are placed *over* the targeted muscle area. Figure 13-16B shows a pair of electrodes positioned over the targeted quadriceps muscle area.

3. Quadripolar

Four (quadri-) electrodes are placed *over* the targeted muscle area. Figure 13-16C shows two pairs of electrodes positioned over the targeted quadriceps muscle area. Note that this method can also be applied via one channel only if a bifurcated cable is used.

4. Multipolar

In this configuration, *more than four* (multi-) electrodes are placed over the targeted muscle contractile area. In Figure 13-16D, six electrodes are positioned over the quadriceps contractile area by using a multichannel stimulator, to which three pairs of electrodes are connected with three pairs of bipolar cables. Note that this electrode placement method can also be applied using a bi-channel stimulator with two pairs of three electrodes, with each pair connected to the stimulator using a bifurcated cable. Figure 13-17 shows the application of the newer all-in-one garment-type NMES unit for quadriceps, which allows multipolar electrode configuration.

G. ELECTRODE PLACEMENT

When placing an electrode over the target muscle, practitioners should always consider placing it over the muscle's motor points. Why? Because the goal of NMES is to optimize the evoked muscle force output while minimizing discomfort during electrical stimulation. There is a consensus in the literature that one of the major factors limiting the clinical use of NMES is the pain, or discomfort, associated with the delivery of electrical current into

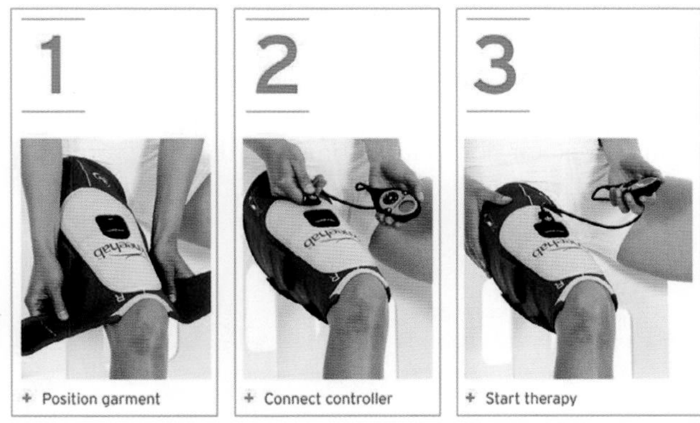

FIGURE 13-17 Application of all-in-one quadriceps garment neuromuscular electrical stimulation unit allowing multipolar electrode configuration. Courtesy of Neurotech Bio-Medical Research Ltd.

the soft tissues. By placing the stimulating electrodes over motor points as opposed to elsewhere over the muscle, less current amplitude is used to generate maximum muscle force output, thus making NMES more comfortable and effective.

1. Muscle Motor Point

Anatomically speaking, a *motor point* is defined as the surface entry point of a bundle of motor nerve fibers into a fascicle of muscle fibers. Electrophysiologically speaking, this motor point is defined as a specific skin area where the targeted muscle is best stimulated with the smallest amount of current amplitude. Research has shown that some human muscles may have more than one motor point. How can practitioners identify or locate motor points prior to NMES? They can refer to charts, published in textbooks and corporate brochures, illustrating motor point standard locations, which often quite markedly differ from each other (e.g., see Prentice, 2011; Botter et al., 2011; Gobbo et al., 2011; Starkey, 2013). Practitioners also can use the following motor point identification technique, recently described by Botter et al. (2011) and Gobbo et al. (2011), to perform individual or personalized motor point localization.

2. Motor Point Identification Technique

To identify motor points using the following technique requires less than 10 minutes and needs to be done only once—that is, prior to using NMES. First, set the electrical parameter as follows—waveform: rectangular pulsed biphasic; pulse duration: 0.15 ms; pulse frequency: 2 Hz. Second, use the monopolar electrode configuration—that is, one small-diameter stimulation pen electrode, such as the one shown in Figure 13-18, with one larger reference electrode placed over the antagonist muscle. Third, place the pen electrode somewhere over the targeted muscle area. Slowly increase the current amplitude while manually scanning the skin surface with the pen electrode, until a clear muscle contraction is visualized. Stop scanning and begin to slowly decrease current amplitude until the muscle contraction becomes barely visible. Mark this electrode position, which corresponds to a motor point, with a skin-marking pen. Continue scanning the targeted muscle surface area until another similar muscle contraction is identified, and mark it. Scan the entire targeted muscle area. Note that some muscles may have more than one motor point. Place the surface electrodes over those identified motor points for optimal NMES.

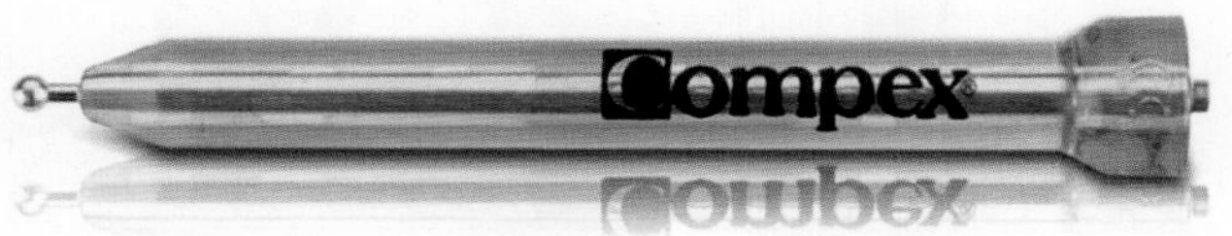

FIGURE 13-18 Motor pen electrode. (Courtesy of DJO Global.)

3. Personalized Motor Point Versus Motor Point from Charts

There is limited evidence in human subjects to show than electrode placement based on personalized motor point identification, rather than on chart locations, elicits significantly greater muscle force output with lower discomfort–pain perception during stimulation (Gobbo et al., 2011). That electrode placement over the personalized motor point is better than electrode placement based on charts may be explained, according to Gobbo and colleagues, by the fact that motor point stimulation triggers maximal motor nerve activation (force output) associated with minimal nerve sensory activation (pain and discomfort). Because discomfort and pain are one the major limiting factor associated with the use of NMES, electrode placement based on personalized motor point identification should be given strong consideration.

4. Motor Point Versus Peripheral Nerve Stimulation Using Monopolar Electrode Configuration

As discussed earlier, the classic monopolar electrode configuration is defined as one electrode (active) placed over the targeted muscle belly with the other electrode (dispersive or indifferent) placed elsewhere (see Fig. 13-16A). In some circumstances, practitioners may want to activate the full muscle group belonging to a given peripheral nerve, as opposed to some specific muscles within the group, as would be the case, for example, with the ankle dorsiflexor muscles innervated by the tibial nerve, or the full knee extensors innervated by the femoral nerve. In such a situation, the active electrode can be placed over the peripheral nerve while keeping dispersive electrode at the same position.

H. STIMULATION MODES

All modern neuromuscular electrical stimulators feature at least two independent channels and a *time-delay switch,* allowing channels to be triggered or activated independently. When such a stimulator is used, manually setting the time-delay switch (D for delay) between channel 1 and channel 2, as illustrated in Figure 13-19, allows practitioners to choose between the following three stimulation modes: synchronous, reciprocal, and overlapping.

1. Synchronous

The synchronous mode is illustrated in Figure 13-19A. It is achieved by setting D at 0 s, with the ON and OFF times of channel 1 equal to the ON and OFF times of channel 2 (e.g., D = 0 s; channel 1: ON = 5 s, OFF 15 s; channel 2: ON = 5 s, OFF = 15 s). Both channels are thus *synchronously* activated (ON) and deactivated (OFF) for the full duration of application. Practically speaking, this mode allows synchronous stimulation of two different muscle groups or two muscle parts within a muscle group.

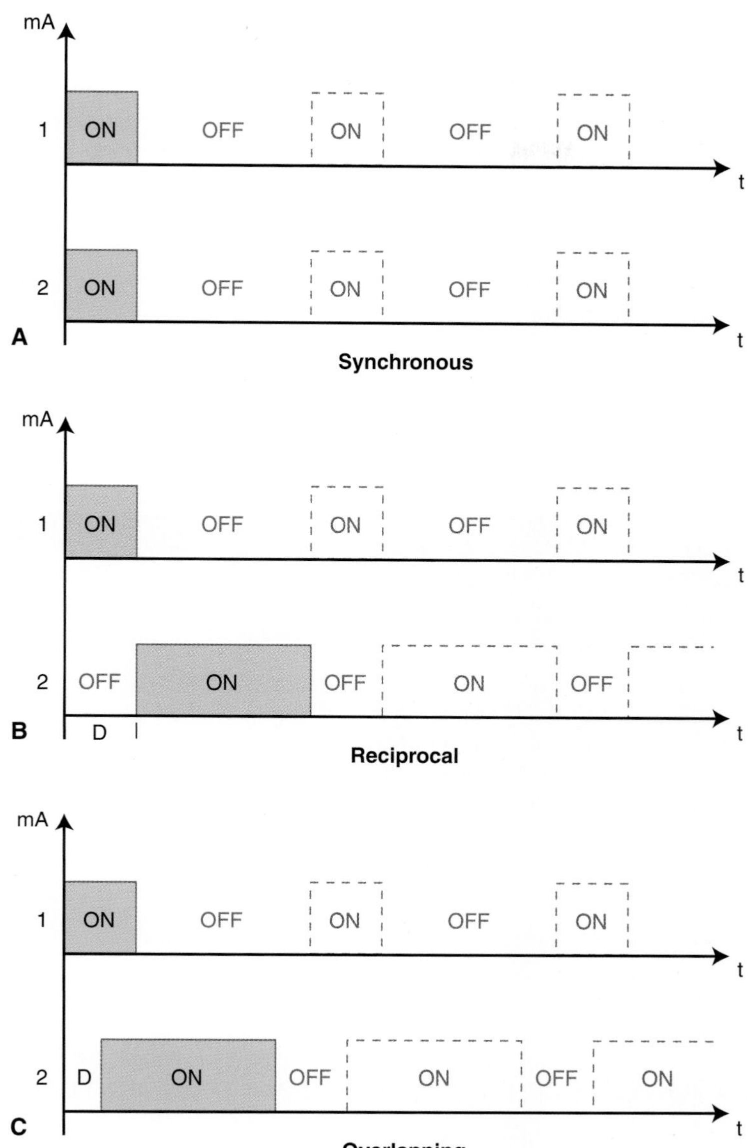

FIGURE 13-19 Synchronous (**A**), reciprocal (**B**), and overlapping (**C**) stimulation modes.

2. Reciprocal

The reciprocal mode, shown in Figure 13-19B, is achieved by setting the D value equivalent to the ON time of channel 1, while setting the ON time of channel 1 equal to the OFF time of channel 2 (e.g., D = 5 s; channel 1: ON = 5 s, OFF = 15 s; channel 2: ON = 15 s, OFF = 5 s). This setting results in a *reciprocal* activation of both channels for the full treatment duration. Clinically speaking, it allows reciprocal, or alternating, stimulation of two different muscles or muscle groups, such as the agonist versus the antagonist.

3. Overlapping

The overlapping mode, illustrated in Figure 13-19C, is achieved by setting the D value greater than 0 s but less than the ON time of channel 1, while keeping the ON and OFF times of both channels identical (e.g., D = 3 s; channel 1: ON = 5 s, OFF = 15 s; channel 2: ON = 5 s, OFF = 15 s). Both channels now *overlap,* as channel 2 is activated 3 seconds after channel 1, for the full duration of the treatment session. Clinically speaking, this mode allows overlapping, or concomitant, stimulation of two different muscles or muscle groups.

I. TRAINING METHODS

There are two methods to deliver NMES: NMES and NMES plus volition. *NMES* implies that that muscle contraction results solely from the electrical energy delivered to the target muscle. Conversely, *NMES plus volition* means that NMES is applied over a voluntarily contracting muscle or muscle group. In other words, this method consists of *superimposing* the electrical current on the patient's voluntary muscle contraction. The resulting muscle contraction reflects the combined effect of both the electrical energy delivered to the muscle and the volitional energy generated by the brain. The body of evidence presented in this chapter reveals that neither method is better than the other in enhancing muscle strength. If the goal is to educate patients about how to contract their muscles, then the NMES plus volition is the preferred method to use.

J. TRAINING PROTOCOL

Of all dosimetric parameters related to the practice of Russian current therapy, the training protocol originally described by Kots (1971, 1977) has received most attention in the literature. This protocol is known as the *10c/10s/50s protocol*. It stands for 10 electrically evoked contractions (c) per bout, with each contraction lasting 10 seconds and interrupted by a rest period of 50 seconds. In other words, this protocol calls for a series of 10 contractions with an ON:OFF time ratio of 10s:50s. Based on series of experiments on Russian athletes, Kots reported (1971, 1977) that this 10c/10s/50s protocol was the best protocol for achieving maximum strength gain without inducing significant muscle fatigue during training. Most investigators have faithfully applied this Russian protocol in their studies to either support or refute Kots's claims, and to determine the therapeutic effectiveness of Russian current therapy. It is important to set an adequate period of muscle inactivation or relaxation (OFF time) between successive evoked contractions (ON time) to prevent muscle fatigue. Practitioners may vary this ratio during the course of a strength-training program to accommodate muscle fatigability. The more fatigable the muscle, the shorter the ON time and/or the longer the OFF time.

APPLICATION, CONTRAINDICATIONS, AND RISKS

Neuromuscular Electrical Stimulation

IMPORTANT: There is a risk of electronic interference between neuromuscular electrical stimulation (NMES) units and rate-responsive pacemakers or implantable cardioverter-defibrillators (ICDs) (Crevenna et al., 2003, 2004). NMES units can be used with these patients *only if*, after cardiac monitoring during treatment, the electrocardiographic recording reveals no interference. **If no such cardiac monitoring is available in your working facility, obtain authorization from the patient's treating cardiologist before using NMES.** Note that NMES units can be used with patients wearing rate-responsive pacemakers or ICDs *only* if the ICD unit is *turned OFF* during therapy (Glotzer, 1998).

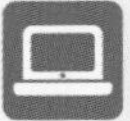

See **online video** for more details.

STEP	RATIONALE AND PROCEDURE
1. Check for contraindications.	*Over anterior cervical area*—stimulation of key organs, such as the vagus nerve, phrenic nerve, and carotid sinuses, results in adverse effects, such as hypotensive reaction and laryngeal spasm *Over thoracic area*—affects normal heart function *Over cranial area*—affects brain function *With patients wearing rate-responsive pacemakers or ICDs*—electronic interference with units (for more details, see Chapter 14). Note that NMES can be used with these patients *only* if the ICD unit is *turned OFF* during therapy. *Over abdominal, pelvic, or lumbar areas with women in their first trimester of pregnancy*—induces labor *Over metal implants*—causes unnecessary pain due to electrical current–induced overheating of implants *In patients with epilepsy*—causes epileptic episode *Over hemorrhagic area*—enhances bleeding due to increased blood flow in the treated area *Over cancerous area*—increases and spreads the tumor due to increased blood flow in the treated area *In patients who are confused and unreliable*—complications during therapy that decrease treatment effectiveness *Over damaged skin*—causes unnecessary and severe pain

STEP	RATIONALE AND PROCEDURE
2. Consider the risks.	*Contact dermatitis and burn*—prolonged use of electrode, electroconductive gel, and adhesive tape over the same skin areas increase the risk of contact dermatitis. Change electrode positions over time. *Stimulator electronic interference*—keep all NMES units at least 3 m (10 ft) away from any functioning shortwave device *Temporary bruising*—the use of a vacuum electrode over fragile skin increases the risk due to the suction force (negative pressure) exerted on such fragile skin *Adverse effects such as fainting, nausea, skin rashes, increased swelling, and pain*—these risks were greater with IFC than with other common electrophysical agents, such as transcutaneous electrical nerve stimulation (TENS) and ultrasound (Partridge et al., 1999). Stimulation of the autonomic system may account for some of these adverse effects. *Muscle damage*—repeated mechanical stress imposed on the same motor units during electrical stimulation (specificity of stimulation) over time may cause muscle damage (Nosaka et al., 2011; Jubeau et al., 2012)
For Muscle Strengthening	
3. Position and instruct patient.	Ensure comfortable body positioning. Instruct not to touch the device, cables, and electrodes and to call for assistance if necessary.
4. Prepare treatment area.	Clean the skin surface in the area of the stimulating electrode with rubbing alcohol to remove impurities and sebum, thus reducing skin impedance. Clip hair to ensure optimal electrode–skin coupling.
5. Select stimulator type.	Choose between a cabinet line-powered or portable battery-operated device (see Fig. 13-1). There is evidence to suggest that portable battery-powered stimulators are as good as cabinet line-powered stimulators to deliver therapeutic NMES. Newer, battery-operated garment-base stimulators, designed for quadriceps muscle strengthening, can also be used (Fig. 13-1E). Plug line-powered stimulators into ground-fault circuit interrupter (GFCI) receptacles to prevent the risk of macroshock leading to electrocution (see Chapter 5).
6. Select current type.	Choose between biphasic pulsed, Russian, and interferential currents.
7. Select electrode type.	Use conventional plate electrodes (see Fig. 13-2A,B). Current density is the ratio of maximum current amplitude to electrode stimulating surface area (mA/cm^2). Research shows that the higher the current density under the electrode, the more discomfort or pain the patient feels beneath that electrode. Larger electrode size is recommended, especially when the current amplitude used to evoke the muscle contraction is relatively high.
8. Prepare stimulating electrode.	Cover surface with a thin and evenly distributed coating of electroconductive gel to optimize conduction at the electrode–skin interface. Note that some electrodes may be pre-gelled.
9. Proceed with electrode configuration and placement.	*Configuration:* Select between the monopolar, bipolar, quadripolar, and multipolar configurations. *Placement:* Localize motor points using electrical stimulation technique or charts. Place electrodes over motor point(s). Note that the distance between a pair of electrodes influences current dispersion within the tissues, which in turn affects the current's penetration depth. The wider the inter-electrode distance, the deeper the current penetration into the tissue. In contrast, the closer the two electrodes, the more superficial the stimulating effect. Positioning electrodes over motor points may decrease discomfort/pain perception during electrical stimulation as well as increase muscle force production (Gobbo et al., 2011). Use a pen electrode to locate motor points (see Fig. 13-18).
10. Attach and connect electrodes.	Attach electrodes to the skin using hypoallergic tape or pre-cut self-adhesive patches. Connect electrodes to the stimulator circuit output using regular or bifurcated lead wires. Optimal skin surface attachment is necessary to ensure that the entire electrode stimulating surface area is in contact with the skin surface to avoid unintentional variations of current density in one region of the skin during the application.

STEP	RATIONALE
11. Select stimulation mode.	Modern electrical stimulators feature at least two independent channels and a time-delay switch, allowing both channels to be triggered or activated independently. When such a stimulator is used, manually setting the time delay between the two channels allows synchronous, reciprocal, or overlapping stimulation modes (see Fig. 13-19). Select the *synchronous mode* when the synchronous or concomitant stimulation of two different muscle groups, or two muscle parts, within a muscle group, is needed. Select the *reciprocal mode* if reciprocal, or alternating, stimulation of two different muscles or muscle groups, such as the agonist versus the antagonist, is required. Select the *overlapping mode* if overlapping stimulation of two different muscles or muscle groups is needed.
12. Select stimulation method.	Choose between *NMES* and *NMES plus volition.*
13. Set dosimetry. 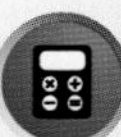	Set pulse/burst/beat duration, frequency, current amplitude, ON time, OFF time, ON:OFF ratio, duty cycle, and ramp up and down times (see Table 13-2 as a guideline). Increase current amplitude with patients who are overweight or obese because more current is needed to reach muscle motor points or motor nerve fibers (Miller et al., 2008). **Use the Online Dosage Calculator: Neuromuscular Electrical Stimulation.**
14. Determine training protocol.	The most common training protocol used to strengthen skeletal muscle, originally introduced by Kots is *10c/10s/50s,* which means 10 consecutive electrically evoked contractions, each lasting 10 seconds (ON time) and separated by a resting interval of 50 seconds (OFF time). Adapt this protocol to the case under treatment. Determine the number of training bouts per training session.
15. Apply treatment.	Ensure adequate monitoring. If home treatment, make sure that the patient is using a battery-operated stimulator and give a written sheet of directives to follow with regard to the overall application.
16. Conduct post-treatment inspection.	Remove the electrodes. Inspect the skin area exposed to the electrodes for any unexpected response. Wash and dry the treated surface areas. In the patient's file, document any unusual sensation that the patient felt during treatment. Wash and dry reusable electrodes.
17. Ensure post-treatment equipment maintenance.	Follow manufacturer recommendations. Immediately report any defects or malfunctions to technical maintenance staff. Routine use of common electrodes requires that clinicians adopt a strict maintenance program, including frequent visual inspection and periodic measurements using a basic multimeter device. Wash and dry reusable electrodes after each treatment to ensure optimal efficacy. Check cables and electrodes regularly for visible wear and tear to ensure optimal efficacy and prevent macroshock, if line-powered stimulators are used. Check electrode impedance monthly to ensure optimal electric conduction, because electrodes will deteriorate with use and time. Use an ohmmeter to check impedance. Discard all reusable electrodes after 6 months of use. Because transmission of microorganisms is likely if suction electrodes and sponges are used, these should be disinfected with 70% isopropyl alcohol after treatment of each patient to avoid cross-infection from one patient to another (Lambert et al., 2000).

For Pelvic Floor Muscle Strengthening

Contrary to most skeletal muscles (see earlier discussion), NMES of pelvic floor muscles is difficult because they lie deep under the genital organs. It is suggested that the preferred method to stimulate these muscles is to use vacuum interferential stimulator with suction cup electrodes (see Fig. 13-1D). The quadripolar, or true interferential mode, with or without scan, is often recommended. Place wet sponges in the cups, and moisten the edge for better adherence. Position the four suction electrodes to focus the resulting clover-shaped current field over the pelvic floor muscle area. Adjust the vacuum pressure level to ensure adequate fixation on the body.

For Gut Stimulation

It is suggested that the preferred method to stimulate the gut or intestinal area is to use an interferential stimulator with either plate or suction electrodes. The quadripolar, or true mode, with or without scan, is recommended because of its penetrating and focused electrical field. Position the four suction electrodes to focus the resulting clover-shaped current field over the gut area. Position the electrodes such that maximum current inference triggers parasympathetic stimulation.

CASE STUDIES

Presented are two case studies summarizing the concepts, principles, and applications of NMES discussed in this chapter. Case Study 13-1 addresses the use of NMES for quadriceps weakness following ACL reconstruction. Case Study 13-2 is concerned with the application of NMES for genuine stress incontinence. Each case is structured in line with the concepts of evidence-based practice (EBP), the International Classification of Functioning, Disability, and Health (ICF) disablement model, and SOAP (*s*ubjective, *o*bjective, *a*ssessment, *p*lan) note format (see Chapter 2 for details).

CASE STUDY 13-1: QUADRICEPS WEAKNESS AFTER ACL RECONSTRUCTION

EVIDENCE-BASED CLINICAL DECISION MAKING PROTOCOL

1. Formulate the Case History

A 26-year-old man is referred by his treating orthopedic surgeon for lasting problems related to decreased quadriceps muscle strength and function following right anterior cruciate ligament (ACL) knee reconstruction, done 12 weeks ago, following a ski accident. At discharge from the hospital, the patient was given a full home voluntary quadriceps muscle-strengthening program. Questioned about his compliance with the program over the past 8 weeks, the patient readily admits very poor compliance, thinking that doing his regular daily activities will be enough to regain full knee extension strength. The patient's chief complaints are right quadriceps muscle weakness and atrophy, combined with difficulty squatting, climbing stairs, and running. He is also frustrated with not being able to ski. Physical examination of the injured knee shows no sign of inflammation and complete range of motion. Measurements reveal a quadriceps force deficit of 40% and a thigh girth deficit of 1.5 cm on the affected side. The patient's goal is to rebuild the bulk and strength in his right quadriceps so that he can ski safely and effectively once again. He is now well motivated, realizing that just doing his daily activities will not restore full knee strength and function. To compensate for his lack of motivation and training, you propose NMES therapy.

2. Outline the Case Based on the ICF Framework

QUADRICEPS WEAKNESS AFTER ACL RECONSTRUCTION		
BODY STRUCTURES AND FUNCTIONS	**ACTIVITIES**	**PARTICIPATION**
Quadriceps muscle weakness	Difficulty squatting	Unable to ski
	Difficulty climbing stairs	
	Difficulty running	

PERSONAL FACTORS	ENVIRONMENTAL FACTORS
Young man	Recreational sports
Athletic character	Fitness and leisure
Competitive	

3. Outline Therapeutic Goals and Outcome Measurements

GOAL	OUTCOME MEASUREMENT
Increase muscle force	Dynamometry
Decrease muscle atrophy	Measuring tape
Increase ability to squat, climb, and run, and accelerate return to skiing	Knee Outcome Survey, which includes the Activities of Daily Living Scale (ADLS) and the Sports Activity Scale (SAS)

4. Justify the Use of Neuromuscular Electrical Stimulation Based on the EBP Framework

PRACTITIONER'S EXPERIENCE	RESEARCH-BASED INDICATIONS	PATIENT'S EXPECTATION
Experienced in NMES	*Strength:* Moderate	No opinion of NMES
Has used NMES in similar cases	*Effectiveness:* Substantiated	Hopes for good results
Is convinced that NMES will be beneficial		

5. Outline Key Intervention Parameters

- **Treatment base:** Private clinic
- **Electrical current:** Russian or burst-modulated alternating sinusoidal current
- **Stimulator type:** Cabinet, line-powered, multi-current electrical stimulator with two output channels
- **Current carrier frequency:** 2,500 Hz sinusoidal alternating current
- **Application protocol:** Follow the suggested application protocol presented for muscle strengthening in *Application, Contraindications, and Risks* box, and make the necessary adjustments for this case.
- **Patient's positioning:** Sitting on the training chair with hips at 90 degrees flexion; knee positioned at 70 degrees of flexion; isometric condition with ankle attached to the dynamometer
- **Application site:** Over right quadriceps muscle
- **Burst duration:** 10 ms
- **Burst frequency:** 50 bups
- **Current amplitude:** Amplitude (mA) set to evoke a muscle contraction force equivalent to approximately 60% of maximum voluntary force (MVF) developed by the affected muscle group (% MVF)
- **ON time:** 10 s; includes ramp up (RU) and down (RD) times because muscle contraction occurs during these two ramp times; RU time: 2 s; RD time: 2 s
- **OFF time:** 40 s
- **ON:OFF time ratio:** 10 s:40 s
- **Duty cycle:** 20%
- **Electrode type, shape, and size:** Plate carbon rubber electrodes covered with electroconductive gel; square; 2.5 × 2.5 cm (1 × 1 in)
- **Electrode configuration:** Quadripolar
- **Electrode placement:** Over motor points located with probe stimulation technique (see text)
- **Stimulation method:** Synchronous
- **Training method:** NMES alone
- **Training protocol:** 10 c/10 s/40 s × 3, meaning a bout of 10 evoked muscle contractions, each lasting 10 s and separated by a 40-s rest period, repeated 3 times. This is equivalent to an ON:OFF time ratio of 10 s:40 s that corresponds to a duty cycle of 20%. The duration of this exercise bout is 8.33 minutes or 500 s [(10 s + 40 s) × 10 c)]. The training regimen is composed of 3 consecutive bouts within a training session, each separated by a 5-minute (300-s) rest period. The full training session thus consists of 30 evoked muscle contractions induced over a 35-minute (2,100 s) period (500 s + 300 s + 500 s + 300 s + 500 s).
- **Number of treatment session per week:** 3 (Mon-Wed-Fri)
- **Concomitant therapy:** Home quadriceps strengthening in between NMES training (Tue and Thurs)
- Use the **Online Dosage Calculator: Neuromuscular Electrical Stimulation.**

6. Report Pre- and Post-Intervention Outcomes

OUTCOME	PRE	POST
Quadriceps force (% of deficit)	28%	10%
Muscle atrophy	1.5 cm	0.5 cm
Knee functional status (ADLS)	72%	95%
Knee functional status (SAS)	65%	90%
Scale: 100% = no difficulty		

7. Document Case Intervention Using the SOAP Note Format

S: Young active male Pt complains about R knee muscle weakness and poor function following ACL reconstruction. Frustrated with his therapeutic progress; well motivated to engage in therapy again.

O: *Intervention:* NMES applied over R quadriceps; Russian current with 2,500 Hz carrier frequency; burst duration: 10 ms; burst frequency: 50 bups; current amplitude equivalent to 60% MVF; ON:OFF ratio:

10s:40s; duty cycle: 30%; plate carbon rubber electrodes, quadripolar electrode configuration; electrode placement over motor points; synchronous 2 channel stimulation; training bout: 10c/10s/40s; 3 bouts per training session, NMES 3 times per week for 3 weeks. *Pre–post comparison:* Decreased muscle force deficit, decrease muscle atrophy, and improved R knee functional status.

A: No adverse effect. Treatment well tolerated with improved quadriceps function.

P: Pt advised to continue home quadriceps strengthening program and slowly resume skiing.

CASE STUDY 13-2: GENUINE STRESS INCONTINENCE

EVIDENCE-BASED CLINICAL DECISION MAKING PROTOCOL

1. Formulate the Case History

A 42-year-old healthy woman and mother to three young children is referred by her gynecologist for the management of genuine stress incontinence. This condition began 2 years ago after the birth of her third child. Her main complaint over the past 6 months is frequent urine loss, particularly with sneezing, coughing, or laughing and when doing strenuous physical home and recreational activities. Physical examination reveals severe pelvic floor muscle weakness of grade 1 on the Modified Oxford Scale palpation, leading to incomplete urethral closure. Muscle recruitment is slow, and the ability to hold is poor. She has difficulty in working out how to tighten or contract her pelvic floor muscle correctly and to hold on for more than a few seconds. The patient's goal is to regain control of her micturition. She wants to avoid the use of medication. She feels socially embarrassed with regard to this problem.

2. Outline the Case Based on the ICF Framework

GENUINE STRESS INCONTINENCE		
BODY STRUCTURES AND FUNCTIONS	**ACTIVITIES**	**PARTICIPATION**
Pelvic floor muscle weakness	Difficulty in controlling micturition	Difficulty with strenuous home activities
		Difficulty with strenuous recreational activities

PERSONAL FACTORS	ENVIRONMENTAL FACTORS
Middle-aged woman	Family
Mother	Home
Housewife	Recreation

3. Outline Therapeutic Goals and Outcome Measurements

GOAL	OUTCOME MEASUREMENT
Increase pelvic floor muscle strength Increase sphincter strength and control, thus enhancing urethral control	Force grading using palpation (Modified Oxford Scale)
Decrease episodes and severity of incontinence, thus decreasing social embarrassment and accelerating return to normal life	Daily voiding diary/continence chart

4. Justify the Use of Neuromuscular Electrical Stimulation Based on the EBP Framework

PRACTITIONER'S EXPERIENCE	RESEARCH-BASED INDICATIONS	PATIENT'S EXPECTATION
Moderate experience in NMES	*Strength:* Moderate	Wants to avoid medication
Has used NMES in a few similar cases	*Effectiveness:* Substantiated	Is looking for a noninvasive treatment
Believes that NMES will be beneficial		

5. Outline Key Intervention Parameters

- **Treatment base:** Private clinic
- **Electrical current:** Interferential or beat amplitude-modulated alternating sinusoidal current
- **Stimulator type:** Cabinet, line-powered, vacuum interferential
- **Application protocol:** Follow the suggested application protocol presented for pelvic floor muscles, and make the necessary adjustments for this case.
- **Patient's positioning:** Semi-supine, knees flexed, with thighs open, giving access to the perineum for electrode placement
- **Stimulation mode:** Quadripolar or true interferential
- **Stimulation method:** NMES superimposed onto voluntary contraction
- **Beat duration:** 10 ms
- **Beat frequency sweep:** 40 to 120 beps
- **Current amplitude:** At the level (mA) where the patient reports a strong but comfortable sensation
- **ON time:** 8 s; includes ramp up (RU) and down (RD) times because muscle contraction occurs during these two ramp times; RU time: 1 s, RD time: 1 s
- **OFF time:** 24 s
- **ON:OFF time ratio:** 8s:24s
- **Duty cycle:** 25%
- **Electrode type, shape surface area:** 4 circular cone suction electrodes; 12 cm^2 (4 in^2)
- **Electrode configuration:** Quadripolar
- **Electrode placement:** Electrodes placed around the perineum as follows: 2 electrodes adjacent to pubic symphysis, and 2 electrodes adjacent to each ischial tuberosity. With this quadripolar placement, the current of each channel is crossing (focused interference) the pelvic floor muscle and bladder areas for optimal stimulation. Suction electrodes kept in place over the skin using minimal suction or vacuum force.
- **Training regimen:** 12c/8s/24s × 3, meaning a bout made of 15 evoked muscle contractions superimposed onto voluntary pelvic floor muscle contractions, each lasting 8 s and separated by a 24-s rest period. This is equivalent to an ON:OFF time ratio of 8s:24s, which corresponds to a duty cycle of 25%. The duration of this exercise is 8 minutes or 480 s [(8 s + 24 s) × 15 c)]. The training regimen is composed of 3 consecutive bouts within a training session, each separated by a 5-minute (300-s) rest period. The full training session thus consists of 45 evoked muscle contractions, each superimposed on 45 voluntary contractions, produced over a 34-minute (2,040-s) period (480 s + 300 s + 480 s + 300 s +480 s).
- **Treatment frequency:** Daily
- **Concomitant therapy:** Daily home pelvic floor muscle strengthening exercises (Kegels).
- **Treatment duration:** 10 days
- Use the **Online Dosage Calculator: Neuromuscular Electrical Stimulation.**

6. Report Pre- and Post-Intervention Outcomes

OUTCOME	PRE	POST
Pelvic floor muscle strength (Modified Oxford Score)	1	3
Continence chart		Improved by 70%

7. Document Case Intervention Using the SOAP Note Format

S: Middle-aged active Pt, diagnosed with stress incontinence causing problem with bladder control and social embarrassment. Pt wants to avoid medication and surgery.

O: *Intervention:* NMES for urinary incontinence using quadripolar IFC; beat frequency sweep: 40 to 120 Hz; ON:OFF time ratio: 8s:24s; duty cycle: 25%; suction electrodes; quadripolar electrode configuration surrounding the perineum; training regimen: 12c/8s/24s × 3 bouts; treatment schedule: daily for 10 days. *Pre-Post Compraison:* NMES, applied concomitantly with a home regimen of Kegels, led to increase PFM force (1 to 3) and decreased micturition (70% improvement).

A: No adverse effect. Treatment well tolerated. By contraction during electrical stimulation, PT can now better contract her pelvic floor muscles and control the incontinence problem.

P: Pt strongly advised to continue her Kegel exercise regimen on a regular basis.

VI. THE BOTTOM LINE

- There is unquestionable scientific evidence to show that NMES can restore and increase muscle strength in patients and healthy individuals.
- NMES cannot be considered as a surrogate training method, but as an adjunct to voluntary muscle training.
- NMES is the delivery of electrical current through the skin causing motor nerve depolarization, which in turn evokes muscle contraction.
- NMES is commonly applied using three types of electrical current: biphasic pulsed, Russian, and interferential currents.
- Biphasic pulsed current may be pulse- or burst modulated. Russian current is burst modulated, and IFC is beat- or amplitude modulated.
- Electrically speaking, there is minimal difference between biphasic burst-, Russian burst- and interferential beat modulation. Given similar parameter settings, all three currents generate similar amounts of current per second.
- During NMES, and contrary to voluntary contraction, MU activation is synchronous and occurs in a reverse order, thus causing rapid onset of muscle fatigue.
- Of all dosimetric parameters, both pulse/burst/beat frequency (temporal recruitment) and current amplitude (spatial recruitment) may be the most important.
- Setting proper ON and OFF times, as well as ramp up and down times, is necessary for the electrically evoked muscle contraction to mimic voluntary contraction as closely as possible.
- Electrode placement over muscle motor point(s) is recommended. Identification of motor points can be personalized using motor point stimulation technique or based on published motor point charts.
- All line-powered neuromuscular electrical stimulators should be plugged into ground-fault circuit interrupter (GFCI) receptacles to prevent macroshock.
- Skin surface preparation before each treatment and periodic calibration of electric stimulators, including electrode resistance and cable continuity checks using a multimeter, are strongly recommended to ensure optimal treatment efficacy.

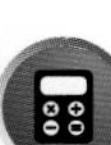

- Use of the **Online Dosage Calculator: Neuromuscular Electrical Stimulation** removes the burden of hand calculation and promotes the adoption of quantitative dosimetry.
- The overall body of evidence reported in this chapter shows the strength of evidence behind NMES to be *moderate* and its level of therapeutic effectiveness *substantiated.*
- As a modern training method, NMES or EMS training represents a promising alternative to traditional strength training for systematically enhancing strength parameters and motor abilities in patients as well as in healthy untrained and trained subjects, including elite athletes.

VII. CRITICAL THINKING QUESTIONS

Clarification: What is meant by neuromuscular electrical stimulation (NMES)?

Assumptions: Many of your colleagues assume that the use of Russian current stimulation causes less discomfort and generates greater tetanic force, and that IFC is more penetrating than the other current because it lowers skin impedance. How would you verify or disprove this assumption?

Reasons and evidence: What leads you to believe that MU recruitment during electrical stimulation is synchronous and occurs in a reverse size order?

Viewpoints or perspectives: How will you respond to a colleague who says that IFC is better than Russian current or biphasic pulse current for enhancing muscle strength?

Implications and consequences: What are the potential implications and consequences related to the following parameter settings: (1) increasing the ON time while keeping the OFF time the same during the course of the training program; (2) using 20 bups as opposed to 50 bups; and (3) setting no ramp up and down times?

About the question: Why is setting current frequency and current amplitude so important for optimal strength training using NMES? Why do you think I ask this question?

VIII. REFERENCES

Articles

Adedoyin RA, Olaogun MO, Fagbeja OO (2002) Effects of interferential current stimulation in management of osteoarthritic knee pain. Physiotherapy, 88: 493–499

Anderson AF, Lipscomb AB (1989) Analysis of rehabilitation technique after anterior cruciate reconstruction. Am J Sports Med, 17: 154–160

APTA (2001). Electrotherapeutic Terminology in Physical Therapy. Alexandria, VA. American Physical Therapy Association.

Avramidis K, Strike PW, Taylor PN, Swain ID (2003) Effectiveness of electric stimulation of the vastus medialis muscle in the rehabilitation of patients after total knee arthroplasty. Arch Phys Med Rehabil, 84: 1850–1853

Behm DG, St-Pierre DM, Perez D (1996) Muscle inactivation: Assessment of interpolated twitch technique. J Appl Physiol, 81: 2267–2273

Belanger AY, Allen ME, Chapman AE (1992) Cutaneous versus muscular perception of electrically evoked tetanic pain. J Orthop Sports Phys Ther, 16: 162–168

Belanger AY, McComas AJ (1981) Extent of motor unit activation during effort. J Appl Physiol Respir Environ Exerc, 51: 1131–1135

Bellew JW, Beiswanger Z, Freeman E, Gaerte C, Trafton J (2012) Interferential and burst-modulated biphasic pulsed currents yield greater muscle force than Russian current. Physiother Thory Pract, 28: 384–390

Bircan S, Senocak O, Kaya PO, Tamci SA, Gulbahar A, Akalin E (2002) Efficacy of two forms of electrical stimulation in increasing quadriceps strength: A randomized controlled trial. Clin Rehabil, 16: 194–199

Botter A, Oprandi G, Lanfranco F, Allasia S, Maffiuletti NA, Minetto MA (2011) Atlas of the muscle motor points for the lower limbs: Implications for electrical stimulation procedures and electrode positioning. Eur J Appl Physiol, 111: 2461–2471

Boutelle D, Smith B, Malone T (1985) A strength study utilizing the Electro-Stim 180. J Orthop Sports Phys Ther, 7: 50–53

Brooks ME, Smith EM, Currier DP (1990) Effect of longitudinal versus transverse electrode placement on torque production by the quadriceps femoris muscle during neuromuscular electrical stimulation. J Orthop Sports Phys Ther, 11: 530–534

Burch FX, Tarro JN, Greenberg JJ, Carroll WJ (2008) Evaluating the benefits of patterned stimulation in the treatment of osteoarthritis of the knee: A multiple-center, randomized, single-blind, controlled study with an independent masked evaluator. Osteoarthritis Cartilage, 16: 895–872

Cabric M, Appell HJ, Resic A (1987) Effects of electrical stimulation of different frequencies on the myonuclei and fiber size in human muscle. Int J Sports Med, 8: 323–326

Caggiano E, Emrey T, Shirley S (1994) Effects of electrical stimulation or voluntary contraction for strengthening the quadriceps femoris muscles in an aged male population. J Orthop Sports Phys Ther, 20: 22–28

Callaghan MJ, Oldham JA, Winstanley J (2001) A comparison of two types of electrical stimulation of the quadriceps in the treatment of patellofemoral pain syndrome. A pilot study. Clin Rehabil, 15: 637–646

Chase J, Robertson VJ, Southwell B, Hutson J, Gibb S (2005) Pilot study using transcutaneous electrical stimulation (interferential current) to treat chronic treatment-resistant constipation and soiling in children. J Gastroenterol Hepatol, 20: 1054–1061

Cheing GL, Hui-Chan CW (2003) Analgesic effects of transcutaneous electrical nerve stimulation and interferential currents on heat pain in healthy subjects. J Rehabil Med, 35: 15–19

Cheing GL, So EM, Chao CY (2008) Effectiveness of electroacupuncture and interferential electrotherapy in the management of frozen shoulder. J Rehabil Med, 40: 166–170

Clarke MC, Chase JW, Gibb S, Hutson JM, Southwell BR (2009a) Improvement of quality of life in children with slow transit constipation after treatment with transcutaneous electrical stimulation. J Pediatr Surg, 44: 1268–1272

Clarke MC, Chase JW, Gibb S, Robertson VJ, Catto-Smith A, Hutson JM, Southwell BR (2009b) Decreased colonic transit time after transcutaneous interferential electric stimulation in children with slow transit constipation. J Pediatr Surg, 44: 408–412

Crevenna R, Mayr W, Keilani M, Pleiner J, Nurh M, Quittan M, Pacher R, Pialka-Moser V, Wolzt M (2003) Safety of a combined strength and endurance training using neuromuscular electrical stimulation of thigh muscles in patients with heart failure and bipolar sensing cardiac pacemakers. Wien Klin Wochenschr, 115: 710–714

Crevenna R, Wolzt M, Fialka-Moser V, Keilani M, Nurh M, Paternostro-Sluga T, Pacher R, Mayr W, Quittan M (2004) Long-term transcutaneous neuromuscular electrical stimulation in patients with bipolar sensing implantable cadioverter defibrillators: A pilot safety study. Artif Organs, 28: 99–102

Currier DP, Mann R (1983) Muscle strength development by electrical stimulation in healthy individuals. Phys Ther, 63: 915–921

Currier DP, Mann R (1984) Pain complaint: Comparison of isometric stimulation with conventional isometric exercise. J Orthop Sports Phys Ther, 5: 318–323

Curwin S, Stanish WD, Valinat G (1980) Clinical applications and biochemical effects of high frequency electrical stimulation. Can Athl Assoc J, 7: 15–16

Defrin R, Ariel E, Paretz C (2005) Segmental noxious versus innocuous electrical stimulation for chronic pain relief and the effect of fading sensation during treatment. Pain, 115: 152–160

Delitto A (2002) Russian electrical stimulation: Putting this perspective into perspective. Phys Ther, 82: 1017–1018

Delitto A, Brown M, Strube MJ, Rose SJ, Lehman RC (1989) Electrical stimulation of quadriceps femoris in an elite weight lifter: A single subject experiment. In J Sports Med, 3: 187–191

Delitto A, McKowen JM, McCarthy JA, Shively RA, Rose SJ (1988a) Electrically elicited co-contraction of a thigh muscular after anterior cruciate ligament surgery. A description and single-case experiment. Phys Ther, 68: 45–50

Delitto A, Rose SJ (1986a) Comparative comfort of three waveforms used in electrically eliciting quadriceps femoris muscle contractions. Phys Ther, 66: 1704–1707

Delitto A, Rose SJ (1986b) Electrically eliciting quadriceps femoris muscle contractions. Phys Ther, 66: 1704–1707

Delitto A, Rose SJ, McKowen JM, Lehman RC, Thomas JA, Shively RA (1988b) Electrical stimulation versus voluntary exercise in strengthening thigh musculature after anterior cruciate ligament surgery. Phys Ther, 68: 663–666

Delitto A, Snyder-Mackler L (1990) Two theories of muscle strength augmentation using percutaneous electrical stimulation. Phys Ther, 70: 158–164

Delitto A, Strube MJ, Shulman AD, Minor SD (1992) A study of discomfort with electrical stimulation. Phys Ther, 72: 410–421

Demirturk F, Akbayrak T, Karakaya IC, Yuksel I, Kirdi N, Demirturk F, Kaya S, Ergen A, Beksac S (2008) Interferential current versus biofeedback results in urinary stress incontinence. Swiss Med Wkly, 138: 317–321

Dobsak P, Novakova M, Fiser B, Siegelova J, Balcarkova P, Spinarova L, Vitovec J, Minami N, Nagasaka M, Kohzuki M, Yambe T, Imachi K, Nitta S, Eicher JC, Wolf JE (2006) Electrical stimulation of skeletal muscles. An alternative to aerobic exercise training in patients with chronic heart failure? Int Heart J, 47: 441–453

Dougall D (1985) The effects of interferential therapy in incontinence and frequency of micturition. Physiotherapy, 71: 135–136

Dowling JJ, Konert E, Ljucovic P, Andrews DM (1994) Are humans able to voluntary elicit maximum force? Neurosci Lett, 179: 25–28

Draper V, Ballard L (1991) Electrical stimulation versus electromyographic biofeedback in the recovery of quadriceps femoris muscle function following anterior cruciate ligament surgery. Phys Ther, 71: 455–461

Dumoulin C, Seabore DE, Quirion-de-Girardi C, Sullivan SJ (1995a) Pelvic-floor rehabilitation. Part 1: Comparison of two surface electrode placements during stimulation of the pelvic-floor musculature in women who are continent using bipolar interferential currents. Phys Ther, 75: 1067–1074

Dumoulin C, Seabore DE, Quirion-de-Girardi C, Sullivan SJ (1995b) Pelvic-floor rehabilitation. Part 2: Pelvic-floor reeducation with interferential currents and exercise in the treatment of genuine stress incontinence in postpartum women—a cohort study. Phys Ther, 75: 1075–1081

Emmerson C (1987) A preliminary study of the effect of interferential current therapy on detrusor instability in patients with multiple sclerosis. Aust J Physioth, 33: 64–65

Eriksson E, Haggmark T (1979) Comparison of isometric muscle training and electrical stimulation supplementing isometric muscle training in the recovery after major knee ligament surgery. Am J Sports Med, 17: 169–171

Eriksson E, Haggmark T, Kiessling KH, Karlsson J (1981) Effect of electrical stimulation on human skeletal muscle. Int J Sports Med, 2: 18–22

Fahey TD, Harvey M, Schroeder RV, Ferguson F (1985) Influence of sex difference and knee joint position on electrical stimulation-modulated strength increases. Med Sci Sports Exerc, 17: 144–147

Feil S, Newell J, Minogue C, Paessler HH (2011) The effectiveness of supplementing a standard rehabilitation program with superimposed neuromuscular electrical stimulation after anterior cruciate ligament reconstruction. Am J Sports Med, 39: 1238–1247

Ferguson JP, Blackley MW, Knight RD, Sutlive TG, Underwood FB, Greathouse DG (1989) Effects of varying electrode site placements on the torque output of an electrically stimulated involuntary quadriceps femoris muscle contraction. J Orthop Sports Phys Ther, 11: 24–29

Fitzgerald GK, Piva SR, Irrgang JJ (2003) A modified neuromuscular electrical stimulation protocol for quadriceps strength training following anterior cruciate ligament reconstruction. J Orthop Sports Phys Ther, 33: 492–501

Franklin ME, Currier DP, Smith ST, Mitts K, Werrell LM, Chenier TC (1991) Effect of varying the ratio of electrically induced muscle contraction time to rest time on serum creatine kinase and perceived soreness. J Orthop Sports Phys Ther, 13: 310–315

Fuentes J, Armijo-Olivo S, Magee DJ, Cross D (2010) Does amplitude-modulated frequency have a role in the hypoalgesic response of interferential current on pressure pain sensitivity in healthy subjects? A randomized crossover study. Physiotherapy, 96: 22–29

Fuentes J, Armijo-Olivo S, Magee DJ, Cross D (2011) A preliminary investigation into the effects of active interferential current therapy and placebo on pressure pain sensitivity: A randomized crossover placebo controlled study. Physiotherapy, 97: 291–301

Gaines JM, Metter EJ, Talbot LA (2004) The effect of neuromuscular electrical stimulation on arthritis knee pain in older adults with osteoarthritis of the knee. Appl Nurs Res, 17: 201–206

Glotzer TV, Gordon M, Sparta M, Radoslovich G, Zimmerman J (1998) Electromagnetic interference from a muscle stimulation device causing discharge of an implantable cardioverter defibrillator: Epicardial bipolar and endocardial bipolar sensing circuits are compared. Pacing Clin Electrophysiol, 21: 1996–1998

Gobbo M, Gaffurini P, Bissolotti L, Esposito F, Orizio C (2011) Transcutaneous neuromuscular stimulation: Influence of electrode positioning and stimulus amplitude settings on muscle response. Eur J Appl Physiol, 111: 2451–2454

Gondin J, Guette M, Ballay Y, Martin A (2005) Electromyostimulation training effects on neural drive and muscle architecture. Med Sci Sports Exerc, 37: 1291–1299

Grimby G, Wigerstad-Lossing I (1989) Comparison of high- and low-frequency muscle stimulators. Arch Phys Med Rehab, 70: 835–838

Gundog M, Atamaz F, Kanylmaz S, Kirazli Y, Celepoglu G (2011) Interferential current therapy in patients with knee osteoarthritis. Am J Phys Med, 91: 107–113

Hallback J, Straus D (1980) Comparison of electro-myo stimulation to isokinetic training in increasing power of the knee extensor mechanism. J Orhtop Sports Phys Ther, 2: 20–24

Hartsell HD (1986) Electrical muscle stimulation and isometric exercises effects on selected quadriceps parameters. J Orthop Sports Phys Ther, 8: 203–209

Harris S, LeMaitre JP, Mackenzie G, Fox KA, Denvir MA (2003) A randomized study of home-based electrical stimulation of the legs and conventional bicycle exercise training for patients with chronic heart failure. Eur Heart J, 24: 871–878

Hartsell HD, Kramer JK (1992) A comparison of the effects of electrode placement, muscle tension, and isometric torque of the knee extensors. J Orthop Sports Phys Ther, 15: 168–174

Henella SM, Hutchins CJ, Castleden CM (1987) Conservative management of urethral sphincter incompetence. Neurourol Urodyn, 6: 191–192

Henneman E, Somjen G, Carpenter DG (1965) Functional significance of cell size spinal motoneurons. J Neurophysiol, 28: 560–580

Herrero AJ, Martin J, Martin T, Abadia O, Fernandez B, Garcia-Lopez D (2010a) Short-term effect of strength training with and without superimposed electrical stimulation on muscle strength and anaerobic performance: A randomized controlled trial. Part I. J Strength Cond Res, 24: 1616–1622

Herrero AJ, Martin J, Martin T, Abadia O, Fernandez B, Garcia-Lopez D (2010b) Short-term effect of plyometrics and strength training with and without superimposed electrical stimulation on muscle strength and anaerobic performance: A randomized controlled trial. Part II. Strength Cond Res, 24: 1616–1622

Hortobagyi T, Lambert NJ, Tracy C (1992) Voluntary and electromyostimulation forces in trained and untrained men. Med Sci Sports Exerc, 24: 702–707

Hurley DA, Minder PH, McDonough SM, Walsh DM, Moore AP, Baxter DG (2001) Interferential therapy electrode placement technique in acute low back pain: A preliminary investigation. Arch Phys Med Rehabil, 82: 485–493

Jarit GK, Mohr KJ, Waller R, Glousman RE (2003) The effects of home interferential therapy on postoperative pain, edema, and range of motion of the knee. Clin J Sports Med, 13: 16–20

Johnson MI, Tabasam G (1999) A double blind placebo-controlled investigation into the analgesic effects of interferential effects (IFC) and transcutaneous electrical nerve stimulation (TENS) on cold-induced pain in healthy subjects. Physioth Theor Pract, 15: 217–233

Johnson MI, Tabasam G (2003a) A single blind investigation into the hypoanalgesic effects of different swing patterns of interferential currents on cold-induced pain in healthy subjects. Arch Phys Med Rehabil, 84: 350–357

Johnson MI, Tabasam G (2003b) An investigation into the analgesic effects of interferential currents and transcutaneous electrical nerve stimulation on experimentally induced ischemic pain in otherwise pain-free volunteers. Phys Ther, 83: 208–223

Johnson MI, Tabasan G (2003c) An investigation into the analgesic effects of different frequencies of the amplitude-modulated wave of interferential current therapy on cold-induced pain in normal subjects. Arch Phys Med Rehabil, 84: 1387–1394

Johnson MI, Wilson H (1997) The analgesic effects of different swing patterns of interferential currents on cold-induced pain. Physiotherapy, 83: 461–467

Jubeau M, Muthalib M, Millet GY, Maffiuletti NA, Nosaka K (2012) Comparison in muscle damage between maximal voluntary and electrically evoked isometric contractions of the elbow flexors. Eur J Appl Physiol, 112: 429–438

Kajbafzadeh AM, Sharifi-Rad L, Baradaram N, Nejat F (2009) Effect of pelvic floor interferential electrostimulation on urodynamic parameters and incontinency of children with myelomeningocele and detrusor overactivity. Urology, 74: 324–329

Kajbafzadeh AM, Sharifi-Rad L, Nejat F, Kajbafzadeth M, Talaei HR (2011) Transcutaneous interferential electrical stimulation for management of neurologic bowel dysfunction in children with myomeningocele. In J Colorectal Dis, 27: 453–458

Koklu S, Koklu G, Ozguclu E, Kayani GU, Akbal E, Hascelik Z (2010) Clinical trial: Interferential electric stimulation in functional dyspepsia patients—a prospective randomized study. Aliment Pharmacol Ther, 31: 961–968

Kots YM (1971) Training with the method of electric tetanic stimulation of muscle by orthogonal impulses. Theory Pract Phys Cult, 4: 66–72 (Translated from Russian and French)

Kots YM (1977) Electrostimulation. Babkin I, Timentsko N (Translators). Paper presented at the Symposium on Electrostimulation of Skeletal Muscles. Canadian–Soviet Exchange Symposium, Concordia University, December 6–10

Kubiak RJ, Whitman KM, Jonhson RM (1987) Changes in quadriceps femoris muscle strength using isometric exercise versus electrical stimulation. J Orthop Sports Phys Ther, 8: 537–541

Lai HS, De Domineco G, Strauss GR (1988) The effect of different electro-motor stimulation training intensities on strength improvement. Aust J Physiother, 34: 151–164

Lambert I, Tebbs SE, Hill D, Moss HA, Davies AJ, Elliott TS (2000) Interferential therapy machines as possible vehicles for cross-infection. J Hosp Infect, 44: 59–64

Lambert JL, Vanderstreaten GG, De Cuyper HJ (1993) Electric current distribution during interferential therapy, Eur J Phys Med Rehab 3: 6–10

Laufer Y, Ries JD, Leininger PM, Alon G (2001) Quadriceps femoris muscle torques and fatigue generated by neuromuscular electrical stimulation with three different waveforms. Phys Ther, 81: 1307–1316

Laughman RK, Youdas JW, Garrett TR, Chao EY (1983) Strength changes in the normal quadriceps femoris muscle as a result of electrical stimulation. Phys Ther, 63: 494–499

Laycock J, Green RJ (1988) Interferential therapy in the treatment of incontinence. Physiotherapy, 74: 161–164

Laycock J, Jerwood D (1993) Does premodulated interferential therapy cure genuine stress incontinence? Physiotherapy, 79: 553–560

Lewek M, Stevens J, Snyder-Mackler L (2001) The use of electrical stimulation to increase quadriceps femoris muscle force in an elderly patient following a total knee arthroplasty. Phys Ther, 81: 1565–1571

Lieber RL, Silva PD, Daniel DM (1996) Equal effectiveness of electrical and volitional strength training for quadriceps femoris muscles after anterior cruciate ligament surgery. J Orthop Res, 14: 131–138

Lyons CL, Robb JB, Irrgang JJ, Fitzgerald GK (2005) Differences in quadriceps femoris torque when using a clinical electrical stimulator versus a portable electrical stimulator. Phys Ther, 85: 44–51

Man IO, Morrissey MC, Cywinski JK (2007) Effect of neuromuscular electrical stimulation on ankle swelling in the early period after ankle sprain. Phys Ther, 87: 53–65

Martin TP, Gundersen LA, Blevins FT, Coutts RD (1991) The influence of functional electrical stimulation on the properties of vastus lateralis fibres following total knee arthroplasty. Scand J Rehabil Med, 23: 207–210

McManus FJ, Ward AR, Robertson VJ (2006) The analgesic effects of interferential therapy on two experimental pain models: Cold and mechanically induced pain. Physiotherapy, 92: 95–102

McMiken DF, Todd-Smith M, Thompson C (1983) Strengthening of human quadriceps muscles by cutaneous electrical stimulation. Scand J Rehabil Med, 15: 25–28

McQuire WA (1975) Electrotherapy and exercises for stress incontinence and urinary frequency. Physiotherapy, 61: 305–307

Miller MG, Cheatham CC, Holcomb WR, Ganschow R, Micheal TJ, Rubbley MD (2008) Subcutaneous tissue thickness alters the effect of NMES. J Sports Rehabil, 17: 68–75

Minder PM, Noble JG, Alves-Guerreiro J, Hill ID, Lowe AS, Walsh DM, Baxter GD (2002) Interferential therapy: Lack of effect upon experimentally induced delayed onset muscle soreness. Clin Physiol Funct Imaging, 22: 339–347

Mintken PE, Carpenter KJ, Eckhoff D, Kohrt WM, Stevens JE (2007) Early neuromuscular electrical stimulation to optimize quadriceps muscle function following total knee arthroplasty: A case report. J Orthop Sports Phys Ther, 37: 364–371

Nemec H (1959) Interferential therapy: A new approach in physical medicine. Br J Physiother, 12: 9–12

Ni Chiosig F, Hendricks O, Malone J (1994) A pilot study of the therapeutic effects of bipolar and quadripolar interferential therapy, using bipolar osteoarthritis as a model. Physiother Ire, 15: 3–7

Nitz AJ, Dobner JJ (1987) High-intensity electrical stimulation effect on thigh musculature during immobilization for knee sprain. A case report. Phys Ther, 67: 219–222

Nobbs LA, Rhodes EC (1986) The effect of electrical stimulation on isokinetic exercise on muscular power of the quadriceps femoris. J Orthop Sports Phys Ther, 8: 260–268

Nosaka K, Aldayel A, Jubeau M, Chen TC (2011) Muscle damage induced by electrical stimulation. Eu J Appl Physiol, 111: 2427–2437

Nuhr MJ, Pette D, Berger R, Quittan M, Crevenna R, Huelsman M, Wiesinger GF, Moser P, Fialka-Moser V, Pacher R (2004) Beneficial effects of chronic low-frequency stimulation of thigh muscles in patients with advanced chronic heart failure. Eur Heart J, 25: 136–143

Oh-oka H (2008) Efficacy of interferential low frequency therapy for elderly wet overactive bladder patients. Indian J Urol, 24: 178–181

Olah KS, Bridges N, Denning J, Farrar DJ (1990) The conservative management of patients with symptoms of stress incontinence: A randomized, prospective study comparing weighted vaginal cones and interferential therapy. Am J Obstet Gynecol, 162: 87–92

Owens J, Malone T (1983) Treatment parameters of high frequency electrical stimulation as established on the Electro-Stim 180. J Orthop Sports Phys Ther, 4: 162–168

Parker MG, Bennett MJ, Hieb MA, Hollar AC, Roe AA (2003) Strength response in human femoris muscle during 2 neuromuscular electrical stimulation programs. J Orthop Sports Phys Ther, 33: 719–726

Parker MG, Keller L, Evenson J (2005) Torque responses in human quadriceps to burst-modulated alternating current at 3 carrier frequencies. J Orthop Sports Phys Ther, 35: 239–245

Partridge CJ, Kitchen SS (1999) Adverse effects of electrotherapy used by physiotherapists. Physiotherapy, 85: 298–303

Petterson S, Snyder-Mackler L (2006) The use of neuromuscular electrical stimulation to improve activation deficits in a patient with chronic quadriceps strength impairments following total knee arthroplasty. J Orthop Sports Phys Ther, 36: 678–685

Pfeifer AM, Cranfield T, Wagner S, Craik RL (1997) Muscle strength: A comparison of electrical stimulation and volitional isometric contractions in adults over 65 years. Physiother Can, 49: 32–39

Philipp A, Wolf GK, Rzany B, Dertinger H, Jung EG (2000) Interferential current is effective in palmar psoriasis: An open prospective trial. Eur J Dermatol, 10: 195–198

Quirk A, Newham RJ, Newham KJ (1985) An evaluation of interferential therapy, shortwave diathermy and exercise in the treatment of osteoarthrosis of the knee. Physiotherapy, 71: 55–57

Quittan M, Wiesinger GF, Sturm B, Puig S, Mayr W, Sochor A, Paternostro T, Resch KL, Pacher R, Fialka-Moser V (2001) Improvement of thigh muscles by neuromuscular electrical stimulation in patients with refractory heart failure. Am J Phys Med Rehabil, 80: 206–214

Romero JA, Sanford TL, Schroeder RV (1982) The effects of electrical stimulation on normal quadriceps on strength and girth. Med Sci Sports Exerc, 14: 194–197

Rooney JG, Currier DP, Nitz AJ (1992) Effect of variation in the burst and carrier frequency modes of neuromuscular electrical stimulation on pain perception of healthy subjects. Phys Ther, 72: 800–806

Ruther CL, Golden CL, Harris RT, Dudley GA (1995) Hypertrophy, resistance training, and the nature of skeletal muscle activation. J Strength Cond Res, 9: 155–159

Rutherford O, Jones DA, Newham DJ (1986) Clinical and experimental application of the percutaneous twitch superimposition technique for the study of human muscle activation. J Neurol Neurosurg Psych, 49: 1288–1291

St-Pierre D, Taylor AW, Lavoie M, Sellers W, Kots YM (1986) Effects of 2500 Hz sinusoidal current on fiber area and strength of the quadriceps femoris. J Sports Med Phys Fitness, 26: 60–66

Selkowitz DM (1985) Improvement in isometric strength of the quadriceps femoris muscle after training with electrical stimulation. Phys Ther, 65: 186–196

Shafshak TS, El-Sheshai AM, Soltan, HE (1991) Personality traits in the mechanisms of interferential therapy for osteoarthritic knee pain. Arch Phys Med Rehab, 72: 579–581

Shanahan C, Ward AR, Robertson VJ (2006) Comparison of the analgesic efficacy of interferential therapy and transcutaneous electric nerve stimulation. Physiotherapy, 92: 247–253

Sinacore DR, Delitto A, King DS, Rose SJ (1990) Type II fiber activation with electrical stimulation: A preliminary report. Phys Ther, 70: 416–422

Sisk TD, Stralka SW, Deering MB, Griffin JW (1987) Effect of electrical stimulation on quadriceps strength after reconstructive surgery of the anterior cruciate ligament. Am J Sports Med, 15: 215–220

Snyder-Mackler L, Delitto A, Baily SL, Stralka SW (1995) Strength of the quadriceps femoris muscle and functional recovery after reconstruction of the anterior cruciate ligament. A prospective, randomized clinical trial of electrical stimulation. J Bone Joint Surg (A), 77: 1166–1173

Snyder-Mackler L, Delitto A, Stralka SW, Bailey SL (1994) Use of electrical stimulation to enhance recovery of quadriceps femoris muscle production in patients following anterior cruciate ligament reconstruction. Phy Ther, 74: 901–907

Snyder-Mackler L, Garrett M, Roberts M (1989) A comparison of torque generating capabilities of three different electrical stimulating currents. J Orthop Sports Phys Ther, 10: 297–301

Snyder-Mackler L, Ladin Z, Schepsis AA, Young JC (1991) Electrical stimulation of the thigh muscles after reconstruction of the anterior cruciate ligament. Effects of electrically elicited contraction of the quadriceps femoris and hamstring muscles on gait and on strength of the thigh muscles. J Bone Joint Surg (A), 73: 49–54

Soo CL, Currier DP, Threlkeld AJ (1988) Augmenting voluntary torque of healthy muscle by optimization of electrical stimulation. Phys Ther, 68: 333–337

Stephenson R, Johnson M (1995) The analgesic effects of interferential therapy on cold-induced pain in healthy subjects: A preliminary report. Physiother Theory Pract, 11: 89–95

Stephenson R, Walker EM (2003) The analgesic effects of interferential (IF) current on cold-pressor pain in healthy subjects: A single blind trial of three IF currents against sham IF and control. Physiother Theory Pract, 19: 99–107

Stevens JE, Mizner RL, Snyder-Mackler L (2004) Neuromuscular electrical stimulation for quadriceps muscle strengthening after bilateral total knee arthroplasty: A case series. J Orthop Sports Phys Ther, 34: 21–29

Switzer D, Hendricks O (1988) Interferential therapy for treatment of stress and urge incontinence. Ir Med J, 81: 30–31

Sylvester KL, Keilty SEJ (1987) A pilot study to investigate the use of interferential in the treatment of anorectal incontinence. Physiotherapy, 73: 207–208

Taylor K, Newton R, Personius W, Bush F (1987) Effect of interferential current stimulation for treatment of subjects with recurrent jaw pain. Phys Ther, 67: 346–350

Trimble MH, Enoka RM (1991) Mechanisms underlying the training effects associated with neuromuscular electrical stimulation. Phys Ther, 71: 273–280

Tugay N, Akbayrak T, Demirturk F, Karakaya IC, Kocaacar O, Tugay U, Karakaya MG, Demirturk F (2007) Effectiveness of transcutaneous electrical nerve stimulation and interferential current in primary dysmenorrhea. Pain Med, 8: 295–300

Turkan A, Inci Y, Fazli D (2005) The short-term effects of physical therapy in different intensities of urodynamic stress incontinence. Gynecol Obstet Invest, 59: 43–48

Underwood FB, Kremser GL, Finstuen K, Greathouse DG (1990) Increasing involuntary torque production by using TENS. J Orthop Sports Phys Ther, 12: 101–104

Vahtera T, Haaranen M, Viramo-Koskela AL, Ruutiainen J (1997) Pelvic floor rehabilitation is effective in patients with multiple sclerosis. Clin Rehab, 11: 211–219

Van der Heijden G, Leffers P, Wolters P, Verheijden J, van Mameren H, Houben JP, Bouter LM, Knipschild PG (1999) No effect of bipolar interferential electrotherapy and pulsed ultrasound for soft tissue shoulder disorders: A randomized controlled trial. Ann Rheum Dis, 58: 530–540

Van Poppel H, Ketelaer P, Van-Deweerd A (1985) Interferential therapy for detrusor hyperreflexia in multiple sclerosis. Urology, 25: 607–612

Walker UA, Uhl M, Weiner SM, Warnatz K, Lange-Nolde A, Dertinger H, Peter HH, Jurenz SA (2006) Analgesic and disease modifying effects of interferential current in psoriatic arthritis. Rheumatol Int, 26: 904–907

Werners R, Pynsent PB, Bulstrode CJ (1999) Randomized trial comparing interferential therapy with motorized lumbar traction and massage in the management of low back pain in a primary care settings. Spine, 24: 1579–1584

Wigerstad-Lossing I, Grimby G, Jonsson T, Morelli B, Peterson L, Renstrom P (1988) Effects of electrical muscle stimulation combined with voluntary contraction after knee ligament surgery. Med Sci Sports Exerc, 20: 93–98

Williams RA, Morrissey MC, Brewster CE (1986) The effect of electrical stimulation on quadriceps strength and thigh circumference in menisectomy patients. J Orthop Sports Phys Ther, 8: 143–146

Wilson PD, Al-Samarrai T, Deakin M, Kolbe E, Brown AD (1987) An objective assessment of physiotherapy for female genuine stress incontinence. Br J Obstet Gyneacol, 94: 575–582

Zambito A, Bianchini D, Gatti D, Rossini M, Adami S, Viapiana O (2007) Interference and horizontal therapies in chronic low back pain due to multiple vertebral fractures: A randomized, double blind, clinical study. Osteoporos Int, 18: 1541–1545

Zambito A, Bianchini D, Gatti D, Viapiana O, Rossini M, Adami S (2006) Interferential and horizontal therapies in chronic low back pain: A randomized, double blind, clinical study. Clin Exp Rheumatol, 24: 534–539

Review Articles

Bax L, Staes F, Verhagen A (2005) Does neuromuscular electrical stimulation strengthen the quadriceps femoris? A systematic review of randomized controlled trials. Sports Med, 35: 191–212

Beatti A, Rayner A, Souvlis T, Chipchase L (2010) The analgesic effect of interferential therapy on clinical and experimental induced pain. Phys Ther Rev, 15: 243–252

Filipovic A, Kleinoder H, Dormann U, Mester J (2011) Electromyostimulation—a systematic review of the influence of training regimens and stimulation parameters on effectiveness in electromyostimulation training of selected strength parameters. J Strength Cond Res, 25: 3218–3238

Filipovic A, Kleinoder H, Dormann U, Mester J (2012) Electromyostimulation—a systematic review of the effects of different electromyostimulation methods of selected strength parameters in trained and elite athletes. J Strength Cond Res, 26: 2600–2614

Fuentes JP, Armijo-Olivo S, Magee DJ, Gross DP (2010) Effectiveness of interferential current therapy in the management of musculoskeletal pain: A systematic review and meta-analysis. Phys Ther, 90: 1219–1238

Glinsky J, Harvey L, van Es P (2007) Efficacy of electrical stimulation to increase muscle strength in people with neurological conditions: A systematic review. Phys Res Int, 12: 175–194

Gondin J, Cozzone PJ, Bendahan D (2011) Is high-frequency neuromuscular electrical stimulation a suitable tool of muscle performance improvement in both healthy humans and athletes? Eur J Appl Physiol, 111: 2473–2487

Hortobagyi T, Maffiuletti NA (2011) Neural adaptations to electrical stimulation strength training. Eur J Appl Physiol, 111: 2439–2449

Kim KM, Croy T, Hertel J, Saliba S (2010) Effects of neuromuscular electrical stimulation after anterior cruciate ligament reconstruction on quadriceps strength, function, and patient-oriented outcomes: A systematic review. J Orthop Sports Phys Ther, 40: 383–391

Maffiuletti NA (2010) Physiological and methodological considerations for the use of neuromuscular electrical stimulation. Eur J Appl Physiol, 110: 223–234

Maffiuletti NA, Minetto MA, Farina D, Bottinelli R (2011) Electrical stimulation for neuromuscular testing and training: State-of-the-art and unresolved issues. Eur J Appl Physiol, 111: 2391–239

Oh-oka H (2010) Neuromodulation in the treatment of overactive bladder with a focus on interferential therapy. Curr Bladder Dysfunct Rep, 5: 39–47

Roche A, Laighin GO, Coote S (2009) Surface-applied functional electrical stimulation for orthotic and therapeutic treatment of drop-foot after stroke—a systematic review. Phys Ther Rev, 14: 63–80

Selkowitz DM (2010) Electrical stimulation for enhancing strength and related characteristics of human denervated skeletal muscle. Phys Ther Rev, 15: 327–333

Ward AR, Shkuratova N (2002) Russian electrical stimulation: The early experiments. Phys Ther, 82: 1019–1030

Chapters of Textbooks

Alon G (1999) Principles of electrical stimulation. In: Clinical Electrotherapy, 3rd ed. Nelson RM, Hayes KW, Currier DR (Eds). Appleton & Lange, Stamford, pp 85–87

Hooke DN (1998) Electrical stimulating currents. In: Therapeutic Modalities for Allied Health Professionals. Prentice WE (Ed). McGraw-Hill, New York, pp 114–117

Prentice WE (2011) Location of motor points. In: Therapeutic Modalities in Rehabilitation, 4th ed. Prentice WE (Ed). McGraw-Hill Medical, New-York, pp 584–586

Robinson AJ (2008) Instrumentation in electrotherapy. In: Clinical Electrophysiology. Electrotherapy and Electrophysiological Testing, 3rd ed. Robinson AJ, Snyder-Mackler L (Eds). Lippincott Williams & Wilkins, Philadelphia, pp 57–58

Starkey C (2013) Motor Points. In: Therapeutic Modalities, 4th ed. Starkey C (Ed). FA davis, Philadelphia, pp 397–398

Internet Resource

http://thePoint.lww.com: Online Dosage Calculator: Neuromuscular Electrical Stimulation

Chapter 14

Transcutaneous Electrical Nerve Stimulation

Chapter Outline

Learning Objectives

Remembering: State and describe the five modes to deliver transcutaneous electrical nerve stimulation (TENS) for pain modulation.

Understanding: Distinguish between the spinal gate system and the descending endogenous opiate system of pain modulation.

Applying: Demonstrate the five application modes of TENS therapy.

Analyzing: Explain how TENS can close the spinal gate via the spinal gate and descending endogenous opiate system.

Evaluating: Describe how to achieve preferential nerve depolarization of sensory fibers, sensory-motor fibers, and sensory-motor-nociceptive fibers.

Creating: Discuss the strength of evidence and therapeutic effectiveness of TENS therapy for pain following soft tissue pathology.

I. FOUNDATION

A. DEFINITION

TENS is the acronym for transcutaneous electrical nerve stimulation. Literally speaking, this acronym refers to the use of electrical stimulators, capable of delivering pulsed currents, for stimulating (depolarizing) peripheral nerve fibers through the skin (thus, the term *transcutaneous*) using surface electrodes. In this chapter, TENS is defined as the application of pulsed electrical current for inducing *electroanalgesia*. This definition is consistent with the historic association in both scientific and clinical literatures between the terms *TENS* and *pain management* (see APTA, 2001). Because TENS is fundamentally used for the management of pain, readers are invited to review Chapter 4, which focuses on the topic of pain from soft tissue pathology, prior to considering this chapter.

B. ELECTRICAL CURRENT

The research-based evidence presented in this chapter indicates that TENS is clinically delivered using biphasic pulsed current, which may be pulse- or burst modulated. This current is very similar to the biphasic pulsed current used for neuromuscular electrical stimulation (NMES) (see the Biophysical Characteristics section).

C. ELECTRICAL STIMULATOR

TENS therapy is delivered, as illustrated in Figure 14-1, using cabinet, multi-current, line-powered stimulators, as well as portable, battery-operated, electrical stimulators. Portable TENS stimulators are commonly sold in a plastic carrying case containing reusable electrodes and lead cables.

D. ELECTRODE AND COUPLING MEDIUM

TENS therapy is delivered by using one or several pairs of surface electrodes, shown in Figure 14-2, made of carbon-impregnated silicon rubber or various flexible conductive tissues. These electrodes, which come in various shapes and sizes, may be reusable or for single use. Sterile electrodes are also available for postoperative treatment. Silicon-rubber electrodes are covered with an electroconductive gel, contained in bottles and refilling bags, to optimize the electrical coupling at the electrode–skin interface. Note that the use of custom-made metal electrodes is on the decline because commercial electrodes offer superior performance and are now relatively cheap to purchase.

E. RATIONALE FOR USE

Pain is by far the dominating symptom that prompts people to consult health-care practitioners. The medical approach to pain therapy is to offer drugs and, if drugs are not successful, to consider surgery. These two therapeutic approaches are invasive and present serious side effects. TENS therapy is an attractive therapeutic alternative for managing pain (Berman et al., 2000) because it is noninvasive and has no side effects. TENS therapy can be administered easily at home and at work, which makes it even more attractive. Finally, the lower cost associated with the delivery of TENS, compared with the high cost of drugs and surgery, makes this treatment more affordable to patients (Chabal et al., 1998).

II. BIOPHYSICAL CHARACTERISTICS

To avoid duplication of material, readers are invited to review the previous chapter on NMES, where the concepts of current waveform and frequency are discussed and illustrated. As mentioned earlier, and illustrated in

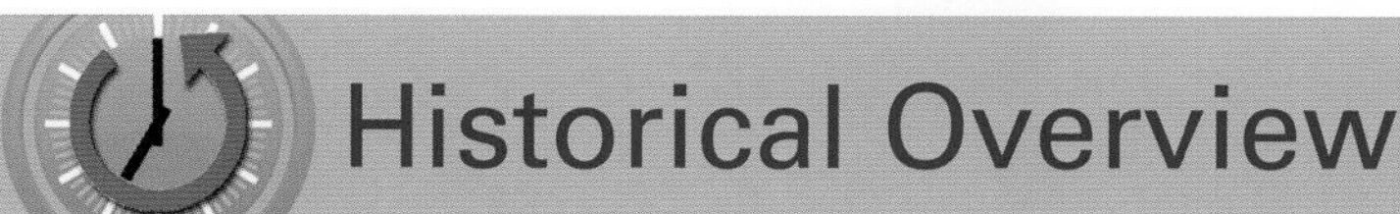

Historical Overview

The use of electrical current for the treatment of pain dates back to the 1st century, when relief of pain from gout was reported after a torpedo fish, or electric ray, was applied against a patient's skin (McMahon et al., 2005). There is consensus in the scientific literature that the discovery of transcutaneous electrical nerve stimulation (TENS) therapy rests on the original work of Canadian psychologist Ronald Melzack and British neuroanatomist Patrick Wall. In 1965, they published a landmark paper describing their newly discovered gate control theory of pain (Melzack et al., 1965). Immediately after publication of this revolutionary pain theory, experiments on humans by American neurosurgeon Norman Shealy and colleagues (Shealy et al., 1967) led to the eventual development of a surgical technique, known as dorsal column stimulation, for pain relief. This technique is based on electrical stimulation of dorsal column nerve fibers. Shealy and colleagues used a transcutaneous battery-operated stimulator, known as Electreat, as a screening device to determine whether patients were good candidates for dorsal column stimulation. Unexpectedly, their preliminary work revealed that some responded better to this simple, noninvasive TENS therapy than to the more technically complicated invasive dorsal column stimulation (Shealy, 1974). This remarkable observation, combined with the work of Melzack and Wall, led to the discovery and clinical application of TENS for pain modulation.

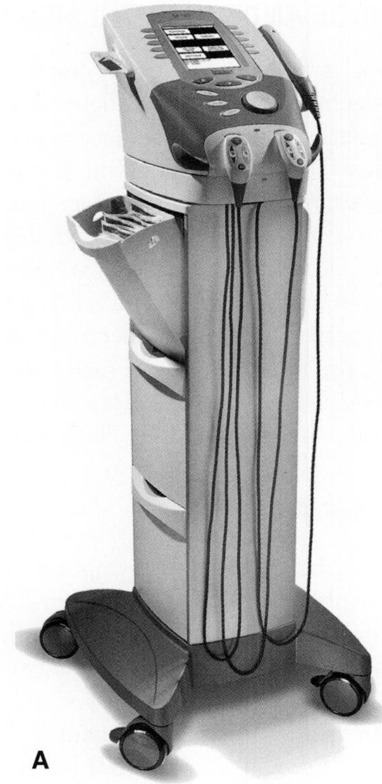

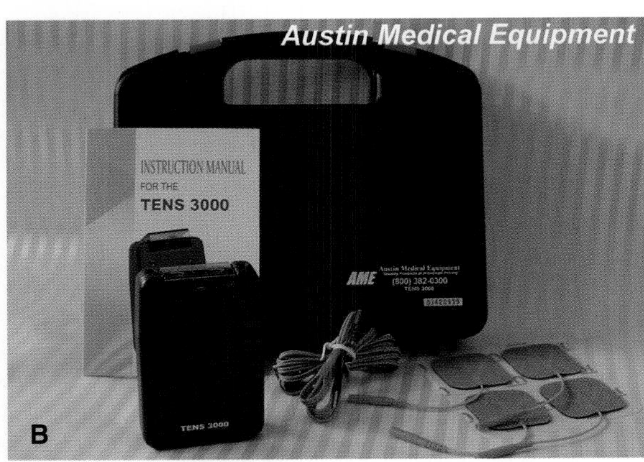

FIGURE 14-1 Typical cabinet (**A**) and portable (**B**) TENS stimulators. (A: Courtesy of DJO Global; B: Courtesy Austin Medical Equipment, Inc.)

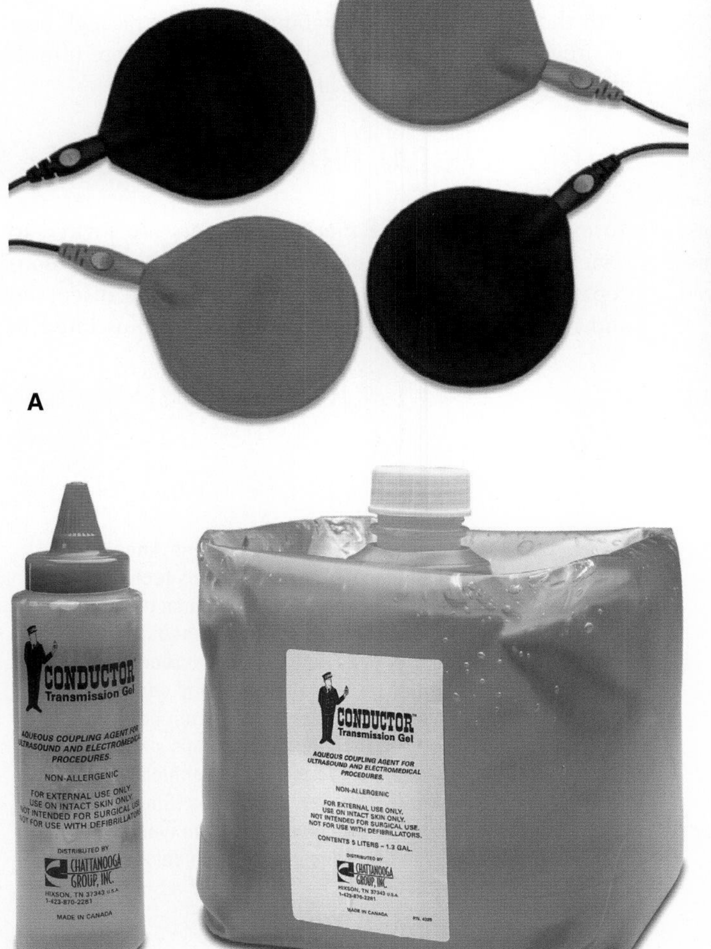

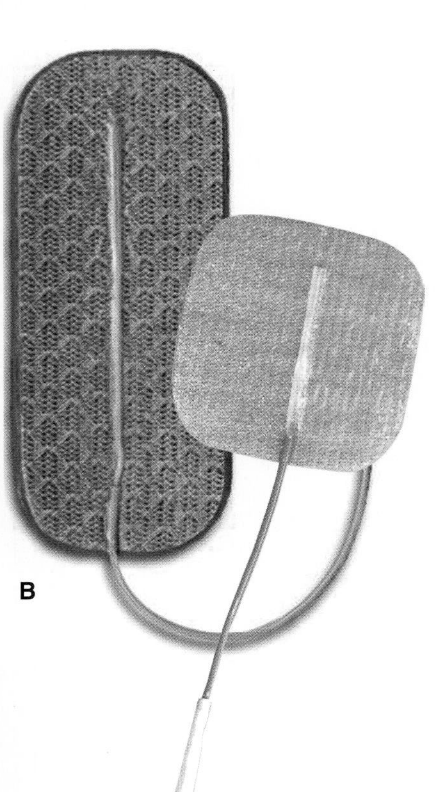

FIGURE 14-2 **A, B:** Typical TENS stimulating electrodes made of carbon-impregnated silicon rubber and flexible conductive materials. **C:** Electroconductive gel to apply under electrodes. (A–C: Courtesy of DJO Global.)

Figure 14-3, the delivery of TENS therapy rests on the use of biphasic pulsed current, which may be pulse- or burst modulated. The process of pulse and burst modulation is identical to the one discussed in Chapter 13. For example, Figure 14-4 illustrates pulse-modulated TENS delivered at a frequency of 3 pps and burst-modulated TENS delivered at 2 bups. The most common TENS waveform is biphasic and symmetrical, thus balanced, with either a square or a rectangular shape. The delivery of a balanced waveform, which has zero net charge, is critical because TENS treatments are often applied daily, for hours at the time, and often over weeks and months.

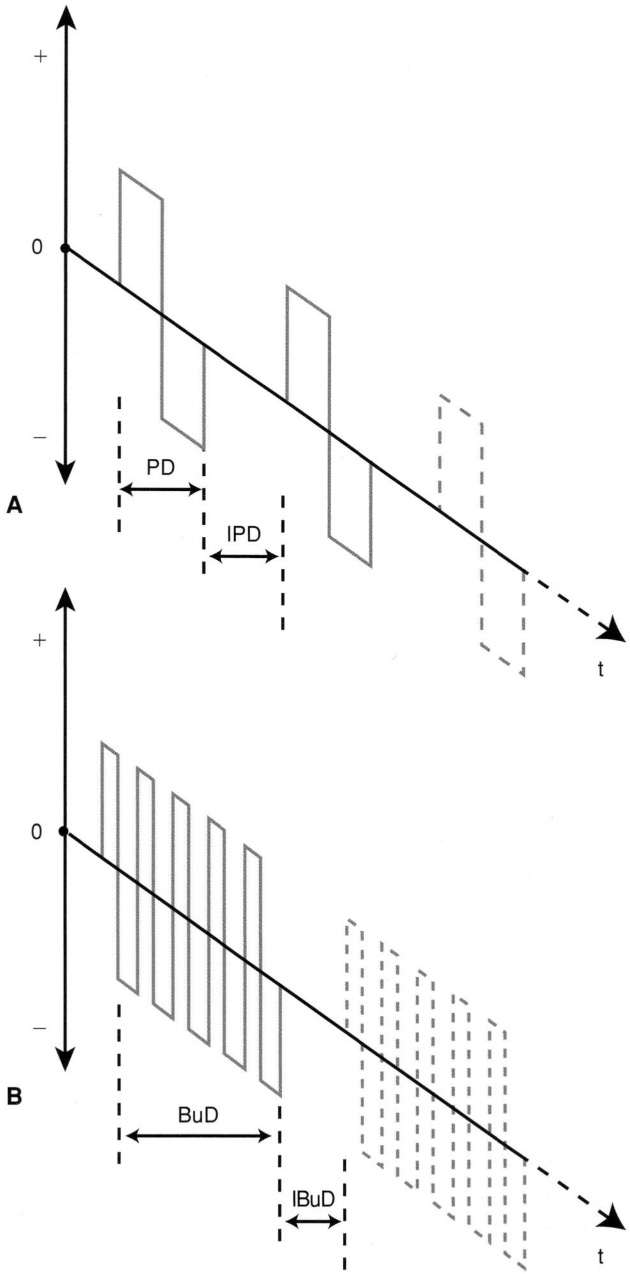

FIGURE 14-3 Pulse- (**A**) and burst-modulated (**B**) biphasic pulsed, symmetrical, and balanced. PD, pulse duration; IPD, interpulse duration; BuD, burst duration; IBuD, interburst duration.

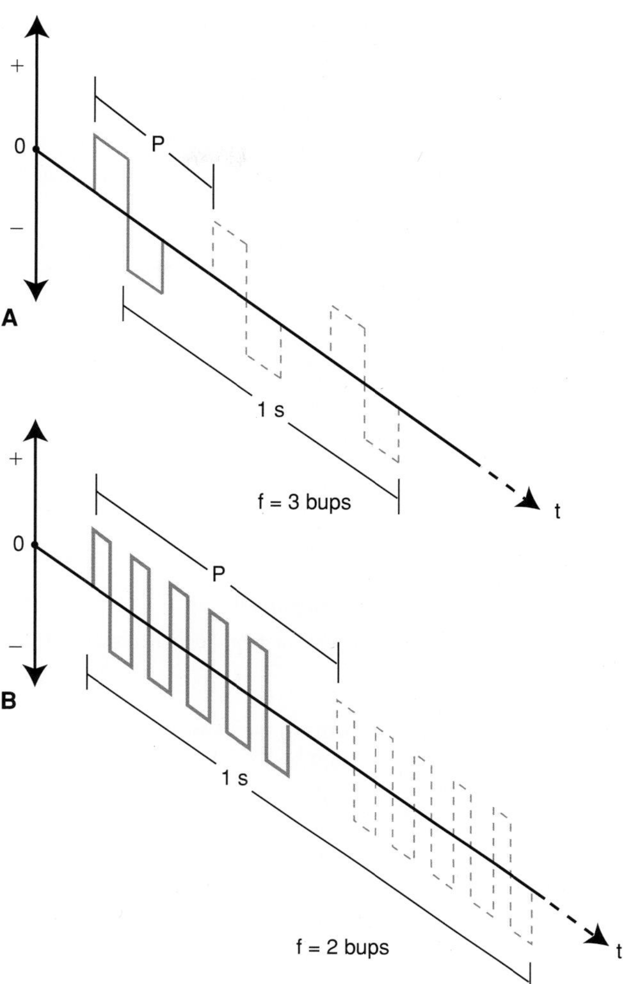

FIGURE 14-4 Frequency(*f*), in which the period (*P*) is equal to either pulse duration (PD) plus the interpulse duration (IPD) for pulse modulation (**A**), or to burst duration (BuD) plus interburst duration (IBuD) for burst modulation (**B**).

In other words, using a balanced waveform prevents the accumulation, or buildup, of electrical charges underneath the electrodes, which, over time, may cause skin irritation and discomfort.

III. THERAPEUTIC EFFECTS AND INDICATIONS

A. PAIN MODULATION

The sole therapeutic effect of TENS, as shown in Figure 14-5, is to modulate or decrease pain through the process of peripheral nerve depolarization by using pulsed electrical current (Bjordal et al., 2003; Sluka et al., 2003; Brosseau et al., 2004; Khadilkar et al., 2005; Miller et al., 2005; Allen, 2006; DeLeo, 2006; Johnson et al., 2007; Ying et al., 2007; Brown et al., 2009; Bedwell et al., 2011; Johnson et al., 2011). This process is *identical* to the one described and illustrated in the previous chapter

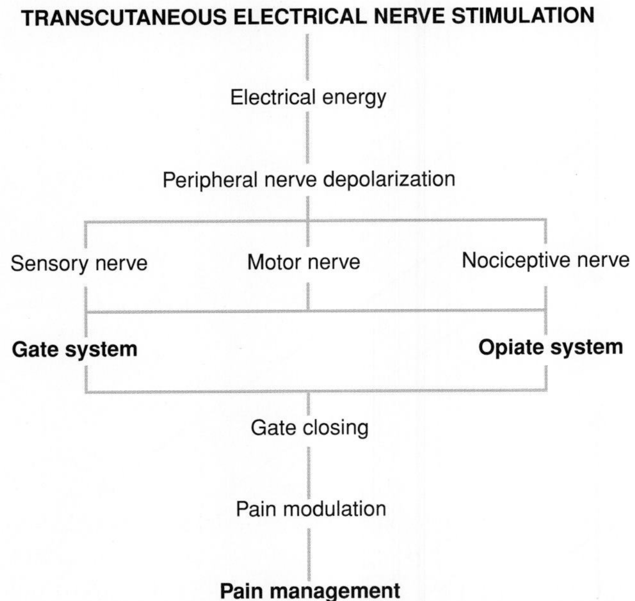

FIGURE 14-5 Proposed physiologic and therapeutic effects of TENS therapy.

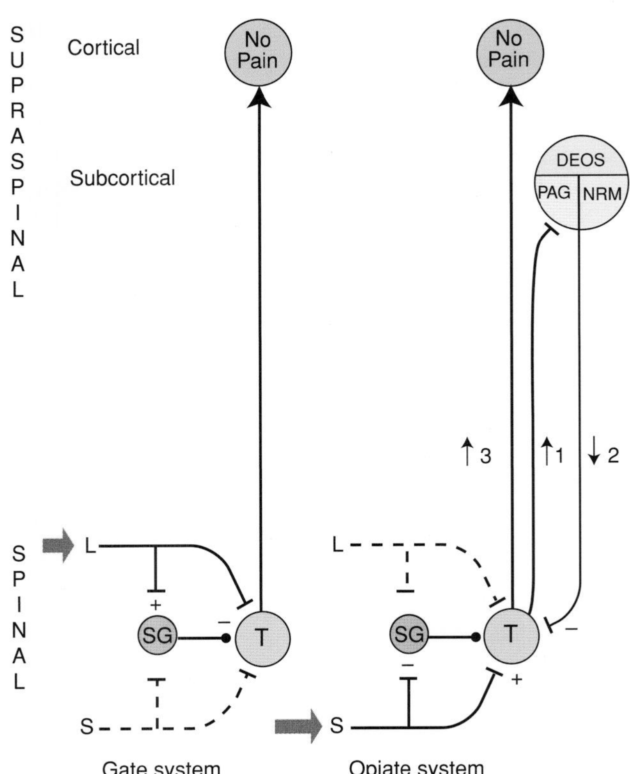

FIGURE 14-6 Schematic representation of both the gate and the opiate system of pain modulation in relation to TENS therapy (see text). L, large fibers; SG, substantia gelatinosa; T, pain-transmitting cells; S, small fibers; DEOS, descending endogenous opiate system; PAG, periaquaductal gray matter; NRM, nucleus raphe magnus; 1, excitatory synapse; 2, inhibitory synapse; arrow L, preferential electrical stimulation of large-diameter sensory fibers (A beta); arrow S, preferential electrical stimulation of small-diameter sensory fibers (A delta and C); arrows 1 and 2, negative feedback loop; arrow 3, pathway to the brain.

on NMES (to avoid duplication, see the Pulse/Burst/Beat Frequency section in Chapter 13). Prior to considering the following material, readers may also want to review Chapter 4, which deals with the topics of pain description, assessment, and scoring. There is a substantial body of evidence to suggest that the selective, or preferential, depolarization of specific groups of afferent nerve fibers affects two key pain modulation systems, known as the gate and opiate systems (see McMahon et al., 2005). Research has shown that three peripheral afferent nerve fibers—namely, the larger-diameter *A-beta* and smaller-diameter *A-delta* and *C* fibers—play a major role, as illustrated in Figure 14-6, in the process of pain modulation (McMahon et al., 2005). The large-diameter A-beta nerve fibers are *mechanosensitive* in nature, carrying information from mechanoreceptors responsible for touch and vibration to the brain (McMahon et al., 2005). The smaller-diameter C and A-delta nerve fibers are *nociceptive* in nature, carrying information from nociceptors (nerve-free endings) buried in soft tissues to the brain (McMahon et al., 2005; DeLeo, 2006). These peripheral afferent nerve fibers travel toward the dorsal horn of the spinal cord to make synaptic contacts with key neurons and interneurons known to play an important role in pain modulation (Melzack et al., 1965; Sluka et al., 2003; McMahon et al., 2005).

B. GATE SYSTEM

The gate control system, proposed by Melzack and Wall in 1965, states that peripheral neural inputs from A-beta, A-delta, and C fibers into the dorsal horn will decrease or increase the flow of impulses to higher processing centers in the brain. In other words, this system implies the action of a spinal gating system, where the gate may be closed (decreased input) or open (increased input), depending on the net neural input coming from the peripheral A-beta, A-delta, and C fibers (see Fig. 14-6). When the gate is closed, it means that no nociceptive inputs can reach the brain, resulting in pain relief. How can TENS close this gate?

1. Gate Closing

Research has shown that gate closing is associated with the preferential evoked depolarization (see bold arrow in Fig. 14-6) of large-diameter (see letter *L*) over small-diameter (see letter *S*) nerve fibers and vice versa (see McMahon et al., 2005). According to the gate control theory of pain, preferential activity in these large fibers is presumed to activate inhibitory interneurons located in the substantia gelatinosa of the dorsal horn of the spinal cord. Activation of these inhibitory interneurons results in the inhibition of pain-transmitting cells, called *T cells,* located in the dorsal horn of the spinal cord. Inhibition of T cells causes the gate to close, thus preventing nociceptive inputs to reach the supraspinal level (subcortical and cortical). The result is no perceived pain.

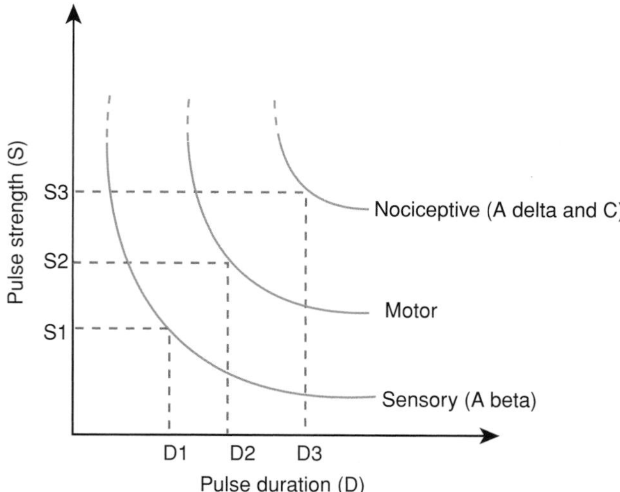

FIGURE 14-7 The classical strength/duration (S/D) curve on which the preferential, electrically evoked depolarization of one group of nerve fibers is made possible during TENS therapy. By selecting a given combination of pulse current amplitude or strength (S) and pulse duration (D), such as seen with S1–D1, S2–D2, and S3–D3 combinations, the preferential depolarization of sensory-only, sensory-motor-only, and sensory-motor-nociceptive nerve fibers can be achieved.

2. Preferential Nerve Fiber Depolarization

Research has shown that selective, or preferential, depolarization of sensory, motor, and nociceptive nerve fibers, using TENS, may be achieved through appropriate settings of the following two key electrical parameters: current amplitude and pulse duration (see McMahon et al., 2005). The interaction between these two stimulation parameters is illustrated in the classical nerve strength/duration (S/D) curve presented in Figure 14-7. The term *strength* (S) is synonymous with current amplitude, measured in milliamperes, and the term *duration* (D) corresponds to pulse duration, measured in microseconds.

a. Sensory-Level Stimulation

With a combination of low current amplitude (S) and short pulse duration (D)—that is, S1–D1 combination—preferential depolarization of large-diameter sensory fibers, such as A-beta fibers, is theoretically possible (see Fig. 14-7). Preferential sensory stimulation (S1–D1) is clinically confirmed when the patient reports sensations of pins and needles and tingling, with no sensation of muscle contraction under the stimulating electrode, and no pain. This sensory stimulation, below the motor and nociceptive threshold, is perceived as comfortable. Sensory threshold stimulation causes the depolarization of large-diameter A-delta fibers.

b. Motor-Level Stimulation

Combinations of higher current amplitudes (S) and longer pulse durations (D)—that is, S2–D2 combination—leads to the concomitant preferential depolarization of large-diameter afferent sensory (A-beta), and large-diameter efferent motor nerve fibers (alpha), causing muscle contraction (see Fig. 14-7). Preferential stimulation of these two types of fibers (S2–D2) can be clinically confirmed when the patient feels a mixed sensation of tingling combined with muscle contraction, without pain. Practitioners can confirm the patient's motor sensation by visualizing or palpating the evoked muscle contraction during stimulation.

c. Noxious-Level Stimulation

Combinations of still higher current amplitudes (S) and longer pulse durations (D), or S3–D3 combination, will lead to the concomitant depolarization of all three nerve fibers—namely, sensory (A-beta), motor (alpha), and nociceptive (A-delta and C fibers). This level of stimulation can be clinically confirmed when the patient experiences a strong and mixed sensation of muscle contraction and pain during stimulation. In other words, this level of stimulation is present when a muscle contraction is clearly apparent and when the patient describes the electrically evoked sensation as being just below the threshold of being intolerable, or too painful.

3. Gate Opening

As stated previously, TENS may either close or open the gate. For a patient to perceive pain, on the basis of Melzack and Wall's gate control theory, the spinal gate must be open—that is, T cells must be depolarized or activated so that nociceptive inputs reach the brain (cortical level), where pain is decoded. How can TENS decrease pain while opening the gate further? Can TENS open the gate, and by what mechanism is pain modulation achieved? The gate control theory stipulates that TENS opens the gate (see Fig. 14-6) through the preferential depolarization (bolded arrow) of the peripheral afferent smaller-diameter A-delta and C fibers (*S*) over the larger-diameter (*L*) A-beta fibers. This opening of the gate allows T cells to depolarize, sending nociceptive inputs to key subcortical neural structures, which activate another pain-modulating system, commonly called the *opiate system*.

C. OPIATE SYSTEM

There is a substantial body of evidence (McMahon et al., 2005) to suggest that the human body possesses its own pain modulation system, known as the descending endogenous opiate system (DEOS). This system, schematized in Figure 14-6, operates at the supraspinal level and involves neurohormonal activity from particular subcortical areas, such as the periaqueductal gray matter and the nucleus raphe magnus.

1. Descending Endogenous Opiate System

The term *descending* indicates that this system operates in a descending fashion, from the supraspinal to the spinal levels. The word *endogenous opiate* indicates that pain modulation occurs through the release of opiate-like substances secreted by the body itself. These endogenous opiate substances are known by the generic term *endorphins*.

2. Preferential A-Delta and C Fiber Depolarization

As shown in Figure 14-6, the preferential depolarization of the nociceptive smaller-diameter (see bold arrow pointing to S) A-delta and C fibers *opens* the spinal gate by inducing a powerful inhibitory effect on the inhibitory neurons contained in the substantia gelatinosa. The resulting T-cell depolarization triggers a negative feedback loop within the DEOS that will lead to pain modulation or relief.

3. Negative Feedback Loop

This feedback loop, represented by arrows 1, 2, and 3 in Figure 14-6, is said to be negative because it begins with T-cell depolarization (arrow 1) and ends with T-cell inhibition (arrow 2) and pain relief (arrow 3) as more and more endogenous opiate substances are secreted within the suffering patient's blood plasma and cerebrospinal fluid (Mayer et al., 1995).

4. Naloxone Test

The modulation of pain through an endogenous opiate system in humans was demonstrated by numerous studies on the use of naloxone—a potent antagonist to exogenous and endogenous opiates (Mannheimer et al., 1984; McMahon et al., 2005). Theoretically speaking, pain modulation is mediated through the opiate system when TENS-induced analgesia is reversed after injection of naloxone. If TENS-induced analgesia is not reversed by naloxone, then pain modulation is presumed to occur through other pain-modulating mechanisms, most likely through the spinal gate system described earlier. In summary, TENS-induced analgesia can occur through the spinal gate system or the DEOS (see Fig. 14-6). Modulation of pain via the spinal gate system implies the closing of the gate by the preferential electrical activation of large-diameter afferent A-beta fibers. Modulation of pain via the opiate system, on the other hand, implies the opening of the spinal gate by the preferential electrical activation of small-diameter A-delta and C fibers. This gate opening triggers the opiate system, which, via its negative loop, closes the gate by releasing more endorphins in the body.

D. RESEARCH-BASED INDICATIONS

The search for evidence behind the use of TENS, displayed in the *Research-Based Indications* box, led to the collection of 199 English peer-reviewed human clinical studies. The methodology and criteria used to assess the strength of evidence and therapeutic effectiveness are described in Chapter 2. As indicated, the strength of evidence is ranked as *strong* for several conditions, including postoperative abdominal pain, labor and post-labor pain, postoperative thoracic pain, osteoarthritis pain, dysmenorrheal pain, and postoperative orthopedic pain. It is *moderate* for low-back pain, neurogenic pain, chronic pain syndromes, stump/phantom pain, rheumatoid arthritis pain, and orofacial pain. Analysis is *pending* for all the other remaining health conditions because fewer than 5 studies could be collected. Over all conditions, the strength of evidence behind the use of TENS is found to be *moderate* and its therapeutic effectiveness *substantiated*.

IV. DOSIMETRY

Dosimetry associated with the application of TENS is based on the selection of one of the following five modes of delivery: conventional, acupuncture like, brief intense, burst, and modulation. Each mode, as described in Table 14-1, is characterized by the setting of three electrical parameters (pulse/burst duration, pulse/burst frequency, and current amplitude, all of which translating into four physiologic and therapeutic correlates (preferential fiber depolarization, preferential mechanism behind pain relief, onset of analgesia, and duration of analgesia).

A. CONVENTIONAL MODE

This mode involves delivery of electrical pulses with relatively short durations, high frequencies, and current amplitudes corresponding to sensory-level stimulation. It is called *conventional* because, by convention or clinical experience, clinicians usually select this mode to begin TENS therapy, as it is perceived by most patients as the most comfortable of all modes. This mode implies the preferential depolarization of large-diameter A-beta fibers using current amplitudes and pulse durations within the sensory-level range. Electrical stimulation is perceived as comfortable (pins and needles; tingling; no muscle contraction), and pain modulation occurs through the gate system. The onset of analgesia is relatively rapid, and analgesia itself is relatively brief.

B. ACUPUNCTURE-LIKE MODE

This mode refers to the delivery of electrical pulses with relatively long durations, low frequencies, and current amplitudes capable of sensory- and motor-level stimulation. It is described as *acupuncture-like* because the pulse frequency is low, resembling traditional needle acupuncture therapy, in which the practitioner slowly rotates the needle in the patient's skin. This mode implies the preferential and concomitant depolarization of afferent large-diameter A-beta and efferent alpha motor fibers innervating skeletal muscles. Electrical stimulation is perceived as tolerable as well as a mixed sensation of tingling and muscle contraction. Pain is presumed to occur via the opiate system. Onset of analgesia

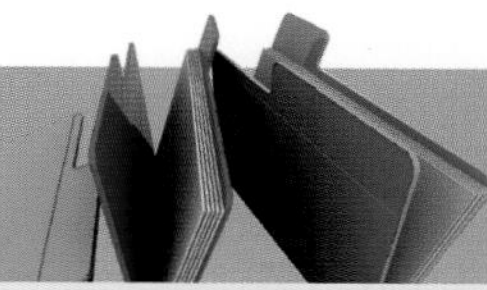

Research-Based Indications

TRANSCUTANEOUS ELECTRICAL NERVE STIMULATION

	Benefit—Yes		Benefit—No	
Health Condition	**Rating**	**Reference**	**Rating**	**Reference**
Postoperative abdominal pain	I	Desantana et al., 2009	I	Galloway et al., 1984
	I	Desantana et al., 2008	I	Cuschieri et al., 1985
	I	Cooperman et al., 1977	I	Conn et al., 1986
	I	Vander Ark et al., 1975	I	Reynolds et al., 1987
	I	Smith et al., 1986	I	Rawat et al., 1991
	I	Hargreaves et al., 1989	I	Taylor et al., 1983
	I	Hollinger, 1986	I	Laitinen et al., 1991
	I	Chen et al., 1998	I	Reuss et al., 1988
	I	Sims, 1991	I	Smedley et al., 1988
	I	Rosenberg et al., 1978	I	Gilbert et al., 1986
	I	Solomon et al., 1980		
	I	Hamza et al., 1999		
	II	Torres et al., 1992		
	II	Hymes et al., 1974		
	II	Caterine et al., 1988		
	II	Ali et al., 1981		
	II	Bussey et al., 1981		
	II	Merrill, 1987		
	II	Merrill, 1988		
	II	Merrill, 1989		
	II	Schomburg et al., 1983		

Strength of evidence: Strong
Therapeutic effectiveness: Substantiated

Health Condition	Rating	Reference	Rating	Reference
Low back pain	I	Melzack et al., 1983	I	Lehmann et al., 1986
	I	Cheing et al., 1999	I	Deyo et al., 1990
	I	Gemignani et al., 1991	I	Melzack et al., 1980
	I	Bertalanffy et al., 2005	I	Marchand et al., 1993
	I	Al-Smadi et al., 2003	I	Herman et al., 1994
	II	Bates et al., 1980	I	Warke et al., 2006
	II	Magora et al., 1978	II	Indeck et al., 1975
	II	Rao et al., 1981	II	Pope et al., 1994
	II	Fried et al., 1984		
	II	Brill et al., 1985		
	II	Fox et al., 1976		
	II	Ersek, 1976		
	II	Laitinen, 1976		
	II	Rutkowski et al., 1977		
	II	Ersek, 1977		
	II	Loeser et al., 1975		
	II	Thorsteinsson et al., 1977		
	II	Ebersold et al., 1975		
	III	Somers et al., 1999		

Strength of evidence: Moderate
Therapeutic effectiveness: Substantiated

Health Condition	Rating	Reference	Rating	Reference
Labor and post-labor pain	I	Harrison et al., 1987	I	Harrison et al., 1986
	I	Mannheimer et al., 1985	I	Lee et al., 1990
	I	Grim et al., 1985	I	Vander Ploeg et al., 1996
	I	Chao et al., 2007	I	Thomas et al., 1988
	II	Bundsen et al., 1981	I	Erkkola et al., 1980
	II	Bundsen et al., 1982	I	Chia et al., 1990
	II	Augustinsson et al., 1977	I	Nesheim, 1981
	II	Kaplan et al., 1998	II	Labrecque et al., 1999
	II	Bortoluzzi, 1989		
	II	Olsen et al., 2007		
	III	Keenan et al., 1985		

Strength of evidence: Strong
Therapeutic effectiveness: Conflicting

Health Condition	Rating	Reference	Rating	Reference
Postoperative thoracic pain	I	Cipriano et al., 2008	I	Foster et al., 1994
	I	Emmiler et al., 2008	I	Stubbing et al., 1988
	I	Bayindir et al., 1991	I	Lim et al., 1983
	I	Navarathnam et al., 1984		
	I	Warfield et al., 1985		
	I	Benedetti et al., 1997		

Health Condition	Benefit—Yes Rating	Benefit—Yes Reference	Benefit—No Rating	Benefit—No Reference
	I	Rooney et al., 1983		
	I	Erdogan et al., 2005		
	II	Solak et al., 2007		
	II	Ho et al., 1987		
	II	Neary, 1981		
	II	Klin et al., 1984		
	III	Carrol et al., 2001		
	III	Thorsen et al., 1997		
Strength of evidence: Strong **Therapeutic effectiveness:** Substantiated				
Osteoarthritis pain	I	Taylor et al., 1981	I	Lewis et al., 1994
	I	Fargas-Babjak et al., 1989	I	Law et al., 2004
	I	Smith et al., 1983a	I	Cheing et al., 2002
	I	Grimmer, 1992	II	Fargas-Babjak et al., 1992
	I	Lewis et al., 1984	II	Jensen et al., 1991
	I	Zizic et al., 1995		
	I	Cheing et al., 2003		
	I	Ng et al., 2003		
	II	Yurtkuran et al., 1999		
	II	Paker et al., 2006		
Strength of evidence: Strong **Therapeutic effectiveness:** Substantiated				
Neurogenic pain	I	Levin et al., 1992	I	Miller et al., 2007
	I	Potisk et al., 1995		
	I	Sonde et al., 1998		
	I	Cheing et al., 2005		
	II	Bajd et al., 1985		
	II	Tekeoglu et al., 1998		
	II	Robaina et al., 1989		
	II	Nathan et al., 1974		
	II	Richardson et al., 1980		
	III	Bodenheim et al., 1983		
	III	Ashwal et al., 1988		
	II	Leijon et al., 1989		
	III	Foley-Nolan et al., 1990		
	III	Frampton, 1996		
Strength of evidence: Moderate **Therapeutic effectiveness:** Substantiated				
Chronic pain syndromes	II	Bates et al., 1980	I	Oosterhof et al., 2006
	II	Fishbain et al., 1996		
	II	Abram et al., 1981		
	II	Tulgar et al., 1991		
	II	Guieu et al., 1991		
	II	Chabal et al., 1998		
	II	Long, 1974		
	II	Meyler et al., 1994		
	II	Eriksson et al., 1979		
	II	Loeser et al., 1975		
	II	Koke et al., 2004		
Strength of evidence: Moderate **Therapeutic effectiveness:** Substantiated				
Stump/phantom pain	I	Finsen et al., 1988		
	II	Katz et al., 1991		
	II	Winnem et al., 1982		
	II	Carabelli et al., 1985		
	II	Miles et al., 1978		
	III	Györi et al., 1977		
	III	Katz et al., 1989		
	III	Giuffrida et al., 2009		
	III	Hirano et al., 1988		
	III	Kawamura et al., 1997		
Strength of evidence: Moderate **Therapeutic effectiveness:** Substantiated				
Dysmenorrheal pain	I	Lundeberg et al., 1985		
	I	Dawood et al., 1990		
	I	Mannheimer et al., 1985		
	I	Milsom et al., 1994		
	I	Neighbors et al., 1987		
	I	Lewers et al., 1989		
	II	Smith et al., 1991		
	II	Kaplan et al., 1994		
	II	Kaplan et al., 1997		
	II	Schietz et al., 2007		
Strength of evidence: Strong **Therapeutic effectiveness:** Substantiated				

Health Condition	Benefit—Yes Rating	Benefit—Yes Reference	Benefit—No Rating	Benefit—No Reference
Postoperative orthopedic pain	I	Arvidsson et al., 1986	I	Walker et al., 1991
	I	Jensen et al., 1985	I	Angulo et al., 1990
	I	Cornell et al., 1984	I	Breit et al., 2004
	I	Lang et al., 2007		
	II	Harvie, 1979		
	II	Smith et al., 1983b		
Strength of evidence: Strong **Therapeutic effectiveness:** Substantiated				
Rheumatoid arthritis pain	I	Abelson et al., 1983	I	Langley et al., 1984
	II	Mannheimer et al., 1979	I	Moystad et al., 1990
	II	Mannheimer et al., 1978		
	II	Bruce et al., 1988		
	II	Kumar et al., 1982		
	II	Vinterberg et al., 1978		
Strength of evidence: Moderate **Therapeutic effectiveness:** Substantiated				
Orofacial pain	I	Hansson et al., 1983		
	II	Hansson et al., 1986		
	II	Pike, 1978		
	II	Stabile et al., 1978		
	II	Eriksson et al., 1984		
	III	Murphy, 1990		
Strength of evidence: Moderate **Therapeutic effectiveness:** Substantiated				
Fewer Than 5 Studies				
Postoperative spinal pain	I	Solomon et al., 1980	II	McCallum et al., 1988
	II	Schuster et al., 1980		
	II	Issenman et al., 1985		
Myofascial pain	I	Graff-Radford et al., 1989	I	Kruger et al., 1998
	I	Hsueh et al., 1997		
Detrusor muscle pain	II	Okada et al., 1998		
	II	Hasan et al., 1996		
Posttraumatic pain	I	Ordog, 1987		
	II	Sloan et al., 1986		
Hemorrhoidectomy pain	I	Chiu et al., 1999		
Painful open perineal lesions	III	Merkel et al., 1999		
Neck pain	I	Nordemar et al., 1981		
Painful shoulder	I	Leandri et al., 1990		
Unstable angina pectoris pain	I	Borjesson et al., 1997		
Chronic intractable angina	II	Nitz et al., 1993		
Temporomandibular pain			II	Linde et al., 1995
Renal colic pain	I	Mora et al., 2006		
Minor rib fracture	I	Oncel et al., 2002		
Strength of evidence: Pending **Therapeutic effectiveness:** Pending				
ALL CONDITIONS **Strength of evidence:** Moderate **Therapeutic effectiveness:** Substantiated				

is relatively slow, and analgesia is sustained for a relatively long period.

C. BRIEF-INTENSE MODE

This mode involves the delivery of electrical pulses with relatively long durations, high frequencies, and current amplitudes capable of noxious stimulation (see Table 14-1). It is described as *brief intense* because durations of application are briefer and current amplitudes much higher, or more intense, than in the other modes, triggering a somewhat brief yet intense, and sometimes painful, stimulation during therapy. This mode implies the preferential depolarization of all nerve fibers (A-beta, A-delta, and C fibers), causing a mixed sensation of strong muscle contraction and maximum tolerable pain. Pain modulation occurs through the opiate system. The onset of analgesia is relatively rapid, and analgesia is sustained for a relatively long period.

D. BURST MODE

This mode refers to the delivery of bursts of pulses of relatively low burst frequencies, with current amplitudes capable of sensory and motor stimulation (see Table 14-1). It is described as *burst* to emphasize the use of bursts of pulses rather than individual pulses. This mode implies the preferential depolarization of sensory A-delta and motor alpha fibers. Electrical stimulation is felt as a mixed sensation of tingling and moderate motor contraction. Pain modulation occurs through the opiate system. The onset of analgesia is relatively slow, and analgesia is sustained for a relatively long period.

TABLE 14-1 MODES OF TRANSCUTANEOUS ELECTRICAL NERVE STIMULATION

	Mode				
Characteristic	**Conventional**	**Acupuncture Like**	**Brief Intense**	**Burst**	**Modulation**
Pulse duration	Short (<150 μs)	Long (>150 μs)	Long (>150 μs)		Variable
Burst duration				Long (>150 μs)	Variable
Frequency	High (>80 pps—Hz)	Low (<10 pps—Hz)	High (>80 pps—Hz)	Low (<10 bups)	Variable
Current amplitude	Comfortable	Comfortable/tolerable	Tolerable	Comfortable	Variable
Perception level	Sensory	Sensory/Motor	Noxious	Sensory/Motor	Variable
Nerve fibers preferentially depolarized	A-beta	A-delta and C	A-delta and C	A-delta and C	Variable
Preferential mechanism for pain modulation	Gate	Opiate	Opiate	Opiate	Variable
Onset of analgesia	Rapid (<30 min)	Slow (>30 min)	Rapid (<30 min)	Slow (>30 min)	Variable
Duration of analgesia	Brief (< few hours)	Long (> few hours)	Long (> few hours)	Long (> few hours)	Variable
Application duration			From 30–180 min		
Treatment frequency			Single to multiple applications per day, over weeks and sometimes months		

See the **Online Dosage Calculator: Transcutaneous Electrical Nerve Stimulation.**

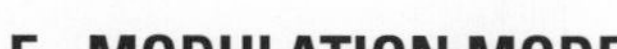

E. MODULATION MODE

This last mode calls upon the random electronic modulation of pulse duration, pulse frequency, and current amplitude (see Table 14-1). It is called *modulation* because one, or two, or all three stimulation parameters are electronically, and randomly, modulated at the same time during therapy, as illustrated in Figure 14-8. This mode is presumed to decrease brain (sensation) and nerve (depolarization) *habituation* to electrical input. Because there is a variable modulation (cycles of increasing and decreasing values), variability is expected to occur with regard to the types of fibers preferentially depolarized and the pain modulation present, as well as the onset and duration of analgesia.

F. APPLICATION DURATION AND TREATMENT FREQUENCY

Two other dosimetric parameters to consider are *application duration* and *treatment frequency* (see Table 14-1). The literature suggests that the application duration of TENS may range between 30 minutes and 3 hours depending of the severity of pain. The golden rule is that TENS should be applied until the patient reports satisfactory pain relief. If no pain relief is achieved using a given mode, another mode of stimulation should be used instead of prolonging the application duration of the initial mode. Treatment frequency may range between single and multiple applications per day, again depending of the severity of pain. Because there is no side effect associated with the application of TENS, patients may receive multiple daily applications over several weeks and months for the management of their pain conditions.

G. WHICH MODE IS BEST?

The current body of evidence does not support the view that one mode of TENS delivery is better than any other for any painful pathologic conditions. Evidence obtained from long-term users of TENS therapy reveals no correlation between patient, site, and cause of pain versus TENS mode selection (Johnson et al., 1991; Persson et al., 2010). The selection of one mode in preference to the other, therefore, is still based on trial and error and

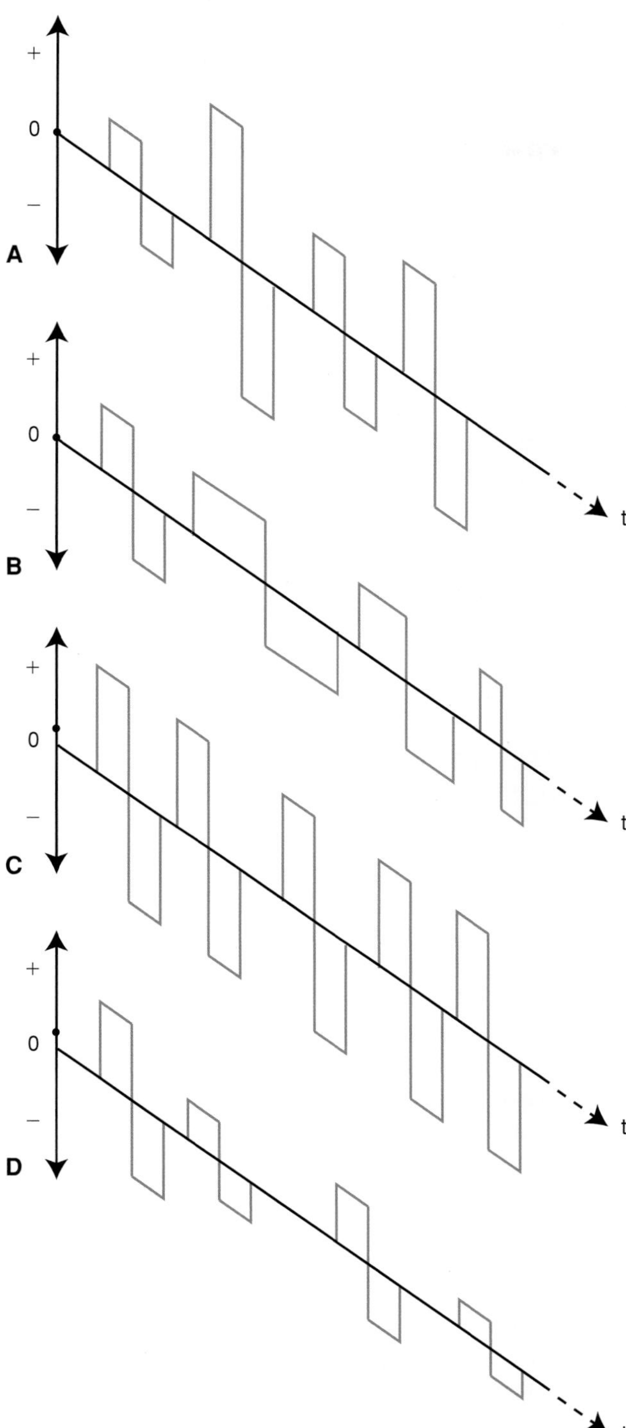

FIGURE 14-8 Modulation mode showing examples of current amplitude modulation (**A**), pulse duration modulation (**B**), pulse frequency modulation (**C**), and pulse amplitude combined with pulse frequency modulation (**D**).

the patient's comfort during therapy (Johnson et al., 1991; Persson et al., 2010). This explains why the general recommendation is to begin therapy with the conventional mode, because it is perceived as being more comfortable than the other four modes of TENS. Articles by Bjordal et al. (2003), Johnson et al. (2007), and Persson et al. (2010) suggest that TENS therapy, regardless of mode of delivery, can provide significant pain relief and, as a result, presents as a viable alternative to drug and surgical therapy.

H. ONLINE DOSAGE CALCULATOR: TRANSCUTANEOUS ELECTRICAL NERVE STIMULATION

As presented earlier, to set up the multiple dosimetric parameters related to the application of TENS requires the use of several formulas and implies multiple calculations. To facilitate dosimetry, this textbook offers the **Online Dosage Calculator: Transcutaneous Electrical Nerve Stimulation.** Log on, select the type of current, enter parameters, and let the calculator do the work for you!

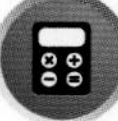

V. APPLICATION, CONTRAINDICATIONS, AND RISKS

Prior to considering the application of TENS, practitioners must first check for contraindications, consider the risks, and then go through key application steps and procedures designed to optimize treatment safety, efficacy, and effectiveness. As discussed next, several important elements need to be taken into consideration to achieve optimal application. The issue related to the application of TENS on people wearing implanted pacemakers and implantable cardioverter-defibrillators (ICDs) deserves particular attention, because of the continued controversy (Eriksson et al., 1978; Kimberley et al., 1987; Hauptman et al., 1992; Sliwa et al., 1996; Weitz et al., 1997; Glotzer et al., 1998; Philbin et al., 1998; Curwin et al., 1999; Broadley, 2000).

A. PACEMAKERS

These electronic devices are prescribed for people of all ages who have an abnormal heart rate (e.g., slower or faster than average, or irregular beating patterns). Their purpose is to ensure a normal heart rate, or to pace the heart. There are several models of pacemakers on the market today. For example, Medtronic Inc., one of the leading manufacturers of pacemakers in the world, offers six different categories of pacemakers that cardiologists and heart surgeons can choose from to treat their cardiac patients. There are presently two basic types of pacemakers commonly implanted in cardiac patients: fixed and rate responsive.

1. Fixed Type

Early pacemakers were of the *fixed* type, also known as asynchronous type, in that they continuously paced the heart at a set fixed rate. These pacemakers have been shown to be *unaffected* by TENS application (Jones, 1976; Eriksson et al., 1978; Shade, 1985; Rasmussen et al., 1988; Chen et al., 1990). The use of TENS, therefore, is not contraindicated in patients with implanted fixed-type pacemakers.

2. Rate-Responsive Type

Newer pacemakers are of the *rate-responsive* type, also known as synchronous or demand type. This type of pacemaker is needed when the heart cannot appropriately increases it own rate according to a person's needs. This pacemaker varies the pacing rate depending on a person's level of activity, respiration, or other factors. Most pacemakers implanted today are rate responsive because they respond to the body's needs, similar to how a healthy heart works. The pacemaker automatically adjusts the pacing rate to match the level of activity, including periods of time during which the patient is at rest or sleeping. **Rate-responsive pacemakers, unfortunately, can be affected by TENS** (Jones, 1976; Eriksson et al., 1978; Chen et al., 1990). Medtronic Inc. (www.medtronic.com) lists the use of TENS under precaution, meaning that there could be electronic interference in the pacemaker due to the electrical field generated by the TENS unit. This interference means that no pacing beat, or extra pacing beats, may be generated by the pacemaker that can seriously affecting heart function. Considering that the patient's safety always come first, this textbook states that the use of TENS on patients wearing rate-responsive pacemakers is *contraindicated, unless* a screening heart monitoring test, using electrocardiography (ECG), reveals no interference during TENS application (see the Application, Contraindications, and Risks box). Although testing heart and pacemaker functions by monitoring ECG during TENS application must be done as a screening test, research has shown that TENS may cause ECG artifacts that may be *wrongly* interpreted as pacemaker dysfunction (Kimberley et al., 1987; Hauptman et al., 1992; Sliwa et al., 1996; Weitz et al., 1997; Marples, 2000). This finding only reinforces the need to have the treating cardiologist's authorization before considering TENS therapy in these patients.

B. CARDIOVERTER-DEFIBRILLATORS

ICDs are prescribed for people who have a faster-than-normal heart rate, or tachycardia, as well as for patients suffering from ventricular fibrillation. For example, when tachycardia occurs, the ICD device immediately delivers a mild shock to the heart, redirecting its rhythm to a normal beating pattern. Interference between TENS units and ICD devices has been reported in numerous case reports (Glotzer et al., 1998; Philbin et al., 1998; Pyatt et al., 2003; Siu et al., 2005; Occhetta et al., 2006; Holmgren et al., 2008). Consequently, the use of TENS in patients with ICDs is *contraindicated, unless* the unit is turned off during the application (see the Application, Contraindications, and Risks box). To ensure maximal safety during TENS therapy with patients wearing pacemakers or ICDs, practitioners should always refer to the manufacturers' lists of contraindications, precautions, and warnings regarding the use of this therapeutic agent with such devices.

C. CONTACT DERMATITIS

One of the most common risks associated with TENS therapy is the development of skin contact dermatitis caused by repeated electrode applications over the same skin areas. A precaution to take in such a case is to change electrode placement from week or week, thus avoiding constant application over the same skin surface area. Another important precaution to take is to monitor the patient's analgesic drug intake in order to determine which of the two treatments, TENS or analgesic drug, best modulates pain.

D. SKIN PREPARATION AND ELECTRODE CONSIDERATIONS

As is the case for the application of NMES, important application issues such as skin preparation, electrode and cable, electrode coupling, electrode current density, and electrode spacing need consideration. To avoid duplication of this information, see the Therapeutic Effects and Indications section in Chapter 13 for further discussion.

E. ELECTRODE CONFIGURATION AND PLACEMENT

Much has been written and discussed about electrode configuration and placement relative to the treatment of pain using TENS therapy. The controversy still exists as to which configuration and placement are best to use for pain modulation. Evidence from the published literature indicates that bipolar, quadripolar, and multipolar electrode configurations are routinely used in clinics (see the Electrode Configuration section in Chapter 13). Practically speaking, the larger the painful area, the greater the number of electrodes used for treatment. As far as electrode placement is concerned, the evidence suggests the following four options. First, electrode placement may be over, or on top of, the painful area. Second, placement may be around the painful area. Third, electrode placement may be along the dermatome(s) associated with the painful area. Fourth, placement may over acupuncture points and trigger points. There is still no evidence to show that one placement is better than the other. Until more evidence is provided, practitioners must continue to rely on trial and error when considering the best electrode placement with their patients.

F. ELECTRODE AND CABLE MAINTENANCE

As is the case with the application of NMES, electrodes and cables, over time and with repeated use, will become less flexible and show signs of degradation (e.g., breaks, cracks). Visual inspection and periodic checks of electrode electric resistance and cable electric continuity, using a multimeter, are highly recommended in order to optimize treatment efficacy.

APPLICATION, CONTRAINDICATIONS, AND RISKS

Transcutaneous Electrical Nerve Stimulation

IMPORTANT: There is a risk of electronic interference between transcutaneous electrical nerve stimulation (TENS) units and rate-responsive pacemakers or implanted cardioverter-defibrillators (ICDs) (Eriksson et al., 1978; Rasmussen et al., 1988; Glotzer et al., 1998; Philbin et al., 1998; Marples, 2000; Pyatt et al., 2003; Siu et al., 2005; Occheta et al., 2006; Holmgren et al., 2008). TENS can be used with these patients *only if,* after cardiac monitoring during treatment, the electrocardiography (ECG) recording reveals no interference (Chen et al., 1990). **If no such cardiac monitoring is available in your working facility, obtain authorization from the patient's treating cardiologist before using TENS.** Note that TENS can be used with patients wearing rate-responsive pacemakers or ICDs **only** if the ICD unit is *turned off during* therapy (Glotzer et al., 1998). Monitor the patient's analgesic drug intake throughout TENS therapy to determine if pain modulation is more attributable to TENS than to drug therapy. Discuss with the treating physician if your patient should continue or discontinue intake of painkillers during the course of TENS therapy.

 See **online video.**

STEP	RATIONALE
1. Check for contraindications.	*Over anterior cervical area*—stimulation of key organs, such as the vagus nerve, phrenic nerve, and carotid sinuses, resulting in adverse effects such as hypotensive reaction and laryngeal spasm
	Over thoracic area—affects normal heart function
	Over cranial area—affects normal brain function
	With patients wearing rate-responsive or demand-type pacemakers or ICDs—risk of interference with normal functioning of the device (Eriksson et al., 1978; Rasmussen et al., 1988; Glotzer et al., 1998; Philbin et al., 1998; Marples, 2000; Pyatt et al., 2003; Siu et al., 2005; Occheta et al., 2006; Holmgren et al., 2008). Note that TENS can be used with these patients *only* after cardiac monitoring during TENS, by means of ECG, reveals no interference (Chen et al., 1990). If no such cardiac monitoring is available in your working facility, obtain authorization from the patient's treating cardiologist before using TENS. Furthermore, TENS can be used with these patients *only* if the ICD unit is *turned off* during therapy (Glotzer et al., 1998).
	Over abdominal, pelvic, or lumbar areas of pregnant women in their first trimester—induces labor
	Over metal implants—causes unnecessary pain due to electrical current-induced overheating of implants
	In patients who are epileptic—causes epileptic episode (Scherder et al., 1999)
	Over hemorrhagic area—enhances bleeding due to increased blood flow in the treated area
	Over cancerous areas—increases and spreads the tumor due to increased blood flow in the treated area
	In patients who are confused and unreliable—complications during therapy that decrease treatment effectiveness
	Over damaged skin—causes unnecessary and severe pain
2. Consider the risks.	*Contact dermatitis and burn*—prolonged use of electrode, electroconductive gel, and adhesive tape over the same skin areas increases the risk of causing contact dermatitis from the materials of which the electrode, gel, and adhesive tape are composed (Fisher, 1978; Zugerman, 1982; Castelain et al., 1986; Marren et al., 1991; Dwyer et al., 1994; Meuleman et al., 1996; Corazza et al., 1999)
	Stimulator electronic interference—keep all TENS units at least 3 m (10 ft) away from any functioning shortwave diathermy device

STEP	RATIONALE
3. Position and instruct patient.	Ensure comfortable body positioning. Instruct the patient not to touch the device, cables, and applicators and to call for assistance if necessary.
4. Prepare treated area.	Clean the skin surface in the area of the stimulating electrodes with rubbing alcohol, or water and soap, to remove impurities and reduce skin impedance. Clip hair to ensure optimal electrode–skin coupling.
5. Select stimulator type.	Choose between cabinet (in clinic therapy) or portable (bedside or home therapy) device. Plug line-powered stimulators into ground-fault circuit interrupter (GFCI) receptacles to prevent the risk of macroshock leading to electrocution (see Chapter 5).
6. Select mode of delivery.	Select between the following modes: conventional, acupuncture like, brief intense, burst, or modulation (see Table 14-1). *Conventional mode* is often selected to begin therapy because the sensation of electrical stimulation is felt as comfortable. If this mode fails to decrease pain after a few treatments, select another mode. Note that there is no evidence to suggest that one mode of delivery is better than the other for the treatment of any given pathology.
7. Select electrode type.	*For postoperative conditions:* Use sterile, disposable electrodes. *For all the other conditions:* Use reusable, nonsterile electrodes. Use electrodes that best suit the localization and size of the treated area.
8. Prepare stimulating electrode.	Cover surface with a thin and evenly distributed coating of electroconductive gel to optimize conduction at the electrode–skin interface. Note that sterile electrodes are pre-gelled. Nonsterile electrodes can also be pre-gelled and ready for use.
9. Place the electrodes.	Select one the following electrode placements: (1) on top of the painful area, (2) around the painful area, (3) along the dermatome(s) corresponding to the painful area, (4) over acupuncture points, and (5) over trigger points. Regularly change electrode placement to avoid contact dermatitis.
10. Attach and connect electrodes.	Attach the electrode to the skin using hypoallergic tapes or pre-cut self-adhesive patches. Connect the electrodes to the stimulator circuit outputs using either regular or bifurcated lead wires or cables of various lengths.
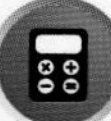 **11. Set dosimetry.**	Set pulse/burst duration, pulse/burst frequency and current amplitude based on the biophysical and physiologic elements presented in Table 14-1. Settings will depend of your choice of mode of delivery. Use the **Online Dosage Calculator: Transcutaneous Electrical Nerve Stimulation.**
12. Apply treatment.	Ensure adequate monitoring. If home treatment, use a portable battery-operated device, and make sure to give to your patient a written sheet of directives to follow with regard to the overall application of TENS.
13. Conduct post-treatment inspection.	Remove the electrodes. Inspect the skin area exposed to the electrodes for any unexpected response. Wash and dry the treated surface areas. Wash and dry reusable electrodes.
14. Ensure post-treatment equipment maintenance.	Follow manufacturer recommendations. Immediately report defects or malfunctions to technical maintenance staff. Routine use of reusable electrodes requires that clinicians adopt a strict maintenance program, including frequent visual inspection and periodic measurement of electrode resistance and cable continuity using a multimeter. Wash and dry reusable electrodes after each treatment to ensure optimal efficacy. Check cables and electrodes regularly for visible wear and tear to ensure optimal efficacy and prevent macroshock if line-powered stimulators are used. Check electrode impedance monthly to ensure optimal electric conduction, because electrodes will deteriorate with use and time. Use an ohmmeter to check impedance. Discard all reusable electrodes after 6 months of use. Transmission of microorganisms is likely if suction electrodes and sponges are used; these should be disinfected with 70% isopropyl alcohol after treatment of each patient to avoid cross-infection from one patient to another.

CASE STUDIES

Presented are two case studies that summarize the concepts, principles, and applications of TENS discussed in this chapter. Case Study 14-1 addresses its use for labor pain. Case Study 14-2 is concerned with the application of TENS for postoperative abdominal pain following cholecystectomy. Each case is structured in line with the concepts of evidence-based practice (EBP), the International Classification of Functioning, Disability, and Health (ICF) disablement model, and SOAP (*s*ubjective, *o*bjective, *a*ssessment, *p*lan) note format (see Chapter 2 for details).

CASE STUDY 14-1: LABOR PAIN

EVIDENCE-BASED CLINICAL DECISION MAKING PROTOCOL

1. Formulate Case History

A healthy 24-year-old woman just arrived at the maternity ward, ready to deliver her first child. Her main wish is to deliver normally—that is, without epidural analgesia. A close girlfriend told her about the benefit of using TENS for labor pain management. She wants this noninvasive pain treatment during all stages of labor.

2. Outline the Case Based on the ICF Framework

LABOR PAIN		
BODY STRUCTURES AND FUNCTIONS	**ACTIVITIES**	**PARTICIPATION**
Labor pain	Wants normal delivery	Fully dedicated to the labor task

PERSONAL FACTORS	ENVIRONMENTAL FACTORS
Healthy young woman	Housewife
Normal pregnancy—minimal risk	Family and work
	Maternity ward

3. Outline Therapeutic Goals and Outcome Measurements

GOAL	OUTCOME MEASUREMENT
Decrease pain	Visual Analogue Scale (VAS)
Satisfaction with pain relief	Self-reported 24h00 after birth—scale of 10 (10 maximum satisfaction and willingness)

4. Justify the Use of Transcutaneous Electrical Nerve Stimulation Based on the EBP Framework

PRACTITIONER'S EXPERIENCE	RESEARCH-BASED INDICATIONS	PATIENT'S EXPECTATION
Experienced in TENS	*Strength:* Conflicting	Is convinced that TENS will be beneficial
Has used TENS occasionally in similar cases	*Effectiveness:* Conflicting	Wants to avoid epidural analgesia
Believes that TENS may be beneficial		Willingness to use TENS during next pregnancy

5. Outline Key Intervention Parameters

- **Treatment base:** Hospital based
- **Electrical current:** Biphasic burst modulated; symmetrical and balanced waveform (see Fig. 14-4B)
- **Stimulator type:** Portable battery-operated device for bedside application (maternity ward)
- **TENS mode:** Burst (see Table 14-1). This mode is chosen because it can enhance the endogenous opiate system, triggering endorphin release and a longer-lasting period of analgesia.
- **Application protocol:** Follow the suggested application protocol in *Application, Contraindications, and Risks* box, and make the necessary adjustments for this case.
- **Patient's positioning:** Patient is free to adopt any position she likes during treatment because she carries the stimulator in her hand.
- **Burst duration:** 250 μs
- **Burst frequency:** 5 bups
- **Current amplitude:** To comfortable level, below visible contraction
- **Electrode type:** Nonsterile, disposable, pre-gelled, auto-adhesive; electrode
- **Electrode number and size:** 4 electrodes (2 pairs); 5 × 10 cm (2 × 4 in)
- **Electrode placement:** Bilaterally at T10 and S2, respectively
- **Application duration:** 30 minutes
- **Treatment frequency:** Multiple applications; as needed until end of labor (complete cervical dilatation)
- **Concomitant therapies:** None
- Use the **Online Dosage Calculator: Transcutaneous Electrical Nerve Stimulation.**

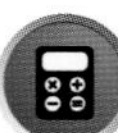

6. Report Pre- and Post-Intervention Outcomes

OUTCOME	PRE	POST
Pain (VAS score)	7/10	2/10
Satisfaction with pain relief and willingness to reuse TENS (score)		8/10

7. Document Case Intervention Using the SOAP Note Format

S: Young woman ready to deliver her first child in the maternity ward. Pt wants normal delivery and also wants to avoid epidural analgesia.

O: *Intervention*: TENS applied over the lower back area; biphasic burst-modulated current; burst duration: 250 μs; burst frequency: 5 bups; current amplitude to comfortable level, electrode placement: 4 electrodes placed bilaterally at T10 and S2; application duration: 30 min; repeated applications as needed until end of labor. *Pre–post comparison*: Decrease pain VAS score (7/10 to 2/10). Pt reported high satisfaction (8/10) with TENS-induced pain relief, and expressed the desire to use it again in her next pregnancy.

A: No adverse effect. Treatment very well tolerated. Pt very satisfied with results.

P: No further treatment required. Patient discharged.

CASE STUDY 14-2: POSTOPERATIVE ABDOMINAL PAIN

EVIDENCE-BASED CLINICAL DECISION MAKING PROTOCOL

1. Formulate the Case History

A 58-year-old man wearing an ICD is resting in his hospital room following an open cholecystectomy (gallbladder removal), performed a few hours ago. Postoperative pain management is done using a patient-controlled analgesia device. The device is programmed to deliver set boluses of morphine at different lockout intervals. The surgeon is aware that this patient has a history of experiencing opiate-related side effects, such as nausea, vomiting, dizziness, and depressed respiration. His goal is to provide the patient with adequate postoperative abdominal pain relief while minimizing the opiate-related side effects. The patient is instructed to request the prescribed narcotics when needed. The surgeon consults you to see if an additional nonpharmacologic pain therapy, with no side effects, can be used to manage the patient's postoperative abdominal pain. You propose using TENS therapy until the patient is discharged from the hospital. Your main goal is to decrease postoperative opiate analgesic requirements and opiate-related side effects while providing adequate pain relief. Your secondary goal is to increase patient's alertness, mobility, and return to work.

2. Outline the Case Based on the ICF Framework

POSTOPERATIVE ABDOMINAL PAIN		
BODY STRUCTURES AND FUNCTIONS	**ACTIVITIES**	**PARTICIPATION**
Acute pain	Difficulty with trunk mobility, sitting, and walking	Hospitalized; unable to perform activities of daily living (ADLs) and work

PERSONAL FACTORS	ENVIRONMENTAL FACTORS
Middle-aged woman	Housewife
History of heart problems	Family and work
Low education	Hospitalized

3. Outline Therapeutic Goals and Outcome Measurements

GOAL	OUTCOME MEASUREMENT
Decrease pain	Visual Analogue Scale (VAS)
Decrease opiate boluses	Monitoring daily number of nausea and vomiting episodes
Decrease pain disability	Pain Disability Index (PDI)

4. Justify the Use of Transcutaneous Electrical Nerve Stimulation Based on the EBP Framework

PRACTITIONER'S EXPERIENCE	RESEARCH-BASED INDICATIONS	PATIENT'S EXPECTATION
Experienced in TENS	*Strength:* Strong	No opinion on TENS
Has used TENS in similar cases	*Effectiveness:* Substantiated	Just wants pain relief with minimal side effects
Is convinced that TENS can be beneficial		

5. Outline Key Intervention Parameters

- **Treatment base:** Hospital
- **Electrical current:** Biphasic pulse modulated; symmetrical, balanced with rectangular shape (see Fig. 14-4A)
- **Stimulator type:** Portable battery-operated device for bedside application
- **Contraindication?:** Although the patient wears an ICD, TENS is not contraindicated here because the treating cardiologist has authorized the *deactivation* of the ICD during each treatment session.
- **TENS mode:** Acupuncture like (see Table 14-1). This mode is chosen because it can enhance the endogenous opiate system, triggering endorphin release and a longer-lasting period of analgesia. Sterile disposable electrodes are used in order to minimize wound infection. Electrodes are kept in place during the whole period, separating wound bandaging, and are replaced with each bandaging session.
- **Application protocol:** Follow the suggested application protocol in *Application, Contraindications, and Risks* box, and make the necessary adjustments for this case.
- **Patient's positioning:** Lying supine in bed—bedside treatment
- **Pulse duration:** 200 μs
- **Pulse frequency:** 8 pps (Hz)
- **Current amplitude:** To comfortable level, below visible contraction
- **Electrode type:** Sterile, disposable, pre-gelled, auto-adhesive; electrode removed and reapplied every 24 hours
- **Electrode number and size:** 2 electrodes; 2.5 × 5 cm (1 × 2 in)
- **Electrode placement:** Around the painful area; in this case para-incisional (i.e., above and below the surgical incision)

- **Application duration:** Approximately 90 minutes, sometimes longer, or until satisfactory pain relief is achieved
- **Treatment frequency:** Daily, every 4 to 6 hours, or when pain relief is needed; until released from hospital
- **Concomitant therapies:** Narcotic bolus infusion
- Use the **Online Dosage Calculator: Transcutaneous Electrical Nerve Stimulation.**

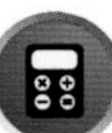

6. Report Pre- and Post-Intervention Outcomes

OUTCOME	PRE	POST
Pain (VAS score)	8/10	4/10
Narcotic intake		Decrease by 70%
Narcotic-related side effect episodes		Decreased by 80%
Pain Disability Index (PDI)		Decreased by 85%

7. Document Case Intervention Using the SOAP Note Format

S: Middle-aged male Pt wearing an ICD is resting in bed after cholecystectomy. Pt presents severe reactions to narcotics. The objective is to decrease the side effects of morphine-induced analgesia by modulating pain with TENS.

O: *Intervention:* TENS applied over the abdominal area; biphasic pulse-modulated current; pulse duration: 200 µs; pulse frequency: 8 pps; current amplitude to comfortable level; electrode placement: 2 electrodes placed above and below the incision area, respectively; application duration and frequency: repeated application until satisfactory pain relief. *Pre–post comparison:* Decrease pain (8/10 to 4/10), decrease narcotic intake (70%), decrease narcotic-related side effects (80%), and decrease pain disability index (85%).

A: No adverse effect. Treatment very well tolerated. Pt satisfied with results.

P: Pt discharged from hospital. Pt will continue TENS therapy at home until satisfactory pain relief is obtained.

VI. THE BOTTOM LINE

- There is moderate to strong scientific evidence to show that TENS can induce significant pain modulation for several pain conditions, including post-surgical conditions.
- TENS is the delivery of electrical current through the skin, causing sensory, motor, and nociceptive nerve depolarization, which in turn trigger the gate and opiate systems for pain modulation.
- TENS is commonly applied using biphasic pulsed current; the current may be pulse- or burst modulated.
- TENS is delivered using the following modes: conventional, acupuncture like, brief intense, burst, and modulation. There is no evidence to show that one mode is better than the other.
- Of all dosimetric parameters and based on the S/D curve, pulse/burst duration (D) and current amplitude (S) may be the most important because their settings allow the preferential depolarization of either sensory, sensory-motor, or sensory-motor-nociceptive nerve fibers.
- Electrode placement may be as follows: on top of the painful area, around the painful area, along the dermatome(s) corresponding to the painful area, over acupuncture points, or over trigger points. There is no evidence to show that one electrode placement is better than the other.
- All line-powered TENS devices must be plugged into ground fault circuit interrupter (GFCI) receptacles to prevent macroshock.
- Skin surface preparation before each treatment and periodic calibration of electric stimulators, including electrode resistance and cable continuity checks using a multimeter, are strongly recommended to ensure optimal treatment efficacy.
- Using the **Online Dosage Calculator: Transcutaneous Electrical Nerve Stimulation** removes the burden of hand calculation and promotes the adoption of quantitative dosimetry.
- The overall body of evidence reported in this chapter shows the strength of evidence behind TENS to be *moderate* and its level of therapeutic effectiveness *substantiated.*

VII. CRITICAL THINKING QUESTIONS

Clarification: What is meant by transcutaneous electrical nerve stimulation (TENS) therapy?

Assumptions: You assume that the TENS stimulator can be programmed such that it will trigger the spinal gate system without simultaneously triggering the DEOS. How do you justify making that assumption?

Reasons and evidence: What leads you to believe that TENS therapy could decrease pain without any side effects?

Viewpoints or perspectives: How would you respond to a colleague who says that there is no way to scientifically determine whether the analgesic effect caused by TENS therapy is modulated or not via the release of endorphins in the body?

Implications and consequences: What are the implications and consequences of using TENS therapy in (1) a patient implanted with a rate-responsive–type pacemaker and (2) in a patient with an ICD?

About the question: Why is it that the electrical waveforms generated by TENS units can be delivered daily, for a few hours at a time, and for several weeks, with a minimal risk of causing contact dermatitis? Why do you think I ask this question?

VIII. REFERENCES

Articles

Abelson K, Langley GB, Sheppeard H, Vlieg M, Wigley RD (1983) Transcutaneous electrical nerve stimulation in rheumatoid arthritis. N Z Med J, 96: 156–158

Abram SE, Reynolds AC, Cusick JF (1981) Failure of naloxone to reverse analgesia from transcutaneous electrical stimulation in patients with chronic pain. Anesth Analg, 60: 81–84

Ali J, Yaffe CS, Serrette C (1981) The effect of transcutaneous electric nerve stimulation on postoperative pain and pulmonary function. Surgery, 89: 507–512

Al-Smadi J, Warke K, Wilson I, Cramp AF, Noble G, Walsh DM (2003). A pilot investigation of the hypoalgesic effects of transcutaneous electrical nerve stimulation upon low back pain in people with multiple sclerosis. Clin Rehabil, 17: 742–749

Angulo DL, Colwell CW (1990) Use of postoperative TENS and continuous passive motion following total knee replacement. J Orthop Sports Phys Ther, 11: 599–604

Arvidsson J, Eriksson E (1986) Postoperative TENS pain relief after knee surgery: Objective evaluation. Orthopedics, 9: 1346–1351

Ashwal S, Tomasi L, Neumann M, Schneider S (1988) Reflex sympathetic dystrophy syndrome in children. Pediatr Neurol, 4: 38–42

Augustinsson LE, Bohlin P, Bundsen P, Carlsson CA, Forssman L, Sjöberg P, Tyreman NO (1977) Pain relief during delivery by transcutaneous electrical nerve stimulation. Pain, 4: 59–65

Bajd T, Gregoric M, Vodovnik L, Benko H (1985) Electrical stimulation in treating spasticity resulting from spinal cord injury. Arch Phys Med Rehab, 66: 515–517

Bates JAV, Nathan PW (1980) Transcutaneous electrical nerve stimulation for chronic pain. Anaesthesia, 35: 817–822

Bayindir O, Paker, T, Akpinar B, Erenturk S, Askin D, Aytac A (1991) Use of transcutaneous electrical nerve stimulation in the control of postoperative chest pain after cardiac surgery. J Cardiothorac Vasc Anesth, 5: 589–591

Benedetti F, Amanzio M, Casadio C, Cavallo A, Gianci R, Giobbe R, Mancusso M, Ruffini E, Maggi C (1997) Control of postoperative pain by transcutaneous electrical nerve stimulation after thoracic operations. Ann Thorac Surg, 63: 773–776

Berman BM, Bausell RB (2000) The use of non-pharmacological therapies by pain specialists. Pain, 85: 313–315

Bertalanffy A, Kober A, Bertalanffy P, Gustroff B, Gore O, Adel S, Hoerauf K (2005) Transcutaneous electrical nerve stimulation reduces acute low back pain during emergency transport. Acad Emerg Med, 12: 607–611

Bodenheim R, Bennett JH (1983) Reversal of a Sudeck's atrophy by the adjunctive use of transcutaneous electrical nerve stimulation. A case report. Phys Ther, 63: 1287–1288

Bolton L (1983) TENS electrode irritation. J Am Acad Dermatol, 8: 134–135

Borjesson M, Eriksson P, Dellborg M, Eliason T, Mannkeimer C (1997) Transcutaneous electrical nerve stimulation in unstable angina pectoris. Coronary Artery Dis, 8: 543–550

Bortoluzzi G (1989) Transcutaneous electrical nerve stimulation in labour: Practicality and effectiveness in a public hospital ward. Austr J Physiother, 35: 81–87

Breit R, Van der Wall H (2004) Transcutaneous electrical stimulation for postoperative pain relief after total knee arthroplasty. J Arthroplasty, 19: 45–48

Brill MM, Whiffen JR (1985) Application of 24-hour burst TENS in a back school. Phys Ther, 65: 1355–1357

Broadley AJ (2000) The diagnostic dilemma of "pseudopacemaker spikes." Pacing Clin Electrophysiol, 23: 286–288

Bruce JR, Riggin CS, Parker JC (1988) Pain management in rheumatoid arthritis: Cognitive behavior modification and transcutaneous neural stimulation. Arthritis Care Res, 32: 1178–1184

Bundsen P, Ericson K, Peterson LE, Thiringer K (1982) Pain relief in labor by transcutaneous electrical nerve stimulation. Acta Obstet Gynaecol Scand, 61: 129–136

Bundsen P, Peterson LE, Selstam U (1981) Pain relief in labor by transcutaneous electrical nerve stimulation. Acta Obstet Gynaecol Scand, 60: 459–468

Bussey JG, Jackson A (1981) TENS for postsurgical analgesia. Contemp Surg, 18: 35–41

Carabelli RA, Kellerman WC (1985) Phantom limb pain: Relief by application of TENS to contralateral extremity. Arch Phys Med Rehab, 66: 466–467

Carrol EN, Badura AS (2001) Focal intense brief transcutaneous electric nerve stimulation for treatment of radicular and postthoracotomy pain. Arch Phys Med Rehabil, 82: 262–264

Castelain PY, Chabeau G (1986) Contact dermatitis after transcutaneous electric analgesia. Contact Dermatitis, 15: 32–35

Caterine JM, Smith DC, Olivencia J (1988) TENS for postsurgical analgesia following gastroplasty. Iowa Med, 78: 369–371

Chabal C, Fishbain DA, Weaver M, Heine LW (1998) Long-term transcutaneous electrical nerve stimulation (TENS) use: Impact on medication and physical therapy costs. Clin J Pain, 14: 66–73

Chao AS, Chao A, Wang TH, Chang YC, Peng HH, Chang SD, Chao A, Chang CJ, Lai CH, Wong AM (2007) Pain relief by applying transcutaneous electrical nerve stimulation (TENS) on acupuncture points during the first stage of labor: A randomized double-blind placebo-controlled trial. Pain, 127: 214–220

Cheing GL, Hui-Chan CW (1999) Transcutaneous electrical nerve stimulation: Nonparallel antinociceptive effects on chronic pain and acute experimental pain. Arch Phys Med Rehab, 80: 305–312

Cheing GL, Hui-Chan CW, Chan KM (2002) Does four weeks of TENS and/or isometric exercise produce cumulative reduction of osteoarthritis knee pain? Clin Rehabil, 16: 749–760

Cheing GL, Luk ML (2005) Transcutaneous electrical nerve stimulation for neuropathic pain. J Hand Surg Br, 30: 50–55

Cheing GL, Tsui AY, Lo SK, Hui-Chan CW (2003) Optimal stimulation duration of TENS in the management of osteoarthritis knee pain. J Rehabil Med, 35: 62–68

Chen D, Philip M, Philip PA, Monga TN (1990) Cardiac pacemaker inhibition by transcutaneous electrical nerve stimulation. Arch Phys Med Rehab, 71: 27–30

Chen L, Tang J, White PF, Sloninsky A, Wender RH, Naruse R, Kariger R (1998) The effect of location on transcutaneous electrical nerve stimulation on postoperative opioid analgesic requirement: Acupoint versus nonacupoint stimulation. Anaesth Analg, 87: 1129–1234

Chia YT, Arulkumaran S, Chua S, Ratnam SS (1990) Effectiveness of transcutaneous electric nerve stimulator for pain relief in labour. Asia Oceania J Obstet Gynecol, 16: 145–151

Chiu JH, Chen WS, Chen CH, Jiang JK, Tang GJ, Lui WY, Lin JK (1999) Effect of transcutaneous electrical nerve stimulation for pain relief on patients undergoing hemorrhoidectomy: Prospective, randomized, controlled trial. Dis Colon Rectum, 42: 180–185

Cipriano G, de Camargo Carvalho AC, Bernardelli GF, Tayar Peres PA (2008) Short-term transcutaneous nerve stimulation after cardiac surgery: Effect on pain, pulmonary function and electrical muscle activity. Interact Cardiovasc Thorac Surg, 7: 539–543

Conn IG, Marshall AH, Yadav SN, Daly JC, Jaffer M (1986) Transcutaneous electrical nerve stimulation following appendicectomy: The placebo effect. Ann R Coll Surg Engl, 68: 191–192

Cooperman AM, Hall B, Mikalacki K, Hardy R, Sardar E (1977) Use of transcutaneous electrical stimulation in the control of postoperative pain: Results of a prospective, randomized, controlled study. Am J Surg, 133: 185–187

Corazza M, Maranini C, Bacilieri S, Virgili A (1999) Accelerated allergic contact dermatitis to a transcutaenous electric nerve stimulation device. Dermatology, 199: 281

Cornell PE, Lopez AL, Malofsky H (1984) Pain reduction with transcutaneous electrical nerve stimulation after foot surgery. J Foot Surg, 23: 326–333

Curwin JH, Coyne RF, Winters SL (1999) Inappropriate defibrillator (ICD) shocks caused by transcutaneous electronic nerve stimulation (TENS) units. Pacing Clin Electrophysiol, 22: 692–693

Cuschieri RJ, Morran CG, McArdle CS (1985) Transcutaneous electrical stimulation for postoperative pain. Ann R Coll Surg Engl, 67: 127–129

Dawood MY, Ramos J (1990) Transcutaneous electrical nerve stimulation (TENS) for the treatment of primary dysmenorrhea: A randomized crossover comparison with placebo TENS and ibuprofen. Obstet Gynecol, 75: 656–660

Desantana JM, Santana-Filho VJ, Guerra DR, Sluka KA, da Silva WM (2008) Hypoalgesic effect of transcutaneous electrical nerve stimulation following inguinal herniorrhaphy: A randomized, controlled trial. J Pain, 9: 623–629

Desantana JM, Sluka K, Lauretti GR (2009) High and low frequency TENS reduce postoperative pain intensity after laparoscopic tubal ligation: A randomized controlled trial. Clin J Pain, 25: 12–19

Deyo RA, Walsh NE, Martin DC, Schoenfeld LS, Ramamurthy S (1990) A controlled trial of transcutaneous electrical nerve stimulation (TENS) and exercise for chronic low back pain. N Engl J Med, 322: 1627–1634

Dwyer CM, Chapman RS, Forsyth A (1994) Allergic contact dermatitis from TENS gel. Contact Dermatitis, 30: 305

Ebersold MJ, Laws EK, Stonnington H, Stillwell GK (1975) Transcutaneous electrical stimulation for treatment of chronic pain: A preliminary report. Surg Neurol, 4: 96–99

Emmiler M, Solak O, Kocogullari C, Dundar U, Ayva E, Ela Y, Cekirdekci A, Kavuncu V (2008) Control of acute postoperative pain by transcutaneous electrical nerve stimulation after open cardiac operations: A randomized placebo-controlled prospective study. Heart Surg Forum, 11: E3000–E3003

Erdogan M, Erdogan A, Erbil N, Karakaya HK, Demircan A (2005) Prospective, randomized, placebo-controlled study of the effect of TENS on postthoracotomy pain and pulmonary function. World J Surg, 29: 1563–1570

Eriksson M, Schuller H, Sjolund B (1978) Hazard from transcutaneous nerve stimulation in patients with pacemakers. Lancet, 1: 1319 (Letter)

Eriksson MB, Sjölund B, Nielzen S (1979) Long term results of peripheral conditioning stimulation as an analgesic measure in chronic pain. Pain, 6: 335–347

Eriksson MB, Sjölund BH, Sundbärg G (1984) Pain relief from peripheral conditioning stimulation in patients with chronic facial pain. J Neurosurg, 61: 149–155

Erkkola R, Pikkola P, Kanto J (1980) Transcutaneous nerve stimulation for pain relief during labour: A controlled study. Ann Chir Gynaecol, 69: 273–277

Ersek RA (1976) Low back pain: Prompt relief with transcutaneous neuro-stimulation—a report of 35 consecutive patients. Orthop Rev, 5: 27–31

Ersek RA (1977) Transcutaneous electrical neurostimulation: A new therapeutic modality for controlling pain. Clin Orthop, 128: 314–323

Fargas-Babjak A, Pomeranz B, Rooney PJ (1992) Acupuncture-like stimulation with Codetron for rehabilitation of patients with chronic pain syndrome and osteoarthritis. Acupunct Electrother Res, 17: 99–105

Fargas-Babjak A, Rooney P, Gerecz E (1989) Randomized trial of Codetron for pain control in osteoarthritis of the hip/knee. Clin J Pain, 5: 137–141

Finsen V, Persen L, Lovlien M, Veslegaard EK, Simensen M, Gasvann AK, Benum P (1988) Transcutaneous electrical nerve stimulation after major amputation. J Bone Joint Surg, 70B: 109–112

Fishbain DA, Chabal C, Abbot A, Heine LW, Cutler R (1996) Transcutaneous electrical nerve stimulation (TENS) treatment outcome in long-term users. Clin J Pain, 12: 201–214

Fisher AA (1978) Dermatitis associated with transcutaneous electrical stimulation current. Cutis, 21: 24–47

Foley-Nolan D, Kinirons M, Coughlan RJ, O'Connor P (1990) Post-whiplash dystonia well controlled by transcutaneous electrical nerve stimulation (TENS): Case report. J Trauma, 30: 909–910

Foster EL, Kramer JF, Lucy SD, Scudds RA, Novick RJ (1994) Effect of TENS on pain, medications, and pulmonary function following coronary artery bypass graft surgery. Chest, 106: 1343–1348

Fox EJ, Melzack R (1976) Transcutaneous electrical stimulation and acupuncture: Comparison of treatment for low back pain. Pain, 2: 141–148

Frampton V (1996) Management of pain in brachial plexus lesions. J Hand Ther, 9: 339–343

Fried T, Johnson R, McCracken W (1984) Transcutaneous electrical nerve stimulation: Its role in the control of chronic pain. Arch Phys Med Rehab, 65: 228–231

Galloway DJ, Boyle P, Burns HJ, Davidson PM, George WD (1984) A clinical assessment of electroanalgesia following abdominal operations. Surg Gynecol Obstet, 159: 453–456

Gemignani G, Olivieri L, Ruju G, Pasero G (1991) Transcutaneous electrical nerve stimulation in ankylosing spondylitis: A double-blind study. Arthritis Rheum, 34: 788–789

Gilbert JM, Gledhill T, Law N, George C (1986) Controlled trial of transcutaneous electrical nerve stimulation (TENS) for postoperative pain relief following inguinal herniorrhaphy. Br J Surg, 73: 749–751

Giuffrida O, Simpson L, Halligan PW (2009) Contralateral stimulation using TENS, of phantom pain. Two confirmatory cases. Pain Med, 11: 133–141

Glotzer TV, Gordon M, Sparta M, Radoslovich G, Zimmerman J (1998) Electromagnetic interference from a muscle stimulation device causing discharge of an implantable cardioverter defibrillator: Epicardial bipolar and endocardial bipolar sensing circuits are compared. Pacing Clin Electrophysiol, 21: 1996–1998

Graff-Radford SB, Reeves JL, Baker RL, Chiu D (1989) Effects of transcutaneous electrical nerve stimulation on myofascial pain and trigger point sensitivity. Pain, 37: 1–5

Grim LC, Morey SH (1985) Transcutaneous electrical nerve stimulation for relief of parturition pain: A clinical report. Phys Ther, 65: 337–340

Grimmer K (1992) A controlled double-blind study comparing the effects of strong burst mode TENS and high rate TENS on painful osteoarthritic knees. Austr J Physiother, 38: 49–56

Guieu R, Tardy-Gervet MF, Roll JP (1991) Analgesic effects of vibration and transcutaneous electrical nerve stimulation applied separately and simultaneously to patients with chronic pain. Can J Neurol Sci, 18: 115–119

Györy AN, Caine DC (1977) Electrical pain control (EPC) of a painful forearm amputation stump. Med J Austr, 2: 156–158

Hamza MA, White PF, Ahmed HE, Ghoname EA (1999) Effect of the frequency of transcutaneous electrical nerve stimulation on the postoperative opioid analgesic requirement and recovery profile. Anesthesiology, 91: 1232–1238

Hansson P, Ekblom A (1983) Transcutaneous electrical nerve stimulation (TENS) as compared to placebo TENS for the relief of acute oro-facial pain. Pain, 15: 157–165

Hansson P, Ekblom A, Thomsson M, Fjellner B (1986) Influence of naloxone on relief of acute oro-facial pain by transcutaneous electrical nerve stimulation (TENS) or vibration. Pain, 24: 323–329

Hargreaves A, Lander J (1989) Use of transcutaneous electrical nerve stimulation for postoperative pain. Nurs Res, 38: 159–161

Harrison RF, Shore M, Woods T, Mathews G, Gardiner J, Unwin A (1987) A comparative study of transcutaneous electrical nerve stimulation (TENS), entonox, pethidine plus promazine and lumbar epidural for pain relief in labor. Acta Obstet Gynaecol Scand, 66: 9–14

Harrison RF, Woods T, Shore M, Mathews G, Unwin A (1986) Pain relief in labour using transcutaneous electrical nerve stimulation (TENS): A TENS/TENS placebo controlled study in two parity groups. Br J Obstet Gynaecol, 93: 739–746

Harvie KW (1979) A major advance in the control of postoperative knee pain. Orthopedics, 2: 26–27

Hasan ST, Robson WA, Pridie AK, Neal DE (1996) Transcutaneous electrical nerve stimulation and temporary S3 neuromodulation of idiopathic detrusor instability. J Urol, 155: 2005–2011

Hauptman PJ, Raza M (1992) Electrocardiographic artifact with a transcutaneous electrical nerve stimulation unit. Int J Cardiol, 34: 110–112

Herman E, Williams R, Stratford P, Fargas-Babjak A, Trott M (1994) A randomized controlled trial of transcutaneous electrical nerve stimulation (CODETRON) to determine its benefits in a rehabilitation program for acute occupational low back pain. Spine, 19: 561–568

Hirano K, Yamashiro H, Maeda N, Takeuchi T (1988) A case of long-standing phantom limb pain: Complete relief of pain. Jap J Anesthesiol, 37: 222–225

Ho A, Hui PW, Cheung J, Cheung C (1987) Effectiveness of transcutaneous electrical nerve stimulation in relieving pain following thoracotomy. Physiotherapy, 73: 33–35

Hollinger JL (1986) Transcutaneous electrical nerve stimulation after cesarean birth. Phys Ther, 66: 36–38

Holmgren C, Carlsson T, Mannheimer C, Edvardsson N (2008) Risk of interference from transcutaneous electrical nerve stimulation on the sensing function of implantable defibrillators. PACE, 31: 151–158

Hsueh T, Cheng P, Kuan T, Hong C (1997) The immediate effectiveness of electrical nerve stimulation and electrical muscle stimulation on myofascial trigger pain. Am J Phys Med Rehabil, 76: 471–476

Hymes AC, Raab DE, Yonehiro EG, Nelson GD, Printy AL (1974). Electrical surface stimulation for control of acute postoperative pain and prevention of ileus. Surg Forum, 24: 447–449

Indeck W, Printy A (1975) Skin application of electrical impulses for relief of pain in chronic orthopedic conditions. Minn Med, 58: 305–309

Issenman J, Nolan MF, Rowley J, Hobby R (1985) Transcutaneous electrical nerve stimulation for pain control after spinal fusion with Harrington rods. Phys Ther, 65: 1517–1520

Jensen H, Zesler R, Christensen T (1991) Transcutaneous electrical nerve stimulation (TENS) for painful osteoarthritis of the knee. Int J Rehab Res, 14: 356–358

Jensen JE, Conn RR, Hazelrigg G, Hewett JE (1985) The use of transcutaneous neural stimulation and isokinetic testing in arthroscopic knee surgery. Am J Sports Med, 13: 27–33

Johnson MI, Asthon CH, Thompson JW (1991) An in-depth study of long term users of transcutaneous electrical nerve stimulation (TENS). Implications for clinical users of TENS. Pain, 44: 221–229

Jones SL (1976) Electromagnetic field interference and cardiac pacemakers. Phys Ther, 56: 1013–1018

Kaplan B, Peled Y, Pardo J, Rabinerson D, Hirsh M, Ovadia J, Neri A (1994) Transcutaneous electrical nerve stimulation (TENS) as a relief for dysmenorrhea. Clin Exp Obstet Gynecol, 21: 87–90

Kaplan B, Rabinerson D, Lurie S, Bar J, Krieser UR, Neri A (1998) Transcutaneous electrical nerve stimulation (TENS) for adjuvant pain-relief during labor and delivery. Int J Gynaecol Obstet, 60: 251–255

Kaplan B, Rabinerson D, Lurie S, Peled Y, Royburt M, Neri A (1997) Clinical evaluation of a new model of a transcutaneous electrical nerve stimulation device for the management of primary dysmenorrhea. Gynecol Obstet Invest, 44: 255–259

Katz J, France C, Melzack R (1989) An association between phantom pain sensations and stump skin conductance during transcutaneous electrical nerve stimulation (TENS) applied to the contralateral leg: A case study. Pain, 36: 367–377

Katz J, Melzack R (1991) Auricular transcutaneous electrical nerve stimulation (TENS) reduces phantom limb pain. J Pain Symptom Manage, 6: 73–83

Kawamura HIK, Yamamoto M, Yamamoto H, Yamamoto M, Ishida K, Kawakami T (1997). The transcutaneous electrical nerve stimulation applied to the contralateral limbs for the phantom limb pain. J Phys Ther Science, 9: 71–76

Keenan DL, Simonsen L, McCrann DJ (1985) Transcutaneous electrical nerve stimulation for pain control during labor and delivery: A case report. Phys Ther, 65: 1363–1364

Kimberley AP, Soni N, Williams TR (1987) Transcutaneous nerve stimulation and the electrocardiograph. Anaesth Intens Care, 15: 358–359

Klin B, Uretzky G, Magora F (1984) Transcutaneous electrical nerve stimulation (TENS) after open heart surgery. J Cardiovasc Surg (Torino), 25: 445–448

Koke AJ, Schouten JS, Lamerichs-Geelen MJ, Lipsch JS, Waltje EM, van Kleef M, Pa J (2004) Pain reducing effects of three types of transcutanenous electrical nerve stimulation in patients with chronic pain: A randomized crossover trial. Pain, 108: 36–42

Kruger LR, van der Linden WJ, Cleaton-Jones PE (1998) Transcutaneous electrical nerve stimulation in the treatment of myofascial pain dysfunction. S Afr J Surg, 36: 35–38

Kumar VN, Redford JB (1982) Transcutaneous electrical nerve stimulation in rheumatoid arthritis. Arch Phys Med Rehab, 63: 595–596

Labrecque M, Nouwen A, Bergeron M, Rancourt JF (1999) A randomized controlled trial of nonpharmacologic approaches for relief of low back pain during labor. J Fam Pract, 48: 259–263

Laitinen J (1976) Acupuncture and transcutaneous electrical stimulation in the treatment of chronic sacrolumbalgia and ischialgia. Am J Chin Med, 4: 169–175

Laitinen J, Nuutinen L (1991) Failure of transcutaneous electrical nerve stimulation and indomethacin to reduce opiate requirement following cholecystectomy. Acta Anaesthesiol Scand, 35: 700–705

Lang T, Barker R, Steinlechner B, Gustorff B, Puskas T, Gore O, Kober A (2007) TENS relieves acute posttraumatic hip pain during emergency transport. J Trauma, 62: 184–188

Langley GB, Sheppeard H, Johnson M, Wigley RD (1984) The analgesic effects of transcutaneous electrical nerve stimulation and placebo in chronic pain patients: A double-blind non-crossover comparison. Rheumatol Int, 4: 119–123

Law PP, Cheing GL, Tsui AY (2004) Does transcutaneous electrical nerve stimulation improve the physical performance of people with knee osteoarthritis? J Clin Rheumatol, 10: 295–299

Leandri M, Parodi CI, Corrieri N, Rigardo S (1990) Comparison of TENS treatments in hemiplegic shoulder pain. Scand J Rehab Med, 22: 69–72

Lee EW, Chung IW, Lee JY, Lam PW, Chin RK (1990) The role of transcutaneous electrical nerve stimulation in management of labour in obstetric patients. Asia Oceania J Obstet Gynaecol, 16: 247–254

Lehmann TR, Russell DW, Spratt KF, Colby H, King Liu Y, Fairchild ML, Christensen S (1986) Efficacy of electroacupuncture and TENS in the rehabilitation of chronic low back pain patients. Pain, 26: 277–290

Leijon G, Boivie J (1989) Central post-stroke pain—the effect of high and low frequency TENS. Pain, 38: 187–191

Levin MF, Hui-Chan CW (1992) Relief of hemiparetic spasticity by TENS is associated with improvement in reflex and voluntary motor functions. Electroencephalogr Clin Neurophysiol, 85: 131–142

Lewers D, Clelland JA, Jackson JR, Varner RE, Bergman J (1989) Transcutaneous electrical nerve stimulation in the relief of primary dysmenorrhea. Phys Ther, 69: 277–290

Lewis B, Lewis D, Cumming G (1994) The comparative analgesic efficacy of transcutaneous electrical nerve stimulation and non-steroidal anti-inflammatory drug for painful osteoarthritis. Br J Rheumatol, 33: 455–460

Lewis D, Lewis B, Sturrock R (1984) Transcutaneous electrical nerve stimulation in osteoarthritis: A therapeutic alternative? Ann Rheum Dis, 43: 47–49

Lim AT, Edis G, Kranz H, Mendelson G, Selwood T, Scott DF (1983) Postoperative pain control: Contribution of psychological factors and transcutaneous electrical stimulation. Pain, 17: 179–188

Linde C, Isacsson G, Jonsson BG (1995) Outcome of 6-week treatment with transcutaneous electrical nerve stimulation compared with splint on symptomatic temporomandibular joint disk displacement without reduction. Acta Odontol Scand, 53: 92–98

Loeser JD, Black RG, Christman RA (1975) Relief of pain by transcutaneous stimulation. J Neurosurg, 42: 308–314

Long DM (1974) External electrical stimulation as a treatment of chronic pain. Minn Med, 5: 195–198

Lundeberg T, Bondesson L, Lundström V (1985) Relief of primary dysmenorrhea by transcutaneous electrical nerve stimulation. Acta Obstet Gynaecol Scand, 64: 491–497

Magora F, Aladjemoff L, Tannenbaum J, Magora A (1978) Treatment of pain by transcutaneous electrical stimulation. Acta Anaesthesiol Scand, 22: 589–592

Mannheimer C, Carlsson CA (1979) The analgesic effect of transcutaneous electrical nerve stimulation (TENS) in patients with rheumatoid arthritis. A comparative study of different pulse patterns. Pain, 6: 329–334

Mannheimer C, Lund S, Carlsson CA (1978) The effect of transcutaneous electrical nerve stimulation (TNS) on joint pain in patients with rheumatoid arthritis. Scand J Rheumatol, 7: 13–16

Mannheimer JS, Whalen EC (1985) The efficacy of transcutaneous electrical nerve stimulation in dysmenorrhea. Clin J Pain, 1: 75–83

Marchand S, Li J, Charest J (1995) Letter to the Editor. Effects of caffeine on analgesia from transcutaneous electrical nerve stimulation. N Engl J Med, 333: 325

Marples IL (2000) Transcutaneous electrical nerve stimulation (TENS): An unusual source of electrocardiogram artifact. Anaesthesia, 55: 719–720

Marren P, DeBerker D, Powell S (1991) Methacrylate sensitivity and transcutaneous electrical nerve stimulation (TENS). Contact Dermatitis, 25: 190–191

McCallum MI, Glynn CJ, Moore RA, Lammer P, Phillips AM (1988) Transcutaneous electrical nerve stimulation in the management of acute postoperative pain. Br J Anaesth, 61: 308–312

Melzack R, Jeans ME, Stratford JG, Monks RC (1980) Ice massage and transcutaneous electrical stimulation: Comparison of treatment for low-back pain. Pain, 9: 209–217

Melzack R, Vetere P, Finch L (1983) Transcutaneous electrical nerve stimulation for low back pain: A comparison of TENS and massage for pain and range of motion. Phys Ther, 63: 489–493

Melzack R, Wall PD (1965) Pain mechanisms: A new theory. Science, 150: 971–979

Merkel SI, Gutstein HB, Malviya S (1999) Use of transcutaneous electrical nerve stimulation in a young child with pain from open perineal lesions. J Pain Symptom Manage, 18: 376–381

Merrill DC (1987) Electroanalgesia in urologic surgery. Urology, 29: 494–497

Merrill DC (1988) FasTENS—a disposable transcutaneous electrical nerve stimulator designed specifically for use in postoperative pain. Urology, 31: 78–79

Merrill DC (1989) Clinical evaluation of FasTENS, an inexpensive, disposable transcutaneous electrical nerve stimulator designed specifically for postoperative electroanalgesia. Urology, 33: 27–30

Meuleman V, Busschots AM, Dooms-Goossens A (1996) Contact allergy to a device for transcutaneous electrical neural stimulation (TENS). Contact Dermatitis. 35: 52–54

Meyler WJ, de Jongste MJ, Rolf CA (1994) Clinical evaluation of pain treatment with electrostimulation: A study on TENS in patients with different pain syndromes. Clin J Pain, 10: 22–27

Miles J, Lipton S (1978) Phantom limb pain treated by electrical stimulation. Pain, 5: 373–382

Miller L, Mattison P, Paul L, Wood L (2007) The effects of transcutaneous electrical nerve stimulation (TENS) on spasticity in multiple sclerosis. Mult Scler, 13: 527–533

Milsom I, Hedner N, Mannheimer C (1994) A comparative study of the effect of high-intensity transcutaneous nerve stimulation and oral naproxen on intrauterine pressure and menstrual pain in patients with primary dysmenorrhea. Am J Obstet Gynecol, 170: 123–129

Mora B, Giorni E, Dobrovits M, Barker R, Lang T, Gore C, Kober A (2006) Transcutaneous electrical nerve stimulation: An effective treatment for pain caused by renal colic in emergency care. J Urol, 175: 1737–1741

Moystad A, Krogstard BS, Larheim TA (1990) Transcutaneous electrical nerve stimulation in a group of patients with rheumatic disease involving the temporomandibular joint. J Prosthet Dent, 64: 596–600

Murphy GJ (1990) Utilization of transcutaneous electrical nerve stimulation in managing craniofacial pain. Clin J Pain, 6: 64–69

Nathan PW, Wall PD (1974) Treatment for post-herpetic neuralgia by prolonged electrical stimulation. Br Med J, 3: 645–647

Navarathnam RG, Wang IY, Thomas D, Klineberg PL (1984) Evaluation of the transcutaneous electrical nerve stimulator for postoperative analgesia following cardiac surgery. Anaesth Intensive Care, 12: 345–350

Neary JM (1981) Transcutaneous electrical nerve stimulation for the relief of post-incisional pain. Am Assoc Nurs J, 49: 151–155

Neighbors LE, Clelland J, Jackson JR, Begman J, Orr J (1987) Transcutaneous electrical nerve stimulation for pain relief in primary dysmenorrhea. Clin J Pain, 3: 17–22

Nesheim BI (1981) The use of transcutaneous nerve stimulation for pain relief during labor. A controlled clinical study. Acta Obstet Gynaecol Scand, 60: 13–16

Ng MM, Leung M, Poon DM (2003) The effects of electro-acupuncture and transcutaneous electrical nerve stimulation on patients with painful osteoarthritic knees: A randomized controlled trial with follow-up evaluation. J Altern Complement Med, 9: 641–649

Nitz J, Cheras F (1993) Transcutaneous electrical nerve stimulation and chronic intractable angina pectoris. Austr J Physiother, 39: 109–113

Nordemar R, Thörner C (1981) Treatment of acute cervical pain—a comparative group study. Pain, 10: 93–101

Occhetta E, Bortnik M, Magnami A, Francalacci G, Marino P (2006) Inappropriate implantable cardioverter-defibrillator discharges unrelated to supraventricular tachyarrythmias. Europace, 8: 863–869

Okada N, Igawa Y, Ogawa A, Nishizawa O (1998) Transcutaneous electrical stimulation of thigh muscles in the treatment of detrusor overactivity. Br J Urol, 81: 560–564

Olsen MF, Elden H, Janson ED, Lilja H, Stener-Victorin E (2007) A comparison of high- versus low-intensity, high-frequency transcutaneous electric nerve stimulation for painful postpartum uterine contractions. Acta Obstet Gynecol Scand, 86: 310–314

Oncel M, Sencan S, Yildiz H, Kurt N (2002) Transcutaneous electrical nerve stimulation for pain management in patients with uncomplicated minor rib fractures. Eur J Cardiothorac Surg, 22: 13–17

Oosterhof J, De Boo TM, Oostendorp BA, Wilder-Smith OG, Crul BJ (2006) Outcome of transcutaneous electrical nerve stimulation in chronic pain: Short-term results of a double-blind, randomized, placebo-controlled trial. J Headache Pain, 7: 196–205

Ordog GJ (1987) Transcutaneous electrical nerve stimulation versus oral analgesic: A randomized double-blind controlled study in acute traumatic pain. Am J Emerg Med, 5: 6–10

Paker N, Tekdos D, Kesiktas N, Soy D (2006) Comparison of the therapeutic efficacy of TENS versus intra-articular hyaluronic acid injection in patients with knee osteoarthritis: A prospective randomized study. Adv Ther, 23: 342–353

Persson AL, Loyd-Pugh M, Sahlstrom J (2010) Trained long-term TENS users with chronic non-malignant pain. A retrospective questionnaire study of TENS usage and patient's experiences. Phys Ther Rev, 15: 294–301

Philbin DM, Marieb MA, Aithal KH, Schoenfeld MH (1998) Inappropriate shocks delivered by an ICD as a result of sensed potentials from a transcutaneous electronic nerve stimulation unit. Pacing Clin Electrophysiol, 21: 2010–2011

Pike PM (1978) Transcutaneous electrical stimulation: Its use in the management of postoperative pain. Anaesthesia, 33: 165–171

Pope MH, Philips RB, Haugh LD (1994) A prospective randomized three-week trial of spinal manipulation, transcutaneous muscle stimulation, massage and corset in the treatment of subacute low-back pain. Spine, 19: 2571–2577

Potisk KP, Gregoric M, Vodovnik L (1995) Effects of transcutaneous electrical stimulation (TENS) on spasticity in patients with hemiplegia. Scand J Rehab Med, 27: 168–174

Pyatt JR, Trenbath D, Chester M, Connelly DT (2003) The simultaneous use of a biventricular implantable defibrillator (ICD) and transcutaneous electrical nerve stimulation (TENS) unit: Implication for device interaction. Europace, 5: 91–103

Rao VR, Wolf SL, Gersh MR (1981) Examination of electrode placements and stimulating parameters in treating chronic pain with conventional transcutaneous electrical nerve stimulation (TENS). Pain, 11: 37–47

Rasmussen MJ, Hayes DL, Vlietstra RE, Thorsteinsson G (1988) Can transcutaneous electrical nerve stimulation be safely used in patients with permanent cardiac pacemakers? Mayo Clin Proc, 63: 443–445

Rawat B, Genz A, Fache JS, Ong M, Coldman AJ, Burhenne HJ (1991) Effectiveness of transcutaneous electrical nerve stimulation (TENS) for analgesia during biliary lithotripsy. Invest Radiat, 26: 866–869

Reuss R, Cronen P, Abplanalp L (1988) Transcutaneous electrical nerve stimulation for pain control after cholecystectomy: Lack of expected benefits. South Med J, 81: 1361–1363

Reynolds RA, Gladstone N, Ansari AH (1987) Transcutaneous electrical nerve stimulation for reducing narcotic use after cesarean section. J Reprod Med, 32: 843–846

Richardson RR, Meyer PR, Cerullo LJ (1980) Neurostimulation in the modulation of intractable paraplegic and traumatic neuroma pains. Pain, 8: 75–84

Robaina FJ, Rodriguez JL, de Vera JA, Martin MA (1989) Transcutaneous electrical nerve stimulation and spinal cord stimulation for pain relief in reflex sympathetic dystrophy. Stereotact Funct Neurosurg, 52: 53–62

Rooney SM, Jain S, Goldiner PL (1983) Effect of transcutaneous nerve stimulation on postoperative pain after thoracotomy. Anesth Analg, 62: 1010–1012

Rosenberg M, Curtis L, Bourke DL (1978) Transcutaneous electrical nerve stimulation for the relief of postoperative pain. Pain, 5: 129–133

Rutkowski B, Niedzialkowska J (1977) Electrical stimulation in low-back pain. Br J Anaesth, 49: 629–632

Scherder E, Van Someren E, Swaab D (1999) Epilepsy: A possible contraindication for transcutaneous electrical nerve stimulation. J Pain Sympt Manag, 17: 151–153

Schietz HA, Jettestad M, Al-Heeti D (2007) Treatment of dysmenorrhoea with a new TENS device (OVA). J Obstet Gynaecol, 27: 726–728

Schomburg FL, Carter-Baker SA (1983) Transcutaneous electrical nerve stimulation for postlaparotomy pain. Phys Ther, 63: 188–193

Schuster GD, Infante MC (1980) Pain relief after low back surgery: The efficacy of transcutaneous electrical nerve stimulation. Pain, 8: 299–302

Shade SK (1985) Use of transcutaneous electrical nerve stimulation for a patient with a cardiac pacemaker. A case report. Phys Ther, 65: 206–208

Shealy CN (1974) Six years' experience with electrical stimulation for control of pain. Adv Neurol, 4: 775–782

Shealy CN, Mortimer JT, Reswick JB (1967) Electrical inhibition of pain by stimulation of the dorsal column: Preliminary clinical report. Anesth Analg, 46: 489–491

Sims DT (1991) Effectiveness of transcutaneous electrical nerve stimulation following cholecystectomy. Physiotherapy, 77: 715–722

Siu CW, Tse HF, Lau CP (2005) Inappropriate implantable defibrillator shock from a transcutaneous muscle stimulation device therapy. J Interv Card Electrophysiol, 13: 73–75

Sliwa JA, Marinko MS (1996) Transcutaneous electrical nerve stimulation-induced electrocardiogram artifact. A brief report. Am J Phys Med Rehab, 75: 307–309

Sloan JP, Muwanga CL, Waters EA, Dove AF, Dave SH (1986) Multiple rib fractures: Transcutaneous nerve stimulation versus conventional analgesia. J Trauma, 26: 1120–1122

Smedley F, Taube M, Wastell C (1988) Transcutaneous electrical nerve stimulation for pain relief following inguinal hernia repair: A controlled trial. Eur Surg Res, 20: 233–237

Smith CM, Guralnick MS, Gelfand MM, Jeans ME (1986) The effects of transcutaneous electrical nerve stimulation on post-cesarean pain. Pain, 27: 181–193

Smith CR, Lewith GT, Machin D (1983a) TENS and osteoarthritis: Preliminary study to establish a controlled method of assessing transcutaneous electrical nerve stimulation as a treatment for pain caused by osteoarthritis. Physiotherapy, 69: 266–268

Smith MJ, Hutchins RC, Hehenberger D (1983b) Transcutaneous electrical nerve stimulation in postoperative knee rehabilitation. Am J Sports Med, 11: 75–81

Smith RP, Heltzel JA (1991) Interrelation of analgesia and uterine activity in women with primary dysmenorrhea. A preliminary report. J Reprod Med, 36: 260–264

Solak O, Turna A, Pekcolaklar A, Metin M, Sayar A, Solak O, Gurses A (2007) Transcutaneous electrical nerve stimulation for the treatment of postthoracotomy pain: A randomized prospective study. Thorac Cardiovasc Surg, 55: 182–185

Solomon RA, Viernstein MC, Long DM (1980) Reduction of postoperative pain and narcotic use by transcutaneous electrical nerve stimulation. Surgery, 87: 142–146

Somers DL, Somers MF (1999) Treatment of neuropathic pain in a patient with diabetic neuropathy using transcutaneous electrical nerve stimulation applied to the skin of the lumbar region. Phys Ther, 79: 767–777

Sonde L, Gip C, Fernaeus SE, Nilsson CG, Viitanen M (1998) Stimulation with low frequency (1.7 Hz) transcutaneous electric nerve stimulation (low-TENS) increases motor function of the post-stroke paretic arm. Scand J Rehab Med, 30: 95–99

Stabile ML, Mallory TH (1978) The management of postoperative pain in total joint replacement. Orthop Rev, 7: 121–123

Stubbing JF, Jellicoe JA (1988) Transcutaneous electrical nerve stimulation after thoracotomy. Pain relief and peak expiratory flow rate: A trial of transcutaneous electrical nerve stimulation. Anaesthesia, 43: 296–298

Taylor AG, West BA, Simon B, Sketon J, Rowlingson JC (1983) How effective is TENS for acute pain? Am J Nurs, 83: 1171–1174

Taylor P, Hallett M, Flaherty L (1981) Treatment of osteoarthritis of the knee with transcutaneous electrical nerve stimulation. Pain, 11: 233–240

Tekeoglu Y, Adak B, Goksoy T (1998) Effect of transcutaneous electrical nerve stimulation (TENS) in Barthel Activities of Daily Living (ADL) index score following stroke. Clin Rehab, 12: 277–280

Thomas IL, Tyle V, Webster J, Neilson A (1988) An evaluation of transcutaneous electrical nerve stimulation for pain relief in labour. Aust N Z J Obstet Gynaecol, 28: 182–189

Thorsen SW, Lumsden SG (1997) Trigeminal neuralgia: Sudden and long-term remission with transcutaneous electrical nerve stimulation. J Manipulative Physiol Ther, 20: 415–419

Thorsteinsson G, Stonnington HH, Stillwell GK, Elveback LR (1977) Transcutaneous electrical stimulation: A double-blind trial of its efficacy for pain. Arch Phys Med Rehab, 58: 8–13

Torres WE, Fraser NP, Baumgartner BR, Nelson RC, Evans GR, Jones V, Peterson J (1992) The use of transcutaneous electrical nerve stimulation during the biliary lithotripsy procedure. J Stone Dis, 4: 41–45

Tulgar M, McGlone F, Bowsher D, Miles J (1991) Comparative effectiveness of different stimulation modes in relieving pain. Part II: A double blind controlled long-term clinical trial. Pain, 47: 157–162

Vander Ark GD, McGrath KA (1975) Transcutaneous electrical stimulation in treatment of postoperative pain. Am J Surg, 130: 338–340

Vander Ploeg JM, Vervest HA, Liem AL, Schagen van Leewen JH (1996) Electrical nerve stimulation (TENS) during the first stage of labour: A randomized clinical trial. Pain, 68: 75–78

Vinterberg H, Donde R, Anderson RB (1978) Transcutaneous electrical nerve stimulation for relief of pain in patients with rheumatoid arthritis. Ugeskr Laeger, 140: 1149–1150

Walker RH, Morris BA, Angulo DL, Schneider J, Colwell CW (1991) Postoperative use of continuous passive motion, transcutaneous electrical nerve stimulation, and continuous cooling pad following total knee arthroplasty. J Arthroplasty, 6: 151–156

Warfield CA, Stein JM, Frank HA (1985) The effect of transcutaneous electrical nerve stimulation on pain after thoracotomy. Ann Thorac Surg, 39: 462–465

Warke K, Al-Smadi J, Baxter D, Walsh DM, Lowe-Strong AS (2006) Efficacy of transcutaneous electrical nerve stimulation (TENS) for chronic low-back pain in multiple sclerosis population: A randomized, placebo-controlled clinical trial. Clin J Pain, 22: 812–819

Weitz SH, Tunick PA, McElhinney L, Mitchell T, Kronzon I (1997) Pseudoatrial flutter: Artifact simulating atrial flutter coursed by a transcutaneous electrical nerve stimulation (TENS). Pacing Clin Electrophysiol, 20: 3010–3011

Winnem MF, Amundsen T (1982) Treatment of phantom limb pain with TENS. Pain, 12: 299–300

Yurtkuran M, Kocagil T (1999) TENS, electroacupuncture and ice massage: Comparison of treatment for osteoarthritis of the knee. Am J Acupunct, 27: 133–140

Zizic TM, Hoffman KC, Holt PA, Hungerford DS, Odell JR, Jacobs MA, Lewis CG, Deal CL, Caldwell JR, Cholewczuski JG, Free SM (1995) The treatment of osteoarthritis of the knee with pulsed electrical stimulation. J Rheumatol, 22: 1757–1761

Zugerman C (1982) Dermatitis from transcutaneous electrical nerve stimulation. J Am Acad Dermatol, 6: 936–939

Review Articles

Allen RJ (2006) Physical agents used in the management of chronic pain by physical therapists. Phys Med Rehabil Clin N Am, 17: 315–345

Bedwell C, Dowswell T, Neilson JP, Lavender T (2011) The use of transcutaneous electrical nerve stimulation (TENS) for pain relief in labour: A review of the evidence. Midwifery, 27: e141–e148

Bjordal JM, Johnson MI, Ljunggreen AE (2003) Transcutaneous electrical nerve stimulation (TENS) can reduce postoperative analgesics consumption. A meta-analysis with assessment of optimal treatment parameters for postoperative pain. Eur J Pain, 7: 181–188

Brosseau L, Yonge K, Marchand S, Robinson V, Osiri M, Wells G, Tugwell P (2004) Efficacy of transcutaneous electrical nerve stimulation for osteoarthritis of the lower extremities: A meta-analysis. Phys Ther Rev, 9: 213–233

Brown L, Holmes M, Jones A (2009) The application of transcutaneous electrical nerve stimulation to acupuncture points (Acu-Tens) for pain relief: A discussion of efficacy and potential mechanisms. Phys Ther Rev, 14: 93–103

DeLeo JA (2006) Basic science of pain. J Bone Joint Surg (A), 88: 58–62

Johnson M, Martinson M (2007) Efficacy of electrical nerve stimulation for chronic musculoskeletal pain: A meta-analysis of randomized controlled trials. Pain, 130: 157–165

Johnson MI, Bjordal JM (2011) Transcutaneous electrical nerve stimulation for the management of painful conditions: Focus on neuropathic pain. Expert Rev Neurother, 11: 735–753

Khadilkar A, Milne S, Brosseau L, Wells G, Tugwell P, Robinson V, Shea B, Saginur M (2005) Transcutaneous electrical nerve stimulation for the treatment of chronic low back pain: A systematic review. Spine, 30: 2657–2666

Miller L, Mattison P, Paul L, Wood L (2005) The effects of transcutaneous electrical nerve stimulation on spasticity. Phys Ther Rev, 10: 201–208

Sluka KA, Walsh D (2003) Transcutaneous electrical nerve stimulation: Basic science mechanisms and clinical effectiveness. J Pain, 4: 109–121

Ying KN, While A (2007) Pain relief in osteoarthritis and rheumatoid arthritis. Br J Community Nurs, 12: 364–371

Monograph

American Physical Therapy Association (2001) Electrotherapeutic Terminology in Physical Therapy. APTA Publication, Alexandria

Textbooks

Mannheimer JS, Lampe GN (1984) Clinical Transcutaneous Electrical Stimulation. FA Davis, Philadelphia

McMahon S, Koltzenburg M (2005) Wall and Melzack's Textbook of Pain. Churchill Livingstone, London

Internet Resources

www.iasp-pain.org: International Association for the Study of Pain

www.ampainsoc.org: American Pain Society

http://thePoint.lww.com: Online Dosage Calculator: Transcutaneous Electrical Nerve Stimulation

Chapter 15

Electrical Stimulation for Tissue Healing and Repair

Chapter Outline

Learning Objectives

Remembering: Describe the biophysical characteristics associated with microcurrent and high-voltage pulsed current.

Understanding: Distinguish between the concept of skin battery and current of injury.

Applying: Demonstrate the over-the-wound and around-the-wound electrode configurations.

Analyzing: Explain the galvanotaxic and germicidal effects of electrical currents used for wound healing.

Evaluating: Formulate the dosimetric parameters that practitioners need to consider to deliver safe and effective electrical stimulation for wound healing.

Creating: Discuss the place that electrical stimulation should have in the management of slow-to-heal dermal wounds.

I. FOUNDATION

A. DEFINITION

Electrical stimulation for tissue healing and repair, designated by the acronym ESTHR, is defined as the use of surface electrical current for enhancing soft-tissue repair and healing. More specifically, ESTHR is used to promote and accelerate the healing process of slow-to-heal cutaneous wounds (APTA, 2001). ESTRH, therefore, can be renamed *electrical stimulation for wound healing*. Its clinical use is approved in the United States

Historical Overview

The delivery of electrical current into refractory wounds to enhance tissue healing is not new. Several reports dating from the 17th century describe the use of electrostatically charged gold leaf to treat various skin lesions (see Kloth, 2005a,b and Sussman et al., 2007). The first published peer-reviewed articles of microcurrent therapy for wound healing in humans were those of Assimacopoulos (1968) for venous ulcers and Wolcott et al. (1969) for diabetic ulcers. A study by Thurman et al. (1971) appears to be the first publication on the therapeutic use of high-voltage pulsed current (HVPC) on humans, reporting benefit for the treatment of a purulent septic diabetic abscess in a single patient. Electrical stimulation for tissue healing and repair (ESTHR) rests on the concept of current of injury, driven by skin batteries, originally proposed in the late 1960s by Robert O. Becker, following his research on animal soft-tissue healing and limb regeneration mechanisms. Becker theorized that a so-called *current of injury,* in the microampere range, driven by so-called *skin battery,* is present in human tissues after trauma and diseases and that such an endogenous current may be important in soft-tissue repair (Becker et al., 1967; Becker et al., 1987; Borgens et al., 1977, 1984). Inspired by findings in animals, similar studies were conducted on humans during the early 1980s to identify and measure such skin-battery voltages and currents of injury. Illingsworth et al. (1980) reported endogenous electrical currents in children at the stump surface of fingers, the tips of which had been accidentally amputated. Two years later, Barker et al. (1982) reported microcurrents leaving a wound in human skin immersed in saline. Then Foulds et al. (1983) set up an experiment to determine whether normal, or noninjured, human skin possessed battery potentials similar to those demonstrated in amphibians. Their results, obtained from 17 healthy subjects, revealed that there are skin batteries in healthy human cutaneous tissue with voltages comparable to those of animal skin batteries. Injured cells originating from tissues such as skin, muscle, and nerve are believed to possess their own injury currents, and these endogenous electrical currents may play a major role in tissue repair. It logically follows that if human tissue repair is mediated, at least in part, by electrical signals, then an exogenous electrical current delivered at the site of wounds may enhance the healing process.

for the treatment of various lower extremity ulcers caused by pressure, vascular insufficiency, and diabetes (Centers for Medicare and Medicaid Services, 2004).

B. ELECTRICAL CURRENTS

Two types of monophasic electrical currents are commonly used to deliver ESTHR. The first current is known as *microcurrent,* designated under different acronyms such as MES (microcurrent electrical stimulation), MCT (microcurrent therapy), and LIDC (low-intensity direct current). *Microcurrent* is defined as the surface delivery of continuous and pulsed monophasic current waveforms, of amplitudes within the microamperage range (thus, the name *micro*)—that is, from 1 to 999 μA, or amplitude of less than 1 mA (APTA, 2001). The second current is *high-voltage pulsed current,* known by the acronym HVPC. This electrical current is defined as the delivery of pulsed, twin-peak, monophasic pulses at a high-driving peak voltage (thus, the name *high-voltage pulsed*), ranging from 150 to 500 volts (APTA, 2001). The biophysical characteristics of these two electrical currents are described in the Biophysical Characteristics section.

C. ELECTRICAL STIMULATORS

Electrical stimulation for wound healing is applied using a variety of electrical stimulators. Figure 15-1 illustrates a cabinet-type, multi-current, line-powered stimulator capable of generating microcurrent and HVPCs simply by pushing a button on the stimulator's console. Also illustrated are a portable, battery-powered HVPC stimulator and two small, wearable and battery-powered HVPC stimulators.

D. ELECTRODE AND COUPLING MEDIUM

Electrical stimulation for wound healing is applied by using a variety of reusable and disposable electrodes. Figure 15-2 illustrates commercial reusable carbon-impregnated rubber electrodes and disposable homemade aluminum foil electrodes. Unlike commercial carbon electrodes, aluminum foil electrodes are very cost-effective and time efficient for treatment of open wounds (Sussman et al., 2012). They are very good conductors of electricity, are nontoxic, and can easily be molded to fit the wound size and configuration. Also illustrated are a flexible, self-adhesive electrode and a garment-type electrode to which a portable stimulator is attached. To optimize electrical conduction at the electrode–skin interface, commercial electrodes are covered with a thin layer of electroconductive gel. Homemade aluminum foil electrodes, on the other hand, are wrapped with layers of sterile gauze pads saturated with Ringer or saline solution.

E. RATIONALE FOR USE

The treatment of slow-to-heal chronic cutaneous wounds remains a significant health problem especially in the aging population (Kloth, 2002, 2005a,b; Sussman et al., 2012). Various therapeutic interventions are available to treat

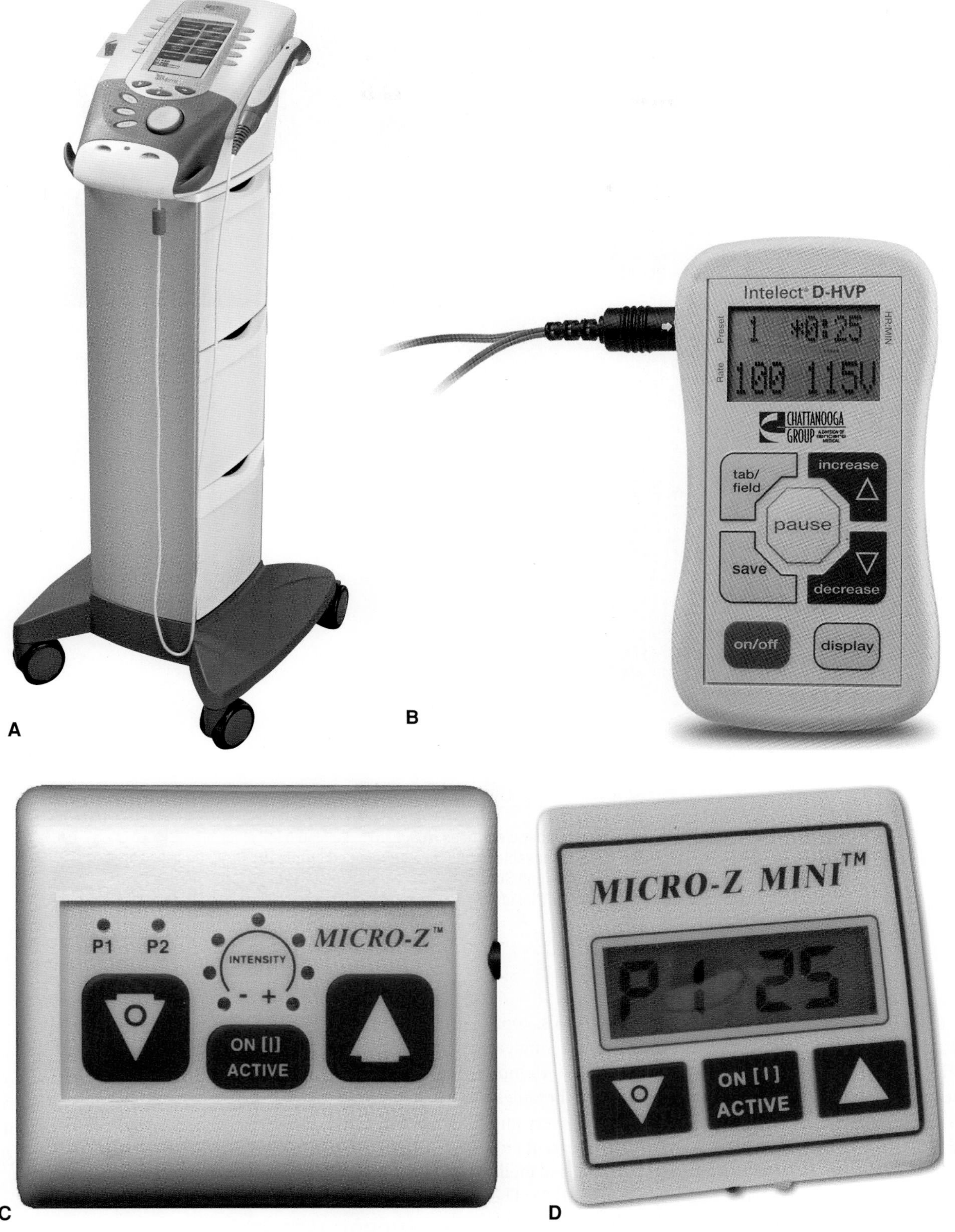

FIGURE 15-1 **A:** Cabinet-type, line powered, electrical stimulator capable of generating microcurrent and high-voltage pulsed current (HVPC). **B:** Portable HVPC stimulator. **C, D:** Wearable and reusable HVPC stimulators. (A, B: Courtesy of DJO Global; C, D: Courtesy of Prizm Medical Inc.)

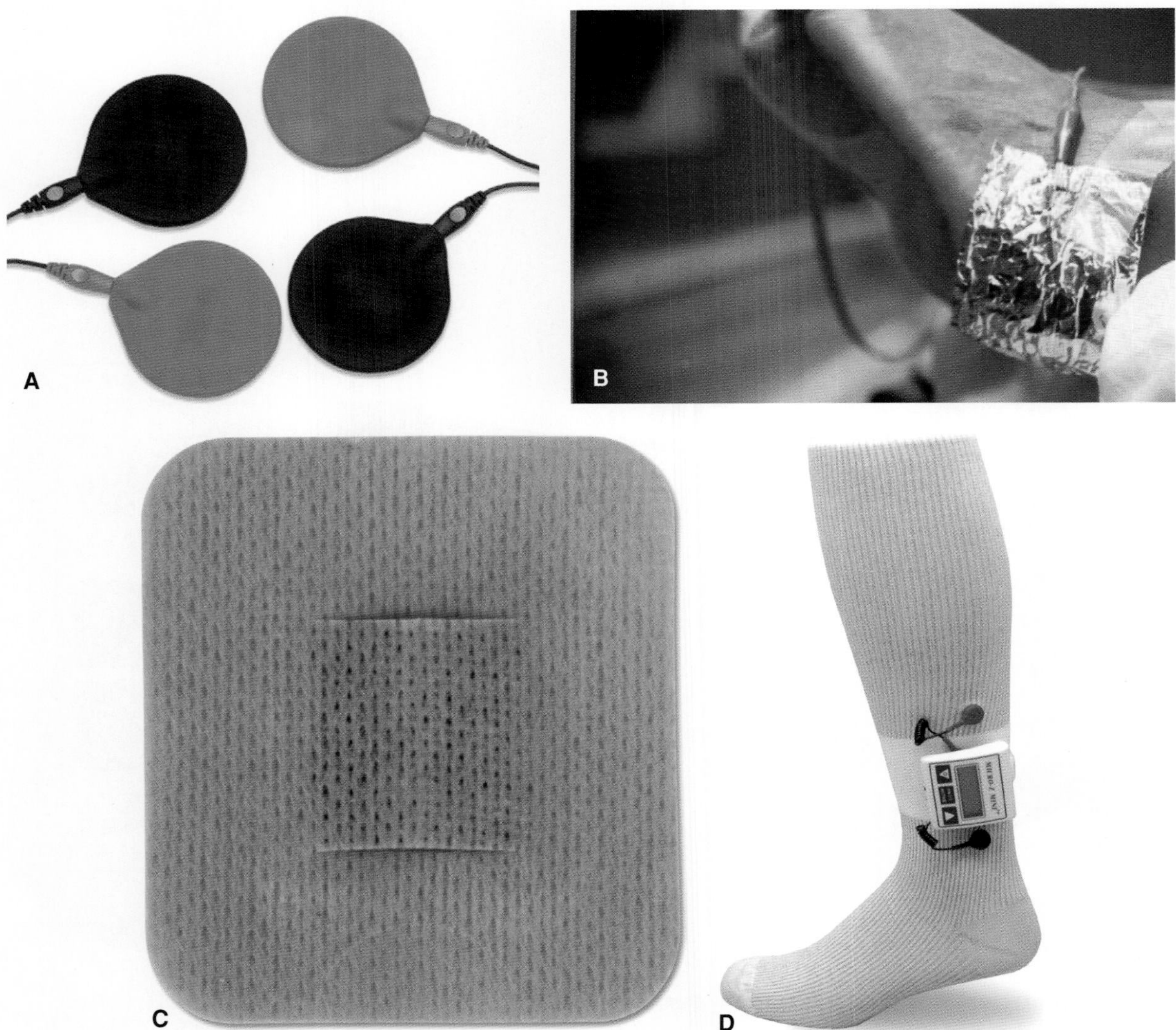

FIGURE 15-2 Typical reusable carbon rubber electrodes (**A**); custom aluminum foil electrode (**B**); pre-gelled, self-adhesive electrodes (**C**); and reusable conductive garment electrode (**D**). (A, C: Courtesy of DJO Global; B: Reprinted with permission from Sussman C, Bartes-Jenson B. *Wound Care: A Collaborative Practice Manual for Health Professionals.* Philadelphia: Lippincott Williams & Wilkins, 2007; D: Courtesy of Prizm Medical Inc.)

wounds, including topical and systemic antibiotics, topical antiseptics and dressings, hydrotherapy, and surgical skin grafting (Kloth, 2005a). Unfortunately, many wounds worsen or do not heal despite the use of such therapies. Research for alternative therapies led to the discovery and application of electrical current, such as microcurrent and HVPC (Becker et al., 1987; Kloth et al., 2002; Falabella et al., 2005; Shai et al., 2005; Sussman et al., 2012). The use of electrical stimulation for wound healing rests on the fact that the human body has an endogenous bioelectric system that enhances soft-tissue wound healing. When a patient's own endogenous bioelectric system fails to contribute to the wound-healing process, therapeutic electrical stimulation is delivered externally to the wound to boost the weak endogenous healing system, thus enhancing and accelerating the wound-healing process.

II. BIOPHYSICAL CHARACTERISTICS

As mentioned earlier, electrical stimulation for wound healing rests on the delivery of two types of currents: microcurrent and HVPC. To avoid duplication of material on the concepts of waveform and frequency, readers are invited to review Chapter 13.

A. MICROCURRENT

As shown in Figure 15-3, a microcurrent is characterized by a monophasic waveform, which can be continuous or pulse modulated, with polarity reversal, and delivered at a peak amplitude of 999 microamperes (μA)—that is, less than 1 mA. A monophasic current has one phase, travels in one direction from the isoelectric line, and returns to

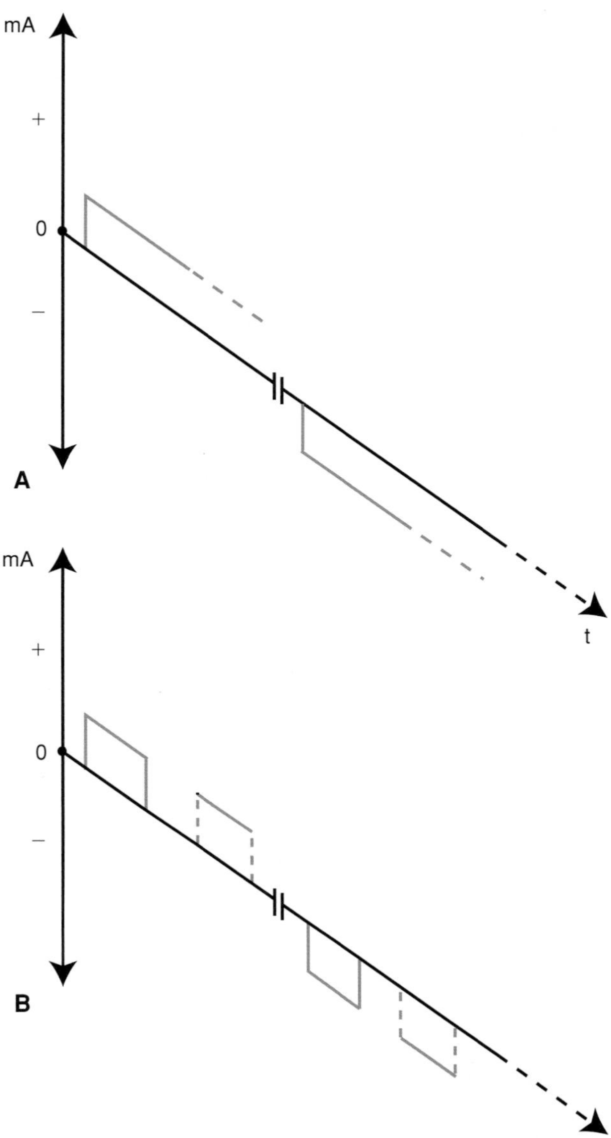

FIGURE 15-3 Typical microcurrent with its characteristic continuous (**A**) or pulsed (**B**) monophasic waveform with polarity reversal. Current amplitude may range between 0 and 999 microamperes (μA).

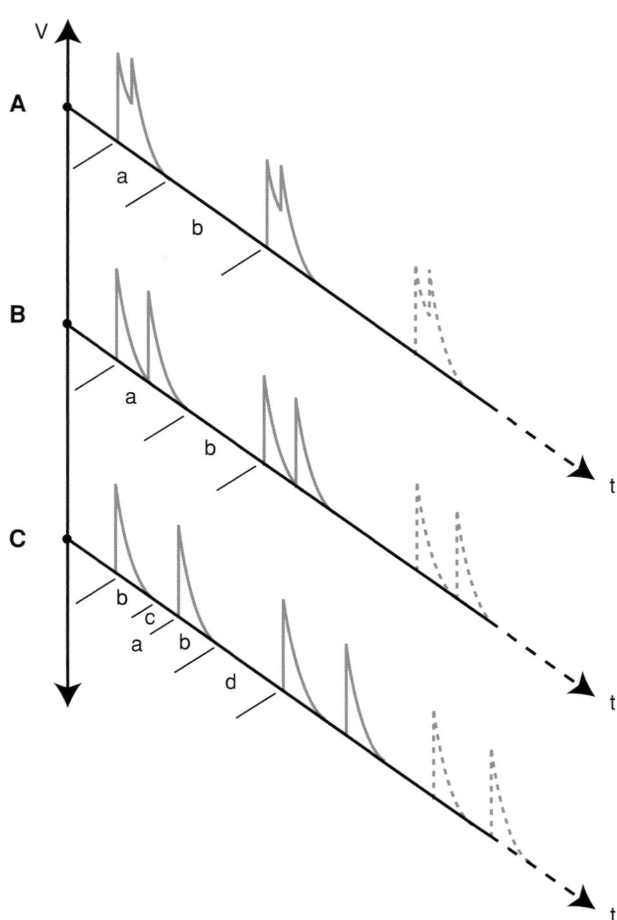

FIGURE 15-4 Typical monophasic, twin-peak pulse patterns generated by a commercial high-voltage pulsed current (HVPC) stimulator. Some stimulators include a control switch that allows the operator to set the time between the first spike waveform and the beginning of the second waveform. **A:** The time between the two spikes is set so that the two waveforms overlap: (*a*) pulse duration, (*b*) interpulse duration. **B:** The time is adjusted so that the second spike waveform begins immediately after the end of the first waveform: (*a*) pulse duration, (*b*) interpulse duration. **C:** The time is adjusted so that an interpulse duration occurs between each twin-peak pulse. Note that pulse duration (*a*) is made of the summation of both spike duration (*b, b*) and interspike duration (*c*); interpulse duration (*d*). Voltage amplitude may range between 150 and 500 volts (*V*).

the isoelectric line after a finite time period. Microcurrent stimulators are *constant current–type* (CC-type) stimulators because they deliver electrical current at constant amplitude (A) regardless of changes in soft tissue impedance (Z) over time. According to Ohm's law, voltage (V) varies proportionally to impedance (Z) to maintain current at a constant level ($V = A \times Z$). Providing constant current amplitude throughout the application makes therapy comfortable for the patient and predictable for the clinician.

B. HIGH-VOLTAGE PULSED CURRENT

1. Waveform

HVPC, illustrated in Figure 15-4, is characterized by twin-peak monophasic pulses, delivered at peak voltage of 500 V (thus, the term *high voltage;* see later discussion).

Each pulse is made of a pair of spike-like waveforms that have an almost instantaneous rise and extremely short peak voltage, followed by an exponential decline. Pulse duration (PD) corresponds to the phase duration of both spikes plus, if applicable, the interspike duration. PD is characteristically very short, ranging from 10 to 100 microseconds (μs), and are usually fixed by the manufacturer. The interspike duration may vary between HVPC stimulators and may be programmable by the operator. Pairs of monophasic, spike-like pulses are generated at frequencies ranging from 1 to 200 pulses per second (pps), or hertz (Hz), through automatic adjustment of interpulse duration (IPD). For example, manually selecting a pulse frequency (f) of 100 Hz, with a fixed pulse duration (PD) of 100 μs, yields an automatic interpulse duration (IPD) of 9,900 μs: $f = 1/(PD + IPD)$; 100 Hz = 1,000,000 μs/

100 μs + 9,900 μs. Do not confuse the terms *pulse* and *peak* when discussing HVPC. Pulse refers to the waveform, not to the number of peaks within the waveform. For example, the display of an HVPC having a 60-pps frequency on the oscilloscope screen will show 60 monophasic pulses and 120 peaks, because each pulse has twin peaks.

2. High Voltage

Contrary to microcurrent stimulators, HVPC stimulators are *constant-voltage type* (CV-type) stimulators because voltage is kept constant regardless of changes in soft tissue impedance (Z) over time. As its name implies, the HVPC stimulator delivers high voltages, usually between 150 and 500 V. Why is a high-driving peak voltage necessary? Because pulse duration is extremely short (less than 100 μs), with a peak spike voltage duration lasting only a fraction of a microsecond (see Fig. 15-4). According to Ohm's law ($V = A \times Z$), current amplitude (A) is directly related to voltage (V). Therefore, for current amplitude (A) to be effective, voltage (V) has to be high enough to compensate for the very short pulse duration, and extremely short spike voltage duration, associated with HVPC. In other words, the shorter the pulse duration, the greater the driving voltage should be in order to generate enough current for therapeutic purposes.

III. THERAPEUTIC EFFECTS AND INDICATIONS

A. SKIN BATTERY AND CURRENTS OF INJURY

The principle behind the use of ESTHR is illustrated in Figure 15-5. Typical *skin battery,* located at the interface between the stratum corneum and the dermis, in normal human skin tissue is illustrated in Figure 15-5A. Becker hypothesized that a direct current bioelectrical system is present in the human body and that this system is responsible for maintaining tissue health (Becker et al., 1987). Figure 15-5B illustrates currents of injury, driven by those skin batteries located at the wound site after trauma or disease. Becker further hypothesized that when the body is injured, a disturbance within the body's electrical system causes a shift in the current flow at the site of injury, which he labeled *current of injury* (Becker et al., 1987). Figure 15-5C presents Becker's fundamental proposition that an exogenous source of electrical current, such as microcurrent or HVPC, applied over the wound would enhance the healing process. In other words, the application of monophasic electrical current is believed to *mimic* and *amplify* those endogenous, weak human skin batteries at the wound site to thus enhance and maintain, with repeated applications over time, the skin healing process.

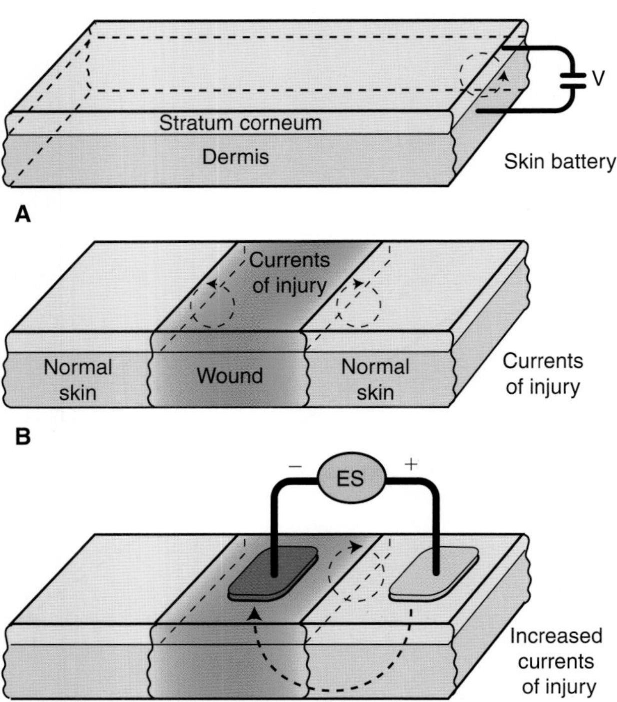

FIGURE 15-5 Schematic representation of a normal skin battery. Continuous flow of endogenous current (*circling arrow*), which is driven by the skin battery, is presumed to sustain the normal repair process of skin tissue in the absence of injury (**A**). Currents of injury flow after a wound to the skin. Injury to the skin (wound) causes the flow of this endogenous current, now called *currents of injury,* to flow at the interface between the damaged and the normal skin tissue (**B**). Increased currents of injury amplitude caused by the application of microcurrent, or high-voltage pulsed current, at the wound site (**C**). ES, electrical stimulation.

B. ENHANCED CURRENTS OF INJURY

The rationale behind ESTHR is the fact that animals as a whole, and amphibians in particular, have a much greater capacity for tissue self-healing than humans. This concept suggests that through the evolutionary process, human currents of injury have become less efficient—hence, the need to mimic and amplify those weak skin batteries to obtain stronger, more efficient currents of injury to enhance soft-tissue repair. In other words, by providing an external current to the wound, MES mimics and augments those weak, natural bioelectric currents to enhance wound repair (Taradaj, 2003; Poltawski et al., 2009).

C. GALVANOTAXIS EFFECTS

Figure 15-6 presents the proposed physiologic and therapeutic effects underlying the use of ESTHR (Kloth, 2005a,b; Robinson, 2008). Electrical stimulation, using those continuous or pulsed monophasic currents (microcurrent and HVPC), is presumed to induce galvanotaxic and bacterial growth inhibition effects on dermal wounds, thus enhancing wound repair.

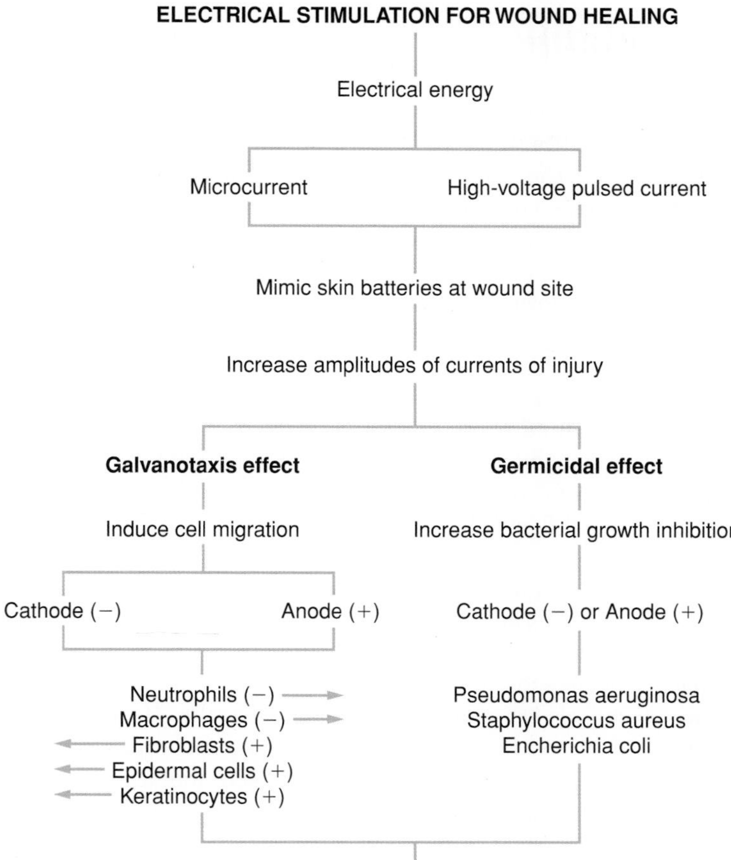

FIGURE 15-6 Proposed physiologic and therapeutic effects of electrical stimulation for wound healing. Negatively and positively charged cells migrate (see *arrows*) toward the anode and cathode, respectively, during electrical stimulation.

1. Monophasic Current

The monophasic nature associated with microcurrent and HVPC implies that their respective waveforms are *unbalanced,* meaning that a net amount of electrical charges (negatively charged electrons) will accumulate under the electrodes over time during therapy. This accumulation of charges introduces the concept of electrode polarity. *Polarity* is the property of having charges, either negative or positive. Practically speaking, the electrode with the greater number of electrons or negative charges is called the *negative electrode* or *cathode* (–), and that with the lower number is called the *positive electrode* or *anode* (+). Based on Coulomb's law of electrical interaction between charged objects or particles, unlike charges (+/–) attract each other, and like charges (+/+; –/–) repel one another. It thus follows that during the application of a monophasic current into soft tissue, the negatively charged cathode will attract positively charged ions, whereas the positively charged anode will attract negatively charged ions. This ionic migration under the electrodes, induced by the passage of a monophasic current, underlies the principle of galvanotaxis.

2. Galvanotaxis

Because many key cells involved in the process of wound healing carry either a negative or a positive charge, (Kloth, 2005a,b) hypothesized that the monophasic nature of those two electrical currents would facilitate *galvanotaxic* attraction of these cells into the wound, thereby promoting the different phases of wound healing. The term *galvanotaxis* stems from the word *galvano* (meaning "galvanic, direct, or continuous current") and the word *taxis,* which refers to orderly arrangement of motile organisms in response to a stimulus either toward the cathode (positively charged cells) or the anode (negatively charged cells).

a. Inflammatory Phase

There is experimental evidence to suggest that negatively charged cells, such as macrophages (–) and neutrophils (–), will migrate, as illustrated in Figure 15-6, toward the anode (+), thus promoting the inflammatory phase (phagocytosis and autolysis) of wound healing (Kloth, 2005a,b; Robinson, 2008). This makes anodal stimulation the treatment option of choice for the management of inflamed wounds.

b. Proliferative Phase

There is also experimental evidence to suggest that positively charged cells, such as fibroblasts (+), will migrate toward the cathode (−) during electrical stimulation, thus promoting the proliferative (collagen formation) phase of wound healing (Kloth, 2005a,b; Robinson, 2008). Cathodal stimulation may therefore be the treatment option of choice for the management of wounds in their proliferative phase.

c. Remodeling/Maturation Phase

There is also experimental evidence to also suggest that positively charged cells, such as keratinocytes (+) and epidermal (+) cells, will migrate toward the cathode (−), thus promoting the remodeling/maturation phase of wound healing. Once again, cathodal stimulation is seen as the preferred treatment option for the management of wounds in this phase of repair.

D. GERMICIDAL EFFECT

There is limited experimental evidence to suggest that passing a monophasic electrical current, such as microcurrent and HVPC, will induce a *germicidal effect* into the wound. In other words, the passing of such electrical current is presumed to treat wound infection by inhibiting the growth of action of microorganisms such as such as *Escherichia coli, Pseudomonas aeruginosa,* and *Staphylococcus aureus* (Merriman et al., 2004; Kloth, 2005a,b; Sussman et al., 2007; Robinson, 2008). This effect is presumed to occur under both electrodes (see Fig. 15-6). Maximal germicidal effects were found using HVPC in vitro, with a voltage of 250 V at the cathode, for a period of 2 hours (Kincaid et al., 1989; Weiss et al., 1989). Guffey et al. (1989) found that an application of at least 30 minutes was necessary to produce a germicidal effect in vitro using HVPC.

E. OTHER PROPOSED EFFECTS ATTRIBUTED TO HIGH-VOLTAGE PULSED CURRENT

There is research-based evidence, as shown next, to suggest that the passing of HVPC into human tissues may trigger additional physiologic and therapeutic effects on soft tissues. Is there scientific evidence to support these effects?

1. Retard Posttraumatic Edema Formation—Conflicting

It is postulated that HVPC may retard edema formation associated with acute inflammatory response to soft-tissue injury. Some have theorized that HVPC may curb edema by reducing microvascular cellular permeability—that is, decreased permeability between cell membranes and interstitial space (Mendel et al., 2010). Edema formation is related to the leakage of negatively charged plasma proteins in cell membranes into interstitial spaces after injury, resulting in an increase of fluid accumulation in the affected area. One possible mechanism may be that the passage of HVPC, through the cathode electrode placed over the swollen area, will repel the negatively charged proteins, thus preventing them from moving out of blood vessels. The evidence from the human scientific literature reveals *conflicting* results, with some studies reporting beneficial effect (Ross et al., 1981; Lamboni et al., 1983; Voight, 1984;) and some showing no effect on swelling (Michlovitz et al., 1988; Griffin et al., 1990; Sandoval et al., 2010; Mendel et al., 2010).

2. Increase Muscle Strength and Blood Flow—Not Supported

Some authors have suggested that pulsed HVPC may be used for muscle strengthening and for increasing muscle blood flow (Alon, 1985; Mohr et al. 1985; Wong, 1986). Only one article was found in the English-language, peer-reviewed literature on the muscle-strengthening effect of HVPC. The controlled study by Mohr et al. (1985) found HVPC stimulation to be *ineffective* for increasing quadriceps muscle force compared with a voluntary isometric muscle contraction regimen. As far as the effect of HVPC on blood flow is concerned, only two peer-reviewed articles, involving healthy subjects, were found in the English-language literature. These two studies report *conflicting* results. Carlson-Walker et al. (1988) found *no increase* of blood flow in the popliteal artery after HVPC stimulation, whereas Heath et al. (1992) did find an *increase* in blood flow that correlated with the voltage amplitude used to contract the calf muscle.

3. Decrease Pelvic Floor Muscle Spasm—Supported

It has been suggested that HVPC may have an *antispasmodic* effect on pelvic floor muscles, particularly for the treatment of levator ani syndrome. There is some evidence to support the fact that prolonged, or long-lasting, evoked contraction of the levator ani muscle using pulsed HVPC can induce muscle fatigue to exhaustion, which in turn promotes its relaxation (no contraction, no spasm) by breaking the muscle spasm–pain cycle (Sohn et al., 1982; Nicosia et al., 1985; Oliver et al., 1985; Billingham et al., 1987; Morris et al., 1987; Hull et al., 1993; Park et al., 2005). Note that this effect is not specific to the use of HVPC. Any other pulsed electrical currents, such as biphasic pulsed, Russian, or interferential (see Chapter 13), can induce the same muscle-exhausting neuromuscular electrical stimulation effect if programmed accordingly.

4. Decrease Delayed-Onset Muscle Soreness—Not Supported

It has also been suggested that HVPC may be beneficial for delayed-onset muscle soreness following bouts of muscle contractions. The evidence from the literature shows no support for the use of this current for this condition, with only one study showing benefit (McLoughlin

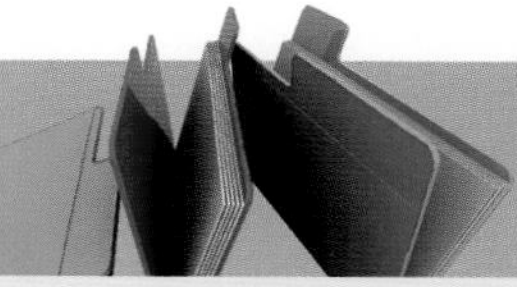

Research-Based Indications

ELECTRICAL STIMULATION FOR TISSUE HEALING AND REPAIR

Health Condition	Benefit—Yes Rating	Benefit—Yes Reference	Benefit—No Rating	Benefit—No Reference
Dermal wound	I	Huckfeldt et al., 2007		
	I	Wood et al., 1993		
	I	Gault et al., 1976		
	I	Carley et al., 1985		
	I	Houghton et al., 2003		
	I	Ahmad, 2008		
	I	Peters et al., 2001		
	I	Unger, 1985		
	I	Kloth et al., 1988		
	I	Goldman et al., 2004		
	I	Feedar et al., 1991		
	II	Burdge et al., 2009		
	II	Mulder, 1991		
	II	Gilcreast et al., 1998		
	II	Houghton et al., 2010		

Health Condition	Benefit—Yes Rating	Benefit—Yes Reference	Benefit—No Rating	Benefit—No Reference
Dermal wounds	II	Griffin et al., 1991		
	II	Akers et al., 1984		
	II	Franek et al., 2000		
	II	Goldman et al., 2003		
	II	Wolcott et al., 1969		
	II	Assimacopoulos, 1968		
	II	Young et al., 2011		
	III	Chapman-Jones et al., 2010		
	III	Barron et al., 1985		
	III	Weiss et al., 1989		
	III	Mawson et al., 1993		
	III	Goldman et al., 2002		
	III	Thurman et al., 1971		
	III	Fitzgerald et al., 1993		

Strength of evidence: Moderate
Therapeutic effectiveness: Substantiated

et al., 2004) and seven other studies revealing no benefit (Denegar et al., 1992; Weber et al., 1994; Bonacci et al., 1997; Butterfield et al., 1997; Allen et al., 1999; Tourville et al., 2006; Curtis et al., 2010).

5. Decrease Pain—Supported

In addition to all of the earlier proposed physiologic and therapeutic effects, HVPC and microcurrent for pain modulation, applied over a variety of conditions, has also been suggested. Several studies have reported beneficial results (Lerner et al., 1981; Quirion de Girardi et al., 1984; Hatten et al., 1990; Johannsen et al., 1993; Shrode, 1993; Bertolucci et al., 1995; McMakin, 1998; Stralka et al., 1998; Maenpaa et al., 2004; McMakin, 2004; Koopman et al., 2009). To use monophasic pulsed current such as HVPC and microcurrent to modulate pain is *not recommended* because its waveform is unbalanced, causing a polar effect—that is, a net accumulation of charges under the electrodes that may cause discomfort and pain, as well as skin irritation and damage over prolonged and repeated applications. The use of balanced biphasic pulsed current is strongly recommended for pain modulation (see Chapter 14).

F. RESEARCH-BASED INDICATIONS

The search for evidence behind the use of electrical stimulation for wound healing, displaced in the *Research-Based Indications* box, led to the collection of 29 English peer-reviewed human clinical studies. The methodology and criteria used to assess the strength of evidence and therapeutic effectiveness are described in Chapter 2. The strength of evidence behind the use of ESTHR is found to be *moderate* and its therapeutic effectiveness *substantiated* for the management of dermal wounds.

IV. DOSIMETRY

Table 15-1 lists common dosimetric parameters used to treat dermal wounds using electrical stimulation. Let us consider each of them.

TABLE 15-1	RECOMMENDED DOSIMETRIC PARAMETERS FOR WOUND HEALING	
Parameters	**Microcurrent**	**High-Voltage Pulsed Current**
Mode	Continuous Pulsed	Pulsed
Frequency	*Continuous:* 0 Hz *Pulsed:* 1–200 Hz	1–200 Hz
Amplitude	Microcurrent range 1–999 μA Comfortable level	High-voltage range 150–500 V Comfortable level
Electrode polarity*	*Anodal stimulation (+):* For inflammatory phase *Cathodal stimulation (–):* For all other healing phases *Anode (+) or cathode (–):* For wound infection	
Polarity reversal**	Every 3 d	
Application duration	30–90 min	
Treatment frequency	1–3 times daily	
Electrode configuration	Over the wound or around the wound	

*Electrode polarity applies only to the over-the-wound electrode configuration.
**Polarity reversal applies to both electrode configurations.

A. CURRENT TYPE AND MODE OF DELIVERY

Electrical stimulation for wound healing may be delivered using microcurrent or HVPC. Microcurrent can be delivered using continuous- or pulsed mode (see Fig. 15-3), and HVPC is commonly delivered in pulsed mode only (see Fig. 15-4). There is no evidence to show that one current type or mode is more beneficial than another.

B. FREQUENCY AND CURRENT/VOLTAGE AMPLITUDE

If pulse mode is used, frequency may be set between 1 and 200 Hz. Amplitude is set in the microamperes for microcurrent and in high-voltage range for HVPC. There is no evidence to show that one frequency is better than another or that microamperage is better than high-voltage for wound management. Settings of amplitudes will largely be determined by the patient's tolerance to the passing of electrical current for a relatively long period.

C. ELECTRODE CONFIGURATION AND POLARITY

The practitioner may choose between the *over-the-wound or around-the-wound* electrode configurations, as illustrated in Figure 15-7. If the over-the-wound configuration is applied, selecting electrode polarity must be considered, as shown in Table 15-1. *Anodal stimulation* should be used in cases where wound *inflammation* is present because the migration (galvanotaxis) of key cells such as macrophages and neutrophils to the wound site will stimulate the inflammatory response, thus improving tissue repair. After the inflammatory phase has subsided, *cathodal stimulation* should be used in order to facilitate the *proliferative/remodeling/maturation* phases of healing through the migration of key cells such as fibroblasts, keratinocytes, and epidermal cells to the wound site. Practitioners may use either cathodal or anodal stimulation first over the *infected* wound, as the evidence seems to suggest that both electrode polarities may induce germ growth inhibition at the wound site (Merriman et al., 2004). Because the different phases of wound healing overlap over time, it is recommended that electrode polarity *be reversed* after a few treatments to ensure migration of both negatively (anti-inflammatory) and positively (repair) charged cells at the wound site during the entire course of therapy.

D. APPLICATION DURATION AND TREATMENT FREQUENCY

Single-application duration may range from 30 to 90 minutes. There is no evidence on which to base the selection of this parameter. Treatments can range between one and four sessions per day depending of the wound condition. Many electrical stimulators feature a switch that allows presetting of a daily ON:OFF time stimulation regimen. For example, setting a daily ON:OFF time regimen of 1 hour:5 hours over a 12-hour period automatically yields two treatment sessions per day. This feature is practical in that it allows practitioners to program all of the parameters

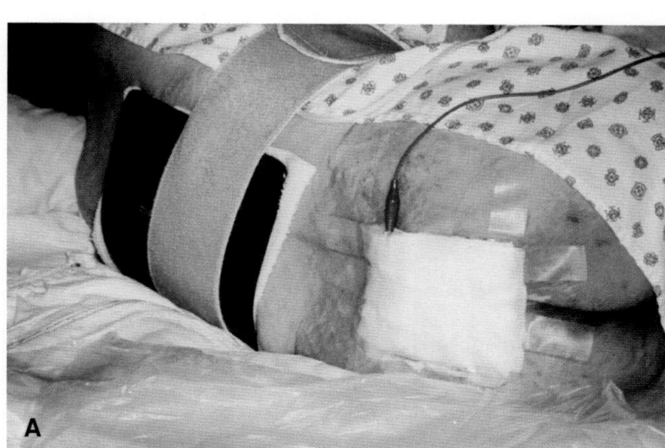

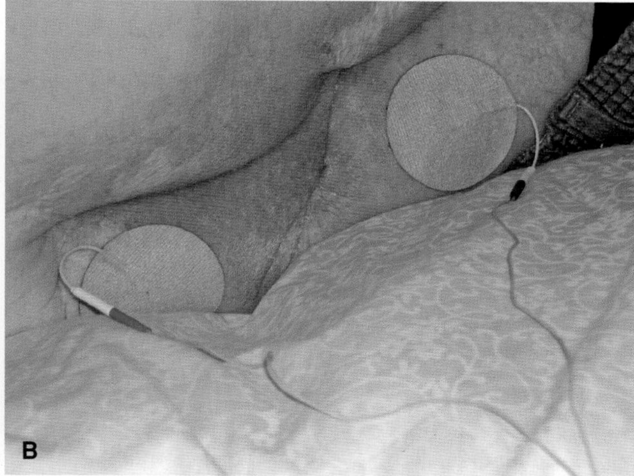

FIGURE 15-7 Electrode placement over the wound (**A**) and around the wound (**B**). (Reprinted with permission from Sussman C, Bates-Jensen B. *Wound Care: A Collaborative Practice Manual for Health Professionals,* 4th ed. Baltimore, Maryland: Lippincott Williams & Wilkins, 2012. Copyright © C. Sussman.)

at one time for half the day, as just mentioned, or for the full day (24-hour period). Treatment days can range from 5 to 7 days per week. There is no evidence on which to base the selection of this parameter.

V. APPLICATION, CONTRAINDICATIONS, AND RISKS

Prior to considering the application of electrical stimulation for tissue healing and repair, practitioners must first check for contraindications, consider the risks, and then go through key application steps and procedures designed to optimize treatment safety, efficacy, and effectiveness. Most contraindications are related to the application of pulsed HVPC. Cross-contamination presents a major risk. A key precaution is to wear protective gown, gloves, mask, and goggles. Research has shown that currents of injury are sustained in a moist wound environment but will shut off when the wound dries out (Kloth, 2005a,b). The clinical implication of this finding is that to facilitate healing, the wound must be covered by occlusive, moisture-retentive dressings at all times (Kloth, 2005a,b; Sussman et al., 2012).

APPLICATION, CONTRAINDICATIONS, AND RISKS

Electrical Stimulation for Wound Healing

Important: To prevent cross-contamination, practitioners *must* adopt protective measures by the wearing of masks, gloves, goggles, and gowns during wound preparation and treatment.

 See **online video** for details.

STEP	RATIONALE AND PROCEDURE
1. Check for contraindications.	*Over osteomyelitic area*—blinding of the site of observation (wound penetration to the bone) because tissue growth after therapy may superficially cover the osteomyelitic area *Over cancerous area*—enhances and spreads the tumor due to increased blood flow into the treated area *Over electronic implants*—interference with normal functioning of these devices *Over the anterior cervical area*—stimulation of key organs adjacent to the skin such as the vagus nerve, phrenic nerve, and carotid sinuses

STEP	RATIONALE AND PROCEDURE
	Over thoracic area—affects normal heart function *Over cranial area*—affects normal brain function *Over metallic implants*—causes unnecessary pain due to electrical current and induces overheating of implants *Over the abdominal pelvic and lumbar areas of women in their first trimester of pregnancy*—induces labor *Over hemorrhagic areas*—further bleeding due to increased blood circulation into the treated areas
2. Consider the risks.	*With infected wounds*—risk of auto- and cross-contamination if adequate measures are not taken *Using a cool coupling media temperature*—risk of chilling the wound, which increases the possibility of slowing down mitotic activity, thus delaying or slowing down wound healing
3. Position and instruct patient.	Ensure comfortable body positioning. Instruct the patient not to touch the device, cables, and electrodes and to call for assistance if necessary. Inform that no sensory sensation may be felt during treatment.
4. Prepare wound.	Wash, cleanse, and debride the wound using mechanical or hydrotherapeutic interventions. Removal of necrotic material, foreign material, heavy metals, and previous topical medication, including petroleum gel or paste, from wounds will prevent penetration, caused by current flow, of foreign materials and medication that may hinder or adversely affect wound healing. Wash normal skin surrounding the wound with rubbing alcohol and then dry the skin.
5. Select device type.	Choose between cabinet (in-clinic therapy) or portable (bedside or home therapy) device. Plug line-powered stimulator into GFCI receptacle to prevent macroshock.
6. Select current type.	Choose between microcurrent and HVPC.
7. Select electrodes.	Disposable electrodes are highly recommended in preference to reusable electrodes, especially if the over-the-wound configuration is used.
8. Select electrode configuration.	Choose between over and around the wound: • *Over the wound:* One electrode is positioned directly on top of the wound and the other a few centimeters away (see Fig. 15-7A). • *Around the wound:* Both electrodes are positioned around the wound, over normal skin area adjacent to the wound margins (see Fig. 15-7B).
9. Prepare and position electrodes.	• *Over the wound:* Wrap electrode with layers of sterile gauze pads, saturate the pads with Ringer solution or normal saline solution, and position the electrode/pad arrangement over the wound (see Fig. 15-7A). Pads must be warmer than the wound before application, but not warmer than 38°C (100°F). Use a portable *infrared thermometer* to record coupling media temperature (see Chapter 7). Cover the other electrode with electroconductive gel. • *Around the wound:* Cover both electrodes with electroconductive gel and then secure to the skin using hypoallergic tape or an adhesive patch (see Fig. 15-7B).
10. Set dosimetry.	Use Table 15-1 as a guideline. Set mode, frequency (if pulsed mode), current or voltage amplitude, and electrode polarity. It is recommended that electrode polarity be *reversed* periodically over the course of therapy to ensure a balanced migration of positively and negatively charged cells at the wound site.
11. Set treatment schedule.	Determine the application duration and the number of treatment sessions per day. The wound may be treated for durations ranging from 30–90 minutes, two or three times a day. Treatments may be delivered daily (see Table 15-1).

STEP	RATIONALE AND PROCEDURE
12. Apply treatment.	Ensure adequate monitoring during treatment.
13. Conduct post-treatment inspection.	Inspect the wound and question the patient on the sensation perceived during treatment. Any unusual sensation felt during treatment should be documented in the patient's file. To optimize treatment effectiveness, *do not remove* the sterile gauze pad covering the wound after treatment. Keep this coupling medium *moist* and in place until the next treatment. Proceed with wound dressing. Discard used material in a biowaste bag.
14. Ensure post-treatment equipment maintenance.	Follow manufacturer recommendations. Immediately report all defects or malfunctions to technical maintenance staff. Conduct regular maintenance and calibration procedures.

CASE STUDIES

Presented are two case studies that summarize the concepts, principles, and applications of electrical stimulation for tissue healing and repair discussed in this chapter. Case Study 15-1 addresses the usage of microcurrent for ischial pressure ulcer affecting an elderly woman. Case Study 15-2 is concerned with the application of HVPC for a venous leg ulcer affecting a senior man. Each case is structured in line with the concepts of evidence-based practice (EBP), the International Classification of Functioning, Disability, and Health (ICF) disablement model, and SOAP (*s*ubjective, *o*bjective, *a*ssessment, *p*lan) note format (see Chapter 2 for details).

CASE STUDY 15-1: ISCHIAL PRESSURE ULCER

EVIDENCE-BASED CLINICAL DECISION MAKING PROTOCOL

1. Formulate the Case History

A well-oriented and underweight 76-year-old woman who shows evidence of poor body hygiene and lives alone in a senior home apartment is referred by her physician for treatment of an infected pressure ulcer over the right ischial tuberosity. The ulcer began approximately 6 months ago. She complains that the wound is slow to heal. Your clinic is located across the street, within 5 minutes walk from this senior home. She presents with difficulty sitting. She enjoys spending long hours sitting on her wooden chair playing cards with friends, knitting, and watching television. Physical examination reveals the presence of a painful stage II pressure ischial ulcer. Wound size is 2 cm^2. The wound is in its proliferative/remodeling/maturation phase of repair. Laboratory results confirm that the ulcer is colonized, or infected, with the bacteria *P. aeruginosa*.

2. Outline the Case Based on the ICF Framework

ISCHIAL PRESSURE ULCER		
BODY STRUCTURES AND FUNCTIONS	**ACTIVITIES**	**PARTICIPATION**
Pain	Difficulty sitting	Difficulty with sitting during leisure activities such as playing cards and watching television
Skin pressure ulcer		
Infected wound		

PERSONAL FACTORS	ENVIRONMENTAL FACTORS
Elderly patient	Leisure and sharing pastimes
Ambulatory	Senior home
Poor body hygiene	

3. Outline Therapeutic Goals and Outcome Measurements

GOAL	OUTCOME MEASUREMENT
Decrease pain	101-point Numerical Rating Scale (NRS-101)
Eliminate wound infection	Bacterial count
Decrease wound size	Digital photograph
Improve ability to sit/accelerate return to leisure activities	Pain Disability Index (PDI)

4. Justify the Use of ESTHR Based on the EBP Framework

PRACTITIONER'S EXPERIENCE	RESEARCH-BASED INDICATIONS	PATIENT'S EXPECTATION
Experienced in electrical stimulation for wound management	*Strength:* Moderate	No opinion on electrical stimulation therapy
Has used electrical stimulation in similar cases	*Effectiveness:* Substantiated	Wants to resume activities of daily living (ADLs) as well as leisure activities
Believes that electrical stimulation will be beneficial		

5. Outline Key Intervention Parameters

- **Treatment base:** Private clinic
- **Electrical current:** Microcurrent
- **Current waveform:** Monophasic
- **Delivery mode:** Pulsed
- **Stimulator type:** Cabinet (see Fig. 15-1A).
- **Risk and precaution:** The open wound is contaminated. To optimize treatment effectiveness, the wound is cleaned, irrigated, and debrided prior to each treatment. To prevent cross-contamination, the practitioner is wearing a protective gown, gloves, mask, and goggles.
- **Application protocol:** Follow the suggested application protocol in *Application, Contraindications, and Risks* box, and make the necessary adjustments for this case.
- **Patient's positioning:** Lying ventral
- **Pulse frequency:** 10 Hz
- **Pulse duration:** 600 μs
- **Current amplitude:** 800 μA
- **Electrode configuration:** Over the wound
- **Active electrode type and size:** Aluminum foil cut to wound size and shape
- **Dispersive electrode type and size:** Carbon rubber (4×8 cm^2 [2×3 in])
- **Coupling media under active electrode:** Sterile saline-soaked gauze packed into the wound
- **Coupling media under dispersive electrode:** Hydrogel pad
- **Active electrode placement:** On top of the wound
- **Dispersive electrode placement:** Over healthy skin, 15 cm away from left gluteal area
- **Active electrode polarity at first treatment:** Negative—cathodal stimulation
- **Electrode polarity reversal:** Every 5 treatments
- **Application duration per session:** 90 minutes
- **Treatment frequency:** Daily; 5 days a week
- **Intervention period:** 3 weeks
- **Concomitant therapies:** Complete daily wound care (cleaning, irrigating, debriding, bandaging)

6. Compare Pre- and Post-Intervention Outcomes

OUTCOME	PRE	POST
Pain (NRS scale)	85/100	22/100
Wound infection (bacterial count)		0
Wound size	2 cm^2	Full closure
Functional activities (PDI)	35/70	5/70

7. Document Case Intervention Using the SOAP Note Format

S: Elderly, well-oriented, and ambulatory female Pt, showing evidence of poor body hygiene, presents with an infected ischial pressure ulcer leading to difficulty with sitting and sitting's leisure activities.

O: *Intervention:* Private clinic based; electrical stimulation applied over the wound; microcurrent; pulsed mode; frequency: 10 Hz; pulse duration 600 µs; current amplitude 800 µA; cathodal stimulation (–) to begin with polarity reversal every 5 days; foil electrode over the wound; daily treatment; 5 days a week for 3 weeks. *Pre–post comparison:* Pain decrease (85/100 to 22/100), elimination of wound infection (0 bacterial count), decrease wound size (2 to 0.5 cm^2), an improved functional capacity (35 to 5/70).

A: No adverse effect. Treatment tolerated.

P: Pt discharged from clinic. Pt advised to minimize prolonged sitting positions and to maintain body hygiene.

CASE STUDY 15-2: VENOUS LEG ULCER

EVIDENCE-BASED CLINICAL DECISION MAKING PROTOCOL

1. Formulate the Case History

An alert 72-year-old male patient who is obese and diabetic, living in his three-floor house with his wife, is referred for treatment of his delayed-healing venous leg ulcer. The ulcer is located 3 cm over the left lateral malleolus. The wound's surface is irregular with a total area of 12 cm^2. Wound duration is of approximately 9 months. No infection is seen. The wound displays light edema. The patient reports having difficulty putting on his shoes, which limits his walking ability and overall ability to do ADLs. He has difficulty moving from one floor to the other. Because of his severe lack of mobility, the patient's strong preference is for home therapy. Having done a brief Internet search on possible noninvasive treatments for his condition, he came across the use of surface electrical stimulation. He wants to avoid surgical treatment at all costs.

2. Outline the Case Based on the ICF Framework

VENOUS LEG ULCER		
BODY STRUCTURES AND FUNCTIONS	**ACTIVITIES**	**PARTICIPATION**
Pain	Difficulty putting shoes on	Difficulty with ambulation
Open venous wound	Difficulty walking	Difficulty with ADLs
Moderate edema		

PERSONAL FACTORS	ENVIRONMENTAL FACTORS
Elderly patient	Daily living
Obese	Home architectural barrier (3 floors)
Diabetic	Ambulation

3. Outline Therapeutic Goals and Outcome Measurements

GOAL	OUTCOME MEASUREMENT
Decrease pain	Visual Analogue Scale (VAS)
Decrease wound size	Digital photograph
Improve ambulation	Patient-Specific Functional Scale (PSFS)

4. Justify the Use of ESTHR Based on the EBP Framework

PRACTITIONER'S EXPERIENCE	RESEARCH-BASED INDICATIONS	PATIENT'S EXPECTATION
Moderately experienced in electrical stimulation	*Strength:* Moderate	Believes that electrical stimulation will be beneficial
Has never used electrical stimulation in similar cases	*Effectiveness:* Substantiated	Wants to avoid surgery and improve ambulation
Hopes that electrical stimulation may be beneficial		

5. Outline Key Intervention Parameters

- **Treatment base:** Home with weekly visit by practitioner
- **Electrical current:** HVPC
- **Current waveform:** Monophasic twin peak
- **Delivery mode:** Pulsed
- **Stimulator type:** Portable (see Fig. 15-1C)
- **Risk and precaution:** The patient is used to caring for his wound. He has done a fine job over the past months considering that no sign of infection is present. The fact that he is obese has no therapeutic relevance here because the target tissue is the skin.
- **Application protocol:** Follow the suggested application protocol in *Application, Contraindications, and Risks* box, and make the necessary adjustments for this case.
- **Patient's positioning:** Sitting with legs extended on bed
- **Pulse frequency:** 125 Hz
- **Pulse duration:** 200 μs (fixed)
- **Voltage amplitude:** 400 V
- **Electrode configuration:** Around the wound
- **Electrode type and size:** One pair of reusable carbon rubber electrodes; circular; 5 cm (2.5 in) in diameter
- **Coupling medium:** Electroconductive gel under both electrodes
- **Electrode placement:** Cathode above and anode below the wound
- **Electrode polarity reversal:** Every 3 treatments
- **Application duration per session:** 120 minutes
- **Treatment frequency:** Daily
- **Intervention period:** 5 weeks
- **Concomitant therapies:** Patient's own daily wound care (cleaning and bandaging) and weekly wound irrigation and debriding by practitioner during home visit

6. Compare Pre- and Post-Intervention Outcomes

OUTCOME	PRE	POST
Pain (VAS)	6/10	2/10
Wound size	12 cm^2	2 cm^2
Functional activities (PSFS)	7/10	3/10

7. Document Case Intervention Using the SOAP Note Format

S: Elderly, alert male Pt who is obese and diabetic presents with a delayed-healing venous leg ulcer leading to difficulty with ambulation and ADLs.

O: *Intervention:* Home based; electrical stimulation applied around the wound; HVPC; pulsed mode; frequency: 125 Hz; pulse duration 200 μs; voltage amplitude 400 V; polarity reversal every 3 days; carbon rubber electrodes covered with electroconductive gel; treatment duration: 120 min; daily treatment for 5 weeks. *Pre–post comparison:* Pain decrease (VAS 6/10 to 2/10), decrease wound size (12 to 2 cm^2), an improved functional capacity (PSFS 7/10 to 3/10).

A: Minimal adverse effect observed (light dermatitis under electrodes). Controlled by rotating electrode placement. Treatment very well tolerated.

P: Pt will continue home daily treatment until full wound closure. Pt is very happy with treatment outcome, and with the possibility of avoiding surgical treatment.

VI. THE BOTTOM LINE

- There is scientific evidence to show that electrical stimulation can significantly enhanced the healing process of slow-to-heal open and closed dermal wounds.
- The human body attempts to maintain a steady state through self-repair.
- Human skin is made of endogenous batteries, which generate microbioelectrical currents. When the skin is injured, endogenous currents of injury, driven by those batteries, flow at the wound site to repair the skin.
- The application of an exogenous source of electrical current, over or around the wound, will mimic and amplify those endogenous currents of injury, thus enhancing or boosting the healing process of those slow-to-heal wounds.
- The healing process is enhanced though the galvanotaxic and germicidal effects of electrical current.
- Electrical stimulation for tissue healing and repair (ESTHR) is delivered by using two types of monophasic currents, namely microcurrent and HVPC.
- Electrode configuration may be over the wound or around the wound.
- Because electrical current is monophasic in nature, electrode polarity becomes an important dosimetric parameter to consider when the over-the-wound electrode configuration is used.
- Application of anodal stimulation is recommended during the inflammatory phase of healing.
- Application of cathodal stimulation is recommended during all remaining phases of healing.
- Both anodal and cathodal stimulation may be used for infected wounds.
- Periodic polarity reversal is recommended for both electrode configurations.
- Keeping the wound moist at all times—that is, during and in between treatments—is crucial to obtain optimal therapeutic effectiveness.
- The wearing of mask, gloves, gown, and goggles is mandatory during wound preparation and treatment to prevent cross-contamination.
- All line-powered electrical stimulators should be plugged into ground-fault circuit interrupter (GFCI) receptacles to prevent macroshock.
- The overall body of evidence reported in this chapter shows the strength of evidence behind electrical stimulation for slow-to-heal wounds to be *moderate* and its level of therapeutic effectiveness *substantiated*.

VII. CRITICAL THINKING QUESTIONS

Clarification: What is meant by electrical stimulation for tissue healing and repair (ESTHR)

Assumptions: You assume that the human body possesses an endogenous bioelectrical system that plays an important role in the process of dermal tissue healing. How do you justify making that assumption?

Reasons and evidence: What leads you to believe that delivering an external source of monophasic electrical current to the wound site can enhance skin repair?

Viewpoints or perspectives: How will you respond to a colleague who says that on the basis of scientific evidence available, HVPC is more effective for wound management than microcurrent?

Implications and consequences: What are the implications or consequences of not maintaining a moist environment for a wound during and in between treatment, and of alternating electrode polarity during the course of treatment?

About the question: Why is the passage of monophasic currents presumed to trigger a galvanotaxic response under the electrodes? Why do you think I ask this question?

VIII. REFERENCES

Articles

Ahmad ET (2008) High-voltage pulsed galvanic stimulation: Effect of treatment duration on healing of chronic pressure ulcers. Ann Burns Fire Disasters, 30: 124–128

Akers TK, Gabrielson AL (1984) The effect of high-voltage galvanic stimulation on the rate of healing of decubitus ulcers. Biomed Sci Instrum, 20: 99–100

Allen JD, Mattacola CG, Perrin DH (1999) Effect of microcurrent stimulation on delayed-onset muscle soreness: A double-blind comparison. J Athl Train, 34: 334–337

Alon G (1985) High-voltage stimulation: Effects of electrode size on basic excitatory responses. Phys Ther, 65: 890–895

Assimacopoulos D (1968) Low-intensity negative electric current in the treatment of ulcers of the leg due to chronic venous insufficiency: Preliminary reports of three cases. Am J Surg, 115: 683–687

Barker AT, Jaffe LF, Vanable JW (1982) The glabrous epidermis of cavies contains a powerful battery. Am J Physiol, 242: 358–366

Barron JJ, Jacobson WE, Tidd G (1985) Treatment of decubitus ulcers: A new approach. Minn Med, 68: 103–106

Becker RO, Murray DG (1967) Method of producing cellular dedifferentiation by means of very small electrical current. Trans N Y Acad Sci, 29: 606–615

Bertolucci LE, Grey T (1995) Clinical comparative study of microcurrent electrical stimulation to mid-laser and placebo treatment in degenerative joint disease of the temporomandibular joint. Cranio, 13: 116–120

Billingham RP, Isler JT, Firend WG, Hostetier J (1987) Treatment of levator syndrome using high-voltage electrogalvanic stimulation. Dis Colon Rectum, 30: 584–587

Bonacci JA, Higbie EJ (1997) Effects of microcurrent treatment on perceived pain and muscle strength following eccentric exercises. J Athl Train, 32: 119–123

Borgens RB, McGinnis ME, Vanable JW, Miles ES (1984) Stump currents in regenerating salamanders and newts. J Exp Zool, 23: 249–256

Borgens RB, Vanable JW, Jaffe LF (1977) Bioelectricity and regeneration: Large currents leave the stumps of regenerating newt limbs. Proc Natl Acad Sci U S A, 74: 4528–4532

Burdge JJ, Hartman JF, Wright ML (2009) A study of HVPC as an adjunctive therapy in limb salvage for chronic diabetic wounds of the lower extremity. Ostomy Wound Manage, 55: 30–38

Butterfield DL, Draper DO, Richard MD (1997) The effects of high-volt pulsed current electrical stimulation on delayed-onset muscle soreness. J Athl Train, 32: 15–20

Carley PJ, Wainapel SF (1985) Electrotherapy for acceleration of wound healing: Low-intensity direct current. Arch Phys Med Rehab, 66: 443–446

Carlson-Walker D, Currier DP, Threlkeld AJ (1988) Effects of high-voltage pulsed electrical stimulation on blood flow. Phys Ther, 68: 481–485

Chapman-Jones D, Young S, Tadej M (2010) Assessment of wound healing following electrical stimulation with Accel-Heal. Wounds, 6: 67–71

Curtis D, Fallows S, Morris M, McMakin C (2010) The efficacy of frequency specific microcurrent therapy on delayed onset muscle soreness. J Bodyw Mov Ther, 14: 272–279

Denegar CR, Yoho AP, Borowicz AJ, Bifulco N (1992) The effects of low-volt microamperage stimulation on delayed onset muscle soreness. J Sport Rehabil, 1: 95–102

Feedar JA, Kloth LC, Gentzkow CD (1991) Chronic dermal ulcer healing enhanced with monophasic pulsed electrical stimulation. Phys Ther, 71: 639–649

Fitzgerald GK, Newsome D (1993) Treatment of a large infected thoracic spine wound using high-voltage pulsed monophasic current. Phys Ther, 73: 355–360

Foulds IS, Barker AT (1983) Human skin battery potentials and their possible role in wound healing. Br J Dermatol, 109: 512–522

Franek A, Polak A, Kucharzewski M (2000) Modern application of high voltage stimulation for enhanced healing of venous crural ulceration. Med Eng Phys, 22: 647–655

Gault WR, Gatens PF (1976) Use of low-intensity direct current in management of ischemic skin ulcers. Phys Ther, 56: 265–269

Gilcreast DM, Stotts NA, Froelicher ES, Baker LL, Moss KM (1998) Effect of electrical stimulation on foot skin perfusion in persons with or at risk for diabetic foot ulcers. Wounds Repair Regen, 6: 434–441

Goldman R, Brewley B, Zhou L, Golden M (2003) Electrotherapy reverses inframalleolar ischemia: A retrospective, observational study. Adv Skin Wound Care, 16: 79–89

Goldman R, Rosen M, Brewley B, Golden M (2004) Electrotherapy promotes healing and microcirculation of infrapopliteal ischemic wounds: A prospective pilot study. Adv Skin Wound Care, 17: 284–294

Goldman RJ, Brewley BI, Golden MA (2002) Electrotherapy reoxygenates inframalleolar ischemic wounds on diabetic patients: A case series. Adv Skin Wound Care, 15: 112–120

Griffin JW, Newsome LS, Stralka SW, Wright PE (1990) Reduction of chronic posttraumatic hand edema: A comparison of high-voltage pulsed current, intermittent pneumatic compression and placebo treatments. Phys Ther, 70: 279–286

Griffin JW, Tooms RE, Mendius RA, Clifft JK, Vander Swaag R, El-Zeky F (1991) Efficacy of high-voltage pulsed current for healing of pressure ulcers in patients with spinal cord injury. Phys Ther, 71: 433–442; discussion 442–444

Guffey JS, Asmussen MD (1989) In vitro bactericidal effects of high voltage pulsed current versus direct current against Staphylococcus aureus. Clin Electrophysiol, 1: 5–9

Hatten E, Hervik JB, Kalheim T, Sundvor T (1990) Pain treatment with Rebox. Fysiotherapeuten, 11: 8–13

Heath ME, Gibbs SB (1992) High-voltage pulsed galvanic stimulation: Effects of frequency of current on blood flow in the human calf muscle. Clin Sci (Lond), 82: 607–613

Houghton PE, Campbell KE, Fraser CH, Harris C, Keast DH, Potter PJ, Hayes KC, Woodbury MG (2010) Electrical stimulation therapy increases rate of healing of pressure ulcers in community-dwelling people with spinal cord injury. Arch Phys Med Rehabil, 91: 669–678

Houghton PE, Kincaid CB, Lovell M, Campbell KE, Keast DH, Woodbury MG, Harris KA (2003) Effect of electrical stimulation on chronic leg ulcer size and appearance. Phys Ther, 83: 17–28

Huckfeldt R, Flick AB, Mikkelson D, Lowe C, Finley PJ (2007) Wound closure after split-thickness skin grafting is accelerated with the use of continuous direct anodal microcurrent applied to silver nylon wound contact dressings. J Burn Care Res, 28: 703–707

Hull Tl, Milsom JW, Church J, Oakley J, Lavery I, Fazio V (1993) Electrogalvanic stimulation for levator syndrome: How effective is it in the long term? Dis Colon Rectum, 36: 731–733

Illingsworth CM, Barker AT (1980) Measurement of electrical currents emerging during the regeneration of amputated finger tips in children. Clin Phys Physiol Meas, 1: 87–89

Johannsen F, Gam A, Haudschild B, Mathiesen B, Jensen L (1993) Rebox: An adjunct in physical medicine? Arch Phys Med Rehab, 74: 438–440

Kincaid CB, Lavoie KH (1989) Inhibition of bacterial growth in vitro following stimulation with high-voltage, monophasic, pulsed current. Phys Ther, 69: 651–655

Kloth LC, Feedar JA (1988) Acceleration of wound healing with high-voltage, monophasic, pulsed current. Phys Ther, 68: 503–508

Koopman JS, Vrinten DH, van Wijck AJ (2009) Efficacy of microcurrent therapy in the treatment of chronic nonspecific back pain. Clin J Pain, 25: 495–499

Lamboni P, Harris B (1983) The use of ice, airsplint, and high-voltage galvanic stimulation in effusion reduction. Athl Train, 118: 23–27

Lerner FN, Kirsh DL (1981) A double blind comparative study of microstimulation and placebo effect in short term treatment of the chronic back pain patient. J Chiropract, 15: 101–106

Maenpaa H, Jaakkola R, Sandstrom M, Von Wendt L (2004) Does microcurrent stimulation increase the range of movement of ankle dorsiflexion in children with cerebral palsy? Disabil Rehabil, 26: 669–677

Mawson AR, Siddiqui FH, Connelly BJ, Sharp CJ, Stewart GW, Summer WR, Biundo JJ (1993) Effect of high-voltage pulsed galvanic stimulation on sacral transcutaneous oxygen tension levels in the spinal cord injured. Paraplegia, 31: 311–319

McLoughlin TJ, Snyder AR, Brolinson PG, Pizza FX (2004) Sensory level electrical muscle stimulation: Effects on markers of muscle injury. Br J Sports Med, 38: 725–729

McMakin C (1998) Microcurrent treatment of myofascial pain in the hand, neck and face. Top Clin Chiropract, 5: 29–35, 73–75

McMakin CR (2004) Microcurrent therapy: A novel treatment method for chronic low back myofacial pain. J Body Mov Ther, 8: 143–153

Mendel FC, Dolan MG, Fish DR, Marzo J, Wilding GE (2010) Effects of high-voltage pulsed current on recovery after grades I and II lateral ankle sprains. J Sports Rehabil, 19: 399–410

Merriman HL, Heygi CA, Albright-Overton, Carlos J, Putnam RW, Mulcare JA (2004) A comparison of four electrical stimulation types on *Staphylococcus aureus* growth in vitro. J Rehab Res Dev, 41: 139–146

Michlovitz S, Smith W, Watkins M (1988) Ice and high-voltage stimulation in treatment of acute lateral ankle sprains. J Orthop Sports Phys Ther, 9: 301–304

Mohr T, Carlson B, Sulentic C, Landry R (1985) Comparison of isometric exercise and high-volt galvanic stimulation on quadriceps femoris muscle strength. Phys Ther, 65: 606–609

Morris L, Newton RA (1987) Use of high-voltage pulsed galvanic stimulation for patients with levator ani syndrome. Phys Ther, 67: 1522–1525

Mulder GD (1991) Treatment of open skin wounds with electric stimulation. Arch Phys Med Rehab, 72: 375–377

Nicosia JF, Abcarian H (1985) Levator syndrome: A treatment that works. Dis Col Rectum, 28: 406–408

Oliver GC, Robin RJ, Salvati EP, Eisentat E (1985) Electrogalvanic stimulation in the treatment of levator syndrome. Dis Col Rectum, 28: 662–663

Park DH, Yoon SG, Kim KU, Hwang DY, Kim HS, Lee JK, Kim KY (2005) Comparison study between electrogalvanic stimulation and local injection therapy in levator ani syndrome. In J Colorectal Dis, 20: 272–276

Peters EJ, Lavery LA, Armstrong DG, Fleischli JG (2001) Electric stimulation as an adjunct to heal diabetic foot ulcers. A randomized clinical trial. Arch Phys Med Rehab, 82: 721–725

Poltawski L, Johnson M, Watson T (2009) Microcurrent therapy in the management of chronic tennis elbow: Pilot studies to optimize parameters. Physioth Res Int, 17: 157–166

Quirion de Girardi CQ, Seaborne D, Savard-Goulet F, Nieto MW, Lambert J (1984) The analgesic effect of high-voltage galvanic stimulation combined with ultrasound in the treatment of low back pain: A one-group pre-test/post-test study. Physiother Can, 36: 327–333

Ross CR, Segal D (1981) High-voltage galvanic stimulation: An aid to postoperative healing. Curr Podiatry, 30: 19–25

Sandoval MC, Ramirez C, Carmago DM, Salvini TF (2010) Effects of high-voltage pulsed current plus conventional treatment on acute ankle spain. Rev Bras Fisioter, 14: 193–199

Shrode LW (1993) Treatment of facial muscles affected by Bell's palsy with high-voltage electrical muscle stimulation. J Manipulative Physiol Ther, 16: 347–352

Sohn N, Weinstein MA, Robbins RD (1982) The levator syndrome and its treatment with high-voltage electrogalvanic stimulation. Am J Surg, 44: 580–582

Stralka SW, Jackson JA, Lewis AR (1998) Treatment of hand and wrist pain. A randomized clinical trial of high-voltage, pulsed, direct current built into a wrist splint. AAOHN J, 46: 233–236

Thurman BF, Christian EL (1971) Response of a serious circulatory lesion to electrical stimulation. A case report. Phys Ther, 51: 1107–1110

Tourville TW, Connelly DA, Reed BV (2006) Effects of sensory-level high-volt pulsed electrical current on delayed-onset muscle soreness. J Sports Sci, 24: 941–949

Unger PG (1985) Wound healing using high-voltage galvanic stimulation. Stimulus, 10: 8–10

Voight ML (1984) Reduction of posttraumatic ankle edema with high-voltage pulsed galvanic stimulation. Athl Train, 19: 278–279, 311

Weber MD, Servedio FJ, Woodall WR (1994) The effect of three modalities on delayed-onset muscle soreness. J Orthop Phys Ther, 20: 236–242

Weiss DS, Eagstein WH, Falanga V (1989) Exogenous electric current can reduce the formation of hypertrophic scars. J Dermatol Surg Oncol, 15: 1272–1275

Wolcott LE, Wheeler PC, Hardwicke HM, Rowley BA (1969) Accelerated healing of skin ulcer by electrotherapy: Preliminary clinical results. South Med J, 62: 795–801

Wong RT (1986) Force of induced muscle contraction and perceived discomfort in healthy subjects. Phys Ther, 66: 1209–1214

Wood JM, Evans PE, Shallreuter KU, Jacobson WE, Sufit R, Newman J, White C, Jacobson M (1993) A multicenter study on the used of pulsed low intensity direct current for healing chronic stage II and III decubitus ulcers. Arch Dermatol, 129: 999–1009

Young S, Hampton S, Tadej M (2011) Study to evaluate the effect of low-intensity pulsed electrical currents on levels of oedema in chronic non-healing wounds. J Wound Care, 38: 368–373

Review Articles

Kloth LC (2005a) Electrical stimulation for wound healing: A review of evidence from in vitro studies, animal experiments, and clinical trials. Int J Low Extrem Wounds, 4: 23–44

Taradaj J (2003) High-voltage stimulation (HVS) for enhanced healing of wounds. Phys Ther Rev, 8: 131–134

Chapters of Textbooks

Kloth LC (2002) Electrical stimulation in tissue repair. In: Wound Healing: Alternatives in Management, 3rd ed. Kloth LC, McCulloch JM (Eds). FA Davis, Philadelphia, pp 271–315

Kloth LC (2005b) Electrical stimulation. In: Wound Healing. Falabella AF, Kirsner RS (Eds). Taylor & Francis, New York, pp 439–479

Robinson AJ (2008) Electrical stimulation to augment healing of chronic wounds. In: Clinical Electrophysiology: Electrotherapy and Electrophysical Testing, 3rd ed. Robinson AJ, Snyder-Mackler L (Eds). Lippincott Williams & Wilkins, Philadelphia, pp 275–299

Monographs

American Physical Therapy Association (2001) Electrotherapeutic Terminology in Physical Therapy. APTA Publications, Alexandria, p 38

Centers for Medicare and Medicaid Services (2004) National Coverage: Determination for Electrical Stimulation and Electromagnetic Therapy for the Treatment of Wounds. NCD 270.1. Washington DC

Textbooks

Becker RO, Selden G (1987) The Body Electric. Electromagnetism and the Foundation of Life. William Morrow, New York

Falabella AF, Kirsner RS (2005) Wound Healing. Taylor & Francis, New York

Kloth LC, McCulloch JM (2002) Wound Healing: Alternatives in Management, 3rd ed., FA Davis, Philadelphia

Shai A, Maibach HI (2005) Wound Healing and Ulcers of the Skin. Springer, Berlin

Sussman C, Bates-Jensen B (2012) Wound Care: A Collaborative Manual for Health Professionals, 4th ed., Lippincott Williams & Wilkins, Philadelphia

Chapter 16

Iontophoresis

Chapter Outline

Learning Objectives

Remembering: List the drug ions, with their related proposed physiologic and therapeutic effects, most commonly used in iontophoresis in the field of rehabilitation.

Understanding: Compare the methods of iontophoresis, needle injection, and oral ingestion for the delivery of drugs into the human body.

Applying: Show the procedural and technical steps necessary to deliver an iontophoretic treatment.

Analyzing: Differentiate between the process of phoresis and electrolysis related to the practice of drug iontophoresis.

Evaluating: Formulate the strength of scientific evidence and therapeutic effectiveness related to the practice of iontophoresis in rehabilitation.

Creating: Defend the use of iontophoresis over oral ingestion and needle injection for local delivery of drugs into the body.

I. FOUNDATION

A. DEFINITION

Iontophoresis is a method of local transfer (*phoresis*), or delivery, of ionized (*ionto*) medicated and nonmedicated substances into the skin and through local microcirculation. Iontophoresis requires the use of electric energy and is implemented using the traditional wire programmable devices and newer wireless nonprogrammable patches.

B. IONTOPHORESORS AND ELECTRODES

Three types of stimulators, also called *iontophoresors,* are commonly used today to deliver iontophoresis. Figure 16-1 illustrates typical portable-, cabinet- and patch-type iontophoresors. Figure 16-2 shows custom reusable metallic and commercial disposable buffered electrodes. The metallic electrode is wrapped with gauze soaked in the therapeutic ion solution. The commercial electrode, on the other hand, is made of a reservoir that is filled with the therapeutic ion solution using a needle. The wireless patch is complete with its battery and electrode unit embedded in the flexible patch material (see Fig. 16-1C). The delivery of iontophoresis for hyperhidrosis (of the hands and feet) is done using electrodes embedded into water trays.

C. IONTOPHORESIS VERSUS OTHER DRUG DELIVERY METHODS

The treatment of soft tissue pathologies very often requires the use of medications such as analgesic drugs to diminish pain and anti-inflammatory drugs to control tissue inflammatory response. In addition to iontophoresis, two other basic methods exist to deliver drugs to injured tissues: oral ingestion and needle injection. Oral ingestion is by far the most utilized for an obvious reason. The only thing the patient needs to do is to swallow the drug tablets. However, drug ingestion involves the gastrointestinal tract in addition to key organs such as the liver for metabolism and the kidneys for elimination. Needle injection, on the other hand, is an invasive technique frequently used by medical specialists. By using a needle to puncture the skin, a given quantity of medication is delivered locally at the site of injury. Just like iontophoresis, and unlike oral ingestion, this method allows the drug to be delivered locally, thus bypassing the systemic route associated with oral ingestion.

D. SYSTEMIC SIDE EFFECTS AND FEAR OF NEEDLES

It is well documented in the literature that most orally ingested drugs can induce light, moderate, or severe side effects depending on their nature, dosage, and duration of

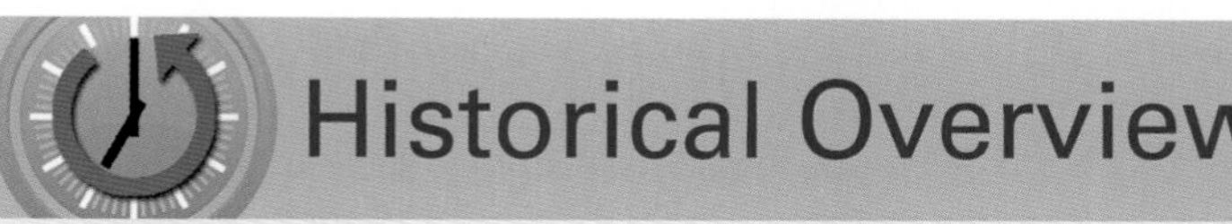

Historical Overview

The idea of medications delivered through the skin via the electromotive force of an electrical current was first proposed in 1747 by Pivati and later, in 1833, by Fabré-Palaprat (Licht, 1983). There is a consensus, however, that the animal experimental work done by Leduc (1900, 1908) contributed most to the worldwide recognition of what was later to be known as iontophoresis therapy (Licht, 1983; Cummings, 1991; Ciccone, 2008). Using the electromotive force of a continuous direct current (DC) generator, after placing a negatively charged potassium cyanide solution (a lethal drug) under the cathode (–) and a positively charged strychnine sulfate solution (a convulsive drug) under the anode (+) with each electrode positioned on a lateral side of two rabbit heads touching one another, Leduc was able to induce, after turning on the current generator for a few minutes, strong tetanic convulsions in one rabbit and death in the other. To test whether these striking physiologic effects resulted from the driving force generated by the electrical current (iontophoresis) or from the passive diffusion of the two drugs across the skin, Leduc repeated the experiment, but this time the polarity of the current was reversed. He placed the positively charged strychnine under the cathode (–) and the negatively charged cyanide under the anode (+). After a few minutes of DC flow through the animal heads, Leduc noticed none of the dramatic and deadly effects that occurred in the earlier experiment. He thus concluded that the flow of electric current was responsible for these physiologic effects and that iontophoresis can occur only if the ionized medication is placed under the electrode with the same charge—that is, negatively charged ions under the cathode and positively charged ions under the anode. This conclusion, made at the beginning of the 20th century, constitutes the scientific foundation under which the basic biophysical principle related to iontophoresis therapy is established (Leduc, 1900, 1908; Nair et al., 1999). The first clinical use of iontophoresis therapy dates back to 1936, when Ishihashi (1936) noted that excessive sweating of the palms (hyperhidrosis) could be reduced by ion transfer of medicated solutions through iontophoretic techniques (Chien et al., 1989). As reported by Stolman (1987), Ishihashi's clinical work went largely unnoticed until 1952, when Bouman et al. (1952) demonstrated the efficacy of tap water–only iontophoresis as an effective therapy for hyperhidrosis.

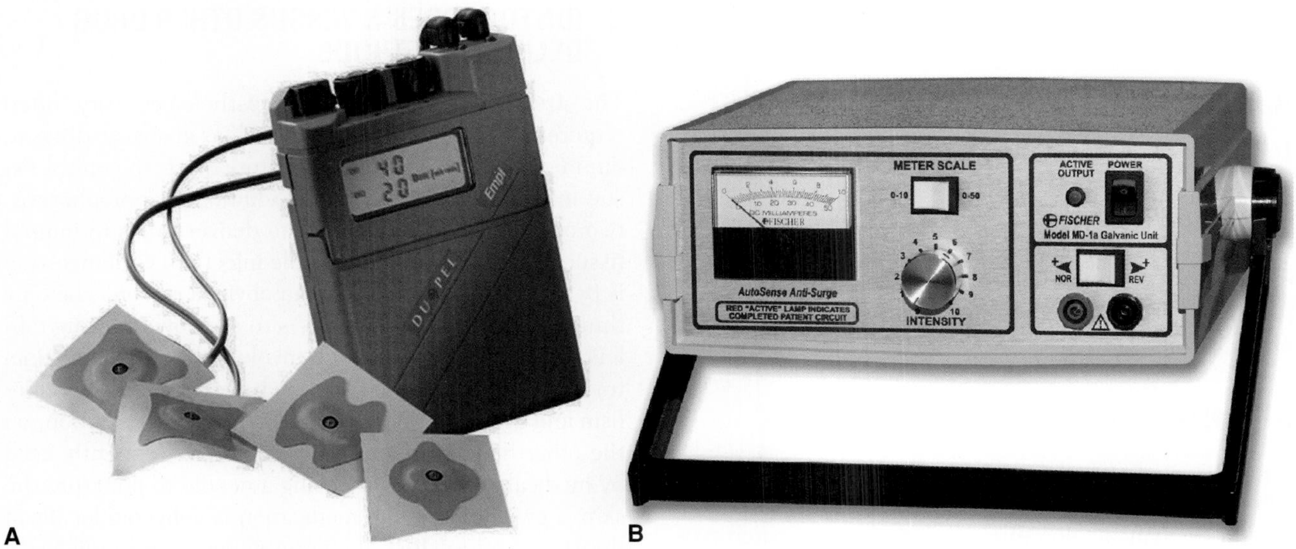

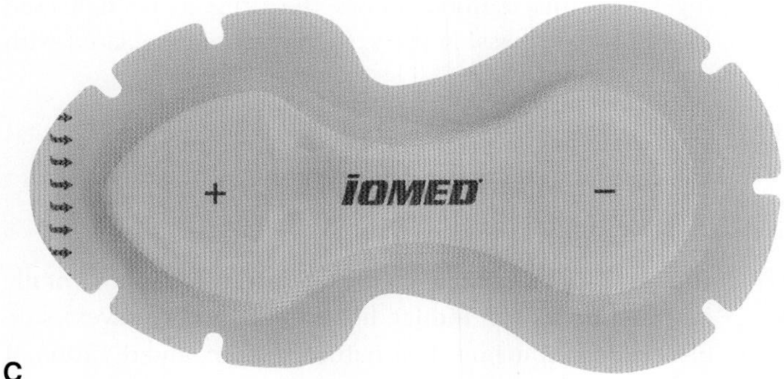

FIGURE 16-1 Typical wire programmable iontophoresors (**A, B**) and wireless nonprogrammable iontophoretic patch (**C**). (A: Courtesy of Empi; B: Courtesy of RA Fischer; C: Courtesy of Iomed Inc.)

consumption. Moreover, it is a common clinical observation that many patients are afraid of needles. What, then, are the advantages and disadvantages of using one method of drug delivery over the other?

E. ADVANTAGES AND DISADVANTAGES

Table 16-1 lists the main advantages and disadvantages associated with each of these three drug delivery methods. Iontophoresis has the main advantage, when compared to needle injection, of being less painful and infection free. It has also the main advantage, when compared to oral ingestion, of bypassing the patient's gastrointestinal tract and liver. Its main disadvantage is that drug delivery is limited to the superficial layers of tissues.

F. RATIONALE FOR USE

The use of iontophoresis is well justified when oral drug ingestion causes significant problems to the patient's

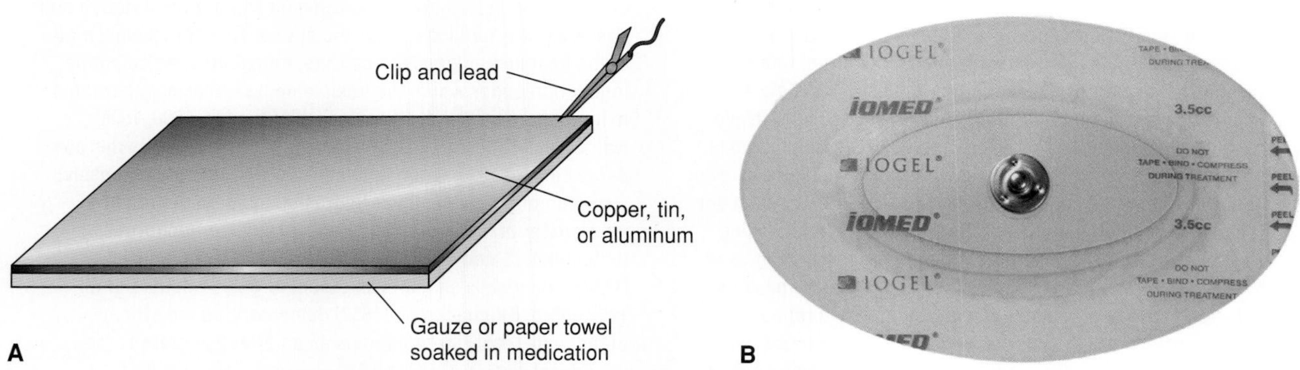

FIGURE 16-2 Custom metallic nonbuffered iontophoretic electrode (**A**). Commercial buffered iontophoretic electrode (**B**). (A: From Robinson et al., *Clinical Electrophysiology*, 3rd ed. Lippincott Williams & Wilkins, Philadelphia, 2008, p. 361; B: Courtesy of Empi.)

TABLE 16-1 IONTOPHORESIS VERSUS ORAL INGESTION AND NEEDLE INJECTION

Method	Advantage	Disadvantage
Oral ingestion	Quick and easy Systemic delivery Noninvasive No professional assistance needed Less costly—drug cost only	Metabolic breakdown by liver Elimination by kidneys Absorption by gastrointestinal tract Potential gastric disorders Amount of drug delivered to the targeted tissue unknown
Needle injection	Precise local delivery Superficial/deep delivery Bypasses gastrointestinal tract Bypasses liver Amount of drug delivered to targeted tissues known	Invasive (skin puncture) Relatively traumatic Relatively painful Potential for infection caused by skin puncture Professional required for delivery More costly than oral ingestion—drug cost plus professional's fee
Iontophoresis	Precise local delivery Noninvasive Bypasses gastrointestinal tract Bypasses liver No skin puncture No risk of infection	Delivery limited to superficial tissues Professional assistance needed More costly than oral ingestion—drug cost plus professional's fee

gastrointestinal tract, liver, or kidneys. It is also indicated when the patient's fear of needles plays an important part in the therapeutic plan. Iontophoresis is widely used around the world not only in rehabilitation but also in the fields of medicine and dentistry (see Henley, 1991; Gangarosa et al., 1995; Banga et al., 1998; Grond et al., 2000; Togel et al., 2002; Ting et al., 2004; Eisenach et al., 2005; Sieg et al., 2009). The scope of this chapter is on the use of iontophoresis for the management of soft tissue pathologies in the field of rehabilitation. More specifically, the emphasis is on the use of therapeutic ions having analgesic, anti-inflammatory, antiseptic, and sclerolytic effects, including the use of nonmedicated and medicated (anticholinergic) tap water.

II. BIOPHYSICAL CHARACTERISTICS

A. CONTINUOUS DIRECT CURRENT

Iontophoresis is described as the use of a continuous, direct electrical current to deliver therapeutically charged ions through the skin and into the systemic circulation (Henley, 1991; Banga et al., 1998; Nair et al., 1999; Ciccone, 2008). Figure 16-3 illustrates the typical continuous direct and monophasic current, flowing over time and having either a positive or a negative polarity, commonly generated by wire programmable and wireless nonprogrammable iontophoresors. Iontophoresors are constant current-type (CC-type) stimulators, meaning that the set current amplitude (say, 80 mA read on the digital meter) remains constant (hence the term *constant current*) during treatment, regardless of changes in tissue impedance over time. The CC concept described is based on Ohm's law, defined by the formula $V = I \times R$, where V = voltage, I = intensity, and R = resistance. In keeping with the American Physical Therapy Association (APTA) monograph (2001), the intensity (I) is replaced here by the amplitude (A), which is the measure of the magnitude of current. Ohm's law is thus rewritten as follows: $V = A \times R$. To keep amplitude (A) constant (CC) when resistance (R) is changing, voltage (V) is automatically adjusted. The main advantage of CC-type stimulators is that they deliver predictable levels of electrical stimulation, making therapy more predictable and comfortable for the patient (no surge of current).

B. ELECTROMIGRATION

Iontophoresis rests on the principle of *electromigration,* which is defined as the movement of ions across the skin under the direct influence of an electrical current (Sieg et al., 2009). From this principle, it follows that the drug, in its ionic form, be placed under the electrode bearing the same charge. Another way to state this principle is that *like poles repel*. As illustrated in Figure 16-4, therapeutic ions are driven through the skin only if a polarity match exists between the charged ions and the electrode under which they are placed—that is, negatively charged ions under the negatively charged electrode (–/–) and positively charged ions under the positively charged electrode (+/+). The *repelling force* set between the current and drug charges having identical polarity is the driving force behind the phoresis phenomenon.

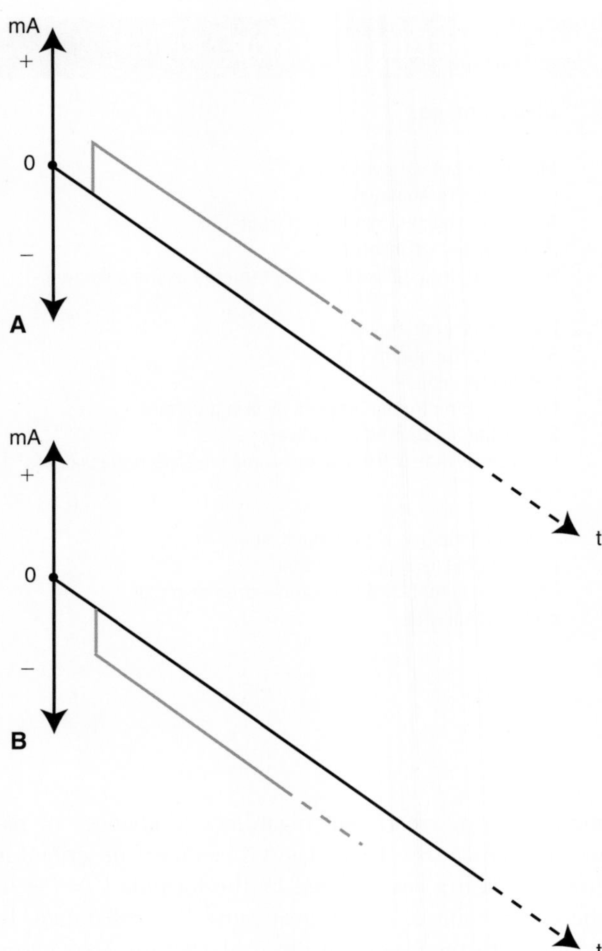

FIGURE 16-3 Continuous, direct, monophasic electrical current waveform, showing positive (**A**) and negative (**B**) polarity.

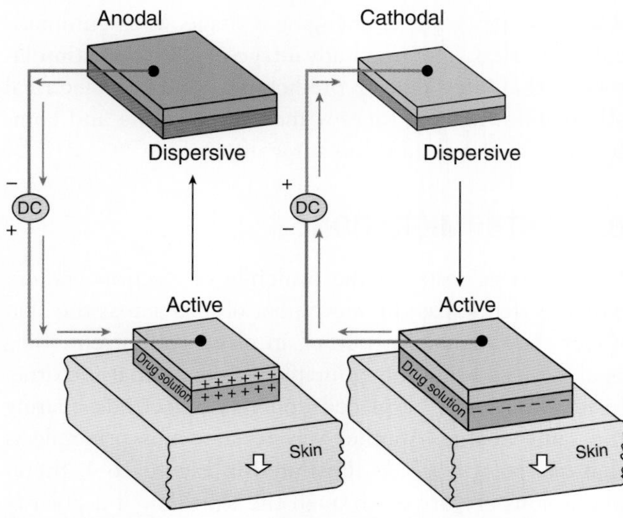

FIGURE 16-4 Illustrated on the left side is *anodal iontophoresis* with the positively charged drug solution placed under the active anode electrode. Illustrated on the right side is *cathodal iontophoresis* with the negatively charged drug solution place under the active cathode electrode. Note that the conductive surface area of the cathode always must be larger than that of the anode, regardless of whether the cathode is used as the active or the dispersive electrode. DC, direct current.

C. ANODAL VERSUS CATHODAL IONTOPHORESIS

The terms *anodal iontophoresis* and *cathodal iontophoresis* refer to phoresis of a positively and a negatively charged drug solution, respectively (Nair et al., 1999).

D. ACTIVE VERSUS DISPERSIVE ELECTRODE

The electrode under which the therapeutic ions are placed is referred to as the active, or delivery, electrode, whereas the other electrode is referred to as the dispersive, or return, electrode (see Fig. 16-4). In this chapter, the terms *active* and *dispersive* are used to denote the electrodes. The use of a dispersive electrode is mandatory for iontophoresis because it closes the electrical circuit.

E. SKIN PATHWAY THROUGH PORES

Convincing scientific evidence suggests that the iontophoretic-driven ion process through the skin is *pore* dependent (Banga et al., 1998). It is paramount to understand that the main barrier to transdermal drug intake is the most superficial avascular stratum corneum layer of the epidermis. Schematically drawn in Figure 16-5 are hair follicles as well as sweat glands, which play a crucial role in providing the main pathways, or pores, through which the charged ions can penetrate first the stratum corneum layer and then the remaining layers of the epidermis and dermis (Kalia et al., 1995; Banga et al., 1998). According to Banga et al. (1998), the diffusional resistance of the skin to permeation of ions is lowest in the hair follicles and sweat gland regions compared with other regions of the epidermis.

F. DRUG PENETRATION DEPTH

Anderson et al., (2003) proposed the following model to explain how drug ions penetrate human tissues during iontophoresis therapy and which key factors may be responsible for such penetration. They first proposed that electrical current causes drug penetration through the stratum corneum and that the rate of penetration of the drug is proportional to the amplitude of this current. They further hypothesize that these drug ions will collect to form a drug depot, or reservoir, within the avascular epidermal layer just under the active electrode. For this to occur, these authors assume that the ionic current is carried by chloride ions, leaving the drug molecules behind, and that the drug delivery rate exceeds the systemic vascular absorption rate. The final proposal of Anderson and colleagues (2003) is that drug absorption from the depot and into the dermis of surrounding tissues occurs by diffusion, suggesting that passive diffusion, not the amplitude of current, governs the depth of drug penetration into the tissues.

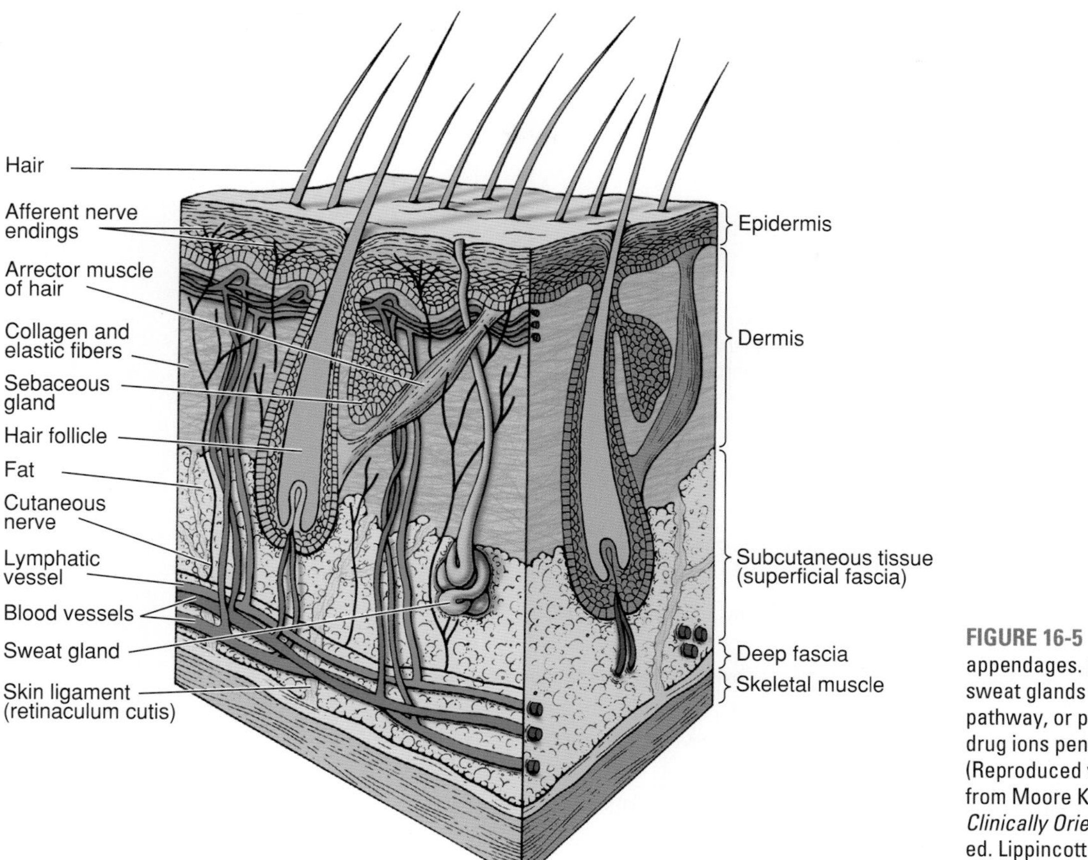

FIGURE 16-5 Human skin and its appendages. Hair follicles and sweat glands provide the main pathway, or pores, though which drug ions penetrate the skin. (Reproduced with permission from Moore KL, Dalley AF (1999), *Clinically Oriented Anatomy*, 4th ed. Lippincott Williams & Wilkins, Philadelphia, p. 13.)

G. EFFECTS OF TIME AND BLOOD FLOW ON PENETRATION DEPTH

Anderson and colleagues (2003) suggest, based on their model described earlier, that for equivalent iontophoretic dosages, it is the factor time (for passive diffusion to occur), not current amplitude, that dictates the ultimate local depth of penetration of the drug. Another key factor to consider, according to these authors, is the state of localized blood flow at the site of injury, indicating that if the local cutaneous capillary beds under the active electrode are dilated, drug penetration depth will be reduced (due to increased clearance). From this model, it appears that electric current is needed only to induce and regulate the penetration rate of drug ions through the stratum corneum layer of the skin. After that, the process of passive diffusion takes over, thus governing the penetration depth of the drug ions into the tissues during iontophoresis.

III. THERAPEUTIC EFFECTS AND INDICATIONS

Figure 16-6 presents the proposed physiologic and therapeutic effects associated with the use of iontophoresis. These iontophoresis effects caused by both cathodal and anodal iontophoresis are phoretic, electrolytic, and pharmacologic in nature.

A. PHORETIC EFFECTS

Drug phoresis (transfer) takes place due to the capacity of electrical current to push drug ions through the skin's first layer (stratum corneum) via the application of one surface electrode (active electrode loaded with ionic drug solution) directly over the treatment area, with the other electrode (dispersive electrode loaded with saline) positioned in the immediate vicinity of the first electrode.

B. ELECTROLYTIC EFFECTS

Because iontophoresis involves the passing of a continuous direct current (DC) into water-soluble drug solutions (electrode system) and human tissues over a certain period, water electrolysis will occur. *Electrolysis* is the process of decomposition of a compound by passing a direct electrical current through it, leading to the formation of electrochemical reactions under both the anode and cathode electrodes.

1. New Compounds

Human tissues are composed of a mixture of approximately 70% sodium chloride (Na^+Cl^-) and water (H_2O). The continuous DC flow through such tissues inevitably leads to electrolysis of this salted water medium at the electrode–skin interface. Over time during therapy, this continuous DC flow will redistribute the sodium and

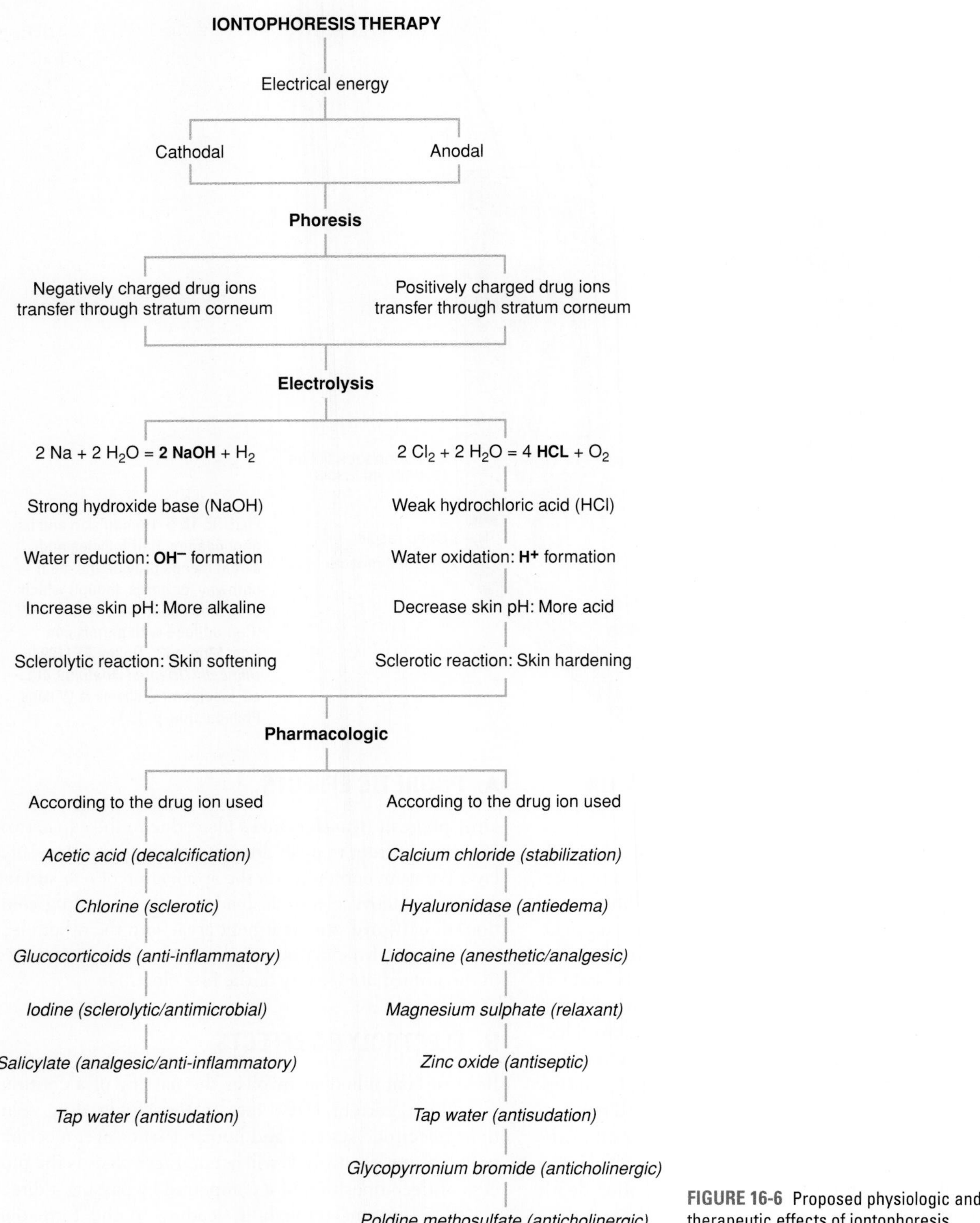

FIGURE 16-6 Proposed physiologic and therapeutic effects of iontophoresis.

chlorine ions with water to form new chemical compounds at the electrode–skin interface.

2. Weak Hydrochloric Acid

As shown in Figure 16-6, the reaction of chlorine with water leads to formation of a *weak hydrochloric acid* (2 Cl_2 + 2 H_2O = 4 HCl + O_2) under the anode, because negatively charged chlorine ions migrate toward this positively charged electrode. This weak acidic reaction produced under the anode is sclerotic and, over time, tends to harden the skin through protein coagulation.

3. Strong Sodium Hydroxide Base

The reaction of sodium with water, on the other hand, leads to formation of a much *stronger sodium hydroxide base* ($2\ Na + 2\ H_2O = 2\ NaOH + H_2$) under the cathode, because the positively charged sodium ions migrate toward this negatively charged electrode (see Fig. 16-6). This stronger alkaline reaction produced under the cathode is sclerolytic in nature and, over time, tends to soften the skin (due to liquefying of proteins), thus exposing it to potential irritation and burn. Such a sclerolytic or caustic reaction is responsible for erythema of the skin and the itching or burning sensation felt under this electrode during therapy (Henley, 1991).

4. Redox

The decomposition of water with electrical current is a *redox* reaction—that is, a reaction that implies the reduction *(red-)* and the oxidation *(-ox)* of water. During electrolysis, water present at the electrode–skin interface is reduced ($4\ H_2O + 4$ electrons $= 2\ H_2 + 4\ OH^-$) at the cathode and oxidized ($2\ H_2O = O_2 + 4\ H^+ + 4$ electrons) at the anode. This electrochemical reaction leads, over time, to a net accumulation of *hydrogen ions* (H^+) under the anode and *hydroxyl ions* (OH^-) under the cathode (see Fig. 16-6).

5. Skin pH Shift

The net accumulation of hydrogen and hydroxyl ions creates a pH instability, or shift, at the electrode–skin interface during iontophoresis. The term *pH* is used to express the hydrogen ion activity of a solution. The average or normal pH value of human skin ranges between 3 and 6, implying that at a physiologic pH, the skin is negatively charged (Guffey et al., 1999; Nair et al., 1999). An accumulation of hydrogen ions (H^+) will induce a *pH drop* (more acid), whereas an accumulation of hydroxyl ions (OH^-) will produce a *pH increase* (more alkaline) under the respective electrodes (see Fig. 16-6).

C. PHARMACOLOGIC EFFECTS

The last therapeutic effect of drug iontophoresis is pharmacologic and relates directly to the specific active ingredient contained in the drug-ionized solution or therapeutic ions. Table 16-2 lists the most common drug ions used in rehabilitation today, including nonmedicated tap water, along with their respective polarities and proposed physiologic and therapeutic effects on soft tissues. The type of medication used will depend on the type of pathology and the desired treatment outcomes (see Case Studies).

1. Getting the Prescribed Drug Solution

Because many of the drugs used for the delivery of iontophoresis require a physician's prescription, such as dexamethasone and lidocaine, nonphysician practitioners must first inform the patient's treating physician of the intention to use iontophoresis and then ask for the drug prescription. With the prescription on hand, nonphysician practitioners can then obtain the desired drug solution, in the form of aqueous solution or ointment, from their pharmacists.

2. Drug Concentration

There is consensus in the literature that the drug ions, listed in Table 16-2, should be delivered to soft tissues within the following ranges of aqueous or ointment concentrations: 2% to 5% aqueous solution; 1% to 5% ointment (for details, see Prentice, 2002; Ciccone, 2008). Medicated ointments are rubbed over the affected area, with the active electrode on top. Medicated aqueous solutions, on the other hand, are injected or impregnated, using a needle, into the electrode reservoir (or gauze) of the active electrode. Commercial electrodes are sold in various sizes, each having a maximum filling capacity of its reservoir, or fiber matrix, ranging between 1 and 5 cc.

D. UNWANTED SIDE EFFECTS

Water electrolysis associated with iontophoresis will cause unwanted electrochemical and electrothermal side effects at the electrode–skin interface if no measures are taken to reduce them. These side effects will manifest themselves in a form of skin irritation or burn under the electrodes, particularly under the cathode (see later discussion). This unwanted reaction is caused as follows. First, during the course of iontophoresis, there is an accumulation of extraneous hydroxyl ions (OH^-) under the cathode and hydrogen ions (H^+) under the anode (see Fig. 16-6). These ions compete with the drug ions of the same charge for the available electrical driving charges, thus reducing drug transfer. Next, this same accumulation of ions, over time, will either raise (at the cathode) or lower (at the anode) skin pH under these electrodes, potentially causing skin irritation and, in some cases, when the net deposit is large enough, a skin burn (Henley, 1991; Banga et al., 1998; Nair et al., 1999).

E. MINIMIZING SIDE EFFECTS

How can practitioners minimize skin irritation and burn during iontophoresis? As discussed earlier and illustrated in Figure 16-6, the risk of inducing skin irritation, and potentially a skin burn, is related to the accumulation of hydroxyl ions (OH^-) under the cathode causing a skin pH increase, which together lead to the formation of a strong alkaline reaction. This alkaline reaction, in turn, causes a strong sclerolytic effect, or softening of the skin, which makes it more susceptible to irritation and burn.

1. Use of Buffered Electrode

One approach to minimize skin irritation and burn during application is to use buffered electrodes. A buffer is any substance that maintains the relative concentrations

TABLE 16-2 COMMONLY USED THERAPEUTIC IONS IN REHABILITATION

Ions	Polarity	Proposed Physiologic and Therapeutic Effects
Acetic acid	–	Decalcifying agent. Increases solubility of calcium deposits in tendons and muscles.
Chlorine	–	Sclerolytic agent. Causes a sclerolytic, softening effect on cutaneous tissues.
Glucocorticoid	–	Anti-inflammatory agent. Reduces tissue inflammation by inhibiting biosynthesis of prostaglandins and other proinflammatory substances. Includes compounds such as dexamethasone (Decadron), hydrocortisone, and prednisone.
Iodine	–	Sclerolytic and antimicrobial agent. Causes a sclerolytic, softening effect on cutaneous tissue in addition to an antimicrobial effect.
Salicylate	–	Analgesic and anti-inflammatory agent. Inhibits the biosynthesis of prostaglandins.
Calcium chloride	+	Membrane-stabilizing agent. Stabilizes excitable cell membranes, thus decreasing excitability threshold in muscles and peripheral nerves.
Hyaluronidase	+	Antiedema agent. Decreases edema by diminishing encapsulation in connective tissues via hydrolization of hyaluronic acid.
Lidocaine	+	Anesthetic and analgesic agent. Decreases local pain through blocking of nerve impulse transmission.
Magnesium sulfate	+	Muscle relaxant agent. Relaxes striated muscles by decreasing the excitability of muscle membranes.
Zinc oxide	+	Antiseptic agent. Enhances tissue healing in addition to acting as a broad antiseptic.
Tap water	+/–	Antisudation/antisweating agent. Suppresses sweating of palms, soles, and armpits by inducing the formation of keratin plugs in the lumen of sweat glands.
Glycopyrronium bromide	+	Anticholinergic agent. Suppresses sweating of palms, soles, and armpits through its anticholinergic effect. Mix with tap water.
Poldine methosulfate	+	Anticholinergic agent. Suppresses sweating of palms, soles, and armpits through its anticholinergic effect. Mix with tap water.

of hydrogen and hydroxyl ions in a solution by neutralizing (binding) any added acid or alkali. Buffering refers to the process by which the hydrogen ion concentration is maintained at a constant level, thus keeping the pH value stable. Figure 16-7 shows a cross-sectional view of one such buffered electrode. The buffered layer of the electrode is capable of neutralizing extraneous hydroxyl and hydrogen ions, thus stabilizing skin pH in addition to maximizing drug delivery (Henley, 1991; Banga et al., 1998; Guffey et al., 1999; Nair et al., 1999). It is important to know that prior to the use of such commercial buffered electrodes, iontophoresis was delivered using noncommercial/nonbuffered electrodes made of some type of malleable metal such as aluminum, tin, and copper covered by layers of gauze (Ciccone, 2008). The main advantages of using noncommercial/nonbuffered electrodes instead of buffered electrodes are that they are much less expensive, are reusable, and can be used to treat much larger body areas.

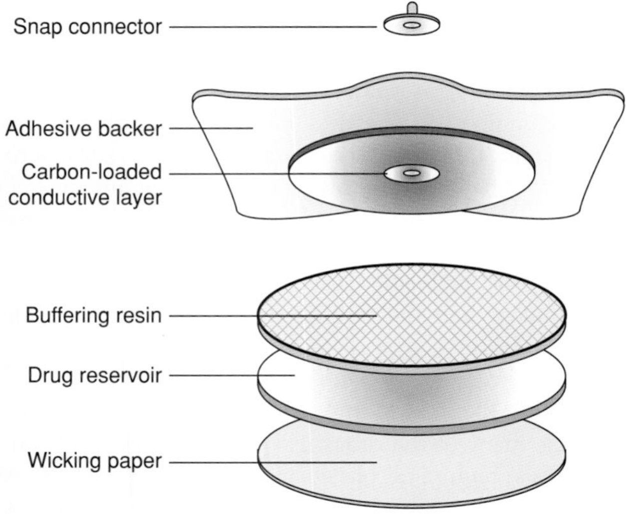

FIGURE 16-7 Three-dimensional view of a buffered electrode.

2. Control Over Electrode Current Density

Another approach to minimize skin irritation and burn is to control the current density (CD). Guffey et al. (1999) showed that subjects who received a dose of 80 milliampers.minute (mA.min) with nonbuffered electrodes demonstrated no visible signs of skin irritation despite the skin pH's being increased by an average of three points (mean, +3.14). These results suggest that changes in skin pH after common therapeutic dosages (range, 1 to 80 mA.min) may not be the prime cause leading to skin irritation or burn and that, perhaps, electrode CD under the electrode may be more to blame.

F. RESEARCH-BASED INDICATIONS

The search for evidence behind the use of iontophoresis, displayed in the *Research-Based Indications* box shown earlier, led to the collection of 66 English peer-reviewed human clinical studies. The methodologies, as well as the criteria, used to assess the strength of evidence and therapeutic effectiveness are described in Chapter 2. As indicated, the strength of evidence behind iontophoresis is ranked as *moderate* for hyperhidrosis, rheumatoid disorders, epicondylitis, Peyronie's disease, temporomandibular joint disorders, and calcifying tendinitis. It may come as a surprise to many practitioners that the application of tap water iontophoresis for hyperhidrosis is common and effective. Hyperhidrosis, a common disorder of excessive sweat, may be generalized over the entire body or focalized over hands, feet, axillae, and face (Solish et al., 2007). This painless condition, when moderate to severe in nature, may have significant effects on patients' lives, including difficulty with certain manual employments (e.g., being a carpenter when affected by palmar hyperhidrosis), activities of daily living, interference with intimacy, and social embarrassment (bad body odor). The results presented support the recommendation made by the Canadian Hyperhidrosis Advisory Committee (Solish et al., 2007) to the effect that tap water iontophoresis should be recognized as a *first-line therapy* for palmar and plantar hyperhidrosis. Therapeutic effectiveness is found to be *substantiated* for all conditions mentioned earlier. Analysis is *pending* for all other health conditions, because fewer than five studies could be collected. Over all conditions treated with iontophoresis, the strength of evidence is found to be *moderate* and its therapeutic effectiveness *substantiated*.

IV. DOSIMETRY

The dosimetry associated with the practice of iontophoresis depends on four parameters: (1) the drug ions selected for the pathology being treated, (2) the polarity of the drug used, (3) the concentration and volume of the ionic drug solution delivered, and (4) the dose used.

A. DRUG SELECTION

Practitioners can choose from a variety of drug agents having specific therapeutic properties (see Table 16-2). The selection is based on the desired therapeutic effects for any given pathology. For example, if the therapeutic goals are to decrease pain or inflammation, analgesic and/or anti-inflammatory drugs will be selected. If the selected drug is under medical control, nonphysician practitioners need to obtain the drug prescription from the treating physician and then the prescribed drug solution or ointment from the pharmacist. Note that nonmedicated and medicated (addition of anticholinergic agents) tap water is selective for the treatment of hand, foot, and armpit hyperhidrosis.

B. DRUG ION POLARITY

Knowledge of the drug ion used is *critical,* because for phoresis to occur at the electrode–skin interface, the negatively charged drug ions *must* be placed under the cathode (negative pole) and the positively charged drug ions under the anode (positive pole). Because tap water has a double polarity (+/–), it can be placed under the cathode or anode. In such a case, it is recommended to inverse the current polarity midway during treatment to ensure an equivalent phoresis of both ions in the skin. Is the simultaneous iontophoresis of two drug ions with the *same polarity* recommended? No, because both ions must compete against each other for their share of the delivery force provided by the DC intensity (Ciccone, 2008). Is the phoresis of two drug ions with *different polarity* recommended? No, because a reversal of polarity is required midway during the application to allow an even or balanced delivery of both drugs, resulting in a half dose of each drug delivered to the soft tissues (Ciccone, 2008). To sum up, the simultaneous phoresis of two drugs, with or without the same polarity, is *not recommended.*

C. DRUG CONCENTRATION AND VOLUME DELIVERY

There is a consensus in the literature that drug concentrations used for iontophoresis usually range within 2% to 5% aqueous solution or ointment. The drug solution should contain relatively low concentrations of medication, because an increased concentration does not appear to increase the amount of drug delivered (Henley, 1991; Ciccone, 2008). The amount or volume (cc) of drug aqueous solution contained in the electrode reservoir or patch varies according to its filling capacity. The fill volume of each electrode is indicated by the manufacturer.

D. DOSE

The amount of drug delivered into the tissues—that is, the dose (D)—is proportional to the current magnitude used

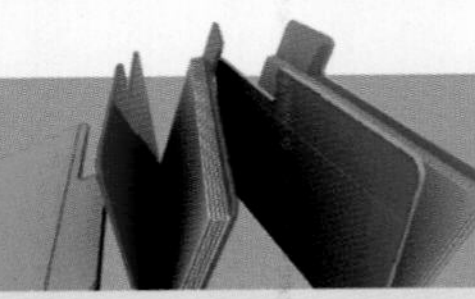

Research-Based Indications

IONTOPHORESIS

Health Condition	Ion	Benefit—Yes Rating	Benefit—Yes Reference	Benefit—No Rating	Benefit—No Reference
Hyperhidrosis	Tap water	I	Stolman, 1987		
		II	Shrivastava et al., 1977		
		II	Akins et al., 1987		
		II	Midtgaard, 1986		
		II	Levit, 1968		
		II	Levit, 1980		
		II	Holzle et al., 1986		
		II	Holzle et al., 1987		
		II	Bouman et al., 1952		
		II	Goh et al., 1996		
		II	Odia et al., 1996		
		II	Karakoç et al., 2002		
		II	Karakoç et al., 2004		
		II	Dolianitis et al., 2004		
		III	Gillick et al., 2004		
		III	Chan et al., 1999		
		III	Elgart et al., 1987		
	Tap water & poldine methosulfate	II	Grice et al., 1972		
		II	Hill, 1976		
	Tap water & glucopyrronium	II	Abell et al., 1974		

Strength of evidence: Moderate
Therapeutic effectiveness: Substantiated

Health Condition	Ion	Benefit—Yes Rating	Benefit—Yes Reference	Benefit—No Rating	Benefit—No Reference
Rheumatoid disorders	Dexamethasone	I	Bertolucci, 1982	II	Li et al., 1996
		II	Harris, 1982		
		II	Pellecchia et al., 1994		
		II	Akinbo et al., 2007		
		III	Hasson et al., 1991		
		III	Hasson et al., 1988		
	Salycilate	II	Aiyejunesie et al., 2007		
Epicondylitis	Dexamethasone	I	Nirsch et al., 2003		
	Diclofenac/ salycilate	II	Demirtas et al., 1998		
	Naproxen	II	Baskurt et al., 2003		
	Lidocaine	III	Yarrobino et al., 2006		
	Cortisone			I	Runeson et al., 2002
	Dexamethasone			III	Panus et al., 1996
Peyronie's disease	Dexamethasone/ lidocaine	I	Montorsi et al., 2000		
	Dexamethasone/ lidocaine	II	Reidl et al., 2000		
	Hydrocortisone	III	Kahn, 1982		
	Glucocorticoids	III	Rothfeld et al., 1967		
Tempo-romandibular joint disorders	Dexamethasone	I	Reid et al., 1994		
	Dexamethasone/ lidocaine	I	Schiffman et al., 1996		
	Dexamathasone	II	Mina et al., 2011		
	Dexamethasone/ lidocaine	III	Braun, 1987		
	Hydrocortisone			III	Kahn, 1980
Calcifying tendinitis	Acetic acid			I	Perron et al, 1997
				I	Leduc et al., 2003
		II	Psaki et al., 1955		

Strength of evidence: Moderate
Therapeutic effectiveness: Substantiated

Fewer Than 5 Studies

Health Condition	Ion	Benefit—Yes Rating	Benefit—Yes Reference	Benefit—No Rating	Benefit—No Reference
Plantar faciitis	Dexamethasone	I	Gudeman et al., 1997		
		II	Chandler, 1998		
Carpal tunnel syndrome	Dexamethasone	II	Banta, 1994		
		II	Gurcay et al., 2012		
Plantar warts	Salicylate	II	Sokoro et al., 2002		
		III	Gordon et al., 1969		
Edema	Hyaluronidase	III	Magistro, 1964		
		III	Boone, 1969		

Health Condition	Ion	Benefit—Yes		Benefit—No	
		Rating	Reference	Rating	Reference
Achilles tendonitis	Dexamethasone	I	Neeter et al., 2003		
Myofascial syndrome	Dexamethasone/ lidocaine	II	Delacerda, 1982		
Postherpetic neuralgia	Prednisone/ lidocaine	II	Ozawa et al., 1999		
Myositis ossificans	Acetic acid	III	Wieder, 1992		
Heel pain	Acetic acid	II	Japour et al., 1999		
Post-surgical hip pain	Salicylate	III	Garzione, 1978		
Lymphedema	Hyaluronidase	III	Schwartz, 1955		
Scar tissue	Iodine	III	Tannenbaum, 1980		

Health Condition	Ion	Benefit—Yes		Benefit—No	
		Rating	Reference	Rating	Reference
Tendon adhesion	Iodine	III	Langley, 1984		
Bacterial wounds	Zinc	III	Balogun et al., 1990		
Ischemic skin ulcers	Zinc	III	Cornwall, 1981		
Subdeltoid bursitis	Magnesium sulfate	II	Weinstein et al., 1958		
Myopathy	Calcium	III	Kahn, 1975		

Strength of evidence: Pending
Therapeutic effectiveness: Pending

ALL CONDITIONS
Strength of evidence: Moderate
Therapeutic effectiveness: Substantiated

(A) and the total application duration (T). This dose is calculated as D (mA.min) = A (mA) × T (min). The literature indicates that the maximum doses used to deliver drug iontophoresis differ significantly from the doses used to deliver tap water iontophoresis. Doses commonly used to deliver drug ions range between 1 and 80 mA.min, with a maximum available current amplitude of 4 mA. Doses commonly used to deliver tap water iontophoresis for hyperhidrosis, using line-powered devices, are much higher than for drugs, ranging between 100 and 500 mA.min, with maximum current amplitude ranging between 10 and 20 mA (see Gillick et al., 2004). A much higher current amplitude is needed because the electrode conductive area (water tray) used is much greater than that used for drug delivery (electrode and patch). In other words, higher current amplitudes can be used safely because current densities under the electrodes are well within the recommended safe values, due to the electrode large conductive areas. To deliver, for example, a prescribed dose of 40 mA.min of dexamethasone for treatment of wrist tendonitis, practitioners may select, using a programmable iontophoresor, one of several combinations of current amplitude and application duration, such as 4.0 mA for 10 minutes, 1.0 mA for 40 minutes, or 2 mA for 20 minutes, simply by turning the knobs on the console. Patch iontophoresors differ from programmable ones in that dosages are preset (40 mA.min or 80 mA.min). Because current delivery will fluctuate over time due to soft tissue impedance changes, manufacturers recommend an application duration, or wearing time, of 12 hours (720 min) for the 40 mA.min patch and 24 hours (1,440 min) for the 80 mA.min patch. The self-contained battery within the patch is activated as soon as the patch is hydrated (i.e., impregnated with the drug solution in one pole of pad and with tap water in the other pad). It will remain activated until the pads are depleted of their solutions. Table 16-3 summarizes key characteristics associated with wire programmable and wireless nonprogrammable iontophoresors.

E. SAFETY ISSUES

There is a limit to the magnitude of current amplitude that can be used within a prescribed dose because of the risk of inducing a skin irritation or burn under the electrodes, particularly under the cathode. The amplitude limit is based on the electrode current density (CD), which is the amount of current amplitude (A) applied against the electrode conductive surface area (S). CD is calculated as follows: CD (mA/cm^2) = A (mA)/S (cm^2). It is important to distinguish between electrode *surface area* and electrode *conductive surface area,* because the latter is always smaller and often unrelated to the former. The maximum safe CD values recommended for iontophoresis are 0.5 mA/cm^2 for the cathode and 1.0 mA/cm^2 for the anode (Cummings, 1991; Ciccone, 2008). These values correspond to 3.3 mA/in^2 for the cathode and 6.6 mA/in^2 for the anode (1 in^2 = 6.452 cm^2). Table 16-4 shows how to determine the maximum current amplitude that can be used in any given application while taking into consideration the recommended safe CD values for each electrode. It is strongly recommended that the conductive surface area of the cathode be larger than that of the anode, regardless of whether the cathode is used as the active or dispersive electrode. This is because a skin burn underneath the cathode is more harmful to the skin than one under the anode. The larger the cathodal conductive surface areas, the smaller the CD, and the lower the risk of cathodal skin burn.

F. ONLINE DOSAGE CALCULATOR: IONTOPHORESIS

As was the case in the previous chapters, an **Online Dosage Calculator** is provided with the objective to lessen the burden associated with recalling formulas and doing hand calculations. Upon entering the dosimetric parameters, the calculator will indicate the precise dose to deliver as

TABLE 16-3 IONTOPHORESORS AND THEIR KEY FEATURES

Wire Programmable	Wireless Nonprogrammable or Patch
Battery-powered electrical stimulator, lead wires, and electrodes	Self-contained system (embedded battery with two poles)
Reusable system; only the electrodes are discarded after single application	Disposable system; patch discarded after single application
Constant current (CC) source—current amplitude and delivery kept constant during therapy despite fluctuations of tissue impedance	Constant voltage (CV) source—current amplitude and delivery vary during therapy due to fluctuations of tissue impedance
Drug dose programmable from 1–80 mA.min	Drug dose fixed by manufacturer; choice of 40 mA.min or 80 mA.min
Tap water dose (hyperhidrosis) programmable from 300–500 mA.min	NA
Current amplitude programmable from 0–5 mA for drugs	Current amplitude prefixed at ~0.1 mA
Current amplitude programmable from 1–20 mA for tap water (hyperhidrosis)	NA
Application duration automatically calculated based on the dosage used	Manufacturers recommend the following continuous wearing time: • 12 h for 40 mA.min patch • 24 h for 80 mA.min patch
No activity allowed during treatment because of electrodes attached to stimulator	Freedom of movement during treatment due to self-contained system

well as the electrode current density and maximum safe current amplitude.

V. APPLICATION, CONTRAINDICATIONS, AND RISKS

Outlined in the *Application, Contraindications, and Risks* box are the contraindications and risks associated with the practice of iontophoresis. It is vital to question the patient about any previous drug sensitivity or allergy before proceeding with therapy. As well, precautions need to be taken during application. For example, the risk of skin irritation or, at worst, skin burn, is the factor that most limits the application of drug iontophoresis. Practitioners should pay close attention to assure that the current device (CD) under the active electrode is always kept within the safe limit.

TABLE 16-4 CALCULATING MAXIMUM SAFE CURRENT AMPLITUDE BASED ON ELECTRODE CURRENT DENSITY

Parameters	Cathode	Anode
Recommended maximum current density (CD)	CD = 0.5 mA/cm^2	CD = 1.0 mA/cm^2
CD = current amplitude (A)/conductive surface area (S)	If A = 2 mA If S = 6 cm^2	If A = 3 mA If S = 4 cm^2
Is the current density (CD) under each electrode safe?	CD = 2 mA/6 cm^2 CD = 0.33 mA/cm^2—safe	CD = 3 mA / 4 cm^2 CD = 0.75 mA/cm^2—safe
What is the maximum safe current amplitude (A) possible under each electrode?	A = CD × S A = 0.5 mA/cm^2 × 6 cm^2 A = 3 mA	A = CD × S A = 1.0 mA/cm^2 × 4 cm^2 A = 4 mA

APPLICATION, CONTRAINDICATIONS, AND RISKS

Iontophoresis

IMPORTANT: Ensure ion/electrode polarity match because polarity mismatch will lead to total ineffectiveness of the iontophoretic treatment because no ion(s) will ever penetrate the skin. The only exception is tap water (+/–), which can be placed under both electrodes irrespective of their polarity. Work in collaboration with the patient's treating physician and your pharmacist. The adequate prescription and preparation of your drug-ionized solutions depends on the collaboration of these two health professionals; never hesitate to consult them. Illustrated are examples of electrode filling with a syringe (Fig. 16-8) and applications of battery- (Fig. 16-9) and line- (Fig. 16-10) powered wire programmable iontophoresors.

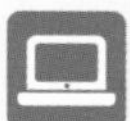

See **online videos.**

ALL AGENTS

STEP	RATIONALE
1. Check for contraindications.	*Over open, damaged, or broken skin*—induces skin irritation, burn, and severe pain (Ciccone, 2008)
	Across temporal and orbicular areas—causes transient visual disturbances
	In cases of known sensitivity or allergy to the therapeutic ions—triggers a life-threatening allergic reaction (Ciccone, 2008)
	Over electronic implants—risk of interference with normal functioning
2. Consider the risks.	*Skin irritation and burn*—risk is increased if the dose is too high, nonbuffered electrodes are used, or current density under the cathode or anode exceeds the recommended safe values
	In the presence of and proximally to flammable sprays or solutions—risk of igniting the flammable materials, thus posing a risk of explosion
	Over skin area showing severe to moderate impaired sensation to heat and pain stimuli—risk of chemical and/or heat burn under the electrodes due to impaired ability to discriminate sensations of heat or pain

WIRE IONTOPHORESOR

STEP	RATIONALE

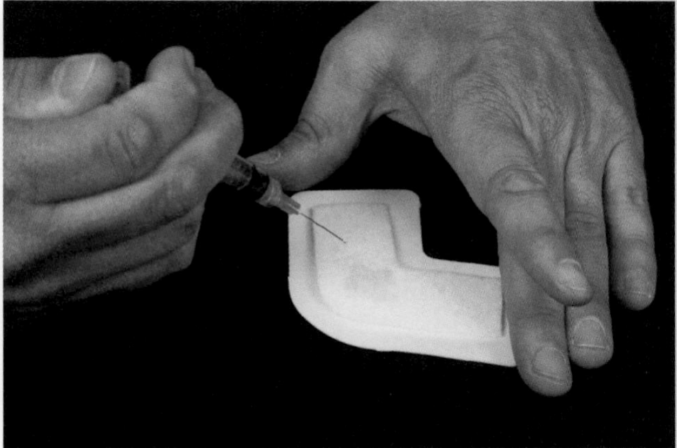

FIGURE 16-8 Electrode filled with a drug solution using a syringe. (Reprinted with permission from Knight, KL and Draper, DO. *Therapeutic Modalities*. Philadelphia: Lippincott Williams and Wilkins, 2008.)

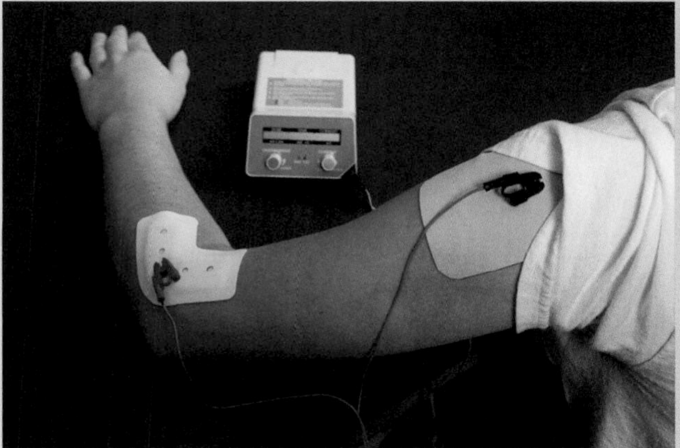

FIGURE 16-9 Application of a wire programmable iontophoresis unit for the treatment of epicondylitis using a portable iontophoresor. (Reprinted with permission from Knight, KL and Draper, DO. *Therapeutic Modalities*. Philadelphia: Lippincott Williams and Wilkins, 2008.)

STEP	RATIONALE
1. Check for contraindications.	See All Agents section.
2. Consider the risks.	See All Agents section.
3. Position and instruct patient.	Ensure comfortable body positioning. Instruct the patient not to touch the device, cables, and electrodes and to immediately report any hot or burning sensation under the electrodes during treatment.
4. Prepare treatment area.	Clean the skin area where the active and dispersive electrodes are to be positioned with rubbing alcohol, or water and soap. If necessary, cut and trim excess hair. Avoid shaving the hair before treatment because of possible skin irritation. The skin area should be free of open wounds.
5. Select device type.	Select wire, reusable and programmable for clinic-based therapy. The wireless type (patch) is the selection of choice for patients who have limited time available for clinical visits and who want to remain active while receiving drug iontophoresis (see later discussion). Plug line-powered devices into ground-fault circuit interrupter (GFCI) receptacles to prevent the occurrence of macroshocks (see Chapter 5).
6. Select electrode type.	Choose between custom nonbuffered or commercial buffered electrodes (see Fig. 16-2 and Table 16-5 below). Buffered electrodes are recommended because they eliminate the adverse effects of iontophoresis.
7. Select therapeutic ion.	Select the appropriate ion according to the condition under treatment (see Table 16-2 and Research-Based Indications box). Note the drug solution polarity. Drug ions are diluted in aqueous solution. Drug concentration may vary between 1% and 10%. Check with the pharmacist and the patient's treating physician for optimal concentration to use.

TABLE 16-5 CUSTOM VERSUS COMMERCIAL IONTOPHORETIC ELECTRODES

Custom	Commercial
Made of malleable metal materials, such as kitchen aluminum foil, under which are applied some layers of absorbent material (gauze or cotton) impregnated with the therapeutic ionic solution	Made of various materials, such as gel matrix, fiber pad (patch), and plastic reservoir-like material all capable of being impregnated with the therapeutic ionic solution
Can be customized to the desired sizes	Come in predetermined sizes
No control over skin pH changes during treatment	Control over skin pH changes due to a buffering agent incorporated within the electrode system. However, some commercial electrodes are sold without a buffering system.
Require more preparation time (customizing of electrodes, gauze, or cloth)	Require less preparation time (precut)
Rather messy to use due to leaking of ionic solution from the impregnated gauze or cloth	Cleaner to use, with no leaking of ionic solution from the electrode system
Require straps, tapes, or elastic bandages to secure electrodes over the skin	Self-adhesive system
Relatively inexpensive system	Relatively more expensive system

STEP	RATIONALE
8. Select method of delivery.	• *Anodal iontophoresis:* Place the positively charged ionic drug solution under the anode (+). • *Cathodal iontophoresis:* Place the negatively charged ionic drug solution under the cathode (–).
9. Prepare electrodes.	• *Active:* Soaked the gauze (custom electrode), or fill the electrode reservoir (commercial) with the drug solution using a syringe. • *Dispersive:* Fill the electrode with tap water or Ringer solution. The filling capacity, or volume (cc), of each electrode is determined by the manufacturer. Do not over- or underfill commercial electrodes.
10. Position electrodes.	• *Active electrode:* Place over the targeted pathologic area. • *Dispersive electrode:* Place a few centimeters away from the active electrode. Avoid rearranging electrodes during treatment—this will affect treatment efficacy and create unpleasant sensations for the patient. Keep adequate distance, or spacing, between the cathode and anode. The distance should be at least equivalent to the diameter of the largest electrode.
11. Set dosimetry.	Set current amplitude (mA) and application duration (min) such that the dosage varies between 1 and 80 mA.min. For both custom or commercial electrodes, make sure that the current density under the cathode and anode is always kept at less than the recommended values of 0.5 and 1.0 mA/cm^2, respectively (Table 16-4). To facilitate dosimetry, use the **Online Dosage Calculator: Iontophoresis**.
12. Apply treatment.	Ensure adequate monitoring.
13. Conduct post-treatment inspection.	Remove the electrodes. Inspect skin integrity for signs of adverse effect. Wash and dry the treated surface areas. Custom metal plate electrodes may be reused only after thorough cleaning and disinfecting. Apply a soothing lotion over the treated skin areas. If *skin irritation* occurs, it will manifest itself as a transient erythema (redness) under one or both electrodes; it should normally disappear within 1–3 hours after treatment. If *skin burn* occurs, *stop* treatment. Periodic application of burn ointments will help to ease the pain while accelerating healing. For severe burn cases that will not heal by themselves, consult a dermatologist.
14. Ensure post-treatment equipment maintenance.	Follow manufacturer recommendations. Immediately report defects or malfunctions to technical maintenance staff. Conduct regular maintenance and calibration procedures.

WIRELESS OR PATCH IONTOPHORESOR

STEP	RATIONALE
1. Check for contraindications.	See All Agents section.
2. Consider the risks.	See All Agents section.
3. Position and instruct patient.	Ensure comfortable body positioning. Instruct the patient not to touch the device, cables, and electrodes and to immediately report any hot or burning sensation under the electrodes during treatment.
4. Prepare treatment area.	Clean the skin area where the active and dispersive electrodes are to be positioned with rubbing alcohol, or water and soap. If necessary, cut and trim excess hair. Avoid shaving the hair before treatment because of possible skin irritation. The skin area should be free of open wounds.
5. Select device type.	Use patch iontophoresors.

STEP	RATIONALE
6. Position patch.	Place the active electrode of the self-adhesive patch over the area to be treated. Ensure even contact between the electrodes and the skin for optimal ion delivery into the treatment area.
7. Set dosimetry.	Dosage is preset by manufacturers. Maximum dosage may be as high as 80 mA.min, and recommended wear or treatment time is 24 hours—see manufacturer recommendations for details.
8. Apply treatment.	The unit is wearable; patients are fully mobile and free to do their activities of daily living.
9. Conduct post-treatment inspection.	Remove the patch. Inspect skin integrity for signs of adverse effect. Wash and dry the treated surface areas. Discard the patch. Apply lotion over the treated skin areas.
10. Ensure post-treatment equipment maintenance.	No maintenance is required because the patch is disposable after single use.

HYPERHIDROSIS IONTOPHORESOR

STEP	RATIONALE
1. Check for contraindications.	See All Agents section.
2. Consider the risks.	See All Agents section.
3. Position and instruct patient.	With the patient sitting, place hands, or feet, in each tray. The water level should be just above the hand or foot level. Instruct the patient to keep hands or feet in the water during treatment and to avoid touching the electrodes built into the bottom of each tray. Touching the electrodes may result in a harmless microshock. Remove all jewelry.
4. Select device type.	Select specially designed iontophoresor for hyperhidrosis (Fig. 16-1B). Such dedicated iontophoresor units are recommended by the International Hyperhidrosis Society (www.sweathelp.org).
5. Set up device.	Fill the tow plastic trays with tap water at room temperature to the top of the built-in electrodes. Connect the trays to the iontophoresor unit using the electrical cables.
6. Select therapeutic ion.	Use tap water at room temperature. Salt or baking soda may be added to tap water to improve electrical conductivity. Anticholinergic agents can also be added to improve treatment effectiveness.

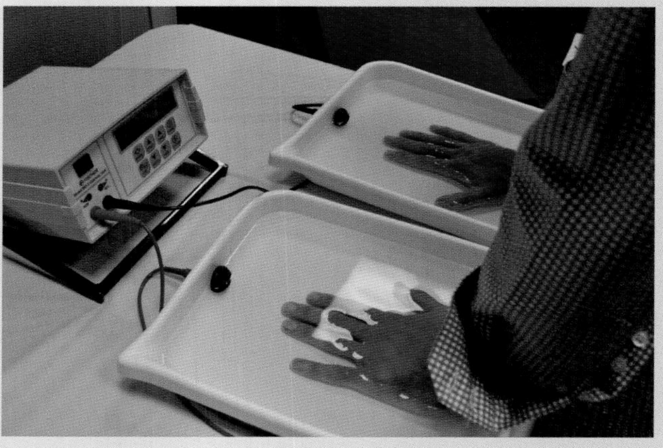

FIGURE 16-10 Application of iontophoresis for hyperhidrosis. (Reprinted with permission, © International Hyperhidrosis Society, www.sweathelp.org.)

STEP	RATIONALE
7. **Set dosimetry.**	Set current amplitude (mA) and application duration (min). Dosage may range between 150 and 300 mA.min (i.e., 15 mA for 20 min). Because large electrode are used, larger current amplitude may be used, keeping the electrode current density within the safe zone (see Table 16-4). Make sure that *electrode polarity* is balanced in both trays by reversing polarity halfway during treatment. To facilitate dosimetry, use the **Online Dosage Calculator: Iontophoresis.**
8. **Apply treatment.**	Ensure adequate monitoring. Patients may need treatments every 2–3 days for 5–10 sessions before a beneficial therapeutic effect is observed.
9. **Conduct post-treatment inspection.**	Inspect skin integrity for signs of adverse effect. Wash and dry the treated surface areas. Discard used water and wash trays.
10. **Ensure post-treatment equipment maintenance.**	Follow manufacturer recommendations. Immediately report defects or malfunctions to technical maintenance staff.

CASE STUDIES

The following two case studies summarize the concepts, principles, and applications of iontophoresis discussed in this chapter. Case Study 16-1 addresses the use of iontophoresis for a traumatic epicondylitis affecting a middle-aged female worker. A portable programmable and wire iontophoresor is used to resolved the case (Fig. 16-9). A wireless nonprogrammable patch iontophoresor could also be used in this case (see Fig. 16-1B). Case Study 16-2 is concerned with the application of iontophoresis for palmar hyperhidrosis affecting a middle-aged male worker. A portable programmable wire iontophoresor is used with a pair of commercial water trays acting as electrodes (Fig. 16-10). Each case is structured in line with the concepts of evidence-based practice (EBP), the International Classification of Functioning, Disability, and Health (ICF) disablement model, and SOAP (*s*ubjective, *o*bjective, *a*ssessment, *p*lan) note format (see Chapter 2 for details).

CASE STUDY 16-1: EPICONDYLITIS

EVIDENCE-BASED CLINICAL DECISION MAKING PROTOCOL

1. Formulate the Case History

A 49-year-old female worker, working full-time for a cleaning company, consults for treatment. She wears a pacemaker, and her present health status is good. She recalls that 3 weeks ago she sustained a major blow to the lateral side of her right elbow while cleaning a container (the container's cover fell on her elbow). The following day she was seen by her physician, who diagnosed the presence of a severe traumatic epicondylitis. After 3 weeks of analgesic and anti-inflammatory oral drug therapy, coupled with rest (absence from work), she reports good improvement. She now experiences no pain at rest and moderate pain during light wrist and hand activities. Physical examination, however, reveals residual signs of inflammation over the lateral epicondyle area. There is moderate swelling, with increasing pain during forceful wrist extension and power grip. She is anxious about prolonging her absenteeism from work. Her goal is to return to work as soon as possible and to stop her oral drug regimen, which is starting to give her some stomach irritation. In other words, she is looking for an alternative treatment to her present oral drug and rest regimen. Finally, she stresses the fact that her physician mentioned that if her condition was to further deteriorate, an injection of drugs into the painful area may be needed. She is afraid of needles and wants to avoid this last treatment approach at all costs.

2. Outline the Case Based on the ICF Framework

EPICONDYLITIS		
BODY STRUCTURES AND FUNCTIONS	**ACTIVITIES**	**PARTICIPATION**
Pain	Difficulty to power grip	Unable to resume full-time work
Decreased grip strength		

PERSONAL FACTORS	ENVIRONMENTAL FACTORS
Middle-aged healthy woman	Factory work
Housewife	Home
	Family

3. Outline Therapeutic Goals and Outcome Measurements

GOAL	OUTCOME MEASUREMENT
Decrease pain	Visual Analogue Scale (VAS)
Increase grip strength	Dynamometry
Improve functional performance	Patient-Specific Functional Scale (PSFS)

4. Justify the Use of Iontophoresis Based on the EBP Framework

PRACTITIONER'S EXPERIENCE	RESEARCH-BASED INDICATIONS	PATIENT'S EXPECTATION
Moderately experienced in iontophoresis	*Strength:* Moderate	No opinion on the use of iontophoresis
Has seldom used iontophoresis in similar cases	*Effectiveness:* Substantiated	Desperate to avoid needle injection
Wants to see if iontophoresis can be beneficial		

5. Outline Key Intervention Parameters

- **Treatment base:** Private clinic
- **Electrical current:** Direct current
- **Current waveform:** Monophasic
- **Delivery mode:** Continuous
- **Stimulator type:** Wire programmable iontophoresor (see Fig. 16-1B or Fig. 16-9)
- **Application protocol:** Follow the suggested application protocol presented for wire iontophoresor in *Application, Contraindications, and Risks* box, and make the necessary adjustments for this case.
- **Patient's positioning:** Sitting with the elbow resting on a table
- **Electrode type:** Commercial buffered electrodes
- **Therapeutic drug ion and polarity:** Dexamethasone (–)
- **Drug concentration:** 4 mg/mL in aqueous solution
- **Electrode placement:** Active cathode over the effected epicondyle area; dispersive anode placed 15 cm away over the arm
- **Active electrode:** Cathode; conductive surface area 4 cm^2; fill volume 2.5 cc—dexamethasone
- **Dispersive electrode:** Anode; conductive surface area 6 cm^2; fill volume 3.5 cc—Ringer solution
- **Dose:** 40 mA.min; delivered using current amplitude of 2 mA for a duration of 20 minutes
- **Treatment frequency:** Daily; 5 consecutive days
- **Intervention period:** 2 weeks
- **Concomitant therapies:** Pain-free progressive regimen of wrist and grip muscle strengthening
- **Use the Online Dosage Calculator: Iontophoresis.**

6. Compare Pre- and Post-Intervention Outcomes

OUTCOME	PRE	POST
Pain (VAS score)	5/10	1/10
Grip force (deficit)	–25%	–10%
Functional performance (PFSF score)	32	12

7. Document Case Intervention Using the SOAP Note Format

S: Middle-aged female worker presents with R chronic epicondylitis causing pain during forceful wrist and grip movements. Previous drug treatment provided adequate pain relief but Pt is still unable to resume full function. Pt wants to stop drug oral ingestion and fears needle drug injection.

O: *Intervention:* Private clinic based; iontophoresis applied over the painful epicondyle area: Pt sitting with elbow resting on table; dexamethasone: 4 mg/mL; cathodal application; dose: 40 mA.min (2 mA × 20 min); treatment schedule: daily, 5-days/week, for 14 days. *Pre–post comparison:* Decrease pain VAS score (5/10 to 1/10), increase grip strength (deficit—25% to 10%), and improved wrist/grip function (PFSF score 32 to 12).

A: Light dermatitis under cathode; disappeared after the fourth treatment. Treatment very well tolerated thereafter. Pt very happy to avoid drug needle injection.

P: No further treatment required. Pt discharged. Pt now working full-time. If condition worsens, consider the possibility of using a wearable iontophoretic patch system while remaining at work.

CASE STUDY 16-2: PALMAR HYPERHIDROSIS

EVIDENCE-BASED CLINICAL DECISION MAKING PROTOCOL

1. Formulate the Case History

A 32-year-old carpenter consults for treatment. His major complaint is excessive sweating of the palmar surface of his hands, which started about a year ago. He explains that his hands are constantly wet and slippery and that the whole thing seems to worsen when he is under pressure at work. He adds that his hand condition led him, over the past 3 months, to improper and unsafe gripping of his hammer and other carpentry tools at work. He indicates that in order to work properly and safely, he has to wear three pairs of cotton gloves a day to absorb the excessive perspiration. He also complains of social embarrassment when he touches his girlfriend and when shaking hands with family members, friends, and coworkers. He reports that he consulted with a physician 2 weeks ago for his hand condition. The physician offered to prescribe an oral anticholinergic drug regimen and added that if the medication did not resolve his condition, he would then refer him to a dermatologist for botulinum toxin injections and, if necessary, for his opinion as to a possible endoscopic thoracic sympathectomy. This young man mentions that before considering any medical or surgical therapeutic interventions, his preference is to undertake a more conservative, and much less invasive, type of treatment. A basic Internet search made him aware that tap water iontophoresis may benefit his condition.

2. Outline the Case Based on the ICF Framework

PALMAR HYPERHIDROSIS		
BODY STRUCTURES AND FUNCTIONS	**ACTIVITIES**	**PARTICIPATION**
Hand hypersudation	Difficulty gripping tools	Social embarrassment (hand touch)
Moist and slippery hands	Inability to work safely and effectively	

PERSONAL FACTORS	ENVIRONMENTAL FACTORS
Young man	Work with tools
Manual worker	Construction site
	Peer pressure

3. Outline Therapeutic Goals and Outcome Measurements

GOAL	OUTCOME MEASUREMENT
Increase hand dryness	Persprint paper
Increase grip firmness and improve safety and effectiveness at work	Count of gloves used per day
Decrease social embarrassment	Personal diary—scale 0 (none) to 10 (maximum)

4. Justify the Use of Iontophoresis Based on the EBP Framework

PRACTITIONER'S EXPERIENCE	RESEARCH-BASED INDICATIONS	PATIENT'S EXPECTATION
Very experienced in iontophoresis	*Strength:* Moderate *Effectiveness:* Substantiated	Believes that iontophoresis can help him
Has used iontophoresis in similar cases		
Very confident that iontophoresis will be beneficial		

5. Outline Key Intervention Parameters

- **Treatment base:** Private clinic
- **Electrical current:** Direct current
- **Current waveform:** Monophasic
- **Delivery mode:** Continuous
- **Stimulator type:** Wire programmable iontophoresor
- **Application protocol:** Follow the suggested application protocol presented for hyperhidrosis iontophoresor in *Application, Contraindications, and Risks* box, and make the necessary adjustments for this case.
- **Patient's positioning:** Sitting with both hands prone
- **Electrode arrangement:** Two commercial electrodes embedded in plastic trays, 40 × 25 × 10 cm each, filled with 2 L of tap water at room temperature (21°C [70°F]). Electrode size: 30 × 20 cm each (600 cm^2). Water level in both trays: at a level sufficient to cover the palmar surfaces of both hands.
- **Therapeutic ion and polarity:** Tap water (+/–) with a teaspoon of salt
- **Electrode polarity:** Automatic reversal (50%–50%)
- **Dose:** 360 mA.min; delivered using current amplitude of 18 mA for a period of 20 minutes
- **Treatment frequency:** Every second day
- **Intervention period:** 4 weeks
- **Concomitant therapies:** None
- **Use the Online Dosage Calculator: Iontophoresis.**

6. Compare Pre- and Post-Intervention Outcomes

OUTCOME	PRE	POST
Hand dryness (Persprint paper; dry surface area)		R hand—increased by 80% L hand—increased by 75%
Handgrip firmness	5 cotton gloves per day	1 cotton glove per day
Social embarrassment (scale; 10 maximum)	7	2

7. Document Case Intervention Using the SOAP Note Format

S: Young male Pt presents with palmar hyperhidrosis causing working issues and social embarrassment.

O: *Intervention:* Private clinic based; iontophoresis; Pt sitting; tap water (+/–) with 1 tsp of salt; both hands soaked in separate trays; dose: 360 mA.min (18 mA × 20 min); treatment schedule: every second day for 4 weeks. *Pre–post comparison:* Improved hand dryness (R hand, 80% increase; L hand, 75% increase), improved hand firmness (from 5 to 1 glove per day), and decreased social embarrassment (7 to 2).

A: Light skin irritation during first few treatments. Treated with hydrocortisone cream. Treatment very well tolerated thereafter.

P: Now that the desired dryness is achieved, Pt decides to purchase the iontophoresis unit for future home-based therapy. Pt advised to a maintenance schedule of 1 treatment per week. To maintain dryness, iontophoresis treatment should be conducted before sweating begins to return.

VI. THE BOTTOM LINE

- There is scientific evidence to show that iontophoresis can induce therapeutic effects on various health conditions.
- Iontophoresis is the delivery of drug ion solutions, as well as tap water, through the skin using continuous direct electrical current.
- For intophoresis to occur, drug ions must be placed under the electrode bearing the same charge or polarity.
- The main pathways, or pores, through which the drug ions can penetrate the skin stratum corneum are hair follicles and sweat glands.
- Iontophoresis is used as a replacement for oral drug ingestion and needle drug injection.

- Iontophoresis causes phoretic, electrolytic, and pharmacologic effects.
- Using buffered electrodes and controlling electrode current densities minimize the unwanted side effects of iontophoresis.
- Iontophoretic dosage is expressed in milliamperes per minute (mA.min).
- Using the **Online Dosage Calculator: Iontophoresis** removes the burden of hand calculation and promotes the adoption of quantitative dosimetry.
- The use of tap water iontophoresis for the treatment of hyperhidrosis is common and recommended as the first line of treatment.
- The overall body of evidence reported in this chapter shows the strength of evidence behind iontophoresis to be *moderate* and its level of therapeutic effectiveness *substantiated.*

VII. CRITICAL THINKING QUESTIONS

Clarification: How would you describe Leduc's contribution to the field of iontophoresis?

Assumptions: Can you explain how the phenomenon of water electrolysis causes unwanted electrochemical reactions to the skin during iontophoresis therapy?

Reasons and evidence: Why is a polarity match between the drug ion and the electrode pole under which it is placed critical to the application of iontophoresis?

Viewpoints or perspectives: What is the relationship between skin irritation/burn, skin pH, the use of buffered electrodes, and the concept of electrode current density?

Implications and consequences: What would happen to the depth of penetration of a given drug if the application duration is short versus long using the same dose in both situations?

About the question: How will you convince a physician that iontophoresis is an effective and safe method for delivering a drug to a localized region of the body? Why do you think I ask this question?

VIII. REFERENCES

Articles

Abell G, Morgan K (1974) Treatment of idiopathic hyperhidrosis by glycopyrronium bromide and tap water iontophoresis. Br J Dermatol, 91: 87–91

Aiyejusunie CB, Kola-Korolo TA, Ajiboye OA (2007) Comparison of the effects of TENS and sodium salicylate iontophoresis in the management of osteoarthritis of the knee. Nig Q J Hosp Med, 17: 30–34

Akinbo SR, Aiyejunusie CB, Akinyemi OA, Adesegun SA, Danesi MA (2007) Comparison of the therapeutic efficacy of phonophoresis and iontophoresis using dexamethasone sodium phosphate in the management of patients with knee osteoarthritis. Niger Postgrad Med, 14: 190–194

Akins DL, Meisenheimer JL, Dobson RL (1987) Efficacy of the Drionic unit in the treatment of hyperhidrosis. J Am Acad Dermatol, 16: 828–833

Anderson CR, Morris RL, Boeh SD, Panus PC, Sembrowich WL (2003) Effects of iontophoresis current magnitude and duration on dexamethasone deposition and localized drug retention. Phys Ther, 83: 161–170

Balogun JA, Abidoye AB, Akala EO (1990) Zinc iontophoresis in the management of bacterial colonized wounds: A case report. Physiother Can, 42: 147–151

Banta CA (1994) A prospective, nonrandomized study of iontophoresis, wrist splinting, and anti-inflammatory medication in the treatment of early mild carpal tunnel syndrome. J Occup Med, 36: 166–168

Baskurt F, Ozcan A, Algun C (2003) Comparison of effects on phonophoresis and iontophoresis of naproxen in the treatment of lateral epicondylitis. Clin Rehab, 17: 96–100

Bertolucci LE (1982) Introduction of anti-inflammatory drugs by iontophoresis: Double-blind study. J Orthop Sports Phys Ther, 4: 103–108

Boone D (1969) Hyaluronidase iontophoresis. Phys Ther, 49: 139–145

Bouman HD, Grunewald Lentzer EM (1952) The treatment of hyperhidrosis of feet with constant current. Am J Phys Med, 31: 158–169

Braun BL (1987) Treatment of an acute anterior disk displacement in the temporomandibular joint: A case report. Phys Ther, 67: 1234–1236

Chan LY, Tang WY, Mok WK, Ly CY, Ip AW (1999) Treatment of palmar hyperhidrosis using tap water iontophoresis: Local experience. Hong Kong Med J, 5: 191–194

Chandler TJ (1998) Iontophoresis of 0.4% dexamethasone for plantar fasciitis. Clin J Sport Med, 8: 68

Cornwall MW (1981) Zinc iontophoresis to treat ischemic skin ulcers. Phys Ther, 61: 359–360

Delacerda FG (1982) A comparative study of three methods of treatment for shoulder girdle myofascial syndrome. J Orthop Sports Phys Ther, 4: 51–54

Demirtas RN, Oner C (1998) The treatment of lateral epicondylitis by iontophoresis of sodium salicylate and sodium diclofenac. Clin Rehab, 12: 23–29

Dolianitis C, Scarff CE, Kelly J, Sinclair R (2004) Iontophoresis with glycopyrrolate for the treatment of palmoplantar hyperiydrosis. Australasian J Dermatol, 45: 208–212

Elgart ML, Puchs G (1987) Tapwater iontophoresis in the treatment of hyperhidrosis. Use of the Drionic device. Int J Dermatol, 26: 194–197

Garzione JE (1978) Salicylate iontophoresis as an alternative treatment for persistent thigh pain following hip surgery. Phys Ther, 58: 570–571

Gillick BT, Kloth LC, Starsky A, Cincinelli-Walker L (2004) Management of postsurgical hyperhidrosis with direct current and tap water. Phys Ther, 84: 262–267

Goh CL, Yoyong K (1996) A comparison of tannic acid versus iontophoresis in the medical treatment of palmar hyperhidrosis. Singapore Med J, 37: 466–488

Gordon AH, Weistein MV (1969) Sodium salicylate iontophoresis in the treatment of plantar warts: Case report. Phys Ther, 49: 869–870

Grice K, Sattar H, Baker H (1972) Treatment of idiopathic hyperhidrosis with iontophoresis of tap water and poldine methosulphate. Br J Dermatol, 86: 72–78

Gudeman SD, Eisele SA, Heidt RS, Colosimo AJ, Sroupe AL (1997) Treatment of plantar fasciitis by iontophoresis of 0.4% dexamethasone. A randomized, double-blind, placebo-controlled study. Am J Sports Med, 25: 312–316

Guffey JS, Rutherford MJ, Payne W, Phillips C (1999) Skin pH changes associated with iontophoresis. J Orthop Sports Phys Ther, 29: 656–660

Gurcay E, Unlu E, Gurcay AG, Tuncay R, Cakci A (2012) Assessment of phonophoresis and iontophoresis in the treatment of carpal tunnel syndrome: A randomized controlled trial. Rheumatol Int, 32: 717–722

Harris PR (1982) Iontophoresis: Clinical research in musculoskeletal inflammatory conditions. J Orthop Sports Phys Ther, 4: 109–112

Hasson SH, Henderson GH, Daniels JC, Schieb DA (1991) Exercise training and dexamethasone iontophoresis in rheumatoid arthritis: A case study. Physiother Can, 43: 11–14

Hasson SM, English SE, Daniels JC, Reich M (1988) Effect of iontophoretically delivered dexamethasone on muscle performance in a rheumatoid arthritic joint: A case study. Arthritis Care Res, 1: 177–182

Hill BH (1976) Poldine iontophoresis in the treatment of palmar and plantar hyperhidrosis. Aust J Dermatol, 17: 92–93

Holzle E, Alberti N (1987) Long-term efficacy and side effects of tap water iontophoresis of palmoplantar hyperhidrosis—the usefulness of home therapy. Dermatologica, 175: 126–135

Holzle E, Ruzicka T (1986) Treatment of hyperhidrosis by a battery-operated iontophoresis device. Dermatologica, 172: 41–47

Ishihashi T (1936) Effects of drugs on the sweat glands by cataphoresis, and an effective method of suppression of local sweating: Observation on the effect of diaphoretics and adiaphoretics. J Orient Med, 25: 101–102

Japour CL, Vohra R, Vohra PK, Garfunkel L, Chin N (1999) Management of heel pain syndrome with acetic acid iontophoresis. J Am Podiatr Med Assoc, 89: 251–257

Kahn J (1975) Calcium iontophoresis in suspected myopathy. Phys Ther, 55: 376–377

Kahn J (1980) Iontophoresis and ultrasound for postsurgical temporomandibular trismus and parasthesia: Case report. Phys Ther, 60: 307–308

Kahn J (1982) Iontophoresis with hydrocortisone for Peyronie's disease. Phys Ther, 62: 975

Kalia YN, Guy RN (1995) The electrical characteristics of human skin in vivo. Pharm Res, 12: 1605–1613

Karakoç Y, Aydemir EH, Kalkan MT (2004) Placebo-controlled evaluation of direct electrical current administration for palmoplantar hyperhidrosis. Int J Dermatol, 43: 503–505

Karakoç Y, Aydemir EH, Kalkan MT, Unal G (2002) Safe control of palmoplantar hyperhidrosis with direct electrical current. Int J Dermatol, 41: 602–605

Langley PL (1984) Iontophoresis to aid in releasing tendon adhesions: Suggestions from the field. Phys Ther, 64: 1395

Leduc BE, Caya J, Tremblay S, Bureau NJ, Dumont M (2003) Treatment of calcifying tendonitis of the shoulder by acetic acid iontophoresis: A double-blind randomized controlled trial. Arch Phys Med Rehab, 84: 1523–1527

Leduc S (1900) Introduction of medicinal substances into depth of tissues by electrical current. Ann Electrobiol, 3: 545–560

Levit F (1968) Simple device for the treatment of hyperhidrosis by iontophoresis. Arch Dermatol, 98: 505–507

Levit F (1980) Treatment of hyperhidrosis by tap water iontophoresis. Cutis, 26: 192–194

Li LC, Scudds RA, Heck CS, Harth M (1996) The efficacy of dexamethasone iontophoresis for the treatment of rheumatoid arthritic knees: A pilot study. Arthritis Care Res, 9: 126–132

Magistro CM (1964) Hyaluronidase by iontophoresis in the treatment of edema: A preliminary clinical report. Phys Ther, 44: 169–175

Midtgaard K (1986) A new device for the treatment of hyperhidrosis by iontophoresis. Br J Dermatol, 114: 485–488

Mina R, Melson P, Owell S, Rao M, Hinze M, Hinze C, Passo M, Graham TB, Brunner HI (2011) Effectiveness of dexamethasone iontophoresis for temporomandibular joint involvement in juvenile idiopathic arthritis. Arthritis Care Res, 63: 1511–1516

Montorsi F, Salonia A, Guazzoni G, Barbieri L, Colombo R, Brausl M, Scattoni V, Rigatti P (2000) Transdermal electromotive multi-drug administration for Peyronie's disease: Preliminary results. J Androl, 21: 85–90

Neeter C, Thomee R, Sillbernagel KG, Thomee P, Karlsson J (2003) Iontophoresis with and without dexamethasone in the treatment of acute Achilles tendon pain. Scand J Med Sci Sports, 13: 376–382

Nirsch RP, Rodin DM, Ochiai DH, Maartmann-Moe C (2003) Iontophoretic administration of dexamethasone sodium phosphate for acute epicondylitis. Am J Sports Med, 31: 189–195

Odia S, Vocks E, Radoski J, Ring J (1996) Successful treatment of dyshidrotic hand eczema using tap water iontophoresis with pulsed direct current. Acta Derm Venereol, 76: 472–474

Ozawa A, Haruki Y, Iwashita K, Sasao Y, Miyahara M, Sugai J, Matsuyama T, Iizuka M, Kawakubo Y, Nakamori M, Ohkido M (1999) Follow-up of clinical efficacy of iontophoresis therapy for postherpetic neuralgia (PHN). J Dermatol, 26: 1–10

Panus PC, Hooper T, Padrones A, Palmer B, Williams D (1996) A case study of exacerbation of lateral epicondylitis by combined use of iontophoresis and phonophoresis. Physiother Can, 48: 27–31

Pellecchia GL, Hamel H, Behnke P (1994) Treatment of infrapatellar tendinitis: A combination of modalities and transverse friction massage versus iontophoresis. J Sports Rehab, 3: 135–145

Perron M, Malouin F (1997) Acetic acid and iontophoresis and ultrasound for the treatment of calcifying tendinitis of the shoulder: A randomized controlled trial. Arch Phys Med Rehab, 78: 379–384

Psaki C, Carol L (1955) Acetic acid ionization: A study to determine the absorptive effects upon calcified tendinitis of the shoulder. Phys Ther, 35: 84–87

Reid KI, Dionne RA, Sicard-Rosenbaum L, Lord D, Dubner RA (1994) Evaluation of iontophoretically applied dexamethasone for painful pathologic temporomandibular joints. Oral Surg Med Pathol, 77: 605–609

Reidl CR, Plas E, Engelhardt P, Daha K, Pfluger H (2000) Iontophoresis for treatment of Peyronie's disease. J Urol, 163: 95–99

Rothfeld SH, Murray W (1967) Treatment of Peyronie's disease by iontophoresis of C21 esterified glucocorticosteroids. J Urol, 97: 874–875

Runeson L, Jaker E (2002) Iontophoresis with cortisone in the treatment of lateral epicondylalgia (tennis elbow)—a double-blind study. Scand J Sci Sports, 12: 136–142

Schiffman EL, Braun BL, Lindgren BR (1996) Temporomandibular joint iontophoresis: A double-blind randomized clinical trial. J Orofac Pain, 10: 157–165

Schwartz MS (1955) The use of hyaluronidase by iontophoresis in the treatment of lymphedema. Arch Intern Med, 95: 662

Shrivastava SN, Sing G (1977) Tap water iontophoresis in palmo-plantar hyperhidrosis. Br J Dermatol, 96: 189–195

Sokoro YT, Repking MC, Clemment JA, Mitchell PL, Berg RL (2002) Treatment of plantar verrucae using 2% sodium salicylate iontophoresis. Phys Ther, 82: 1184–1191

Stolman LP (1987) Treatment of excess sweating of the palms by iontophoresis. Arch Dermatol, 123: 893–896

Tannenbaum M (1980) Iodine iontophoresis in reduction of scar tissue. Phys Ther, 60: 792

Weinstein MV, Gordon A (1958) The use of magnesium sulfate iontophoresis in the treatment of subdeltoid bursitis. Phys Ther, 38: 96–98

Wieder DL (1992) Treatment of traumatic myositis ossificans with acetic acid iontophoresis. Phys Ther, 72: 133–137

Yarrobino TE, Kalbfleisch JH, Ferslew KE, Panus PC (2006) Lidocaine iontophoresis mediates analgesia in lateral epicondylalgia treatment. Phys Res Int, 11: 152–160

Review Articles

Brown M, Marting G, Jones SA, Akomeah FK (2006) Dermal and transdermal drug delivery systems: Current and future prospects. Drug Deliv, 13: 175–187

Chien YW, Banga K (1989) Iontophoretic (transdermal) delivery of drugs: Overview of historical development. J Pharm Sci, 78: 353–354

Dixit N, Bai V, Baboota S, Ahuja A, Ali J (2007) Iontophoresis—an approach for controlled drug delivery: A review. Curr Drug Deliv, 4: 1–10

Eisenach JH, Atkinson JLD, Fealey RD (2005) Hyperhidrosis: Evolving therapies for a well-established phenomenon. Mayo Clin Proc, 80: 657–666

Fischer GA (2005) Iontophoretic drug delivery using IOMED Phoresor system. Expert Opin Drug Deliv, 2: 391–403

Gangarosa LP, Ozawa A, Ohkido M, Shimomura Y, Hill JM (1995) Iontophoresis for enhancing penetration of dermatologic and antiviral drugs. J Dermatol, 11: 865–875

Grond S, Radbrush L, Lehmann KA (2000) Clinical pharmacokinetics of transdermal opioids: Focus on transdermal fentanyl. Clin Pharmacokinet, 38: 59–89

Gurney AB, Washer DC (2008) Absorption of dexamethasone sodium phosphate in human connective tissue using iontophoresis. Am J Sports Med, 36: 753–759

Hamann H, Hodges M, Evans B (2006) Effectiveness of iontophoresis of anti-inflammatory medications in the treatment of common musculoskeletal inflammatory conditions: A systematic review. Phys Ther Rev, 11: 190–194

Hashmonai M, Kopelman D, Assalia A (2000) The treatment of primary palmar hiperhidrosis: A review. Surg Today, 30: 211–218

Henley EJ (1991) Transcutaneous drug delivery: Iontophoresis, phonophoresis. Crit Rev Phys Rehab Med, 2: 139–151

Nair V, Pillai O, Poduri R, Panchagnula R (1999) Transermal iontophoresis. Part I: Basic principles and considerations. Methods Find Exp Clin Pharmacol, 21: 139–151

Semalty A, Semalty M, Singh R, Saraf SK, Saraf S (2007) Iontophoretic drug delivery system: A review. Technol Health Care, 15: 237–245

Sieg A, Wascotte V (2009) Diagnostic and therapeutic applications of iontophoresis. J Drug Target, 17: 690–700

Solish N, Bertucci V, Dansereau A, Hong HC, Lynde C, Lupin M, Smith KC, Storwick G, Canadian Hyperhidrosis Advisory Committee (2007) A comprehensive approach to the recognition, diagnosis, and severity-based treatment of focal hyperhidrosis: Recommendations of the Canadian Hyperhidrosis Advisory Committee. Dermatol Surg, 33: 908–923

Ting WW, Vest CD, Sontheimer RD (2004) Review of traditional and novel modalities of local therapeutics across the stratum corneum. Int J Dermatol, 43: 538–547

Togel B, Greve B, Raulin C (2002) Current therapeutic strategies for hyperhidrosis: A review. Eur J Dermatol, 12: 219–223

Walling HW, Swick BL (2011) Treatment options for hyperhidrosis. Am J Clin Dermatol, 12: 285–295

Chapters of Textbooks

Ciccone CD (2008) Electrical stimulation for the delivery of medication: Iontophoresis. In: Clinical Electrophysiology, 3rd ed. Robinson AJ, Snyder-Mackler L (Eds). Lippincott Williams & Wilkins, Philadelphia, 2007, pp 351–381

Cummings J (1991) Iontophoresis. In: Clinical Electrotherapy, 2nd ed. Nelson RM, Currier DP (Eds). Appleton & Lange, Norwalk, pp 317–327

Licht S (1983) History of electrotherapy. In: Therapeutic Electricity and Ultraviolet Radiation, 3rd ed. Stillwell GK (Ed). Williams & Wilkins, Baltimore, pp 1–64

Prentice WE (2002) Iontophoresis. In: Therapeutic Modalities for Physical Therapists. McGraw–Hill, New York, pp 133–149

Monograph

American Physical Therapy Association (2001) Electrotherapeutic Terminology in Physical Therapy. APTA Publications, Alexandria

Textbook

Leduc S (1908) Electric Ions and Their Use in Medicine. Rebman, Ltd, Liverpool

Internet Resources

www.sweathelp.org: International Hyperhidrosis Society (IHHS)

http://thePoint.lww.com: Online Dosage Calculator: Iontophoresis

PART V

Mechanical Agents

Chapter 17

Spinal Traction

Chapter Outline

Learning Objectives

Remembering: List and describe the various techniques use to deliver spinal traction therapy.
Understanding: Compare the static, intermittent, and intermittent with progression/regression traction modes.
Applying: Demonstrate the applications of cervical and lumbar traction.
Analyzing: Explain the proposed physiologic and therapeutic effects associated with spinal traction therapy.
Evaluating: Formulate the strength of scientific evidence and therapeutic effectiveness related to the practice of spinal traction therapy.
Creating: Defend the use of spinal traction therapy.

I. FOUNDATION

A. DEFINITION

Spinal traction is defined as the use of traction forces applied to the cervical and lumbar spine via various mechanical systems. It is described as the application of traction techniques by using tables, pulleys, cables, and weights for the treatment of cervical and back pain disorders.

B. SPINAL TRACTION TECHNIQUES

Spinal traction is applied by using various traction techniques, which are classified and described in Table 17-1. The body of literature presented in this chapter indicates

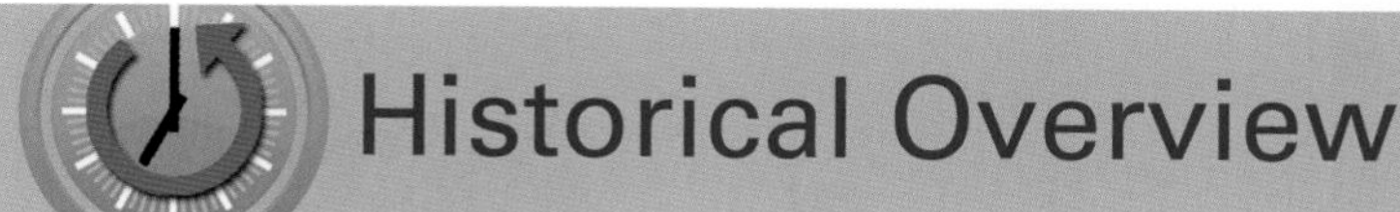

The use of traction force to treat spinal disorders dates back to the time of Hippocrates (400s BC). Application of traction beds and corsets began in the 19th century (Gay et al., 2008). The modern application of traction force for cervical and lumbar disorders began in the 1950s with James Cyriax. Mechanical traction therapy gained further support in the 1960s based on the first studies on humans, which were conducted by Judovich and colleagues (1954, 1955, 1957) and Colachis and Strohm (1965a,b, 1966, 1969). These studies showed that human vertebral separation can be achieved by exerting a mechanical traction force on the vertebral column.

that motorized, pneumatic, weighted, and manual traction are the most common techniques used today by clinicians to treat cervical and lumbar disorders. Less commonly used are the autotractive (self-tractive), positional, and inverted techniques.

C. SCOPE OF CHAPTER

This chapter focuses on the use of motorized, pneumatic, and weighted traction techniques. Manual traction is beyond the scope of this chapter because it falls within the broad field of manual therapy (i.e., mobilization and manipulation techniques), about which several textbooks are written (e.g., see Lederman, 2008; Olson, 2008; Cook, 2010; King et al., 2010). Autotraction and positional traction techniques are also beyond the scope of this chapter because their application is marginal and techniques of application not standardized. Inverted traction is *not recommended* because it may present severe potential adverse effects (see Table 17-1).

TABLE 17-1 SPINAL TRACTION TECHNIQUES

Classification	Description
Motorized	• *Motorized pulley and rope table:* Traction force applied by a pulley and rope assembly, which is driven by an electrical motor. The rope is attached to the pulley at one end and to body harnesses or halters at the other end. • *Motorized split table with cervical assembly:* Traction force applied by built-in electrical motors. For lumbar traction, motorization allows the lumbar section of the split table to move in flexion/extension, rotation, and lateral flexion. For cervical traction, motorization of the cervical assembly causes traction (see Fig. 17-2). • *Motorized computerized table:* Traction force applied by a pulley and rope assembly, which is driven by a computerized programmable electrical motor. The rope is attached to the pulley at one end and to body harnesses or halters at the other end.
Pneumatic	Traction force applied by a manual pump, which inflates a built-in air chamber that causes the mobile section of the device to slide in relation to the fixed section. Traction force is read from the gauge mounted on the pump. Pumping increases traction force, and releasing the blow-off valve decreases it.
Weighted	Traction is applied by a dead weight suspended through a pulley and rope assembly. One end of the rope is attached to the dead weight and the other end to the halter (see Fig. 17-5).
Autotractive	Traction force applied by the patient's own body weight or by pushing and pulling actions. Autotraction implies gravitational lower body suspension using upper limbs.
Positional	Traction force applied by the patient's own body segment weights. The patient adopts and maintains a body position for passively stretching the lumbar or cervical spine.
Inverted	Traction force is applied by suspending the patient's body weight by the ankles, in the *head-down position,* using a purpose-built reclining table. This technique is not recommended because it may cause major side effects such as increased diastolic and systolic blood pressure (Haskvitz et al., 1986), as well as increased ophthalmic pressure (Zito, 1988).
Manual	Traction force is applied manually by the practitioner. Manual traction is part of the whole field of manual therapy, which includes spinal mobilization and manipulation techniques.

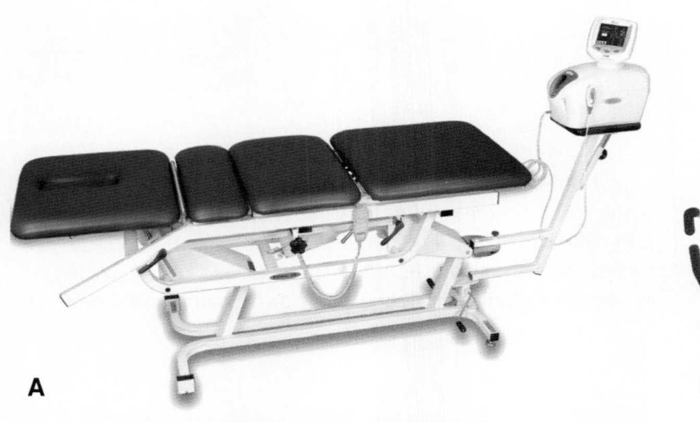

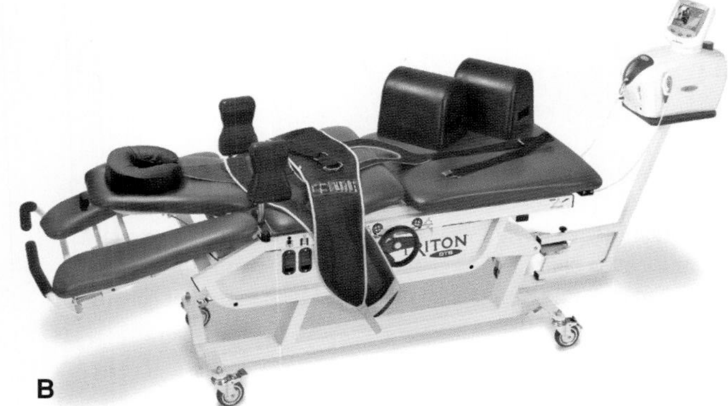

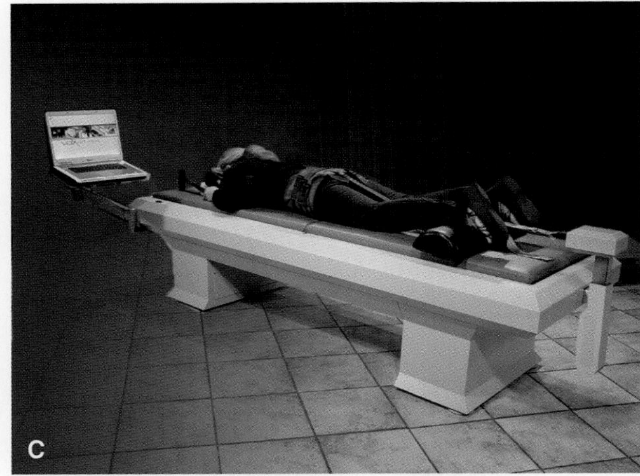

FIGURE 17-1 Typical motorized pulley and cable-type traction tables (**A, B**) and motorized computerized spinal decompression table (**C**). (A, B: Courtesy of DJO Global; C: Courtesy of VAX-D Medical Technologies.)

D. SPINAL TRACTION DEVICES

1. Motorized Tables

Figure 17-1 illustrates typical motorized spinal tables used to treat both the lumbar and cervical spines. Traction force is generated by a programmable electric motor mounted on the traction table. This motor drives a pulley to which is attached a rope or cord (see Fig. 17-1A,B). For lumbar traction, the motorized pulley pulls on the rope attached to adjustable lumbar harnesses, shown in Figure 17-2, thus creating a traction force on the lumbar spine. A thoracic harness holds the thoracic segment of the spine in place during traction. Lumbar and thoracic harnesses may have different shapes and attachments. For cervical traction, a portable traction device (see Fig. 17-2B), made of side wedges or pads with a restraining head strap, is mounted to the traction table. With the rope attached to the cervical traction device, the electrical motor pulls on the sliding section of the device, thus creating traction force at the base of the occiput. Newer, more sophisticated, and more expensive motorized computerized spinal decompression tables are also available to treat spinal disorders (see Fig. 17-1C). These devices, although marketed as being *decompression-type* devices, are in fact akin to the traditional spinal *traction-type* devices presented earlier. The patient is fitted with pelvic harness and lies supine, or prone, on the traction table. The upper body is positioned on the stationary section of the table and is restrained by the patient holding on to adjustable handgrips, or by the use of passive armrest restraints. Motorized traction force, applied via a cable attached to the patient's harnesses, is delivered in a smooth, computerized, controlled fashion on the patient's spine.

2. Motorized Split Table With Cervical Assembly

Motorized split traction tables, mounted with removable cervical assembly, also are used to treat both lumbar and cervical spine disorders. This traction table uses no pulley and cable. *Cervical traction* is applied, with the use of a cervical assembly made of two adjusting neck wedges and a head strap. The patient lies supine with the neck wedges cradling the occiput. The head strap is secured to hold the patient's head and neck in proper position. The motorized cervical traction force is contained within the table. *Lumbar traction* is applied by the motorized separation of the split table, which provides easy adjustments in flexion/extension, rotation, and lateral flexion for treatment in various positions. The patient lies supine or prone with the thoracic harness attached to the fixed section of the table, and the lumbar harness is attached to the movable section of the table. Traction is applied as the lumbar section of the table moves.

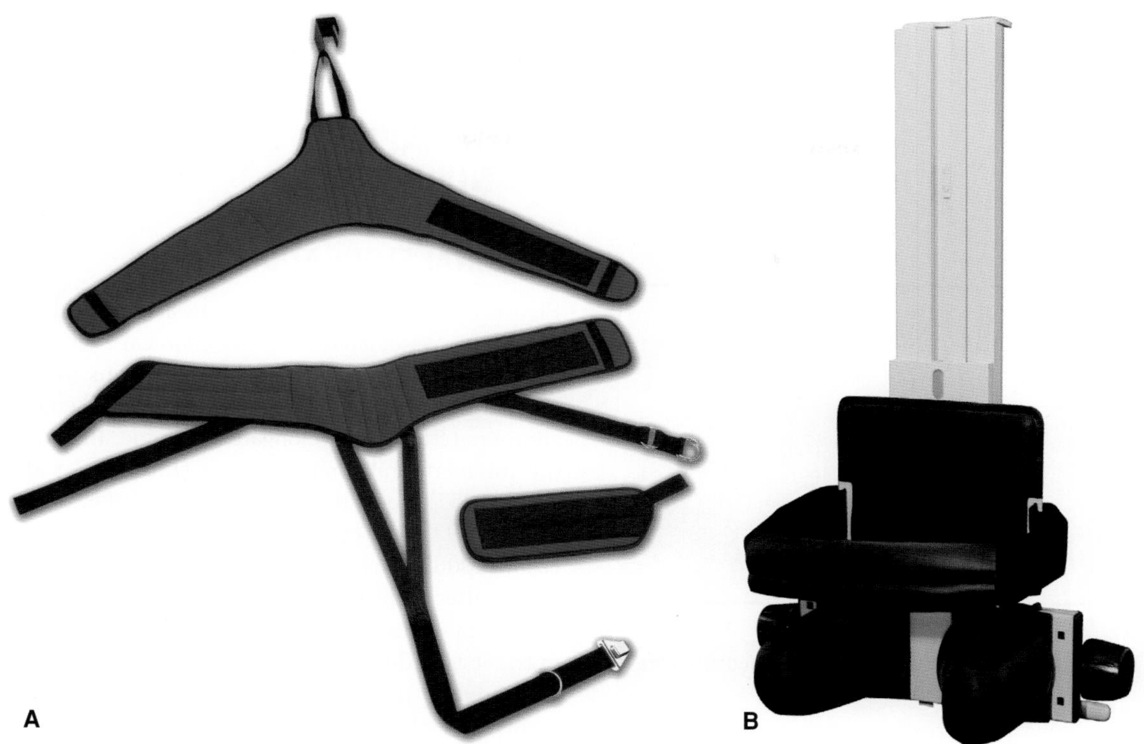

FIGURE 17-2 Adjustable thoracic and lumbar traction harnesses (**A**) and removable cervical traction unit (**B**) (used with motorized pulley and cable-type traction table A, B: Courtesy of DJO Global.)

3. Weighted Device

The device is composed of a portable mechanical pulley system mounted on a door. A rope is attached at one end to a cervical occipito-mandibular halter and at the other end to a plastic bag filled with water, which serves as a dead weight. The suspended dead weight creates traction force on the cervical spine. The use of this device is on the decline because of the unnecessary pressure exerted on the temporomandibular joint (TMJ) during therapy.

4. Pneumatic Devices

Common portable pneumatic cervical and lumbar traction devices are used mainly for home therapy. Traction force is generated by manually inflating a built-in air chamber, which causes it to expand and thus creates a traction force on the movable section of the device.

E. RATIONALE FOR USE

Neck and back disorders are common, disabling to various degrees, and costly to treat. A wide variety of therapeutic interventions are used today to treat these disorders, often resulting from disk herniation, degenerative disk diseases, and nerve root compression. Among all conservative treatments available, mechanical spinal traction plays an important role by providing passive spinal elongation, the key purpose of which is to increase intervertebral spaces. In short, vertebral distraction, or decompression, is presumed to increase the foraminal area, which in turn decreases peripheral nerve and nucleus pulposus pressure, thus reducing pain and disability.

II. BIOPHYSICAL CHARACTERISTICS

A. MECHANICAL PRINCIPLE

The biophysical principle behind spinal traction, regardless of the techniques (see earlier discussion) and modes (see later discussion) used to deliver it, lies in the application of *mechanical energy,* the aim of which is to exert a traction force on the vertebral column that will result in the separation of cervical, or lumbar, vertebrae. Mechanical energy is defined as the combination of *potential* and *kinetic* energy. Potential energy results from the force of gravity, of which force underlies the application of weighted, auto, positional, and inverted traction techniques. Kinetic energy is mechanical energy due to movement. It underlies the application of motorized and pneumatic traction, as well as manual traction.

B. TRACTION FORCE

Force is defined as the capacity to do work or to cause physical change. Spinal traction forces are commonly expressed in units of kilograms (kg) or pounds (lb), where 1 kg equals 2.2 lb. Traction force is also expressed as a percentage of the patient's body weight (% BW). For example, a traction force of 20 kg (44 lb) applied

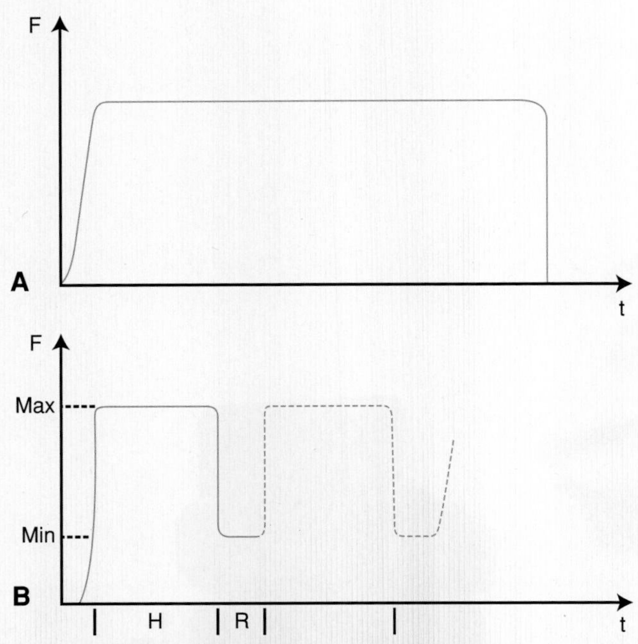

FIGURE 17-3 Static (**A**) and intermittent (**B**) spinal traction modes.

on a patient weighing 100 kg (220 lb) is equivalent to a traction force of 20% BW. For pneumatic traction devices, the applied pressure is automatically converted into units of force on the device's reading gauge (see the Dosimetry section).

C. TRACTION MODES

Spinal traction is applied, as illustrated in Figure 17-3, by using two modes: static and intermittent. Let us consider each of them.

1. Static Mode

This mode denotes the steady, sustained, or continuous application of a fixed traction force for the entire treatment duration (Fig. 17-3A). An example would be the application of a traction force of 10 kg (22 lb) for a period of 20 minutes.

2. Intermittent Mode

This mode refers to the interrupted, alternating, or cycling application of a fixed maximal (MAX) and minimal (MIN) traction force delivered through a preset *cycle* of maximum force application (hold time [H]) and minimal force application period (relax time [R]), of which the cycle (H:R) is repeated for a number of times over the entire treatment duration (Fig. 17-3B). Here is an example of intermittent traction: MAX:MIN—40 kg (88 lb):10 kg (22 lb); H:R (45s:15s). In this case, maximal force is applied for 45 seconds followed by minimal force applied for 15 seconds, for a total cycle duration of 60 seconds. Note that during intermittent traction, the traction force never returns to zero baseline. A minimum traction force is maintained during the relaxation phase, thus always providing a tractive action on the spine during the entire treatment period (Fig. 17-3B).

III. THERAPEUTIC EFFECTS AND INDICATIONS

A. SPINAL ELONGATION

Figure 17-4 lists the proposed physiologic and therapeutic effects associated with mechanical spinal traction. There is undisputable evidence in humans to show that mechanical traction applied on the vertebral column with appropriate force can elongate the spine, thus increasing the intervertebral foraminal area (Judovich et al., 1954, 1955, 1957; Colachis et al., 1965a,b, 1966, 1969; Wong et al., 1992; Sari et al., 2005; Vaughn et al., 2006; Liu et al., 2008). It is postulated that this mechanical elongating effect will increase intervertebral space, decrease intradiscal pressure, increase diffusion of fluids and nutrient into disks, retract bulging disk material, release pressure on nerve roots, stretch intervertebral ligaments, stretch paravertebral muscles, and increase blood flow. Mechanically elongating the spine is presumed to decrease muscle spasm, decrease pain, and improve blood flow in the affected vertebral area. Together, these effects are assumed to enhance spinal mobility and function. To better identify which type of patients are most likely to benefit from cervical and lumbar traction, clinical prediction rules have recently been developed and tested (Raney et al., 2009; Cai et al., 2011). The results suggest that patients older than 55 years who show positive cervical distraction tests, nerve tension tests, shoulder abduction tests, and peripheralization of symptoms are most likely to benefit from cervical traction therapy (Raney et al., 2009). Data also suggest that patients older than 30 years who present with no neurologic deficit are more likely to benefit from lumbar traction (Cai et al., 2011). These rules should serve as guidelines, because further studies are needed to validate them. Overall, spinal traction is considered as one treatment alternative to surgical treatment for herniated disks.

B. RESEARCH-BASED INDICATIONS

The search for evidence behind the use of spinal traction, displayed in the *Research-Based Indications* box, led to the collection of 72 English peer-reviewed human clinical studies. The methodologies and criteria used to assess the strength of evidence and therapeutic effectiveness are described in Chapter 2. As indicated, the strength of evidence behind spinal traction is ranked as *moderate* for both the lumbar and cervical spine. There are a good number of studies showing no beneficial effect following lumbar traction. Over all conditions treated with spinal traction, the strength of evidence is found to be *moderate* and its therapeutic effectiveness *substantiated*.

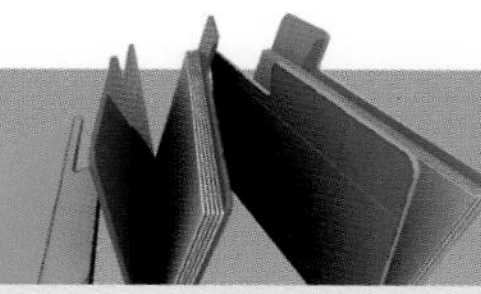

Research-Based Indications

SPINAL TRACTION

Health Condition	Benefit—Yes Rating	Benefit—Yes Reference	Benefit—No Rating	Benefit—No Reference
Back disorders	II	Larsson et al., 1980	I	Mathews et al., 1975
	II	Beattie et al., 2008	I	Schimmel et al., 2009
	II	Macario et al., 2008	II	Coxhead et al., 1981
	II	Lidstrom et al., 1970	II	Borman et al., 2003
	II	Sherry et al., 2001	II	Beurskens et al., 1995
	II	Tesio et al., 1993	II	Beurskens et al., 1997
	II	Letchuman et al., 1993	II	Pal et al., 1986
	II	Oudenhoven, 1978	II	Werners et al., 1999
	II	Harrison et al., 2002a	II	Sweetman et al., 1993
	II	Gionis et al., 2003	II	Van der Heijden et al., 1995
	II	Gose et al., 1998	II	Weber, 1973
	II	Naguszewski et al., 2001	II	Weber et al., 1984
	II	Onel et al., 1989	II	Ljunggren et al., 1992
	II	Tesio et al., 1989	II	Mathews et al., 1987
	II	Guevenol et al., 2000		
	II	Ljunggren et al., 1984		
	II	Moret et al., 1998		
	II	Unlu et al., 2008		
	II	Shealy et al., 1997		
	II	Ramos et al., 2004		
	II	Apfel et al., 2010		
	II	Fritz et al., 2007		
	II	Ozturk et al., 2006		
	II	Macario et al., 2008		
	II	Sari et al., 2005		
	II	Cleland et al., 2005		
	III	Hood et al., 1968		
	III	Gupta et al., 1978		
	III	Corkery, 2001		
	III	Meszaros et al., 2000		

Strength of evidence: Moderate
Therapeutic effectiveness: Substantiated

Health Condition	Benefit—Yes Rating	Benefit—Yes Reference	Benefit—No Rating	Benefit—No Reference
Neck disorders	I	Harrison et al., 2002b	I	Goldie et al., 1970
	II	Lee et al., 1996	I	Klaber-Moffett et al., 1990
	II	Swezey et al., 1999	I	Brewerton et al., 1966
	II	Valtonen et al., 1970	I	Chiu et al., 2011
	II	Hattori et al., 2002	II	Wong et al., 1997
	II	Zylbergold et al., 1985	II	Pennie et al., 1990
	II	Cai et al., 2011	II	Loy, 1983
	II	Mysliwiec et al., 2011	II	Young et al., 2009
	II	Joghataei et al., 2004	III	Jette et al., 1985
	II	Shakoor et al., 2002		
	II	Saal et al., 1996		
	III	Walker, 1986		
	III	Chung et al., 2002		
	III	Constantoyannis et al., 2002		
	III	Browder et al., 2004		
	III	Olson, 1997		
	III	Moeti et al., 2001		
	III	Waldrop, 2006		
	III	Baker et al., 1992		

Strength of evidence: Moderate
Therapeutic effectiveness: Substantiated

ALL CONDITIONS
Strength of evidence: Moderate
Therapeutic effectiveness: Substantiated

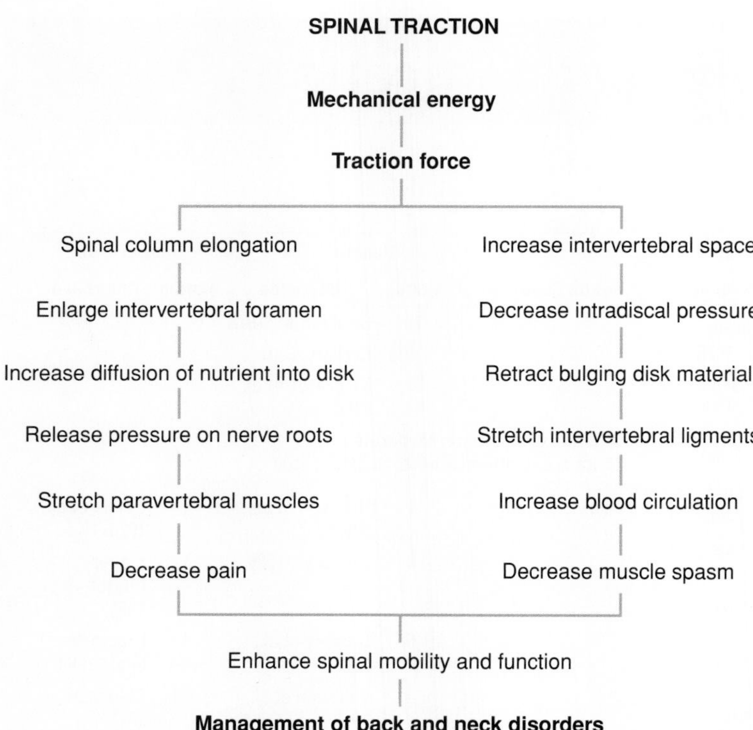

FIGURE 17-4 Proposed physiologic and therapeutic effects of spinal traction.

Note that the percentages of studies showing benefit are relatively low at 67% and 68% for the back and neck disorders, respectively.

IV. DOSIMETRY

Table 17-2 presents recommended dosimetric parameters associated with the application of spinal traction therapy. The guiding principle is that traction force exerted on the spine should be large enough to overcome the resistive forces (weight, friction, and gravity) acting on the displaced spinal segments.

A. TRACTION TECHNIQUE

Selecting one traction technique is often based on the acuity and severity of the spinal condition as well as on

TABLE 17-2 RECOMMENDED DOSIMETRIC PARAMETERS FOR SPINAL TRACTION THERAPY

Parameters	Cervical/Lumbar
Traction technique	Selection is based on the acuity and severity of the spinal condition, as well as on the patient's preference. Select the technique that best induces cervical/lumbar *muscle relaxation* prior and during therapy.
Traction force*	Apply *maximum tolerable but pain-free* traction force, which should be large enough to cause spinal elongation. Traction force may be expressed in kilograms (kg), pounds (lb), or as a percentage of body weight (% BW): • *Cervical force range:* 20% to 30% BW • *Lumbar force range:* 30% to 60% BW
Angle of pull	Range between 0 and 30 degrees
Traction mode	*Static:* Maximal (MAX) traction force applied over the entire treatment duration *Intermittent:* Maximal:Minimal (MAX: MIN) traction force applied during Hold:Relax (H:R) cycles *H:R cycle:* H time: 5–60 s; R time: 5–60 s
Application duration	10–30 min
Treatment frequency	Daily to every other day

*Maximal traction force exerted by clinical-based cervical devices is 22.7 kg (50 lb). Maximal traction force exerted by clinical-based lumbar devices is 181.8 kg (400 lb). Home-based cervical and lumbar traction devices exert approximately 50% of clinical-based maximal force.

the patient's preference. The technique that best induces muscle relaxation prior and during treatment should be used. For example, clinicians are likely to use cervical motorized or pneumatic cervical traction over weighted traction because the latter has the advantage of placing the traction force on the skull's occipital bone rather than on the TMJ, thus greatly improving comfort during therapy. Moreover, cervical traction with the patient in the supine position (motorized and pneumatic techniques) has the advantage of reducing the resistive force offered because it reduces the gravitational force acting on the head while promoting muscle relaxation. This position, in contrast to the seated position, implies that a lower, more comfortable traction force can be used for treatment. There is no evidence to show that one technique, device, or mode is more effective than any other for managing cervical and lumbar disorders. The trial and error method is, unfortunately, inevitable in order to come up with optimal dosimetry.

B. TRACTION FORCE

Optimal traction therapy requires the application of maximal tolerable but pain-free force levels. Too large of a force may cause pain exacerbation, whereas too low of a force may be therapeutically ineffective. As stated earlier, traction force may be expressed in kilograms (kg), pounds (lb), or as a percentage of body weight (% BW). For example, the application of a lumbar traction force of 40 kg (88 lb) on an 80-kg (176 lb) patient is equivalent to using a 50% BW traction force. Conversely, using a 30% BW traction force on the same patient is equivalent to using a traction force of 24 kg (53 lb). Selecting the most appropriate traction force is related to the acuity of the spinal condition as well as to the magnitude of the resistive forces exerted by the body segment during traction. Anthropometric research has shown that the human head accounts for approximately 8.3% of the total BW, meaning that the head of a 90-kg (198 lb) man weighs approximately 7.5 kg (16.5 lb). It has also established that the human pelvis/lower limb segment accounts for approximately 30% of the total body weight, meaning a weight of approximately 27 kg (60 lb) for a man weighing 90 kg (198 lb). Theoretically speaking, it follows from these anthropometric findings that it is *unlikely,* if not *impossible,* for a cervical traction force of less than 8.3% BW to elongate the human cervical spine. So is the case for a lumbar traction force smaller than 30% BW. This is because in order to elongate the spine, or distract the vertebrae, the traction force must first overcome the body segment weight under traction. To express and report dosimetric traction forces in units of kilograms or pounds only is acceptable as long as the patient's body weight is also reported. This is because a traction force of 20 kg (44 lb), for example, will have a much smaller spinal elongating effect on a man weighing 60 kg (132 lb) versus one weighing 130 kg (287 lb). *Consequently, this textbook strongly recommends to express and report traction force in units of percentage of body weight.* As discussed earlier and demonstrated in the literature, traction forces—in order to be effective in elongating the spine in the supine position—should be in the range of 10% to 30% BW for the cervical spine and of 30% to 60% BW for the lumbar spine (see Wong et al., 1992; Joghataei et al., 2004; Cleland et al., 2005; Sari et al., 2005; Vaughn et al., 2006). A study by Liu et al. (2008), using a weighted cervical traction unit on healthy adult volunteers, showed through the use of magnetic resonance that cervical traction forces equivalent to 7%, 13%, and 20% BW caused average increases of 3.7%, 8.7%, and 10% in intervertebral foraminal height, respectively. In other words, this study confirms the general principle that the larger the applied traction force on the spine, the more significant the spinal elongation and physiologic changes. Traction force adjustments or fluctuation during the whole course of treatment will be guided by the patient's response and by the evolution of the spinal disorder during treatment. Contrary to what is written in some electrophysical agent (EPA) textbooks, there is *no scientific evidence* to show that a specific dosimetric traction force range is more efficient than another for the management of pain, muscle spasm, and any other symptoms related to spinal disorders.

C. TRACTION FORCE ANGLE OF PULL

The traction force angle of pull is the angle with which the traction is applied in relation to the long axis of the spine. Angle of pull may range between 0 and 30 degrees (see Table 17-2). An angle of pull of 0 degrees means that traction force pulls the cervical or lumbar segment *in line* with the long axis of the vertebral column (neutral or axial traction). Conversely, an angle of pull greater than 0 degrees means that the cervical or lumbar segment is pulled offline, or *off axial,* with a certain degree of flexion or lateral flexion. There is evidence to show that when using motorized traction for the cervical spine in a supine position in healthy people, the neutral position (0 degrees) yields greater percentages of posterior/anterior intervertebral separation and facet joint separation when compared with angles of pull ranging between 15 and 30 degrees of flexion (Wong et al., 1992; Vaughn et al., 2006).

D. TRACTION MODE

Practitioners may choose between the static and intermittent mode (see Fig. 17-3). There is no evidence to show than one mode is better than the other. Once again, selection should be based on the patient's preference—that is, tolerance and maximal muscle relaxation during therapy. For intermittent traction, the hold (H-MAX traction) and relax (R-MIN traction) time cycle may range between 5 and 90 seconds. For example an H:R cycle of 45s:15s means that maximal traction force is applied for 45 seconds and followed immediately by the application of a minimal force during the relax time, which lasts 15 seconds. The intermittent H:R cycle duration is 60 seconds.

E. APPLICATION DURATION AND TREATMENT FREQUENCY

Application duration may range between 10 and 30 minutes depending of the patient's condition and traction mode used. Treatment frequency may range between daily and every other day depending of the patient's tolerance to treatment and therapeutic progress.

V. APPLICATION, CONTRAINDICATIONS, AND RISKS

Prior to considering the application of spinal traction, practitioners must first check for contraindications, consider the risks, and then go through key application steps and procedures designed to optimize treatment safety, efficacy, and effectiveness. Important elements of this protocol involve the determination of the patient's body weight as well as the application of the harnesses, which should be placed directly over bare skin to avoid slippage (i.e., loss of traction force) during traction. Another important element is to conduct thorough historical, physical, and, if necessary, radiologic examinations prior to considering if this EPA is mandatory. Moreover, the risk of exacerbating pain is always present.

APPLICATIONS, CONTRAINDICATIONS, AND RISKS

Spinal Traction

IMPORTANT: Prior to considering spinal traction therapy, conduct a thorough historical and physical examination of the spine and, if necessary, request radiologic imagery reports in order to *eliminate the contraindications* to spinal traction therapy. To achieve the patient's maximal muscle relaxation prior and during treatment is capital for optimal therapeutic effectiveness. When possible, apply lumbar traction harnesses against the patient's bare skin, or against thin and tight clothing, in order to minimize slipping during therapy. Illustrated, as examples, are the applications of motorized pulley and cable traction (Figs. 17-5 and 17-6A), motorized computerized traction (Fig. 17-6B) and weighted traction (Fig. 17-7).

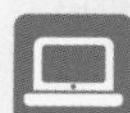

See **online videos.**

ALL AGENTS

STEP	RATIONALE
1. Check for contraindications.	*Spinal disease, infection, inflammation, and tumor*—induces further damage
	Vertebral fracture or dislocation—damages the spinal cord due to increased joint mobility
	Spinal instability or hypermobility—damages the spinal cord due to increased joint mobility
	Severe disk herniation—enhances herniation
	Vertebral arterial dysfunction—creates vascular damage
	Spinal cord stenosis—enhances compression of the spinal cord
	Osteoporosis—vertebral fracture
	Arthritis and rheumatoid arthritis—enhances degeneration
	Aortic aneurysm—hemorrhage
	Abdominal hernia—enhances the condition
	Uncontrolled hypertension—enhances the condition
	Pregnancy (lumbar traction only)—complications

STEP	RATIONALE
2. Consider the risks.	*Pain exacerbation*—traction force may cause sudden and unexpected exacerbation of cervical or lumbar pain (Laban et al., 1992, 2005). If present, stop treatment and reassess the need for traction therapy. *In patients with history of spinal surgery*—may lead to complications *In patients suffering from spondylolysis and spondylolisthesis*—traction may lead to spinal hypermobility. Careful monitoring of the condition throughout treatment is necessary. *In patients with respiratory and hypertensive disorders*—may enhance the conditions. These patients should be observed for signs of distress during initial application (Quain et al., 1985; Balogun et al., 1990; Podein et al., 1998). *In patients with dentures*—may cause undue pressure on the dentures if an occipito-mandibular halter is used. Use only an occipital halter. *In patients with temporomandibular dysfunction*—may aggravate the condition if an occipito-mandibular halter is used. Use only an occipital halter.

LUMBAR TRACTION

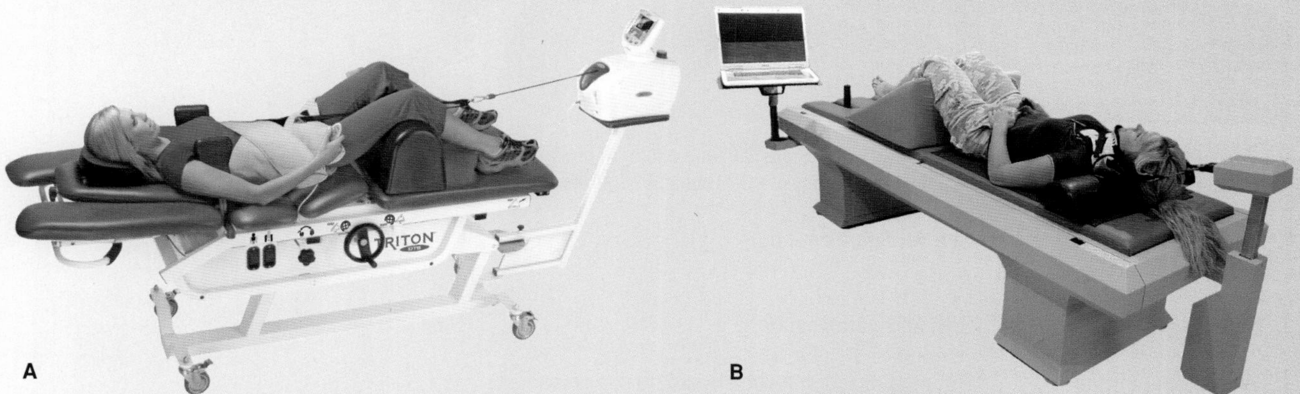

FIGURE 17-5 Application of motorized pulley and cable (**A**) and motorized computerized (**B**) spinal traction tables for lumbar spine. (A: Courtesy of DJO Global; B: Courtesy of VAX-D Medical Technologies.)

STEP	RATIONALE
1. Check for contraindications.	See All Agents section.
2. Consider the risks.	See All Agents section.
3. Weigh the patient.	Because traction force should be expressed as a percentage of body weight (% BW; see later discussion), measure the patient's weight.
4. Position and instruct patient.	Select body position that allows maximum muscle relaxation, thus promoting optimal elongation or vertebral separation. Instruct patient to empty the bladder before treatment because traction force exerted by pelvic belts may trigger urgency for micturition on a relatively full bladder. Also instruct patient to refrain from coughing or sneezing during therapy because increased intra-abdominal pressure may increase intradiscal pressure.
5. Secure patient to traction table.	Fit the thoracic and lumbar harnesses. Secure the thoracic harness to the table. Tighten any slack in the harnesses. Pull the end of the traction rope or cord out from the traction unit. Clip the rope to the lumbar harness. Plug line-powered devices into ground-fault circuit interrupter (GFCI) receptacles to prevent macroshock (see Chapter 5).
6. Set dosimetry.	Use the recommended parameters presented in Table 17-2 as a guideline. Note that lumbar traction force should range between 30% and 60% BW for effective spinal elongation. Apply axial or off-axial traction.

STEP	RATIONALE
7. **Apply treatment.**	Ensure adequate monitoring during treatment. Make sure that the safety switch is in the patient's hands throughout the duration of treatment.
8. **Conduct post-treatment inspection.**	Inspect the skin where the harnesses were positioned, and question the patient on the level of spinal elongation that he or she has perceived during treatment.
9. **Ensure post-treatment equipment maintenance.**	Follow manufacturer recommendations. Immediately report all defects or malfunctions to technical maintenance staff.

CERVICAL TRACTION

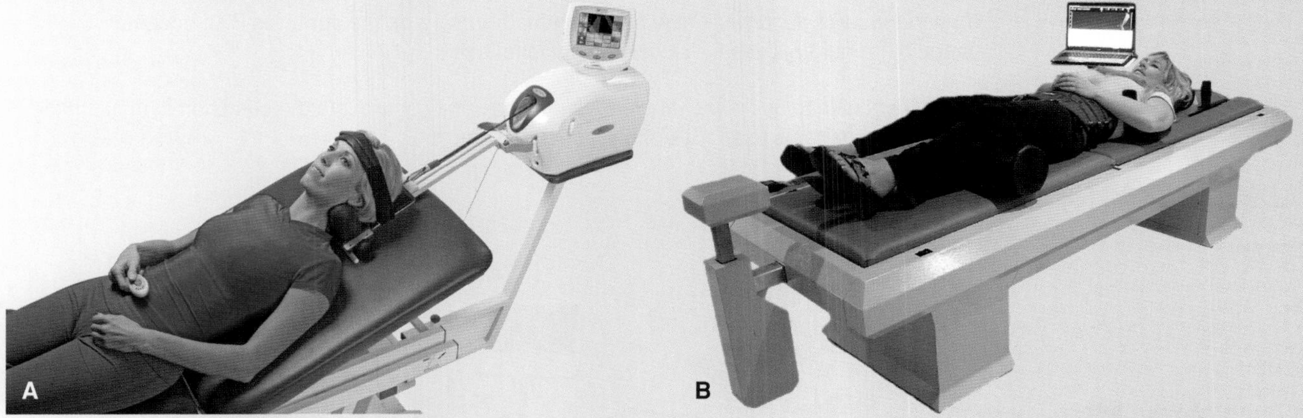

FIGURE 17-6 Application of motorized pulley and cable (**A**) and motorized computerized (**B**) spinal traction tables for cervical spine. (A: Courtesy of DJO Global; B: Courtesy of VAX-D Medical Technologies.)

STEP	RATIONALE
1. **Check for contraindications.**	See All Agents section.
2. **Consider the risks.**	See All Agents section.
3. **Weigh the patient.**	Because traction force should be expressed as a percentage of body weight (% BW; see later discussion), measure the patient's weight.
4. **Position and instruct patient.**	Select body position (sitting or lying) that allows maximum muscle relaxation, thus promoting optimal elongation or vertebral separation. Instruct patient with dentures to keep them in place during cervical traction using an occipito-mandibular halter, because traction force may misalign the temporomandibular joint, causing pain.
5. **Secure patient to traction device.**	Fit halter to patient's head and neck.
6. **Set dosimetry.**	Use the recommended parameters presented in Table 17-2 as a guideline. Note that cervical traction force should range between 20% and 30% BW for effective spinal elongation.
7. **Apply treatment.**	Ensure adequate monitoring during treatment. Make sure that the safety switch is in the patient's hands throughout the duration of treatment.

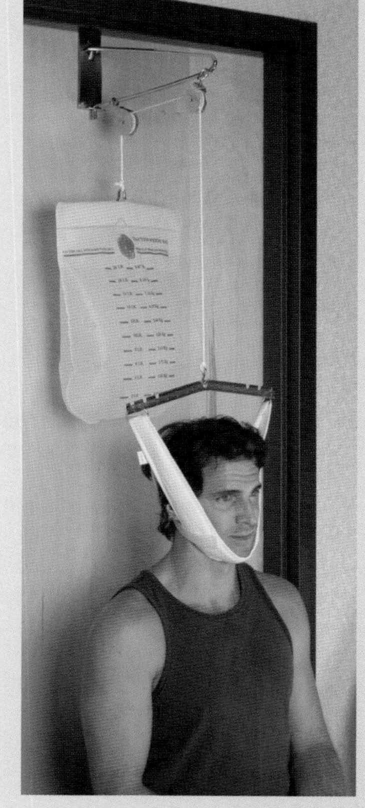

FIGURE 17-7 Application of weighted cervical traction device. (Courtesy of DJO Global.)

STEP	RATIONALE
8. Conduct post-treatment inspection.	Inspect the skin where the harnesses were positioned, and question the patient on the level of spinal elongation that he or she has perceived during treatment.
9. Ensure post-treatment equipment maintenance.	Follow manufacturer recommendations. Immediately report all defects or malfunctions to technical maintenance staff.

CASE STUDIES

Presented are two case studies that summarize the concepts, principles, and applications of spinal traction therapy discussed in this chapter. Case Study 17-1 addresses the use of spinal traction for a cervical radiculopathy affecting a middle-aged female worker. Case Study 17-2 is concerned with the use of spinal traction for the treatment of chronic low back pain affecting a middle-aged male worker. Each case is structured in line with the concepts of evidence-based practice (EBP), the International Classification of Functioning, Disability, and Health (ICF) disablement model, and SOAP (*s*ubjective, *o*bjective, *a*ssessment, *p*lan) note format (see Chapter 2 for details).

CASE STUDY 17-1: CERVICAL RADICULOPATHY

EVIDENCE-BASED CLINICAL DECISION MAKING PROTOCOL

1. Formulate the Case History

A 36-year-old woman, who fell on ice 4 weeks ago while ice skating, is referred for treatment by her physician. Magnetic resonance imaging, taken 2 weeks ago, indicates the presence of a C5–C6 paracentral herniated disk, with mild neural foraminal narrowing. Medical examination revealed that this patient is suffering from a moderate case of cervical radiculopathy caused by this C5–C6 herniated disc. There is no history or presence of atherosclerotic obstruction of the carotid and vertebral arteries. The patient is complaining, today, of pain radiating to the upper extremities that is provoked or exacerbated by cervical active range of motion (ROM). She also complains of limited ROM in her neck and occasional headaches. Physical examination now reveals the presence of a paracervical spasm. There is also myotomal muscle weakness and paresthesia related to the C5–C6 spinal level. This woman has a history of temporomandibular dysfunction, which is currently under control following therapy. Her body weight is 50 kg (110 lb). This patient is limited in her activities of daily living and is presently able to work only part-time. Her past 4-week drug treatment, which consisted of analgesic, anti-inflammatory, and antispasmodic drugs, provided some pain relief. She definitively wants to be treated conservatively before considering surgery as the ultimate therapeutic option. Her goal is to be able to resume her normal daily activities and return to full-time work.

2. Outline the Case Based on the ICF Framework

CERVICAL RADICULOPATHY		
BODY STRUCTURES AND FUNCTIONS	**ACTIVITIES**	**PARTICIPATION**
Bilateral upper limb radicular pain	Difficulty with head movement	Inability to work full-time
Paracervical muscle spasm		
Myotomal weakness		
Dermatomal paresthesia		

PERSONAL FACTORS	ENVIRONMENTAL FACTOR
Middle-aged woman	Mother of 3 children
Healthy	

3. Outline Therapeutic Goals and Outcome Measurements

GOAL	OUTCOME MEASUREMENT
Decrease radicular pain	Visual Analogue Scale (VAS)
Increase cervical ROM	Goniometry
Enhance neck function/accelerated return to full-time work	Neck Disability Index (NDI)

4. Justify the Use of Spinal Traction Based on the EBP Framework

PRACTITIONER'S EXPERIENCE	EVIDENCE-BASED INDICATIONS	PATIENT'S EXPECTATION
Experienced in spinal traction	*Strength:* Moderate	Has no expectation
Has used this EPA in similar cases	*Effectiveness:* Conflicting	Wants to avoid surgery
Believes that spinal traction may be beneficial		

5. Outline Key Intervention Parameters

- **Treatment base:** Hospital
- **Traction technique:** Motorized pulley and cable
- **Traction mode:** Intermittent
- **Risk and precaution:** Patient has a history of TMJ dysfunction. To avoid any traction force on the TMJ, an occipital halter is used.
- **Application protocol:** Follow the suggested application protocol in *Application, Contraindications, and Risks* box, and make the necessary adjustments for this case.
- **Patient's positioning:** Lying supine
- **Patient's body weight:** 50 kg (110 lb)
- **Traction force (MAX:MIN):** Max: 20% BW; MIN: 4% BW
- **Traction force angle of pull:** 0 degrees (neutral or axial)
- **Traction hold/relax time (H:R):** H:90s:R:30s
- **Application duration:** 20 minutes (1,200 seconds), for a total of 10 traction cycles
- **Treatment frequency:** Every second day
- **Intervention period:** 4 weeks
- **Concomitant therapies:** Home daily regimen of pain-free cervical flexibility and strengthening exercises

6. Report Pre- and Post-Intervention Outcomes

OUTCOME	PRE	POST
Pain (VAS score)	6/10	2/10
Cervical ROM	*Bilateral rotation:* 30% restriction *Flexion:* 40% restriction	5% restriction 15% restriction
Neck function (NDI score)	65%	15%
Work status	Part-time	Full-time

7. Document Case Intervention Using the SOAP Note Format

S: Middle-aged female Pt presents with a moderate case of cervical radiculopathy caused by C5–C6 herniated disk.

O: *Intervention:* Intermittent motorized cervical txn; Pt supine; occipital halter; 0-degree angle of pull; Pt's BW 50 kg (110 lb); MAX:MIN traction force: 20% BW:4% BW; H:R time: 90s: 30s; application duration 20 min; treatment frequency: every other day. *Pre–post comparison:* Pain decrease: VAS 6/10 to 2/10. ROM increase: rotation 30% to 5% restriction; flexion

40% to 15% restriction. Improved neck function: NPI score 65% to 15%. Improved work status: part-time to full-time.

A: Treatment difficult to tolerate at the beginning but well tolerated thereafter. No adverse effect. Pt very pleased with therapeutic outcomes.

P: No further treatment required. Prognosis is excellent because a post-therapeutic follow-up magnetic resonance image revealed complete regression of the herniated intervertebral disk. Pt instructed to continue home neck flexibility and strengthening exercise regimen until satisfactory recovery.

CASE STUDY 17-2: CHRONIC LOW BACK PAIN

EVIDENCE-BASED CLINICAL DECISION MAKING PROTOCOL

1. Formulate the Case History

A 46-year-old male carpenter is suffering for chronic low back pain resulting from lifting plywood sheets at work approximately 3 months ago. Magnetic resonance imaging, taken 2 week ago, shows no lumbar disk herniation. The patient has been on a regimen of analgesic, anti-inflammatory, and muscle relaxant drugs since the back pain began. Medication is failing to bring adequate relief and function. He is currently working 3 days a week. He still complains of residual pain over the lower back area, which causes difficulty with lifting. Physical examination reveals moderate back muscle spasm. Straight leg raising (SLR) is normal. Spinal ROM is within the normal range. Patient weighs 100 kg (220 lbs). He wants to stop all medication. He is looking to an alternative and noninvasive treatment. His goal is to return to full time work as soon as possible.

2. Outline the Case Based on the ICF Framework

CHRONIC LOW BACK PAIN		
BODY STRUCTURES AND FUNCTIONS	**ACTIVITIES**	**PARTICIPATION**
Chronic lumbar pain	Difficulty with lifting	Inability to work full-time
Back muscle spasm		

PERSONAL FACTORS	ENVIRONMENTAL FACTORS
Middle-aged man	Carpenter
Healthy	Construction site

3. Outline Therapeutic Goals and Outcome Measurements

GOAL	OUTCOME MEASUREMENT
Decrease lumbar pain	Numerical Pain Rating Scale (NPRS)
Decrease back muscle spasm	Palpation
Enhance back function/accelerate return to full-time work	Modified Oswestry Low Back Pain Disability Questionnaire

4. Justify the Use of Spinal Traction Based on the EBP Framework

PRACTITIONER'S EXPERIENCE	RESEARCH-BASED EVIDENCE	PATIENT'S EXPECTATION
Has minimal experience in spinal traction	*Strength:* Moderate	Wants to stop medication
Has used this EPA in similar cases	*Effectiveness:* Conflicting	Is looking for an alternative therapy
Believes that spinal traction may be beneficial		Wants to return to full-time work

5. Outline Key Intervention Parameters

- **Treatment base:** Private clinic
- **Traction technique:** Motorized split table
- **Traction mode:** Intermittent
- **Risk and precaution:** None
- **Application protocol:** Follow the suggested application protocol in *Application, Contraindications, and Risks* box, and make the necessary adjustments for this case.
- **Patient's positioning:** Lying prone
- **Patient's body weight:** 100 kg (220 lb)
- **Traction force (MAX:MIN):** MAX: 40% BW; MIN: 10% BW
- **Traction force angle of pull:** 0 degrees (neutral or axial)
- **Traction hold/relax time (H:R):** H:50s:R:10s
- **Application duration:** 30 minutes (1,800 seconds), for a total of 30 traction cycles
- **Treatment frequency:** Every day
- **Intervention period:** 2 weeks
- **Concomitant therapies:** Reduction in medications combinee with daily regimen of lower spine flexibility exercise at home

6. Report Pre- and Post-Intervention Outcomes

OUTCOME	PRE	POST
Pain (NPRS score)	4/10	1/10
Muscle spasm	Present	Absent
Low back pain disability (Oswestry score)	42	10
Work status	Part-time	Full-time

7. Document Case Intervention Using the SOAP Note Format

S: Middle-aged male Pt presents with chronic low back pain resulting from heavy lifting at work.

O: *Intervention:* Intermittent motorized split table lumbar txn; Pt prone; Velcro thoracic and lumbar harnesses; 0-degree angle of pull; Pt's BW 100 kg (220 lb); Max:Min traction force: 40% BW:10% BW; H:R time: 50s:10s; application duration: 30 min; treatment frequency: daily. *Pre–post comparison:* Pain decrease: NPRS 4/10 to 1/10. Muscle spasm absent. Improved low back function: Oswestry score 42 to 10. Improved work status: part-time to full-time.

A: Good response. No complaint during therapy.

P: No further treatment required. Pt instructed on the ergonomics of lifting.

VI. THE BOTTOM LINE

- There is scientific evidence to show that spinal traction can induce significant elongation of both the cervical and the lumbar spine.
- Spinal traction rests to the delivery of mechanical energy in the form of traction force applied to the spine.
- Traction force may be expressed in percentage of body weight (% BW), kilograms (kg) or pounds (lb). It is recommended to express traction force in units of percentage of body weight (% BW).
- Maximum but pain-free traction force should be applied.
- Cervical traction force should range between 20% and 30% BW.
- Lumbar traction force should range between 30% and 60% BW.
- Spinal traction is commonly delivered using three techniques: motorized, pneumatic, and weighted.
- Spinal traction is applied using the static and intermittent mode.
- Intermittent traction implies the delivery of maximal force (MAX) during the hold time (H), flowed by a minimal force (MIN) during the relax time (R). H:R cycles are repeated over the entire application duration.
- There is no evidence to show that one technique or mode is therapeutically better than the other.
- The overall body of evidence reported in this chapter shows the strength of evidence behind spinal traction to be *moderate* and its level of therapeutic effectiveness *substantiated*. Note that the percentages of studies showing benefit are low (68% lumbar; 67% cervical) and close to the threshold of being conflicting (60%).

VII. CRITICAL THINKING QUESTIONS

Clarification: What is meant by spinal traction therapy?

Assumptions: You assume that spinal traction therapy is more effective for managing cervical disorders than lumbar disorders. How do you justify making that assumption?

Reasons and evidence: What leads you to believe that spinal traction force can elongate the vertebral column?

Viewpoints or perspectives: How would you respond to a colleague who says that spinal traction therapy is contraindicated in cases of disk herniation?

Implications and consequences: What are the implications of using spinal traction therapy without initially carrying out thorough physical and radiologic examinations?

About the question: What is the rationale for choosing the occipital versus the temporomandibular halter to deliver cervical traction? Why do you think I ask this question?

VIII. REFERENCES

Articles

Apfel C, Cakmakkaya O, Martin W (2010) Restoration of disk height through non-invasive spinal decompression is associated with decreased discogenic low back pain: A retrospective cohort study. BMC Musculoskeletal Dis, 11: 155

Baker P, Marcous BC (1992) The effectiveness of home cervical traction on relief of neck pain and impaired cervical range of motion. Phys Ther Case Reports, 2: 145–152

Balogun JA, Abereoje OK, Olaogun MO, Obajuluwa VA, Okonofua FE (1990) Cardiovascular responses of healthy subjects during cervical traction. Physiother Can, 42: 16–22

Beattie PF, Nelson RM, Michener LA, Cammarata J, Donley J (2008) Outcomes after a prone lumbar traction protocol for patients with activity-limiting low back pain: A prospective case series studies. Arch Phys Med Rehabil, 89: 269–274

Beurskens AJ, de Vet HC, Koke AJ, Lindeman E, Regtop W, van der Heijden GJ, Knipschield PG (1995) Efficacy of traction for non-specific low back pain: A randomized clinical trial. Lancet, 346: 1596–1600

Beurskens AJ, de Vet HC, Koke AJ, Regtop W, van der Heijden GJ, Lindeman E, Knipschield PG (1997) Efficacy of traction for nonspecific low back pain: 12-week and 6-month results of a randomized clinical trial. Spine, 22: 2756–2762

Borman P, Kerskin D, Bodur H (2003) The efficacy of lumbar traction in the management of patients with low back pain. Rheumatol Int, 23: 82–86

Brewerton DA, Beardwell A, Blower PW, Brown MR, Campbell EDR, Cochrane GM (1966) British Association of Physical Medicine. Pain in the neck and arm: A multicenter trial of the effects of physiotherapy. BMJ, 2: 253–258

Browder DA, Erhard RE, Piva SR (2004) Intermittent cervical traction and thoracic manipulation for management of mild cervical compressive myelopathy attributed to cervical herniated disc: A case series. J Orthop Sports Phys Ther, 34: 701–712

Cai C, Ming G, Ng LY (2011) Development of a clinical prediction rule to identify patients with neck pain who are likely to benefit from home-based mechanical cervical traction. Eur Spine, 20: 912–922

Chiu TW, Ng JK, Walther-Zhang B, Lin RJ, Ortelli L, Chua SK (2011) A randomized controlled trial on the efficacy of intermittent cervical traction for patients with chronic neck pain. Clin Rehab, 25: 814–822

Chung TS, Lee YJ, Kang SW, Park CJ, Kang WS, Shim YM (2002) Reducibility of cervical disk herniation: Evaluation at MR imaging during cervical traction with a nonmagnetic traction device. Radiology, 225: 895–900

Cleland JA, Whitman JM, Fritz JM, Palmer JA (2005) Manual physical therapy, cervical traction, and strengthening exercises in patients with cervical radiculopathy: A case series. J Orthop Sports Phys Ther, 35: 802–811

Colachis SC, Strohm BR (1965a) Cervical traction relationship of time to varied tractive force with constant angle of pull. Arch Phys Med Rehab, 46: 815–819

Colachis SC, Strohm BR (1965b) A study of tractive forces and angle of pull on vertebral interspaces in the cervical spine. Arch Phys Med Rehab, 46: 820–830

Colachis SC, Strohm BR (1966) Effect of duration of intermittent cervical traction on vertebral separation. Arch Phys Med Rehab, 47: 353–359

Colachis SC, Strohm BR (1969) Effects of intermittent traction on separation of lumbar vertebrae. Arch Phys Med Rehab, 50: 251–258

Constantoyannis C, Konstantinou D, Kourtopoulos H, Papadakis N (2002) Intermittent cervical traction for cervical radiculopathy caused by large-volume herniated disks. J Man Phys Ther, 25: 188–192

Corkery M (2001) The use of lumbar harness traction to treat a patient with lumbar radicular pain: A case report. J Manual Manipulative Ther, 9: 191–197

Coxhead CE, Inskip H, Meade TW, North WR, Troup JD (1981) Multicentre trial of physiotherapy in the management of sciatic symptoms. Lancet, 1: 1065–1068

Fritz JM, Lindsay W, Matheson JW, Brennan GP, Hunter SJ, Moffit SD, Swalberg A, Rodriguez B (2007) Is there a subgroup of patients with low back pain likely to benefit from mechanical traction? Results of a randomized clinical trial and subgrouping analysis. Spine, 32: E793–E800

Gionis TA, Groteke E (2003) Spinal decompression. Orthopedic Technol Rev, 5: 36–39

Goldie I, Landquist A (1970) Evaluation of the effect of different forms of physiotherapy in cervical pain. Scand J Rehab Med, 2: 117–121

Gose EE, Naguzewski WK, Naguzewski RK (1998) Vertebral axis decompression therapy for pain associated with herniated or degenerated discs or facet syndrome: An outcome study. Neurol Res, 20: 186–190

Guevenol K, Tuzun C, Peker O, Goktay Y (2000) A comparison of inverted spinal traction and conventional traction in the treatment of lumbar disc herniations. Physiother Theory Pract, 16: 151–160

Gupta R, Ramarao S (1978) Epidurography in reduction of lumbar disc prolapsed by traction. Arch Phys Med Rehab, 59: 322–327

Harrison DE, Caillet R, Harrison DD, Janik TJ, Holland B (2002a) Changes in sagittal lumbar configuration with a new method of extension traction: Nonrandomized clinical controlled trial. Arch Phys Med Rehab, 83: 1585–1591

Harrison DE, Caillet R, Harrison DD, Janik TJ, Holland B (2002b) A new 3-point bending traction method of restoring cervical lordosis and cervical manipulation: A nonrandomized clinical controlled trial. Arch Phys Med Rehab, 83: 447–453

Haskvitz EM, Hanten WP (1986) Blood pressure response to inversion traction. Phys Ther, 66: 1361–1364

Hattori M, Shirai Y, Aoki T (2002) Research on the effectiveness of intermittent cervical traction therapy, using short-latency somatosensory evoked potentials. J Orthop Sci, 7: 208–216

Hood LB, Chrisman D (1968) Intermittent pelvic traction in the treatment of the ruptured intervertebral disc. Phys Ther, 48: 21–30

Jette DU, Flakel JE, Trombly C (1985) Effect of intermittent, supine cervical traction on the myoelectric activity of the upper trapezius muscle in subjects with neck pain. Phys Ther, 65: 1173–1176

Joghataei MT, Arab AM, Khaksar H (2004) The effect of cervical traction combined with conventional therapy on grip strength on patients with cervical radiculopathy. Clin Rehab, 18: 879–887

Judovich BD (1954) Lumbar traction therapy and dissipated force factors. Lancet, 74: 411–414

Judovich BD (1955) Lumbar traction therapy. Elimination of physical factors that prevent lumbar stretch. JAMA, 159: 549–550

Judovich BD, Nobel GR (1957) Traction therapy: A study of resistance forces. Preliminary report on a new method of lumbar traction. Am J Surg, 93: 108–114

Klaber-Moffett JA, Hughes GI, Griffiths P (1990) An investigation of the effects of cervical traction. Part 2: The effects on the neck musculature. Clin Rehab, 4: 287–290

Laban MM, Macy JA, Meerschaert JR (1992) Intermittent cervical traction: A progenitor of lumbar radicular pain. Arch Phys Med Rehabil, 73: 295–296

Laban MM, Mahal BS (2005) Intraspinal dural distraction inciting spinal radiculopathy: Cranial to caudal and caudal to cranial. Am J Phys Med Rehabil, 84: 141–144

Larsson U, Choler U, Lindstrom A, Lind G, Nachemson A, Nilsson B, Roslund J (1980) Auto-traction for treatment of lumbago-sciatica. Acta Orthop Scand, 51: 791–798

Lee MY, Wong MK, Tang FT, Chang WH, Chiou WK (1996) Design and assessment of an adaptive intermittent cervical traction modality with EMG biofeedback. J Biomech Eng, 118: 597–600

Letchuman R, Deusinger R (1993) Comparison of sacrospinalis myoelectric activity and pain levels in patients undergoing static and intermittent lumbar traction. Spine, 18: 1361–1365

Lidstrom A, Zachrisson M (1970) Physical therapy on low back pain and sciatica. Scand J Rehab Med, 2: 37–42

Liu J, Ebraheim NA, Sanford CG, Patil V, Elsamaloty H, Treuhaft K, Farrell S (2008) Quantitative changes in the cervical neural foramen resulting from axial traction: In vivo imaging study. Spine J, 8: 619–623

Ljunggren AE, Weber H, Larssen S (1984) Autotraction versus manual traction in patients with prolapsed lumbar intervertebral discs. Scand J Rehab Med, 16: 117

Ljunggren AE, Walker L, Weber H, Amundsen T (1992) Manual traction versus isometric exercises in patients with herniated lumbar discs. Physioth Theory Pract, 8: 207–213

Loy T (1983) Treatment of cervical spondylosis: Electroacupuncture versus physiotherapy. Med J Aust, 2: 32–34

Macario A, Richmond C, Auster M, Pergolizzi JV (2008) Treatment of 94 outpatients with chronic discogenic low back pain with the DRX9000: A retrospective chart review. Pain Pract, 8: 11–17

Mathews JA, Hickling J (1975) Lumbar traction: A double blind controlled study of sciatica. Rheumatol Rehab, 14: 222–225

Mathews JA, Mills SB, Jenkins VM, Grimes SM, Morkel MJ, Mathews W, Scott CM, Sittampalam Y (1987) Back pain and sciatica: Controlled trial of manipulation, traction, sclerosant and epidural injections. Br J Rheumatol, 26: 416–423

Meszaros TF, Olson R, Kulig K, Creighton D, Czarnecki E (2000) Effect of 10%, 30%, and 60% body weight traction on the straight leg raise test of symptomatic patients with low back pain. J Orthop Sports Phys Ther, 30: 595–601

Moeti P, Marchetti G (2001) Clinical outcome from mechanical intermittent cervical traction for the treatment of cervical radiculopathy: A case series. J Orthop Sports Phys Ther, 31: 207–213

Moret MC, van der Stap M, Hagmeijer R, Molenaar A, Koes BW (1998) Design and feasibility of a randomized clinical trial to evaluate the effect of vertical traction in patients with a lumbar radicular syndrome. Man Ther, 3: 203–211

Mysliwiec A, Saulicz E, Kuszewski M, Kokosz M, Wolny T (2011) Assessment of the influence of Saunders traction and transcutaneous electrical nerve stimulation on hand grip force in patients with neck pain. Ortop Traumatol Rehabil, 13: 37–44

Naguszewski WK, Naguszewski RK, Gose EE (2001) Dermatomal somatosensory evoked potential demonstration of nerve root decompression after VAX-D therapy. Neurol Res, 23: 706–714

Olson VL (1997) Whiplash-associated chronic headache treated with home cervical traction. Phys Ther, 77: 417–424

Onel D, Tuzlaci M, Sari H, Demir K (1989) Computed tomographic investigation of the effect of traction on lumbar disc herniations. Spine, 14: 82–90

Oudenhoven RC (1978) Gravitational lumbar traction. Arch Phys Med Rehab, 59: 510–512

Ozturk B, Gunduz OH, Ozoran K, Bostanoglu S (2006) Effect of continuous lumbar traction on the size of herniated disc material in lumbar disk herniation. Rheumatol Int, 26: 622–666

Pal B, Mangion P, Hossain MA, Diffey BL (1986) A controlled trial of continuous lumbar traction in the treatment of back pain and sciatica. Br J Rheumatol, 25: 181–183

Pennie B, Agambar L (1990) Whiplash injuries: A trial of early management. J Bone Joint Surg (B), 72: 277–279

Podein RJ, Iaizzo PA (1998) Applied forces and associated physiological responses induced by axial spinal unloading with the LTX 3000 lumbar rehabilitation system. Arch Phys Med Rehabil, 79: 505–513

Quain MC, Tecklin JS (1985) Lumbar traction: Its effect on respiration. Phys Ther, 65: 1343–1346

Ramos G (2004) Efficacy of vertebral axial decompression on chronic low back pain: Study of dosage regimen. Neurol Res, 26: 320–324

Raney NH, Peterson EJ, Smith TA, Cowan JE, Rendeiro DG, Deyle GD, Childs JD (2009) Development of a clinical prediction rule to identify patients with neck pain likely to benefit from cervical traction and exercise. Eur Spine, 18: 382–391

Saal JS, Saal JA, Yurth EF (1996) Nonoperative management of herniated cervical intervertebral disc with radiculopathy. Spine, 21: 1877–1883

Sari H, Akarirmak U, Karacan I, Akman H (2005) Computed tomographic evaluation of lumbar spinal structures during traction. Physiother Theory Pract, 21: 3–11

Schimmel JJ, de Kleuver M, Horsting PP (2009) No effect of traction in patients with low back pain: A single centre, single blind, randomized controlled trial of Intervertebral Differential Dynamics Therapy. Eur Spine J, 18: 1943–1850

Shakoor MA, Ahmed MS, Kibria G, Khan AA, Mian MA, Hasan SA, Nahar S, Hossain MA (2002) Effect of cervical traction and exercises therapy in cervical spondylosis. Bengladesh Med Res Counc Bull, 28: 61–69

Shealy CN, Borgmeyer V (1997) Decompression, reduction and stabilization of the lumbar spine: A cost-effective treatment for lumbosacral pain. Am J Pain Manage, 7: 63–65

Sherry E, Kitchener P, Smart R (2001) A prospective randomized controlled study of VAX-D and TENS for the treatment of chronic low back pain. J Neurol Res, 23: 780–784

Sweetman BJ, Heinrich I, Anderson JA (1993) A randomized controlled trial of exercises, short wave diathermy, and traction for low back pain, with evidence of diagnosis-related response to treatment. J Orthop Rheumatol, 6: 159–166

Swezey RL, Swezey AM, Warner K (1999) Efficacy of home cervical traction therapy. Am J Phys Med Rehabil, 78: 30–32

Tesio L, Luccarelli G, Fornari M (1989) Natchev's auto-traction for lumbago-sciatica: Effectiveness in lumbar disc herniation. Arch Phys Med Rehabil, 70: 831–834

Tesio L, Merlo A (1993) Autotraction versus passive traction: An open controlled study in lumbar disc herniation. Arch Phys Med Rehabil, 74: 871–876

Unlu Z, Tasci S, Tarhan S, Pabuscu Y, Islak S (2008) Comparison of 3 physical therapy modalities for acute pain in lumbar disc herniation measured by clinical evaluation and magnetic resonance imaging. J Man Physiol Ther, 31: 191–198

Valtonen EJ, Kiuru E (1970) Cervical traction as a therapeutic tool. A clinical analysis based on 212 patients. Scand J Rehabil Med, 2: 29–36

Van der Heijden GJ, Beurskens AJ, Dirx MJ, Bouter LM, Lindeman E (1995) Efficacy of lumbar traction: A randomized clinical trial. Physiotherapy, 81: 29–35

Vaughn HT, Having KM, Rogers JL (2006) Radiologic analysis of intervertebral separation with a 0 degrees and 30 degrees rope angle using the Saunders cervical traction device. Spine, 31: E39–E43

Waldrop MA (2006) Diagnosis and treatment of cervical radiculopathy using a clinical prediction rule and a multimodal intervention approach: A case series. J Orthop Sports Phys Ther, 36: 152–159

Walker GL (1986) Goodley polyaxial cervical traction: A new approach to a traditional treatment. Phys Ther, 66: 1255–1259

Weber H (1973) Traction therapy in sciatica due to disc prolapse. J Oslo City Hosp, 23: 167–176

Weber H, Ljunggren E, Walker L (1984) Traction therapy in patients with herniated lumbar intervertebral discs. J Oslo City Hosp, 34: 61–70

Werners R, Pynsent PB, Bulstrode CJ (1999) Randomized trial comparing interferential therapy with motorized lumbar traction and massage in the management of low back pain in a primary care setting. Spine, 24: 1579–1584

Wong AM, Lee M, Chang W, Tang F (1997) Clinical trial of a cervical traction modality with electromyographic biofeedback. Am J Phys Med Rehabil, 76: 19–25

Wong AM, Leong C, Chen C (1992) The traction angle and cervical intervertebral separation. Spine, 17: 136–138

Young IA, Michener LA, Cleland JA, Aquilera AJ, Snyder AR (2009) Manual therapy, exercise, and traction for patients with cervical radiculopathy: A randomized clinical trial. Phys Ther, 89: 632–642

Zito M (1988) Effect of two gravity inversion methods on heart rate, systolic brachial pressure, and ophthalmic artery pressure. Phys Ther, 68: 20–25

Zylbergold RS, Piper MC (1985) Cervical spine disorders: A comparison of three types of traction. Spine, 10: 867–871

Review Articles

Gay RE, Brault JS (2008) Evidenced-informed management of chronic low back pain with traction therapy. Spine J, 8: 234–242

Macario A, Richmond C, Auster M, Pergolizzi JV (2008) Treatment of 94 outpatients with chronic discogenic low back pain with the RDX9000: A retrospective chart review. Pain Pract, 8: 11–17

Textbooks

Cook C (2010) Orthopedic Manual Therapy, 2nd ed. Prentice Hall, New York

King HH, Janig W, Patterson MM (2010) The Science and Clinical Application of Manual Therapy. Churchill Livingstone, London

Lederman E (2008) The Science & Practice of Manual Therapy, 2nd ed. Churchill Livingstone, London

Li LC, Bombardier C (2001) Physical therapy management of low back pain: An exploratory survey of therapist approaches. Phys Ther, 81: 1018–1028

Olson KA (2008) Manual Physical Therapy of the Spine. Saunders, New York

Chapter 18

Limb Compression

Chapter Outline

Learning Objectives

Remembering: List the key differences between compressive garments and pneumatic pumps for limb compression.

Understanding: Compare the static, sequential, and sequential graded methods of limb compression.

Applying: Demonstrate the application of limb compression therapy.

Analyzing: Explain the mechanical (hemodynamic) and biochemical (hematologic) effects attributed to limb pneumatic compression therapy.

Evaluating: Discuss the rationale for using limb compression therapy, as opposed to a pharmacologic anticoagulation therapy, for the prophylaxis of deep vein thrombosis and venous thromboembolism.

Creating: Show how to improve existing devices and garments for limb compression therapy.

I. FOUNDATION

A. DEFINITION

Limb compression is defined as the application of mechanical external compressive forces over the upper and lower limbs for improving venous, arterial, and lymphatic circulation. Today's most common methods of delivery of limb compression therapy are compression garments made of stretched fabrics and pneumatic pumps connected to air-filled compressive garments wrapped around the limbs. Table 18-1 lists the main characteristics associated with these two limb compression methods. Compression garments, such as bandages, stockings, and sleeves, provide mechanical elastic energy stored in their fabrics to deliver constant pressure gradients, ranging between 10 and 80 mm Hg, on the limbs. Pneumatic pumps, on the other hand, provide intermittent mechanically compressed air into inflatable garments generating pressure gradients ranging from 1 to 130 mm Hg. Both methods are used to treat the upper and lower extremities, either at the hospital, private clinic, or home. Compression garments have the advantage of being wearable while providing therapeutic mobility.

B. COMPRESSION GARMENT

Compression garments are specialized elastic stretch pieces of clothing designed to exert compression, when stretched, on the upper and lower extremities Compressive garments are available in a wide range of styles, sizes, and graded compression gradients. Putting on and removing compressive stockings and sleeves can be difficult. To facilitate their application, donning and doffing aids are available. Relatively cheaper and simpler to use than pneumatic compression devices, graded compression garments are the most popular mechanical method of therapeutic limb compression (Lippi et al., 2011). Unfortunately, a major limitation to their use is improper fitting, which can cause several complications such as pain, skin irritation, and breakdown, and possibly skin ulceration and tourniquet effect that may block arterial and venous flow.

C. COMPRESSION PNEUMATIC PUMP

Figure 18-1 illustrates typical compression pneumatic pumps used with specially designed air-inflatable single- or multiple-chamber garments for the upper and lower extremities, and calf and foot cuffs. Pneumatic pumps present more advantages, when compared to compression garments, by being able to deliver variable intermittent compression (see Table 18-1). Pneumatic garments are available in various shapes, sizes, and number of chambers. Unfortunately, the regular use of those tightly wrapped air-inflatable compression garments around the limbs for prolonged periods often presents several side effects such as sweating, heating sensation, itchiness, and skin irritation, which all lead to discomfort. One alternative, for the lower extremity, is to use a pneumatic foot compression device made of a pump connected to a ventilated air-inflatable rigid pad foot cover. The use of foot pumps is advantageous in high-risk trauma patients who have a contraindication to heparin because of their injuries and who cannot have compressive garments placed on lower extremities secondary to external fixators or large bulky dressings. In other words, the major advantage of this foot pump system is that it only requires access to the foot, which enables it to be used in patients with Jones dressings and casts. Also available in the field of limb compression is a pneumatic foot-calf pump system made of a pneumatic pump connected to foot and calf garment. Such a device is used mainly for improving arterial blood flow in patients suffering from lower limb critical limb ischemia.

D. RATIONALE FOR USE

The rationale behind the development and clinical application of limb compression therapy is to provide practitioners with a therapeutic means, other than walking and voluntary muscle contraction, to enhance peripheral

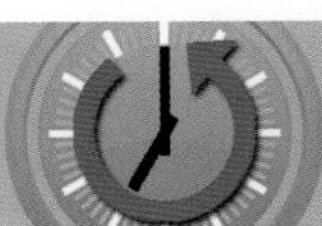

Historical Overview

The history of limb compression is ancient, dating back to around 500 BC (Lippi et al., 2011). The use of elastic compression to treat leg ulcers dates back to the 18th century. Its use as a prophylactic measure against deep vein thrombosis came later in the early 19th century. In the 1930s, a group of investigators noted that intermittent cycles of pressures applied to the lower limbs of patients suffering from various peripheral vascular diseases, such as Raynaud's disease, vascular claudication, and foot ulcers, had a beneficial therapeutic effect by improving arterial circulation (Landis et al., 1933; Reid et al., 1934; Landis, 1935). According to Delis et al. (2005), clinical interest in limb compression therapy remained dormant for approximately four decades until a study by Gaskell and colleagues (1978), which showed a significant improvement in the walking ability of patients with vascular stable intermittent claudication following limb compression therapy. Today, mechanical limb compression therapy is routinely used in hospitals, clinics, and at home, primarily for the prophylaxis of deep vein thrombosis (DVT) and venous thromboembolism (VTE) in patients at risk of bleeding following pharmacologic anticoagulation therapy.

TABLE 18-1 LIMB COMPRESSION METHODS

	Methods	
Characteristic	**Compression Garment**	**Pneumatic Pump**
Material	Bandage/Stocking/Sleeve	Pump and air-inflatable garment
Mechanical principle	Elastic	Pneumatic
Compression mode	Constant	Intermittent
Pressure range	10 to 80 mm Hg	1 to 130 mm Hg
Wear ability	Yes	No
Application	Upper and lower extremities	
Therapeutic base	Hospital/Clinic/Home	

venous, arterial, and lymphatic circulation after injuries and surgery, as well as in the presence of disease and prolonged immobilization. For example, this chapter will show that the main indications for limb compression therapy is to *prevent* both deep venous thrombosis (DVT) and venous thromboembolism (VTE) in bedridden and surgical patients, whether it be at the hospital or at home, and to *treat* edema of traumatic, venous, and lymphatic origin, venous leg ulcers, and patients suffering from vascular intermittent claudication and critical limb ischemia.

II. BIOPHYSICAL CHARACTERISTICS

A. MECHANICAL PRINCIPLE

The two limb compression methods described in Table 18-1 work on the same principle, which is to use *mechanical energy* to compress, or squeeze, blood and lymph from underlying vein and lymphoid vessels, thus creating an upward volumetric displacement, and to push arterial blood into soft tissues, thus enhancing their oxygenization. This mechanical energy may be elastic and pneumatic in

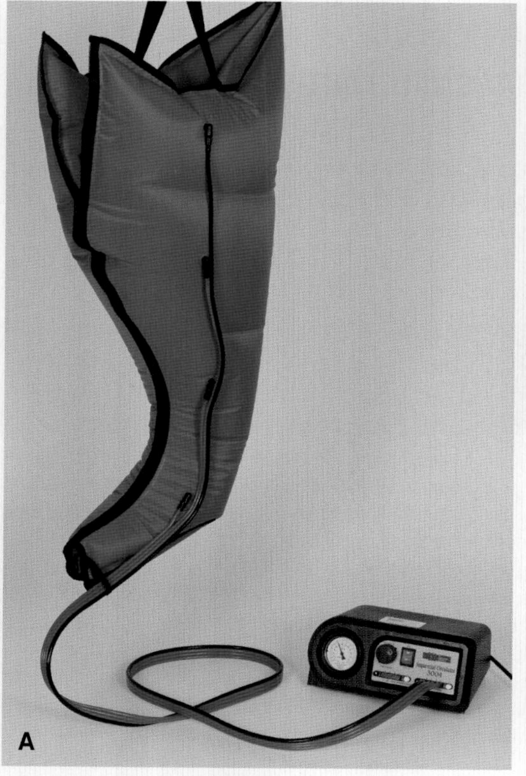

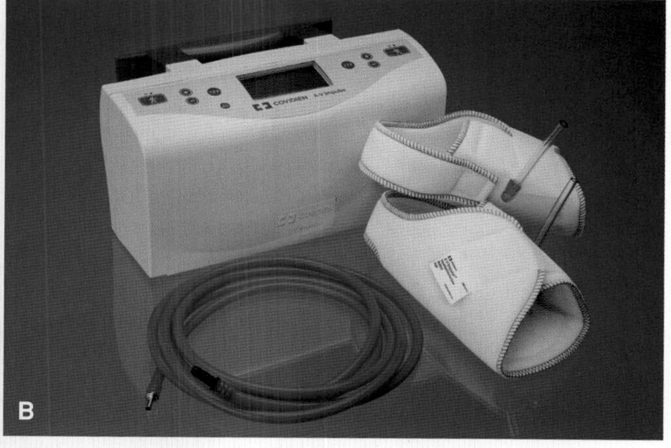

FIGURE 18-1 Typical compression pneumatic systems with limb garment (**A**) and rigid foot sole air-inflated garment (**B**). (Courtesy of Bio Compression Systems; B: A-V Impulse System is a trademark of a Covidien Company © Covidien. All rights reserved.)

nature, exerting constant and intermittent compression on the limbs. All compression garments and pumps are designed to exert a mechanical pressure gradient on the surface of lower and upper extremities (Morris, 2008).

B. PRESSURE

1. Compressive Garment

The pressure developed beneath any garment is based on *Laplace's law* and is governed by the tension (tensile force) in the fabric and the circumference of the limb. It is calculated by using the following simplified formula: $P = T/C$, where P is pressure in millimeters of mercury (mm Hg), T is garment tension or tensile force in kilogram force (kgf), and C is the circumference of the limb in centimeters (cm). Pressure is commonly expressed in units of millimeters of mercury (mm Hg) and in units of kilo pascal (kPa), where 1 mm Hg equals 0.133 kPa. Sub-garment pressure is, therefore, *directly* proportional to garment tensile force but *inversely* proportional to the circumference of the limb over which it is applied. This means that a garment applied with constant tension to a limb of normal proportions will automatically produce *graded* (or graduated) compression. In other words, graded compression means that the pressure gradient will be the highest distally on the limb (lowest circumference), then will gradually decrease up, proximally, as the limb circumference increases.

2. Pneumatic Pump and Air-Inflatable Garment

Pneumatic compression systems are active, programmable systems capable of exerting *intermittent* pressure on the upper and lower extremities by using single- and multiple-chamber garments. The use of a single-chamber garment provides a nonsequential (only one chamber) uniform (non-graded) pressure on the limb. A multiple-chamber garment, on the other hand, can provide sequential uniform, as well as sequential graded, pressure on the limb. Figure 18-2 illustrates the intermittent, sequential, and uniform/graded modes of pneumatic limb compression. The term *intermittent* means that pressure is periodically interrupted, yielding to repeated cycles of air inflation and deflation. The word *sequential* refers to the ordering or sequencing of pressure, which always starts distally and then gradually moves proximally on the limb. Sequential pressure, therefore, is only possible with multi-chamber garments. The term *grade* is in relation to the pressure changes occurring in the garment during therapy. Graded pressure is, therefore, only possible when multiple-chamber garments are used.

a. Intermittent Uniform Mode

Figure 18-2A exemplifies the *intermittent uniform* pressure mode, with inflation (i) and deflation (d) times, generated in a single-chamber garment. The pressure level in each pressure cycle is uniform or identical. Deflation and deflation times are identical in each compression cycle, and the garment starts to deflate as soon as the prescribed maximum pressure is reached.

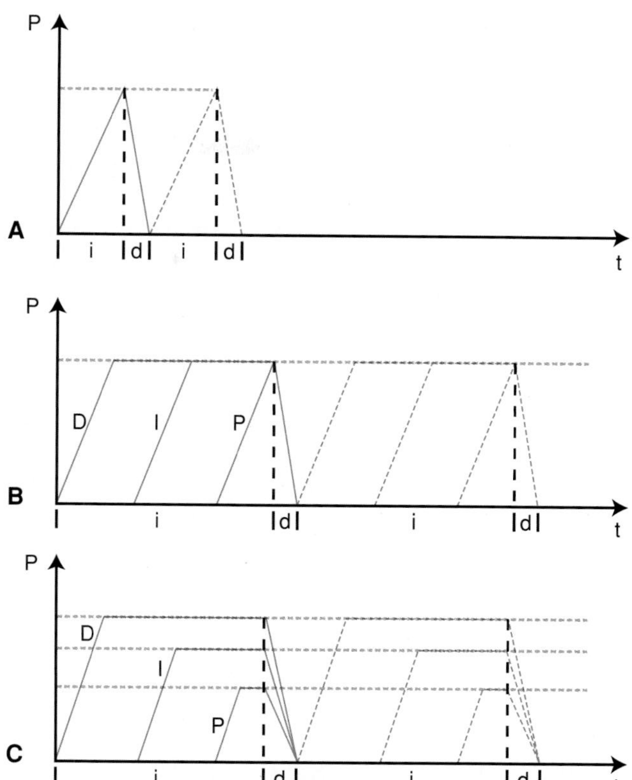

FIGURE 18-2 The intermittent, sequential, and graded nature of pneumatic limb compression. **A:** Intermittent uniform pressure, within a single-chamber garment, with related inflation and deflation cycles. **B:** Intermittent, sequential, and uniform pressure: The three-chamber garment is inflated sequentially—that is, from its distal (*D*) to intermediate (*I*) to proximal (*P*) chambers, and all three chambers deflate simultaneously. **C:** Intermittent, sequential, and graded pressure: The three-chamber garment is inflated sequentially, pressure is graded being higher distally than proximally, and all three chambers deflate simultaneously.

b. Intermittent Sequential Uniform Mode

Figure 18-2B shows the *intermittent sequential uniform* pressure mode developed in a three-chamber garment. In this example, maximum pressure levels are identical (uniform) in all three chambers. Air inflation is sequential beginning in the distal (D) chamber, followed by the inflation of the intermediate (I) and proximal (P) chambers, respectively. The inflation rise time is identical in all three chambers. Maximum pressure is maintained in both the distal and intermediate chamber until the proximal chamber is fully inflated. Pressure is uniform in each chamber and with each cycle, and all three chambers deflate at the same time.

c. Intermittent Sequential Graded Mode

The *intermittent sequential graded* mode is illustrated in Figure 18-2C. Pressure is graded, or graduated, in each chamber. Maximal pressure is developed in the distal chamber, followed by decreasingly lower pressure levels in the intermediate and proximal chambers, respectively. All three chambers deflate at the same time. In this example, the intermittent and sequential parameters are identical to those described in the earlier examples.

III. THERAPEUTIC EFFECTS AND INDICATIONS

Throughout an average day, the body pumps fluids to all of the extremities, and to the heart, by using movement, work, or muscle activity. Venous blood and lymph are pumped proximally toward the heart, whereas arterial blood is pushed distally into the tissues. Unfortunately, trauma, disease, and surgery can significantly disrupt the body's own pumping effect, causing major side effects such as edema, venous thrombosis, ischemia, and skin ulcers. It is in those circumstances that limb compression therapy may play a very important therapeutic role in providing artificial resting and working pressures on the affected limb for the purpose of improving venous, arterial, and lymphatic flow (see Kumar et al., 2002; Morris et al., 2004; Roderick et al., 2005; Urbankova et al., 2005; Kalodiki et al., 2007; Morris et al., 2008; Rinehart-Ayres et al., 2010; Kakkos et al., 2011; Rhan et al., 2011; Feldman et al., 2012; Field et al., 2012; Gould et al., 2012).

A. RESTING AND WORKING PRESSURE

1. Bandages

Compression bandages are *wearable* therapeutic aids. There are three basic types of bandages used in limb compression therapy: inelastic short stretch, elastic long stretch, and semi-elastic multilayer. The extent to which a bandage can be stretched at rest, and during work, specifies its resting and working pressure. Consequently, the pressure exerted by the garment on the tissues at *rest*—that is, without muscle contraction—is known as its resting pressure. Conversely, the pressure exerted by the garment during *work*—that is, during muscle contraction—is defined as its working pressure. Figure 18-3 presents the mechanophysiologic concept behind the resting and working pressure exerted by compression garment and pneumatic pump system. Shown is a simplified anatomic model depicting a vessel (V) placed between a muscle (M) and a bone (B). Under normal conditions—that is, without bandaging and without muscle contraction—the vessel presents a given diameter (see Fig. 18-3A). To apply a bandage over a resting limb (without muscle contraction) causes its resting pressure, of which its action is to squeeze the vessel between the resting muscle and the rigid bony surface, resulting in a decrease in its diameter, coupled with an upward fluid volumetric displacement (see Fig. 18-3B). To apply the same bandage over a working limb (with muscle contraction) causes its working pressure, of which its action is to facilitate the voluntary muscle contraction compressive effect of the vessel (see Fig. 18-3C) against the rigid bony surface. In other words, the bulging of the contracting muscle is counteracted, or opposed, by the bandage's working pressure, thus enhancing the ability of contracting muscle to further squeeze the vessel. The working pressure is determined by the garment resistance provided against the working musculature underneath. Resting pressure is permanent. Working pressure, on the other hand, is temporary or cyclical, and is present only during muscle activity. Governed by Laplace's law, compression bandages provide graded pressure (larger distally than proximally) on the limb.

2. Stocking and Sleeve

Compression stockings and sleeves are also wearable aids. Their application usually follows that of bandages in providing less compression for longer support. These garments are divided into four different compression classes, differentiated according to the magnitude of their *resting pressure*. The compression classes are standardized based on the level of resting pressure at the ankle (stocking) and wrist (sleeve) areas. Additionally governed by Laplace's law, they provide graded compression that is tightest at the ankle and wrist, then gradually becomes less constrictive toward the knee and elbow. Compression stockings and sleeves provide both resting and working pressure on the limb by using the same mechanisms described earlier for bandages (see Fig. 18-3, A to C).

B. MUSCLE AND VENOUS PUMP

Pneumatic compression systems are nonwearable dynamic, programmable systems that are capable of exerting intermittent pressure on the limb (see Fig. 18-3, D to E). They are applied on resting extremities. Contrary to bandages, stockings, and sleeves, which can be applied for several hours and days at the time, pneumatic compression therapy is only applied for a few minutes at a time. Pneumatic compression, through intermittent and repeated cycles of garment inflation and deflation wrapped around the upper and lower extremities, is intended to provide a mechanical means of mimicking or simulating two important physiologic vascular pumps, known in the literature as the calf muscle pump and the venous foot pump (Delis, 2005; Partsch, 2008; Corley et al., 2010).

1. Calf Muscle Pump

The presence of gravity and immobility make venous blood and lymph return to the heart more difficult. The *calf muscle pump,* often referred to as the body's secondary heart, helps to propel venous blood and lymph back to the heart. This muscle pump works only when there is a calf muscle contraction, such as during walking, jogging, and running, or during foot/ankle voluntary exercises. When the calf muscles are resting, this pump shuts down and, consequently, blood return from the lower extremities to the heart is significantly reduced. Complete reversed blood flow (reflux) is prevented by the presence of passive one-way valves in the veins. As illustrated in Figure 18-3C, intermittent pneumatic squeezing of the vein segment occurs when muscle contraction increases the pressure within the muscle compartment. Just like a

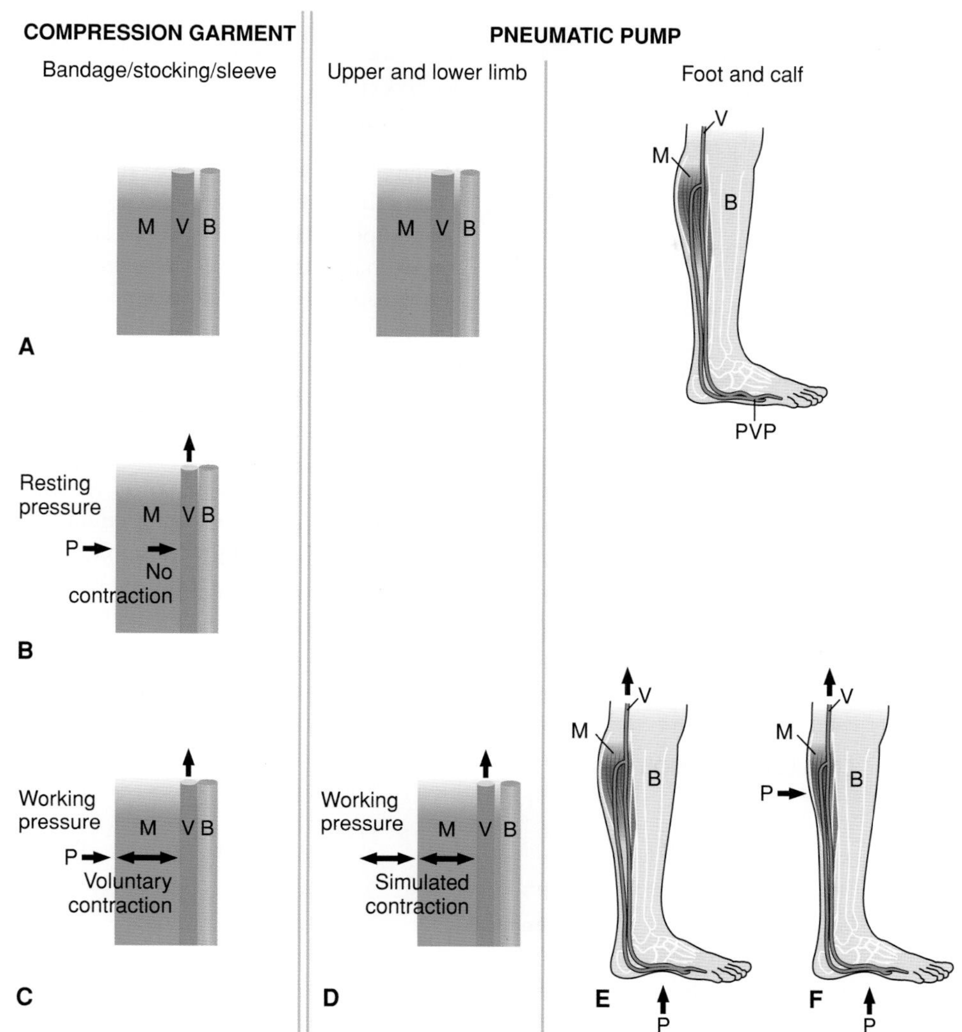

FIGURE 18-3 Schematic model showing mechanical effects of limb compression on the vasculature. **A:** Models showing a vessel (*V*) in between a muscle (*M*) and a bone (*B*) surface, and the plantar venous plexus (*PVP*). **B:** Resting pressure exerted by the garment on the noncontracting muscle compresses the vessel against the rigid bony surface. **C:** Working pressure exerted by the garment against the bulging voluntary contracting muscle compresses the vessel. **D:** Simulated intermittent working pressure exerted by the pneumatic foot pump system on the muscle pump. **E:** Simulated intermittent working pressure exerted by the pneumatic foot pump system on the PVP. **F:** Simulated and sequential intermittent working pressure exerted by the pneumatic calf-foot pump system on both the calf muscle and the plantar venous plexus, respectively.

sphygmomanometer, the calf muscle pump can achieve pumping pressures of several hundred millimeters of mercury before venous valve failure occurs.

2. Foot Pump

In 1983, Gardner and Fox discovered a venous pump on the sole of the human foot, which consists of a plexus of veins that fills by gravity and empties upon weight bearing, thus increasing lower limb blood flow without muscular assistance (see Fig. 18-3A). This large group of veins, called the *plantar venous plexus* (PVP), acts as a built-in return pump (Gardner et al., 1983; Corley et al., 2010). Each time the foot bears weight or hits the ground when walking or running, the plantar venous plexus is flattened, stretched, and squeezed, thus pumping blood back up to the heart (Corley et al., 2010). Unfortunately, the foot pump is completely inactive in the absence of ambulation. *Foot pump* systems (see Fig. 18-1B) are specifically designed to *mimic* weight bearing, thus activating the physiologic foot pump. It does so by inflating and deflating a small air-filled balloon mounted on the rigid foot sole that presses on the bottom of the foot. The pressure from the inflated balloon empties the PVP, thus sending venous blood back up to the heart, as shown in Figure 18-3E. Artificially increasing venous blood circulation in the lower extremities is critical for individuals who spend a considerable amount of time in bed following surgery or disease, because blood can pool in the lower limbs, which increases the risk, for example, of DVT.

3. Calf and Foot Pumps

Limb compression therapy is also used to enhance arterial blood flow into lower limb ischemic tissues, thus preventing amputation. The main purpose of using a *calf/foot pneumatic device,* such as the one shown in Figure 18-1B, is to activate both the muscle (calf) and venous (foot) pumps in order to push arterial blood into the ischemic tissues (see Fig. 18-3F). In doing so, this pneumatic system concomitantly enhances the return of venous blood and lymph to the heart.

C. MECHANICAL AND BIOCHEMICAL EFFECTS

Figure 18-4 summarizes the proposed physiologic and therapeutic effects associated with limb compression therapy. The body of scientific literature indicates that the application of external limb compression exerts both mechanical (hemodynamic) and biochemical (hematologic) effects on the vascular system (Gardner et al., 1983; Chouhan et al., 1999; Chen et al., 2001; Morris et al., 2004).

1. Mechanical Effect

When the extremities are mechanically compressed, venous blood and lymph are squeezed from the underlying superficial and deep vessels and are accelerated in a proximal direction, resulting in significant increases in venous and lymphatic flow (Chen et al., 2001). Concomitantly, arterial blood is pushed distally into the tissues. There is also an increase of hydrostatic pressure in the extracellular space, actively forcing excess fluid (edema) back into the circulation. Together, these mechanical effects prevent blood stasis and enhance revascularization (see Fig. 18-4). The mechanical effects of limb compression underlie the *treatment* for edema, whether it be traumatic, venous, or lymphatic in nature, and the treatment for venous leg ulcer, intermittent claudication, and critical limb ischemia (see later discussion).

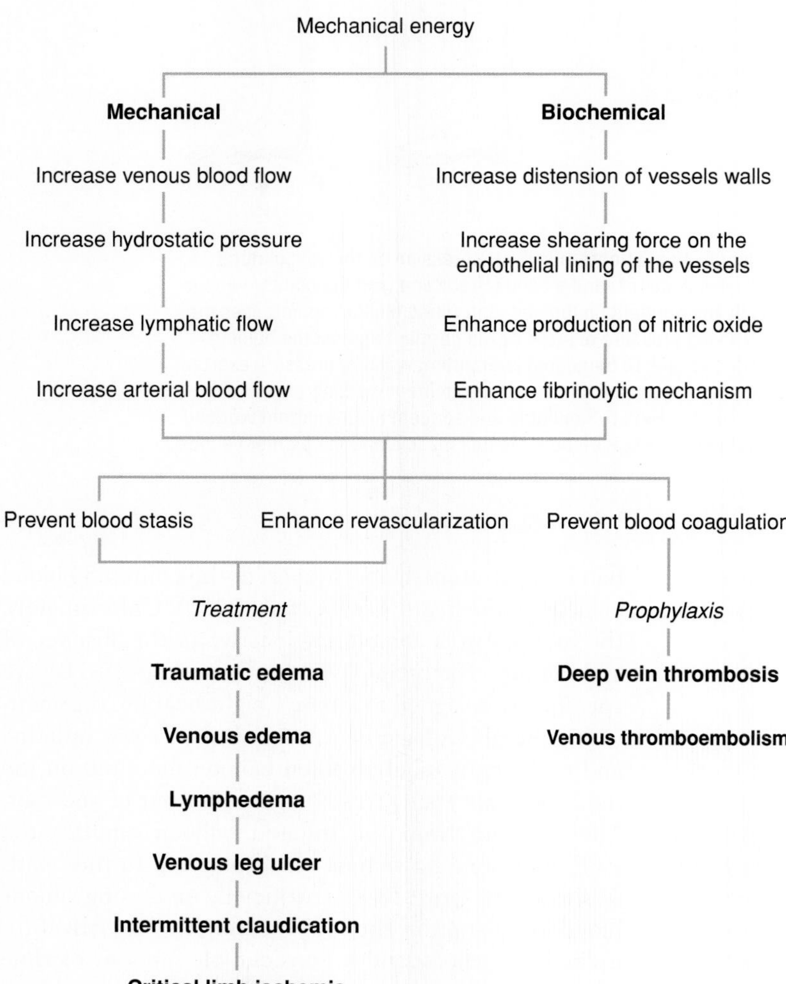

FIGURE 18-4 Proposed physiologic and therapeutic effects of limb compression therapy.

2. Biochemical Effect

Research has also shown that limb compression can cause biochemical (hematologic) effects on the peripheral vasculature. There is undisputable evidence to show that increased blood flow (see earlier discussion) in both arterial and venous systems causes distension of the vessels, resulting in increased shearing force on the endothelial lining (Comerota, 2011). It is postulated that this effect contributes to the antithrombotic effect of limb compression therapy by enhancing the fibrinolytic mechanism, which prevents blood coagulation (see Fig. 18-4). Consequently, mechanical limb compression therapy is believed to play an important role in the **prophylaxis** of DVT and VTE when pharmaceutical anticoagulation therapy (e.g., the use of warfarin [Coumadin] and heparin) is contraindicated because of the risk of increased bleeding (Hull et al., 1990; Fordyce et al., 1992; Woolson, 1996).

D. EFFECT ON EDEMA

Edema is an excessive accumulation of fluid in the interstitial space that causes swelling. The major causes of edema are trauma, venous insufficiency, and impaired lymphatic circulation. *Traumatic edema* results from fluid escaping from injured blood and lymphatic vessels, in which fluid accumulates or pools in the injured area. *Venous edema* is caused by venous insufficiency resulting from dysfunctional valves and lack of activity. *Lymphedema* is an abnormal accumulation of lymph fluid in subcutaneous tissues or body cavities resulting from inefficiency of the lymphatic drainage system. Lymphatic fluid, or lymph, is a colorless fluid that travels through the lymphatic system, which is made of vessels and nodes, carrying cells that help fight infection and disease. Lymphedema may develop following mechanic obstruction of the lymphatics or reduction of lymphatic vessels and nodes following surgery. Limb compression is a particularly useful treatment option for patients suffering from chronic venous insufficiency and lymphedema and have failed other conservative treatments such as compression garments and manual massage. The objective of compression therapy is to force venous blood and lymph out of the extremities and into central body compartments where drainage is preserved. The goals are to decrease swelling, restore function, and enhance the cosmetic aspect of the affected limb.

E. EFFECT ON VENOUS LEG ULCER

A venous leg ulcer is a necrotic crater-like lesion of the skin of the lower leg caused by chronic venous congestion. The ulcer is often associated with venous stasis, which is characterized by the formation of edema and a rise of tissue pressure (Comerota, 2011). Limb compression therapy is a treatment of choice because it can prevent blood stasis and increase venous blood circulation (O'Sullivan-Drombolis et al., 2009).

F. EFFECT ON INTERMITTENT CLAUDICATION AND CRITICAL LIMB ISCHEMIA

Emptying of the venous blood from larger veins and venules of the leg increases the arteriovenous pressure gradient. By taking advantage of this effect, pneumatic compression is presumed to improve arterial blood flow (Delis et al., 2005; Comerota, 2011). There is evidence, as shown next in the *Research-Based Indications* box, that limb compression can benefit patients with arterial occlusive diseases such as intermittent claudication and critical limb ischemia.

G. EFFECT ON DEEP VEIN THROMBOSIS AND VENOUS THROMBOEMBOLISM

DVT is a condition in which a blood clot (thrombus) forms in one or more of the deep veins in the body, usually in the legs. DVT can develop following prolonged immobilization, as well as following certain medical or surgical conditions that affect blood coagulation. DVT is a serious condition because a blood clot that has formed in the vein can break loose, travel through the bloodstream, and lodge in the lungs, blocking blood flow and causing a pulmonary embolism. VTE is a condition that includes both DVT and pulmonary embolism. It is a leading health-care problem that kills thousands of patients annually. VTE is identified as the number one *preventable* cause of death in hospitalized patients (Caprini, 2010; Lippi et al., 2011). In moderate-risk patients when pharmacologic prophylaxis is contraindicated, limb compression therapy is used as an alternative measure. High-risk patients commonly receive both pharmacologic and mechanical prophylaxis to reduce their relative risk (MacLellan et al., 2007). For nonsurgical and acutely ill hospitalized patients at increased risk for thrombosis who are bleeding or are at high risk for major bleeding, mechanical thromboprophylaxis with a compression garment and pneumatic pump is highly recommended (Khan et al., 2012).

H. RESEARCH-BASED INDICATIONS

The search for evidence behind the use of limb compression, displayed in the *Research-Based Indications* box shown earlier, led to the collection of 99 English peer-reviewed human clinical studies. The methodology and criteria used to assess the strength of evidence and therapeutic effectiveness are described in Chapter 2. As indicated, the strength of evidence is ranked as *moderate* for both the *prevention* of DVT and VTE, and for the *treatment* of traumatic and venous edema; lymphedema; venous leg ulcer; intermittent claudication; and critical limb ischemia. Overall—that is, considering all the studied health conditions as a group—the strength of evidence behind the use of limb compression is found to be *moderate* and its therapeutic effectiveness *substantiated*.

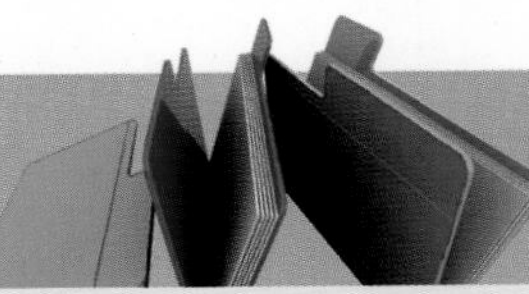

Research-Based Indications

LIMB COMPRESSION

	Benefit—Yes		Benefit—No	
Health Conditions	**Rating**	**Reference**	**Rating**	**Reference**
Deep vein thrombosis and venous thromboembolism	I	Hull et al., 1990	II	Muir et al., 2000
	I	Skillman et al., 1978		
	I	Coe et al., 1978		
	I	Fisher et al., 1995		
	I	Hartman et al., 1982		
	I	Wilson et al., 1992		
	II	Sobieraj-Teague et al., 2012		
	II	Maxell et al., 2001		
	II	Santori et al., 1994		
	II	Pedegana et al., 1977		
	II	Elliott et al., 1999		
	II	Borow et al., 1983		
	II	O'Donnell et al., 2008		
	II	Caprini et al., 1983		
	II	Daniel et al., 2008		
	II	Silbersack et al., 2004		
	II	Hansberry et al., 1991		
	II	Hass et al., 1990		
	II	Ben-Galim et al., 2004		
	II	Scurr et al., 1987		
	II	Clarke-Pearson et al., 1993		
	II	Lachiewicz et al., 2007		
	II	Bradley et al., 1993		
	II	Fordyce et al., 1992		
	II	Woolson, 1996		
	II	Soderdahl et al., 1997		
	II	Nicolaides et al., 1983		
	II	Pidala et al., 1992		
	II	Bailey et al., 1991		
	II	Johansson et al., 1998		
	II	Hooker et al., 1999		
	II	Janssen et al., 1993		
	II	Warwick et al., 1998		
	II	Kamran et al., 1998		
	II	Turpie et al., 1977		
	II	Muhe, 1984		
	II	Nicolaides et al., 1980		
	II	Spain et al., 1998		
	III	Iwama et al., 2004		

Strength of evidence: Moderate
Therapeutic effectiveness: Substantiated

Health Conditions	**Rating**	**Reference**	**Rating**	**Reference**
Traumatic and venous edema	I	Airaksinen, 1989	I	Grieveson, 2003
	I	Airaksinen et al., 1991	II	Roper et al., 1999
	I	Airaksinen et al., 1988		
	I	Jacobs et al., 1986		
	II	Airaksinen et al., 1990		
	II	Vanscheidt et al., 2009		
	II	Gurdal et al., 2012		
	II	Waterman et al., 2012		
	II	Thordarson et al., 1999		
	II	Stockle et al., 1997		
	II	Gardner et al., 1990		

Strength of evidence: Moderate
Therapeutic effectiveness: Substantiated

Health Conditions	**Rating**	**Reference**	**Rating**	**Reference**
Lymphedema	II	Franzeck et al., 1997	I	Dini et al., 1998
	II	Swedborg, 1984		
	II	Haghighat et al., 2010		
	II	Richmand et al., 1985		
	II	Pappas et al., 1992		
	II	Zanolla et al., 1984		

Health Conditions	Benefit—Yes Rating	Benefit—Yes Reference	Benefit—No Rating	Benefit—No Reference
	II	Szuba et al., 2002		
	II	Pilch et al., 2009		
	II	Szolnoky et al., 2009		
	II	Didem et al., 2005		
	III	Swedborg, 1977		
	III	Klein et al., 1988		
	III	Alexander et al., 1983		
	III	Kim-Sing et al., 1987		
Strength of evidence: Moderate **Therapeutic effectiveness:** Substantiated				
Venous leg ulcer	I	Hazarika et al., 1981		
	I	Armstrong et al., 2000		
	II	Nikolovska et al., 2005		
	II	Samson, 1993		
	II	Smith et al., 1990		
	II	Rowland, 2000		
	II	Kumar et al., 2002		
	II	Alpagut et al., 2005		
	II	Pfizenmaier et al., 2005		
	II	McCulloch et al., 1994		
	II	Schuler et al., 1996		
	III	Hofman, 1995		
	III	Mulder et al., 1990		
	III	McCulloch, 1981		
	III	Wunderlich et al., 1998		
Strength of evidence: Moderate **Therapeutic effectiveness:** Substantiated				
Critical limb ischemia and intermittent claudication	I	Delis et al., 2000c		
	I	Delis et al., 2000d		
	I	Delis et al., 2000e		
	I	Kavros et al., 2008		
	II	Delis et al., 2000b		
	II	Delis et al., 2001		
	II	Van Bemmelen et al., 2000		
	II	Van Bemmelen et al., 2001		
	II	Delis et al, 2005		
	II	Ramaswami et al., 2005		
	II	Kakkos et al., 2005		
	II	Louridas et al., 2002		
	II	Gaskell et al., 1978		
	II	Montori et al., 2002		
	II	Sultan et al., 2008		
	II	Sultan et al., 2011		
Strength of evidence: Moderate **Therapeutic effectiveness:** Substantiated				
ALL CONDITIONS **Strength of evidence:** Moderate **Therapeutic effectiveness:** Substantiated				

V. DOSIMETRY

A. COMPRESSION BANDAGES

Table 18-2 lists key dosimetric considerations related to the application of compression bandages. Bandages offer constant graded elastic resting and working pressure on the limb over which they are applied. Sub-bandage pressure is based on Laplace's law. In cases where the bandage width (W) is constant, and only one layer is applied (N), the pressure is thus directly proportional to the bandage tensile force (T) and inversely proportional to the limb circumference (C) over which it is applied. Compression bandages may exert pressure ranging between 10 and 80 mm Hg when correctly wrapped around the limbs following manufacturer recommendations.

1. Inelastic Short Stretch

These bandages present low resting and high working pressure. Low resting pressure prevents the tourniquet effect at rest, and high working pressure provides the necessary counterforce to the contracting muscles during work or movement. Because they are well tolerated due to their low resting pressure, they may be applied for several consecutive days at a time, making them particularly suitable for the treatment of various types of edema and venous leg ulcers in mobile patients (see Table 18-2).

2. Elastic Long Stretch

These bandages have the exact opposite effect. Their low working pressure does not offer adequate resistance against the contracting muscles, and fluid would inevitably accumulate. In addition, their high resting pressure

TABLE 18-2 COMPRESSION BANDAGE DOSIMETRIC CONSIDERATIONS

	Compression Bandage		
	Pressure*		
Type	**Resting**	**Working**	**Indication**
Inelastic short stretch**	Low	High	Edema—traumatic, venous, and lymphatic Venous leg ulcer
Elastic long stretch***	High	Low	Deep vein thrombosis Venous thromboembolism
Semi-elastic multilayer****	Mid	Mid	All the above indications

*Sub-bandage pressure is based on Laplace's law and is calculated as follows: $P = (T \times N) / (C \times W)$, where P is pressure, T is the bandage tensile force, N is the number of layers, C is the limb circumference, and W is the bandage width.
**Well tolerated because of low resting pressure. May be applied for several consecutive days.
***Poorly tolerated because of high resting pressure. Applied for only a few hours at a time.
****Offers compromise between the short- and long-stretch bandages.

could cause a tourniquet effect if applied for too long under no supervision. These bandages, precisely because of their high resting pressure, are indicated for the prophylaxis of DVT and VTE in bedridden patients, thus preventing blood stasis in their extremities. Because they may be particularly uncomfortable due to their high resting pressure, these bandages may need to be removed after a few hours and reapplied later (see Table 18-2).

3. Semi-Elastic Multilayer

These bandages exert moderate resting and working pressure on the limb, thus offering the benefits of both short-stretch and long-stretch bandages.

B. COMPRESSION STOCKING AND SLEEVE

In contrast to short-term treatment with compression bandages, compression stockings and sleeve are designed for the long-term and permanent treatment of venous problems. They are used when the compression bandages have already relieved congestion. The stockings ensure the therapy results achieved so far and prevent any recurrence. Compression stockings and sleeves also offer graded elastic resting and working pressure on the extremities. Table 18-3 lists key dosimetric considerations related to their application. These garments are classified based on the pressure they can exert on the limb, of which pressure is standardized for the ankle (lower limb stocking) and wrist (upper limb sleeve), respectively. For example, selecting a 30 mm Hg stocking for therapy thus implies that this garment, when properly fitted for limb length and circumference, exerts a pressure of 30 mm Hg at the ankle. As indicated in the table, stockings and sleeves are indicated for the treatment of chronic venous insufficiency and lymphedema, where pressure is needed for prolonged periods. The more severe the condition, the higher the garment pressure level should be (see Table 18-3).

TABLE 18-3 COMPRESSION STOCKING AND SLEEVE DOSIMETRIC CONSIDERATIONS

Pressure Classes*			Indication
I	Mild	15–20 mm Hg	Functional venous insufficiency (varicose vein) Light lymphedema
II	Moderate	21–30 mm Hg	Mild chronic vein insufficiency
III	Strong	31–40 mm Hg	More advanced chronic vein insufficiency Venous leg ulcer Moderate lymphedema
IV	Very strong	>41 mm Hg	Severe chronic vein insufficiency Severe lymphedema

*Pressure is based on Laplace's law and is calculated as follows: $P = T/C$, where P is pressure, T is the stocking/sleeve tensile force, and C is the limb circumference. Stocking (lower limb) and sleeve (upper limb) pressure is standardized for the ankle and wrist, respectively. Proper fitting requires precise limb circumferential and length measurements.

TABLE 18-4 COMPRESSION PNEUMATIC PUMP DOSIMETRIC CONSIDERATIONS

System	Pressure	Inflation/Deflation	Indication
Limb	*Upper limb:* 30–60 mm Hg *Lower limb:* 40–80 mm Hg	Slow inflation/deflation cycles mimic normal muscle contraction	Edema—traumatic, venous, and lymphatic Venous leg ulcer Deep vein thrombosis Venous thromboembolism
Foot	Up to 130 mm Hg	Rapid inflation and deflation cycles mimic normal weight bearing during ambulation	Critical limb ischemia Intermittent claudication

C. PNEUMATIC PUMP SYSTEMS

Pneumatic pump systems are made of an electric pump connected to air-inflatable garments using plastic tubing. These pneumatic systems offer intermittent, programmable, uniform, and graded resting and working pressures on the limb (see Fig. 18-2). If the air-inflatable limb garments have more than one chamber, they also offer sequential pressure delivery. Three basic pneumatic systems are available. The first system is designed to treat the entire upper and lower extremities using specially made single- and multiple-chamber garments. Its purpose is to activate the muscle pump through simulated intermittent muscle contractions (see Fig. 18-3D). The second system is made of a pump connected to a specially designed air-inflatable foot cuff. This system activates the venous foot pump by repeatedly flattening the PVP, thus mimicking weight bearing (see Fig. 18-3F). It is indicated when there is dressing or cast, making it impossible to wrap upper and lower garments around the affected limb. The third system is made of a pump connected to a foot and calf air-inflatable cuff. Its purpose is to activate both the calf muscle pump and the foot pump (see Fig. 18-3E–F).

1. Limb Pressure Gradient

There is consensus in the scientific and corporate literature that pressure gradients used for the *upper extremities* should range between 30 and 60 mm Hg—that is, below the patient's resting diastolic pressure, which should be about 80 mm Hg. Because venous pressure is usually higher in the lower extremities, there is also a consensus that pressure gradients used for the *lower extremities* should be between 40 and 80 mm Hg, and as high as 130 mm Hg on some occasions (Delis et al., 2000a) (Table 18-4). Limb compression systems are indicated for the treatment of edema and venous leg ulcers, as well as for the prophylaxis of DVT and VTE.

2. Foot Pressure Gradient

There is evidence to show that in order to effectively empty the PVP, intermittent larger pressure gradients that are similar to those generated during weight bearing, which can be as high as 130 mm Hg, need to be applied under the foot (Morris et al., 2004). Foot and calf-foot compression systems are mainly used for enhancing arterial blood flow in patients suffering from critical limb ischemia and intermittent claudication.

3. Inflation and Deflation Time

The inflation (compression) and deflation (decompression) times of garments are programmable, often ranging between 1 and 120 seconds, yielding slow to more rapid compression cycles. Pressure settings are also programmable. With multiple-chamber garments, pressure settings may yield both uniform and graded pressure (see Fig. 18-2).

4. Treatment Duration and Frequency

Compression garments are wearable agents that may be applied for several hours daily, or applied for a 24-hour period over consecutive days. Compression pump systems, on the other hand, are not wearable and are applied up to 1 hour at the time, one to three times daily.

V. APPLICATION, CONTRAINDICATIONS, AND RISKS

Prior to considering the application of limb compression, practitioners must first check for contraindications, consider the risks, and then go through key application steps and procedures designed to optimize treatment safety, efficacy, and effectiveness. Important elements of this protocol involve the proper fitting of garments, which requires precise limb circumferential and length measurements. It is critical to look for the presence of DVT or VTE prior to considering limb compression therapy. Monitoring of the patient's blood pressure before, during, and after therapy is very important to minimize the occurrence of adverse effects. To visualize and get more details on the application of some compression garments and pneumatic pump systems, readers are invited to view selected **online videos.**

APPLICATION, CONTRAINDICATIONS, AND RISKS

Limb Compression

IMPORTANT: Conduct *thorough* vascular and pulmonary examinations prior to consider limb compression therapy in order to exclude all contraindications. Monitor blood pressure before, during, and at the end of treatment to determine whether the treatment may be harmful. End treatment if significant blood pressure changes occur. Note that limb compression therapy is for the *prevention,* not treatment, of deep vein thrombosis (DVT). Illustrated, as examples, are the applications of a foot (Fig. 18-5) and foot-calf (Fig. 18-6) pump compression systems.

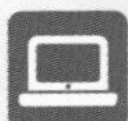

See **online videos.**

ALL AGENTS

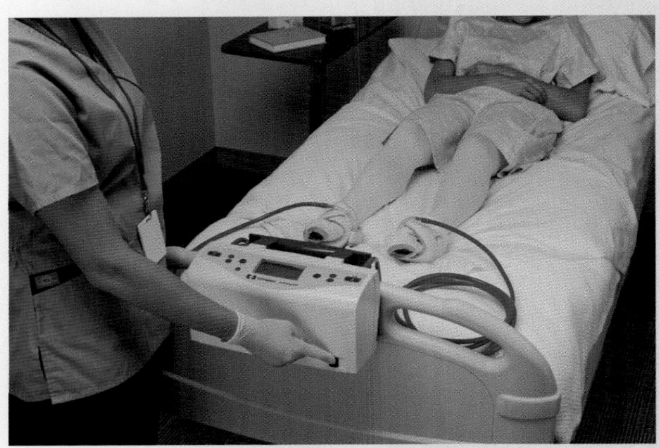

FIGURE 18-5 Application of a compressive foot pump system at bedside. (A-V Impulse System is a trademark of a Covidien company © Covidien. All rights reserved.)

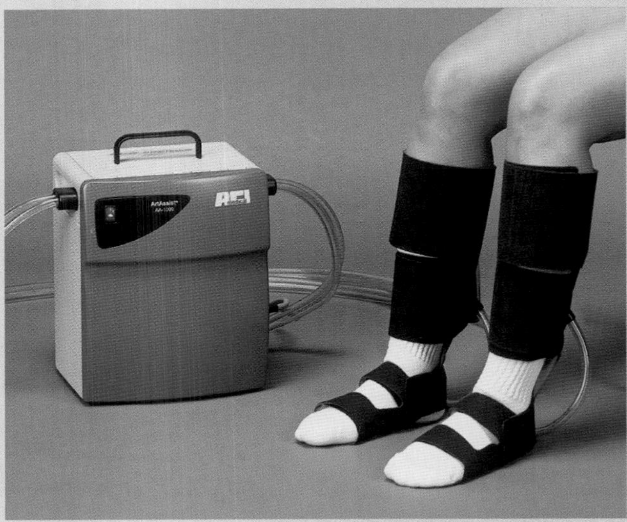

FIGURE 18-6 Application of a compressive foot-calf pump system in seated position. (Courtesy of ACI Medical.)

STEP	RATIONALE
1. Check for contraindications.	*Peripheral arterial insufficiency*—tissue ischemia *Acute dermatitis*—damage to the skin and pain *Acute microbial infection*—promote an environment conductive to infection by increasing moisture and temperature *Malignant tumor*—aggravation from increasing temperature *Neuropathy*—aggravation from further compression of the nerves
2. Consider the risks.	*In cases of occult arterial diseases*—risk of developing a foot ulcer following intermittent pneumatic compression (IPC) treatment, most likely caused by occult arterial disease (Oakley et al., 1998) *Malfunctioning of IPC device*—risk of developing an acute compartment due to malfunctioning of IPC devices (Werbel et al., 1986) *In cases of limb lymphedema*—risk of developing genital edema when the IPC device is used for lower limb lymphedema (Boris et al., 1998)

STEP	RATIONALE
	Peroneal nerve compression—risk of nerve compression at the level of the fibula head. Cases of peroneal nerve palsy have been documented (Pittman, 1989; Lachman et al., 1992; McGrory et al., 2000; Fukuda, 2006). *In-hospital patient falls*—IPC devices are rarely associated with in-hospital patients falls (Boelig et al., 2011)

WEARABLE COMPRESSION GARMENTS

NOTE: In hospital treatment settings (inpatient), these garments (bandages, stockings, and sleeves) are both applied and removed by practitioners themselves with patients playing a passive role. In home-based treatment settings (outpatient), patients play a very active role in that they are asked to put on and remove these garments by themselves by using donning and doffing aids.

STEP	RATIONALE
1. Check for contraindications.	See All Agents section.
2. Consider the risks.	See All Agents section.
3. Instruct patient.	• *Inpatient:* Ensure comfortable position that promote muscle relaxation. • *Outpatient:* Explain that compressive garments need to be worn over the affected area daily according to your treatment schedule.
4. Prepare treatment area.	Remove clothing and jewelry, and inspect the skin area.
5. Select the appropriate garment.	Select between bandages, stockings, or sleeves. See Tables 18-2 and 18-3 for guidelines.
6. Apply the garment.	There are various types of compressive garments on the market, and each requires a special technique of application, often by using donning and doffing aids. To describe the steps related to these various techniques is thus beyond the scope of this textbook. Follow manufacturers' recommended technique of application, and see **online videos.** 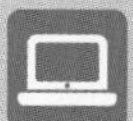
7. Conduct post-treatment procedures.	Remove the garment, and inspect the exposed skin surface and treated area. Question the patient on the level of pressure perceived during treatment.
8. Ensure post-treatment equipment maintenance.	Follow manufacturers' maintenance recommendations. Wash or discard stockinette after therapy to ensure optimal hygiene. To enhance compliance with treatment, educate patients and staff about the importance of compliance with treatment (Anglen et al., 1998; Cornwell et al., 2002; Segers et al., 2002).

PNEUMATIC PUMP

STEP	RATIONALE
1. Check for contraindications.	*Suspected or known DVT and pulmonary embolism*—aggravation because the thrombus may dislodge, or the embolus may travel under the compression force and block arteries to vital organs *Suspected or known acute infections of the skin, such as cellulitis*—aggravation

STEP	RATIONALE
	Suspected or known thrombophlebitis—aggravation *Severe arteriosclerosis or other ischemic vascular disease*—aggravation because the intermittent closing down of the damaged arteries may further impair circulation in the area *Local dermatologic conditions, such as dermatitis and skin grafts*—aggravation by garments *Active metastatic disease affecting the limb*—aggravation *Over unstable fracture*—affects adequate bone union because of bone movement caused by the compressive force *Uncontrolled hypertension*—increases blood pressure to a dangerous level by increasing vascular load on the heart *Congestive heart failure and pulmonary edema*—increases the vascular load on the failing organ system caused by the shifting of blood from the peripheral to the central circulation *Obstructed venous/lymphatic return*—increases load (blood and lymph) on these systems because the obstruction to return flow does not allow adequate circulation
2. Consider the risks.	See All Agents section.
3. Position and instruct the patient.	Ask the patient to empty the bladder. Ensure comfortable body positioning and place the affected extremity in an elevated position. Inform the patient that he or she will feel cycles of limb compression and decompression.
4. Prepare treatment area.	Remove all jewelry and clothing. For sanitation and comfort purposes, cover the treated limb segment with a cylindrical cotton bandage or stockinette. Make sure that it is free of wrinkles before sliding the air-filled garment over it.
5. Select pump and garment system.	*For upper and lower limbs:* Select pump with single- or multiple-chamber garment system. *For foot or foot-calf only:* Select pump with foot only or foot-calf garment system. Check for garment leaks and tears to ensure optimal treatment efficacy.
6. Select compression mode.	Choose between intermittent uniform, intermittent sequential uniform, and intermittent sequential graded mode.
7. Set dosimetry.	See Table 18-3 for guidance.
8. Apply treatment.	Connect garment to pump with tubing. View **online videos** for further details on the techniques of application. Ensure adequate monitoring. Elevate the limb to obtain the gravitational effect. Watch for episodes of numbness and tingling during therapy, because peripheral nerve compression, caused by compressive force, may lead to nerve damage. Plug devices into ground-fault circuit interrupter (GFCI) receptacles to eliminate the risk of electrical shock (see Chapter 5 for details). 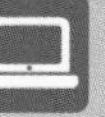
9. Conduct post-treatment procedures.	Inspect the exposed skin surface and limb area. Question the patient about the level of pressure perceived during treatment. Wash the exposed limb (to remove sweat) and the stockinette. Put back the graded compression garment for future use.
10. Ensure post-treatment equipment maintenance.	Follow manufacturer recommendations. Immediately report defects or malfunctions to technical maintenance staff.

CASE STUDIES

Presented are two case studies that summarize the concepts, principles, and applications of limb compression therapy discussed in this chapter. Case Study 18-1 addresses the use of pneumatic compression for the prophylaxis of DVT following total hip replacement surgery in a 58-year-old male patient. Case Study 18-2 is concerned with the treatment of breast cancer–related lymphedema affecting a 63-year-old female patient. Each case is structured in line with the concepts of evidence-based practice (EBP), the International Classification of Functioning, Disability, and Health (ICF) disablement model, and SOAP (*s*ubjective, *o*bjective, *a*ssessment, *p*lan) note format (see Chapter 2 for details).

CASE STUDY 18-1: DEEP VEIN THROMBOSIS

EVIDENCE-BASED CLINICAL DECISION MAKING PROTOCOL

1. Formulate the Case History

A 58-year-old male elite golfer is scheduled for a total replacement of his right hip because of severe osteoarthritis. One of the most potentially lethal complications in the early postoperative period of surgery is deep vein thrombosis (DVT) caused by venous stasis, which may lead to pulmonary embolism. Prevention of DVT is therefore essential in the management of this patient who has a history of thromboembolism and hypertension. His hypertension problem is currently under control. The orthopedic surgeon is well aware that the prevention of DVT using drug anticoagulation therapy (such as warfarin [Coumadin] or heparin) is often associated with a major complication—namely, severe bleeding of soft tissue. The surgeon, considering this possible complication and the patient's history of thromboembolism, decides to manage the risk of DVT by using mechanical intermittent limb compression. The surgeon handles the intraoperative portion of the compression treatment and refers his patient for the postoperative portion of this treatment (day 2 to discharge from hospital). Contrary to all other case studies presented in this textbook, the treatment goal here is the *prevention* of post-surgical DVT.

2. Outline the Case Based on the ICF Framework

PROPHYLAXIS OF DEEP VEIN THROMBOSIS		
BODY STRUCTURES AND FUNCTIONS	**ACTIVITIES**	**PARTICIPATION**
Hip pain	Difficulty walking	Inability to play golf
Decreased hip range of motion (ROM)	Difficulty ascending and descending stairs	

PERSONAL FACTOR	ENVIRONMENTAL FACTOR
Athletic man	Competitive sport

3. Outline Therapeutic Goals and Outcome Measurements

GOAL	OUTCOME MEASUREMENT
Prevent DVT	Clinical monitoring for signs of DVT Doppler ultrasonographic screening

4. Justify the Use of Limb Compression Based on the EBP Framework

PRACTITIONER'S EXPERIENCE	RESEARCH-BASED INDICATIONS	PATIENT'S EXPECTATION
Experienced in limb compression	*Strength:* Moderate	None
Has used this agent occasionally in similar cases	*Effectiveness:* Substantiated	
Is convinced that limb compression will be beneficial		

5. Outline Key Intervention Parameters

- **Treatment base:** Hospital
- **Compression method:** Pneumatic pump with lower limb garment
- **Compression mode:** Intermittent sequential graded
- **Risk and precaution:** Although this patient has a history of hypertension, limb compression therapy can be safely used in this case because his hypertensive condition is under control.
- **Application protocol:** Follow the suggested application protocol for pneumatic pump in *Application, Contraindications and Risks* box, and make the necessary adjustments for this case. See **online videos**.

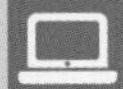

- **Patient's positioning:** Lying supine in bed with the lower extremities elevated
- **Garment type:** 3 chambers—foot (D), leg (I) and thigh (P)
- **Graded pressure gradients (mm Hg):** D: 90; I: 70; P: 50
- **Inflation time (s):** D 80; I 80; P 80
- **Hold time (s):** D: 140; I: 80; P: 20
- **Deflation time (s):** Synchronous 50
- **Application duration:** 18 hours a day with periodic removal of the garment for bathing and sleeping
- **Concomitant therapy:** Daily orthopedic nursing care

6. Report Pre- and Post-Intervention Outcomes

OUTCOME	PRE	POST
DVT	None	None

7. Document Case Intervention Using the SOAP Note Format

S: Senior male Pt referred for the prevention of DVT following total hip replacement surgery.

O: *Intervention:* Pneumatic intermittent sequential graded compression to affected LE; 3-chamber garment; pressure gradients: D 90, I 70, P 50 mm Hg; inflation time: 60 s for each chamber; deflation time: synchronous 50 s; applied for approximately 18 hours daily. *Pre–post comparison:* No sign of DVT as measured by Doppler ultrasonographic screening.

A: Treatment well tolerated. No adverse effect.

P: No further treatment required. Prognosis is excellent if the Pt continues to wear graduated compression stockings at home for a few days and gradually increases his weight-bearing duration and walking distance.

CASE STUDY 18-2: POST-MASTECTOMY LYMPHEDEMA

EVIDENCE-BASED CLINICAL DECISION MAKING PROTOCOL

1. Formulate the Case History

A 63-year-old woman presents with moderate lymphedema, according to the Stillwell classification for lymphedema, affecting her right upper limb 3 months post mastectomy for right breast cancer. The combination of elevation and manual lymphatic drainage at home failed to provide adequate control. She wants a home base treatment that will provide long-term compression while keeping her arm mobility. She is ready to purchase the compression sleeve and the donning and doffing aids. Circumferential measurements on the affected limb, when compared to the contralateral side, are as follows: wrist +6 cm; elbow +10 cm; axilla +5 cm. She is concerned about the limited function of her right arm and about the cosmetic aspect of her condition. Her main goal is to optimize function in her dominant limb in order to do all of her activities of daily living (ADLs). Her dream is to be able to play tennis once again.

2. Outline the Case Based on the ICF Framework

POST-MASTECTOMY LYMPHEDEMA		
BODY STRUCTURES AND FUNCTIONS	**ACTIVITIES**	**PARTICIPATION**
Lymphedema	Difficulty with right upper limb function	Difficulty with ADLs. Inability to play tennis

PERSONAL FACTORS	ENVIRONMENTAL FACTORS
Middle-aged woman	Married
Healthy	Retired
Active	

3. Outline Therapeutic Goals and Outcome Measurements

GOAL	OUTCOME MEASUREMENT
Decrease lymphedema	Circumferential tape measurement
Enhance limb function	American Shoulder and Elbow Surgeons (ASES) Questionnaire

4. Justify the Use of Limb Compression Based on the EBP Framework

PRACTITIONER'S EXPERIENCE	RESEARCH-BASED INDICATIONS	PATIENT'S EXPECTATION
Experienced in the use of compression garments	*Strength:* Moderate	Has no expectation
Has used this agent in similar cases	*Effectiveness:* Substantiated	
Believes that limb compression will be beneficial		

5. Outline Key Intervention Parameters

- **Treatment base:** Home
- **Compression method:** Upper limb sleeve
- **Doffing and donning aids:** Gloves and metallic butler
- **Application protocol:** Follow the suggested application protocol for compressive garments in Application, Contraindications, and Risks, and make the necessary adjustments for this case. See **online videos.**

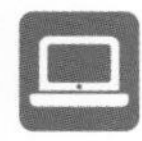

- **Graded pressure gradients (mm Hg):** 35 mm Hg
- **Application duration:** 18 hours a day with periodic removal of the garment for bathing and sleeping
- **Treatment duration:** 6 months
- **Concomitant therapies:** Skin care and self-massage

6. Report Pre- and Post-Intervention Outcomes

OUTCOME	PRE	POST
Edema—arm circumference	*Wrist:* +6 cm *Elbow:* +10 cm *Axilla:* +5 cm	*Wrist:* +2 cm *Elbow:* +3 cm *Axilla:* +1 cm
Upper limb function (ASES score)	10	21

7. Document Case Intervention Using the SOAP Note Format

S: Middle-aged female Pt presents with moderate right upper limb lymphedema following mastectomy.

O: *Intervention:* Compression sleeve; pressure: 35 mm Hg; application duration: approximately 18 hours daily min;

treatment duration: 6 months. *Pre–post comparison:* Lymphedema reduction: wrist from 6 to 2 cm; elbow from 10 to 3 cm; axilla from 5 to 1 cm. Improved upper arm function: ASES score from 10 to 21.

A: Treatment difficult to tolerate at the beginning but well tolerated thereafter. No adverse effect. Pt very pleased with therapeutic outcomes.

P: Treatment continued for another 3 months or until the Pt is satisfied with the results.

VI. THE BOTTOM LINE

- There is strong scientific evidence to show that limb compression can induce significant vascular effects on the venous, arterial, and lymphatic systems.
- Limb compression rests on the delivery of mechanical elastic and pneumatic energy.
- Limb compression therapy is delivered by using wearable compression garments, such as bandages, stockings, and sleeves, and nonwearable programmable pneumatic pumps connected to air-inflatable garments with flexible plastic tubing.
- Compression garments and pneumatic pump systems offer both resting and working pressure on the affected limb.
- Compression garments exert passive, continuous, and graded pressure on the resting and working affected limb.
- Compression pneumatic systems exert an active, intermittent, sequential, uniform, and graded pressure on the resting limb by producing cycles of compression (inflation) and decompression (deflation) that mimic muscle and venous pumps.
- Limb compression plays a major role in the prophylaxis of DVT and VTE.
- Limb compression plays an important role in the treatment of edema (traumatic, venous, lymphatic), venous leg ulcer, intermittent claudication, and critical limb ischemia.
- Dosimetry consists of selecting the required pressure gradient and adequately fitting the garment based on specific and precise limb circumferential and length measurements.
- The overall body of evidence reported in this chapter shows the strength of evidence behind limb compression therapy to be *moderate* and its level of therapeutic effectiveness *substantiated*.

VII. CRITICAL THINKING QUESTIONS

Clarification: What is meant by pneumatic intermittent, sequential, and graded pressure?

Assumptions: You assume that the use of limb compression therapy as an alternative to drugs for the prevention of DVT is well justified. How do you justify making that assumption?

Reasons and evidence: What leads you to believe that limb compression therapy can induce significant mechanical and biochemical changes on the peripheral vascular system?

Viewpoints or perspectives: How will you respond to a colleague who says that there is no difference between the pressure exerted by an elastic garment and that of an air-inflated garment?

Implications and consequences: What are the implications and possible consequences of a failure to record the patient's blood pressure before and during intermittent pneumatic compression treatment?

About the question: Can limb compression therapy be beneficial for patients suffering from vascular intermittent claudication and critical limb ischemia? Why do you think I ask this question?

VIII. REFERENCES

Articles

Airaksinen O (1989) Changes in post traumatic ankle joint mobility, pain, and edema following intermittent pneumatic compression therapy. Arch Phys Med Rehab, 70: 341–344

Airaksinen O, Kolari PJ, Herve R, Holopainen R (1988) Treatment of post traumatic edema in lower legs using intermittent pneumatic compression. Scand J Rehab Med, 20: 25–28

Airaksinen O, Kolari PJ, Miettinen H (1990) Elastic bandages and intermittent pneumatic compression for treatment of acute ankle sprains. Arch Phys Med Rehab, 71: 380–383

Airaksinen O, Partanen K, Kolari PJ, Soimakallio S (1991) Intermittent pneumatic compression therapy in post traumatic lower limb edema: Computed tomography and clinical measurements. Arch Phys Med Rehab, 72: 667–670

Alexander M, Wright E, Wright J, Wright JB, Bikowski JB (1983) Lymphedema treated with linear pump: Pediatric case report. Arch Phys Med Rehab, 64: 132–133

Alpagut U, Davioglu E (2005) Importance and advantages of intermittent external pneumatic compression therapy in venous stasis ulceration. Angiology, 56: 19–23

Anglen JO, Goss K, Edwards J, Huckfeldt RE (1998) Foot pump prophylaxis for deep venous thrombosis: The rate of effective usage in trauma patients. Am J Orthop, 27: 580–582

Armstrong DG, Nguyen HC (2000) Intermittent pneumatic compression promoted healing in foot infections. Arch Surg, 135: 1405–1409

Bailey JP, Kruger MP, Solano FX, Zajko AB, Rubash HE (1991) Prospective randomized trial of sequential compression devices vs low-dose warfarin for deep venous thrombosis prophylaxis in total hip arthroplasty. J Arthroplasty, 6: 29–35

Ben-Galim P, Steinberg EL, Rosenblatt Y, Parnes N, Manehem A, Arbel R (2004) A miniature and mobile intermittent pneumatic compression device for the prevention of deep-vein thrombosis after joint replacement. Acta Orthop Scand, 75: 584–587

Boelig MM, Streiff MB, Hobson DB, Kraus PS, Pronovost PJ, Haut ER (2011) Are sequential compression devices commonly associated with in-hospital falls? A myth-busters review using the patient safety net database. J Patient Saf, 7: 77–79

Boris M, Weindorf S, Lasinski BB (1998) The risk of genital edema after external pump compression for lower limb lymphedema. Lymphology, 31: 15–20

Borow M, Goldson HJ (1983) Prevention of postoperative deep venous thrombosis and pulmonary emboli with combined modalities. Am Surg, 49: 599–605

Bradley JG, Krugener GH, Jager HJ (1993) The effectiveness of intermittent plantar venous compression in prevention of deep venous thrombosis after total hip arthroplasty. J Arthroplasty, 1: 57–61

Caprini JA, Chucker JL, Zukerman L (1983) Thrombosis prophylaxis using external compression. Surg Gynecol Obstet, 156: 599–604

Chouhan VD, Comerota AJ, Sun L, Harada R, Gaughan JP, Rao AK (1999) Inhibition of tissue factor pathway during intermittent pneumatic compression: A possible mechanism for antithrombotic effect. Arterioscler Thromb Vasc Biol, 19: 2812–2817

Clarke-Pearson DL, Synan IS, Dodge R, Soper JT, Berchusk A, Coleman RE (1993) A randomized trial of low-dose heparin and intermittent pneumatic calf compression for the prevention of deep venous thrombosis after gynecologic oncology surgery. Am J Obstet Gynecol, 168: 1146–1154

Coe NP, Collins Re, Klein LA, Bettmann MA, Skillman JJ, Shapiro RM, Salzman EW (1978) Prevention of deep vein thrombosis in urological patients: A controlled randomized trial of low-dose heparin and external pneumatic compression boots. Surgery, 83: 230–234

Corley GJ, Broderick BJ, Nestor SM, Breen PP, Grace PA, Quondamatteo F, Olaighin G (2010) The anatomy and physiology of the venous foot pump. Anat Rec (Hoboken), 293: 370–378

Cornwell EE, Chang D, Velmahos G, Jindal A, Baker D, Phillips J, Bonar J, Campbell K (2002) Compliance with sequential compression device prophylaxis in at-risk trauma patients: A prospective analysis. Am Surg, 68: 470–473

Daniel J, Pradhan A, Pradhan C, Ziaee H, Moss M, Freeman J, McMinn DJ (2008) Multimodal thromboprophylaxis following primary hip arthroplasty: The role of adjuvant intermittent pneumatic compression. J Bone Joint Surg (B), 90: 562–569

Delis KT, Azizi ZA, Stevens RJ, Wolfe JH, Nicolaides AN (2000a) Optimum intermittent pneumatic compression stimulus for lower-limb venous emptying. Eur J Vasc Endovasc Surg, 19: 261–269

Delis KT, Husmann MJ, Cheshire NJ, Nicolaides AN (2001) Effects of intermittent pneumatic compression of the calf and thigh on arterial calf inflow: A study of normals, claudicants, and grafted arteriopaths. Surgery, 129: 188–195

Delis KT, Labropoulos N, Nicolaides AN, Glenville B, Stansby G (2000b) Effect of intermittent pneumatic compression on popliteal artery heamodynamics. Eur J Vasc Endovac Surg, 19: 270–277

Delis KT, Nicolaides AN (2005) Effects of intermittent pneumatic compression of foot and calf on walking distance, hemodynamics, and quality of life in patients with arterial claudication: A prospective randomized controlled study with 1-year follow-up. Ann Surg, 241: 431–441

Delis KT, Nicolaides AN, Labropoulos N, Stansby G (2000c) The acute effects of intermittent pneumatic foot versus calf versus simultaneous foot and calf compression on popliteal artery hemodynamics: A comparative study. J Vasc Surg, 32: 284–292

Delis KT, Nicolaides AN, Wolfe JH, Stansby G (2000d) Improving walking ability and ankle brachial pressure indices in symptomatic peripheral vascular disease with intermittent pneumatic foot compression: A prospective controlled study with a one-year follow-up. J Vasc Surg, 31: 650–651

Delis KT, Slimani G, Hafez HM, Nicolaides AN (2000e) Enhancing venous outflow in the lower limb with intermittent pneumatic compression: A comparative haemodynamic analysis on the effect of foot vs. calf vs. foot and calf compression. Eur J Vasc Endovasc Surg, 19: 250–260

Didem K, Ufuk YS, Serfar S, Zumre A (2005) The comparison of two different physiotherapy methods in treatment of lymphedema after breast surgery. Breast Cancer Res Treat, 93: 49–54

Dini D, Del Mastro L, Gozza A, Lionetto O, Forno G, Vidili G, Bertelli G, Venturini M (1998) The role of pneumatic compression in the treatment of post mastectomy lymphedema: A randomized phase III study. Ann Oncol, 9: 187–190

Elliott CG, Dudney TM, Egger M, Orme JF, Clemmer TP, Horn SD, Waever L, Handrahan D, Thomas F, Merrell S, Kitterman N, Yeates S (1999) Calf-thigh sequential pneumatic compression compared with plantar venous pneumatic compression to prevent deep vein thrombosis after non-lower extremity trauma. J Trauma, 47: 25–32

Fisher CG, Blachut PA, Salvian AJ, Meek RN, O'Brien PJ (1995) Effectiveness of pneumatic compression devices for the prevention of thromboembolic disease in orthopeadic trauma patients: A prospective, randomized study of compression alone versus no prophylaxis. J Orthop Trauma, 9: 1–7

Fordyce MJ, Ling RS (1992) A venous foot pump reduces thrombosis after total hip replacement. J Bone Joint Surg (B), 74: 45–49

Franzeck UK, Spiegel I, Fischer M, Bortzler C, Stahel HU, Bollinger A (1997) Combined physical therapy for lymphedema evaluated by fluorescence microlymphography and lymph capillary pressure measurements. J Vasc Res, 34: 306–311

Fukuda H (2006) Bilateral peroneal nerve palsy caused by intermittent pneumatic compression. Intern Med, 45: 93–94

Gardner AM, Fox RH (1983) The venous pump of the human foot—preliminary report. Bristol Med Chir J, 367: 109–112

Gardner AM, Fox RH, Lawrence C, Bunker TD, Ling RS, McEachen AG (1990) Reduction of posttraumatic swelling and compartment pressure by impulse compression of the foot. J Bone Joint Surg (B), 72: 810–815

Gaskell P, Parrott JC (1978) The effect of a mechanical venous pump on the circulation of the feet in the presence of arterial obstruction. Surg Gynecol Obstet, 146: 583–592

Grieveson G (2003) Intermittent pneumatic compression pump settings for optimum reduction of oedema. J Tissue Viab, 13: 98–110

Gurdal SO, Kostanoglu A, Cavdar I, Ozbas A, Cabioglu N, Ozcinar B, Igci A, Muslumanoglu M, Ozmen V (2012) Comparison of intermittent pneumatic compression with manual lymphatic drainage for treatment of breast cancer-related lymphedema. Lymph Res Biol, 10: 129–135

Haghighat S, Lofti-Tokaldany M, Yunesian M, Akbari ME, Nazemi F, Weiss J (2010) Comparing two treatment methods for post mastectomy lymphedema: Complex decongestive therapy alone and in combination with intermittent pneumatic compression. Lymphology, 43: 25–33

Hansberry KL, Thompson IM, Bauman J, Deppe S, Rodrigez FR (1991) A prospective comparison of thromboembolic stockings, external sequential pneumatic compression stockings and heparin sodium/dihydroergotamine mesylate for the prevention of thromboembolitic complications in urological surgery. J Urol, 145: 1205–1208

Hartman JT, Pugh JL, Smith RD, Robertson WW, Yost RP, Janssen HF (1982) Cyclic sequential compression of the lower limb in prevention of deep venous thrombosis. J Bone Joint Surg (A), 64: 1059–1062

Hass SB, Insall JN, Scuderi GR, Windsor RE, Ghelman B (1990) Pneumatic sequential-compression boots compared with aspirin prophylaxis of deep-vein thrombosis after total knee arthroplasty. J Bone Joint Surg (A), 72: 27–31

Hazarika EZ, Wright DE (1981) Chronic leg ulcers. The effects of pneumatic intermittent compression. Practitioner, 225: 189–192

Hofman D (1995) Intermittent compression treatment for venous leg ulcers. J Wound Care, 4: 163–165

Hooker JA, Lachiewicz PF, Kelley SS (1999) Efficacy of prophylaxis against thromboembolism with intermittent pneumatic compression after primary and revision of total hip arthroplasty. J Bone Joint Surg (A), 81: 690–696

Hull RD, Raskob GE, Gent M, McLoughlin D, Julian D, Smith FC, Dale NI, Reed-Davis R, Lofthouse RN, Anderson C (1990) Effectiveness of intermittent pneumatic leg compression for preventing deep vein thrombosis after total hip replacement. JAMA, 263: 2313–2317

Iwama H, Obara S, Ohmizo H (2004) Changes in femoral vein blood flow velocity by intermittent pneumatic compression: Calf compression device versus plantar-calf sequential compression device. J Anesth, 18: 232–233

Jacobs M, McCance KL, Stewart ML (1986) Leg volume changes with EPIC and posturing in dependent pregnancy edema: External pneumatic intermittent compression. Nurs Res, 35: 86–89

Janssen H, Trevino C, Williams D (1993) Hemodynamic alterations in venous blood flow produced by external pneumatic compression. J Cardiovasc Surg, 34: 441–447

Johansson K, Lie E, Ekdahl C, Lindfeldt J (1998) A randomized study comparing manual lymph drainage with sequential pneumatic compression for treatment of postoperative arm lymphedema. Lymphology, 31: 56–64

Kakkos SK, Geroulakos G, Nicolaides AN (2005) Improvement of the walking ability in intermittent claudication due to superficial femoral artery occlusion with supervised exercise and pneumatic foot and calf compression: A randomized controlled trial. Eur J Vasc Endovasc Surg, 30: 164–175

Kamran SI, Downey D, Ruff RL (1998) Pneumatic sequential compression reduces the risk of deep vein thrombosis in stroke patients. Neurology, 50: 1683–1688

Kavros SJ, Delis KT, Turner NS, Voll AE, Liedl DA, Gloviczki P, Rooke TW (2008) Improving limb salvage in critical ischemia with intermittent pneumatic compression: A controlled study with 18-month follow-up. J Vasc Surg, 47: 543–549

Kim-Sing C, Basco VE (1987) Post mastectomy lymphedema treated with the Wright linear pump. Can J Surg, 30: 368–370

Klein MJ, Alexander MA, Wright JM, Redmond CK, LeGasse AA (1988) Treatment of adult lower extremity lymphedema with the Wright linear pump: Statistical analysis of a clinical trial. Arch Phys Med Rehab, 69: 202–206

Kumar S, Samraj K, Nirujogi V, Budnik J, Walker M (2002) Intermittent pneumatic compression as an adjuvant therapy in venous ulcer disease. J Tissue Viability, 12: 42–50

Lachiewicz PF, Soileau ES (2007) Mechanical calf compression and aspirin prophylaxis for total knee arthroplasty. Clin Orthop Relat Res, 464: 61–64

Lachmann EA, Rook JL, Tunkel R, Nagler W (1992) Complications associated with intermittent pneumatic compression. Arch Phys Med Rehab, 73: 482–485

Landis EM (1935) The treatment of peripheral diseases by means of alternative negative and positive pressure. Penn Med J, 38: 579–583

Landis EM, Gibbon JH (1933) The effects of alternating suction and pressure on blood flow to the lower extremities. J Clin Invest, 12: 925–961

Lourida G, Saadia R, Spelay J, Addoh A, Weighell W, Arneja AS, Tanner J, Guzman R (2002) The ArtAssist device in chronic lower limb ischemia. A pilot study. Int Angiol, 21: 28–35

Maxell GL, Synan I, Dodge R, Carroll B, Clarke-Pearson DL (2001) Pneumatic compression versus low molecular weight heparin in gynecologic oncology surgery: A randomized trial. Obstet Gynecol, 98: 989–995

McCulloch JM (1981) Intermittent compression for the treatment of a chronic stasis ulceration: A case report. Phys Ther, 61: 1452–1453

McCulloch JM, Marler KC, Neal MB, Phifer TJ (1994) Intermittent pneumatic compression improves venous ulcer healing. Adv Wound Care, 7: 22–24, 26

McGrory BJ, Burke DW (2000) Peroneal nerve palsy following intermittent sequential pneumatic compression. Orthopedics, 23: 1103–1105

Montori VM, Kavros SJ, Walsh EE, Rooke TW (2002) Intermittent compression pump for nonhealing wounds in patients with limb ischemia: The Mayo Clinic experience (1998–2000). Int Angiol, 21: 360–366

Muhe E (1984) Intermittent sequential high-pressure compression of the leg: A new method of preventing deep vein thrombosis. Am J Surg, 147: 781–785

Muir KW, Watt A, Baxter G, Grosset DG, Lees KR (2000) Randomized trial of graded compression stockings for prevention of deep vein thrombosis after acute stroke. QJM, 93: 359–364

Mulder G, Robison J, Seely J (1990) Study of sequential compression therapy in the treatment of non-healing chronic venous ulcers. Wounds, 2: 111–115

Nicolaides AN, Fernandes E, Fernandes J, Pollock AV (1980) Intermittent sequential pneumatic compression of the legs in the prevention of venous stasis and postoperative deep venous thrombosis. Surgery, 87: 69–76

Nicolaides AN, Miles C, Hoare M, Jury P, Helmis E, Venniker R (1983) Intermittent sequential pneumatic compression of the legs and thromboembolism-deterrent stockings in the prevention of postoperative deep vein thrombosis. Surgery, 94: 21–25

Nikolovska S, Arsovski A, Damevska K, Gocev G, Pavlova L (2005) Evaluation of two different pneumatic compression cycle settings in the healing of venous ulcers: A randomized trial. Med Sci Monit, 7: 337–343

Oakley MJ, Wheelwright EF, James P (1998) Pneumatic compression boots for prophylaxis against deep vein thrombosis: Beware occult arterial disease. Br Med J, 316: 454–455

O'Donnell MJ, McRea S, Kahn SR, Julian JA, Kearon C, Mackinnon B, Magier D, Strulovich C, Lyons T, Robinson S, Hirsh J, Ginsberg JS (2008) Evaluation of a venous-return assist device to treat severe post-thrombosis syndrome (VENOPTS). Thromb Haemost, 99: 623–629

Pappas CH, O'Donnell TF (1992) Long-term results of compression treatment for lymphedema. J Vasc Surg, 16: 555–564

Partsch H (2008) Intermittent pneumatic compression in immobile patients. Int Wound J, 5: 389–397

Pedegana LR, Burgess EM, Moore AJ, Carpenter ML (1977) Prevention of thromboembolic disease by external pneumatic compression in patients undergoing total hip arthroplasty. Clin Orthop Relat Res, 128: 190–193

Pfizenmaier DH, Kavros SJ, Liedl DA, Cooper LT (2005) Use of intermittent pneumatic compression for treatment of upper extremity vascular ulcers. Angiology, 56: 417–422

Pidala MJ, Donovan DL, Kepley RF (1992) A prospective study on intermittent pneumatic compression in the prevention of deep vein thrombosis in patients undergoing total hip or total knee replacement. Surg Gynecol Obstet, 175: 47–51

Pilch U, Wozniewski M, Szuba A (2009) Influence of compression cycle time and number of sleeve chambers on upper extremity lymphedema volume reduction during intermittent pneumatic compression. Lymphology, 42: 26–35

Pittman GR (1989) Peroneal nerve palsy following sequential pneumatic compression. JAMA, 261: 2201–2202

Rasmaswami G, D'Ayala M, Hollier LH, Deutsch R, McElhinney AJ (2005) Rapid foot and calf compression increases walking distance in patients with intermittent claudication: Results of a randomized study. J Vasc Surg, 41: 794–801

Reid MR, Hermann LG (1934) Passive vascular exercises—treatment of vascular diseases by rhythmic alternation of environmental pressure. Arch Surg, 29: 697–704

Richmand DM, O'Donnell TF, Zelikovski A (1985) Sequential pneumatic compression for lymphedema: A controlled trial. Arch Surg 129: 1116–1119

Roper TA, Redford S, Tallis RC (1999) Intermittent compression for the treatment of the oedematous hand in hemiplegic stroke: A randomized control trial. Age Ageing, 28: 9–13

Rowland J (2000) Intermittent pump versus compression bandages in the treatment of venous leg ulcers. Aust N Z J Surg, 70: 110–113

Samson RH (1993) Compression stockings and non-continuous use of polyurethane foam dressings for the treatment of venous ulceration. A pilot study. J Dermatol Surg Oncol, 19: 68–72

Santori FS, Vitullo A, Stopponi M, Santori N, Ghera S (1994) Prophylaxis against deep-vein thrombosis in total hip replacement. Comparison of heparin and foot impulse pump. J Bone Joint Surg (B), 76: 579–583

Schuler JJ, Maibenco T, Megerman J, Ware M, Montalvo J (1996) Treatment of chronic leg ulcers using sequential gradient intermittent pneumatic compression. Phlebology, 11: 111–116

Scurr JH, Coleridge-Smith PD, Hasty JH (1987) Regimen for improved effectiveness of intermittent pneumatic compression in deep venous thrombosis prophylaxis. Surgery, 102: 816–820

Segers P, Blegrado J, Leduc A, Leduc O, Verdonck P (2002) Excessive pressure in multichambered cuffs used for sequential compression therapy. Phys Ther, 82: 1000–1008

Silbersack Y, Taute BM, Hein W, Podhaisky H (2004) Prevention of deep-vein thrombosis after total hip and knee replacement. Low-molecular-weight heparin in combination with intermittent pneumatic compression. J Bone Joint Surg (B), 86: 809–812

Skillman JJ, Collins RE, Coe RE, Goldstein BS, Shapiro RM, Zervas NT, Bettman MA, Salsman EW (1978) Prevention of deep vein thrombosis in neurosurgical patients: A controlled, randomized trial of external pneumatic compression boots. Surgery, 83: 354–358

Smith PC, Sarin S, Hasty J, Scurr JH (1990) Sequential gradient pneumatic compression enhances venous ulcer healing: A randomized trial. Surgery, 108: 871–875

Sobieraj-Teague M, Hirsh J, Yip G, Gastaldo F, Stokes T, Sloane D, O-Donnell MJ, Eikelboom JW (2012) Randomized controlled trial of a new portable calf compression device (Venowave) for the prevention of venous thrombosis in high-risk neurosurgical patients. J Thromb Hemost, 10: 229–235

Soderdahl DW, Henderson SR, Hansberry KL (1997) A comparison of intermittent pneumatic compression of the calf and whole leg in preventing deep venous thrombosis in urological surgery. J Urol, 157: 1774–1776

Spain DA, Bergamini TM, Hoffmann JF, Carrillo EH, Richardson JD (1998) Comparison of sequential compression devices and foot pumps for prophylaxis of deep venous thrombosis in high-risk trauma patients. Am Surg, 64: 522–525

Stockle U, Hoffmann R, Schutz M, Von Fournier C, Sudkamp NP, Haas N (1997) Fastest reduction of posttraumatic edema: Continuous cryotherapy or intermittent impulse compression? Foot Ankle Int, 18: 432–438

Sultan S, Esan O, Fahy A (2008) Nonoperative active management of critical limb ischemia: Initial experience using a sequential compression device for limb savage. Vascular, 16: 130–139

Sultan S, Hamada N, Soylu E, Fahy A, Hynes N, Tawflick W (2011) Sequential compression biomechanical device in patients with critical limb ischemia and nonreconstructible peripheral vascular disease. J Vasc Surg, 54: 440–446

Swedborg I (1977) Volumetric estimation of the degree of lymphedema and its therapy by pneumatic compression. Scand J Rehab Med, 9: 131–135

Swedborg I (1984) Effects of treatment with an elastic sleeve and intermittent pneumatic compression in post mastectomy patients with lymphoedema of the arm. Scand J Rehab Med, 16: 35–41

Szolnoky G, Lakatos B, Keskeny T, Varga E, Varga M, Dobozy A, Kemeny L (2009) Intermittent pneumatic compression acts synergistically with manual lymphatic drainage in complex decongestive physiotherapy for breast treatment-related lymphedema. Lymphology, 42: 188–194

Szuba A, Achalu R, Rockson SG (2002) Decongestive lymphatic therapy for patients with breast carcinoma-associated lymphedema. A randomized prospective study of a role for adjunctive intermittent pneumatic compression. Cancer, 95: 2260–2267

Thordarson DB, Greene N, Shepherd L, Perlman M (1999) Facilitating edema resolution with a foot pump after calcaneus fracture. J Orthop Trauma, 13: 43–46

Turpie AG, Gallus A, Beattie WS, Hirsh J (1977) Prevention of venous thrombosis in patients with intracranial disease by intermittent pneumatic compression of the calf. Neurology, 27: 435–438

Van Bemmelen PS, Gitlitz DB, Faruqui RM, Weiss-Olmanni J, Brunetti VA, Giron F, Ricotta JJ (2001) Limb salvage using high-pressure intermittent compression arterial assist device in cases unsuitable for surgical revascularization. Arch Surg, 136: 1280–1285

Van Bemmelen PS, Weiss-Olmanni J, Ricotta JJ (2000) Rapid intermittent compression increases skin circulation in chronically ischemic legs with infra-popliteal arterial obstruction. VASA, 29: 47–52

Vanscheidt W, Ukat A, Partsch H (2009) Dose-response of compression therapy for chronic venous edema—higher pressures are associated with greater volume reduction: Two randomized clinical trials. J Vasc Surg, 49: 396–402

Warwick D, Harrison J, Glew D, Mitchelmore A, Peters TJ, Donovan J (1998) Comparison of the use of a foot pump with the use of low-molecular-weight heparin for the prevention of deep-vein thrombosis after total hip replacement: A prospective randomized trial. J Bone Joint Surg (A), 80: 1158–1166

Waterman B, Walker JJ, Swaims C, Shortt M, Tood MS, Machen SM, Owens BD (2012) The efficacy of combined cryotherapy and compression compared with cryotherapy alone following anterior cruciate ligament reconstruction. J Knee Surg, 25: 155–160

Werbel GB, Shybut GT (1986) Acute compartment syndrome caused by a malfunctioning pneumatic compression boot: A case report. J Bone Joint Surg (A), 68: 1445–1446

Wilson NV, Das SK, Kakkar VV, Maurice HD, Smibert JG, Thomas EM, Nixon JE (1992) Thrombo-embolic prophylaxis in total knee replacement. Evaluation of the A-V Impulse System. J Bone Joint Surg (B), 74: 50–52

Woolson ST (1996) Intermittent pneumatic compression prophylaxis for proximal deep vein thrombosis after total hip replacement. J Bone Joint Surg (A), 78: 1735–1740

Wunderlich RP, Armstrong DG, Harkless LB (1998) Is intermittent pulsatile pressure a valuable adjunct in healing the complicated diabetic wound? Ostomy Wound Manage, 44: 70–74, 76

Zanolla R, Mongeglio C, Balzarini A, Martino G (1984) Evaluation of the results of three different methods of postmastectomy lymphedema treatment. J Surg Oncol, 26: 210–213

Review Articles

Caprini JA (2010) Mechanical methods for thrombosis prophylaxis. Clin Appl Throm Hem, 16: 668–673

Chen AH, Frangos SG, Kilaru S, Sumpio BE (2001) Intermittent pneumatic compression devices—physiological mechanisms of action. Eur J Vasc Endovasc Surg, 21: 383–392

Comerota AJ (2011) Intermittent pneumatic compression: Physiologic and clinical basis to improve management of venous leg ulcers. J Vasc Surg, 53:1121–1129

Delis KT (2005) The case for intermittent pneumatic compression of the lower extremity as a novel treatment in arterial claudication. Perspect Vasc Surg Endovasc Ther, 17: 29–42

Feldman SL, Stout NL, Wanchai A, Stewart BR, Cormier JN, Armer JM (2012) Intermittent pneumatic compression therapy: A systematic review. Lymphology, 45: 13–45

Field TS, Hill MD (2012) Prevention of deep vein thrombosis and pulmonary embolism in patients with stroke. Clin Appl Thromb Hemost, 18: 5–19

Gould MK, Garcia DA, Wren SM, Karanicolas PJ, Arcelus JI, Heit JA, Samama CM (2012) Prevention of VTE in nonorthopedic surgical patients: Antithrombotic therapy and prevention of thrombosis, 9th ed: American College of Chest Physicians Evidence-Based Clinical Practice Guidelines. Chest, 141:2 Suppl, e227S–e277S

Kakkos SK, Warwick D, Nicolaides AN, Stansby GP, Tsolakis IA (2011) Combined (mechanical and pharmacological) modalities for the prevention of venous thromboembolism in joint replacement surgery. J Bone Joint Surg (B), 94: 729–734

Kalodiki E (2007) Use of intermittent pneumatic compression in the treatment of venous ulcers. Future Cardiol, 3: 185–191

Khan SR, Lim W, Dunn AS, Cushman M, Dentali F, Akl EA, Cook DJ, Balekian AA, Klein RC, Le H, Schulman S, Murad MH (2012) Prevention of VTE in nonsurgical patients: Antithrombotic therapy and prevention of thrombosis, 9th ed: American College of Chest Physicians Evidence-Based Clinical Practice Guidelines. Chest, 141:2 Suppl, e195S–e226S

Kumar S, Walker MA (2002) The effects of intermittent pneumatic compression on the arterial and venous system of the lower limb: A review. J Tissue Viab, 12: 58–66

Lippi G, Favaloro EJ, Cervellin G (2011) Prevention of venous thromboembolism: Focus on mechanical prophylaxis. Semin Thromb Hemost, 37: 237–251

MacLellan DG, Fletcher JP (2007) Mechanical compression in the prophylaxis of venous thromboembolism. ANZ J Surg, 77: 418–423

Morris RJ (2008) Intermittent pneumatic compression—systems and applications. J Med Eng Tech, 32: 179–188

Morris RJ, Woodcock JP (2004) Evidence-based compression: Prevention of stasis and deep vein thrombosis. Ann Surg, 239: 162–171

Morris RJ, Woodcock JP (2008) Intermittent pneumatic compression of graduated compression stockings for deep vein thrombosis prophylaxis. Ann Surg, 251: 393–396

O'Sullivan-Drombolis DK, Houghton PE (2009) Pneumatic compression in the treatment of chronic ulcers. Phys Ther Rev, 14: 81–92

Rahn DD, Mamik MM, Sanses T, Matteson KA, Aschtenazi SO, Washington BB, Steinberg AC, Harvie HS, Lukban JC, Uhlig K, Balk EM, Sung VW (2011) Venous thromboembolism prophylaxis in gynecologic surgery. A systematic review. Obst Gynecol, 118: 1111–1125

Rinehart-Ayres M, Fish K, Lapp K (2010) Use of compression pumps for treatment of upper extremity lymphedema following treatment for breast cancer: A systematic review. Rehab Oncol, 28: 10–18

Roderick P, Ferris G, Wilson K, Halls H, Jackson D, Collins R, Baigent C (2005) Towards evidence-based guidelines for the prevention of venous thromboembolism: Systematic review of mechanical methods, oral anticoagulation, dextran and regional anaesthesia as thromboprolaxis. Health Technol Assess, 49: 1–78

Urbankova J, Quiroz R, Kucher N, Goldhaber SZ (2005) Intermittent pneumatic compression and deep vein thrombosis prevention. A meta-analysis in postoperative patients. Thromb Haemost, 94: 1181–1185

Chapter 19

Continuous Passive Motion

Chapter Outline

Learning Objectives

Remembering: State the rationale behind the use of continuous passive motion (CPM) therapy.
Understanding: Explain the mechanical principle behind the use of CPM therapy.
Applying: Demonstrate the application of a CPM device.
Analyzing: Summarize the proposed physiologic and therapeutic effects associated with CPM therapy.
Evaluating: Distinguish between key parameters related to the dosimetry of CPM therapy.
Creating: Defend why CPM therapy should be initiated as soon as possible after joint surgery.

I. FOUNDATION

A. DEFINITION

Continuous passive motion, known by the acronym CPM, is defined as a postoperative therapeutic mechanical agent that passively and continuously moves a joint through a prescribed range of motion (ROM) for an extended period of time. CPM therapy is a therapeutic intervention, the key aim of which is to move human joints without the patient's assistance. In other words, CPM provides a motion substitute until the patient is able to actively move the affected joints in the desirable ROM. Practitioners can find, in the current market, commercial CPM devices designed to mobilize several joints such as the hip, knee, ankle, big toe, shoulder, elbow, wrist, and finger joints.

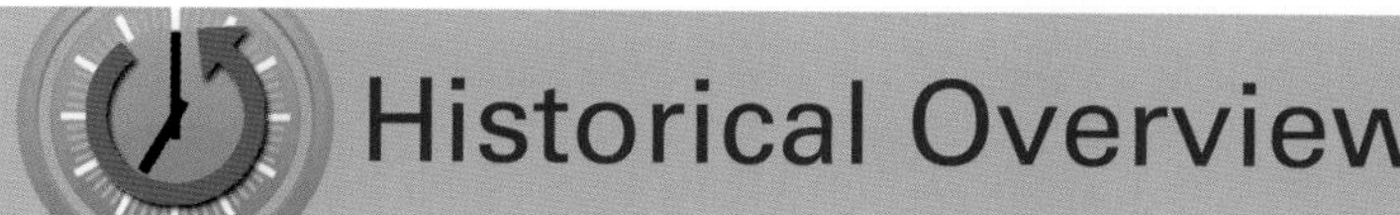

Controversy between the use of rest or movement to treat soft-tissue pathologies dates back to Hippocrates and Aristotle, the former proposing that the best way to heal the body is to rest it, whereas the latter's viewpoint was that movement will best promote healing (McCarthy et al., 1993). The dilemma about using immobilization or motion to treat joint pathologies lasted until the 1960s, when evidence from scientific research began to document the ill effects of using rest or immobilization and the beneficial effects of using early mobilization to treat joint pathologies (Salter et al., 1960). The application of continuos passive motion (CPM) as a therapeutic agent for joint pathologies was originally proposed by Robert Salter and colleagues in the early 1970s (Salter et al., 1982, 1984, 1989, 1994, 1996). The principle underlying Salter's concept is that joint motion is necessary to maintain articular cartilage health. His concept was a blow to the time-honored but unproven dictum that joint pathologies must be rested or immobilized, just as with bones after fractures, in order to heal properly (Salter, 1989). The first clinical documentation on the use of CPM therapy on human joints is that of Salter and colleagues in 1984. They reported on the therapeutic benefits of this treatment on nine individuals affected with various bone and joint pathologies (Salter et al., 1984). Since then, Salter's work has inspired a large body of basic and clinical research on the use and effects of this mechanical therapeutic agent for postoperative management of joint pathologies.

B. CONTINUOUS PASSIVE MOTION DEVICES

Figure 19-1 illustrates typical CPM devices used to mobilize the knee, ankle, elbow, shoulder, and wrist. A typical CPM device is made of three parts: a carriage made of levers on which rests a body's extremity support system; an electrically powered motor-controller unit that mechanically moves metallic levers; and a handheld control system programmable for ROM, speed of motion, and duration of treatment. These devices can be used in hospital, clinical, and home settings.

C. RATIONALE FOR USE

Post-surgical joint management is very often associated with severe pain that prevents patients from actively mobilizing the affected joint in the hours and days after surgery. Research has shown that prolonged rest or immobilization of a joint after surgery significantly increases the risk of joint stiffness, which later may cause significant mobility and functional problems. The rationale behind the use of CPM therapy is thus to provide a substitute for the patient's temporary inability to actively move his or her affected joint by providing controlled passive and continuous joint motion for extended periods of time. The main purpose of this mechanical therapeutic agent is to prevent postoperative joint stiffness, which in turn should enhance soft-tissue healing and accelerate the recovery of joint mobility and function.

II. BIOPHYSICAL CHARACTERISTICS

The biophysical principle underlying CPM therapy is mechanical in nature. A torque, or moment of force, about the affected joint axis of rotation is generated by means of a programmable electrical motor embedded in the device, which moves metal or plastic levers through various angles of the joint ROM. Torque (T) is the product of force (F) perpendicularly applied to a lever arm (d) and is calculated as follows: $T = F \times d$. Torque is expressed in units of newton-meter (N-m) or pound-inch (lb-in), where 1 Nm equals 8.85 lb-in. Figure 19-2 shows a series of photographs that illustrates the basic mechanical principle behind CPM devices. It shows a knee CPM device that passively moves the knee joint from full extension (–3 degrees) to flexion (120 degrees) and back to full extension, thus creating a full cycle of passive knee extension/flexion motion. During this passive cycling of the joint, the patient is instructed to completely relax the musculature around the affected joint.

III. THERAPEUTIC EFFECTS AND INDICATIONS

A. JOINT MOBILIZATION

Figure 19-3 presents the proposed physiologic and therapeutic effects associated with CPM therapy (Salter, 1994; O'Driscoll et al., 2000; Grella, 2008; Du Plessis et al., 2011). The device generates a moment of force (torque) about the joint axis that mimics volitional joint movement. The periodic displacement of the joint stretches the periarticular structures, thus preventing joint stiffness by minimizing both joint hemarthrosis and edema. The continuous passive mechanical stress applied to the joint also compresses meniscal and articular cartilages. Joint compression is presumed to enhance the remodeling (alignment) of collagen in addition to causing a pumping effect that circulates the synovial fluid in the affected joint. It is well established that both meniscal and articular cartilages are relatively avascular structures that derive most

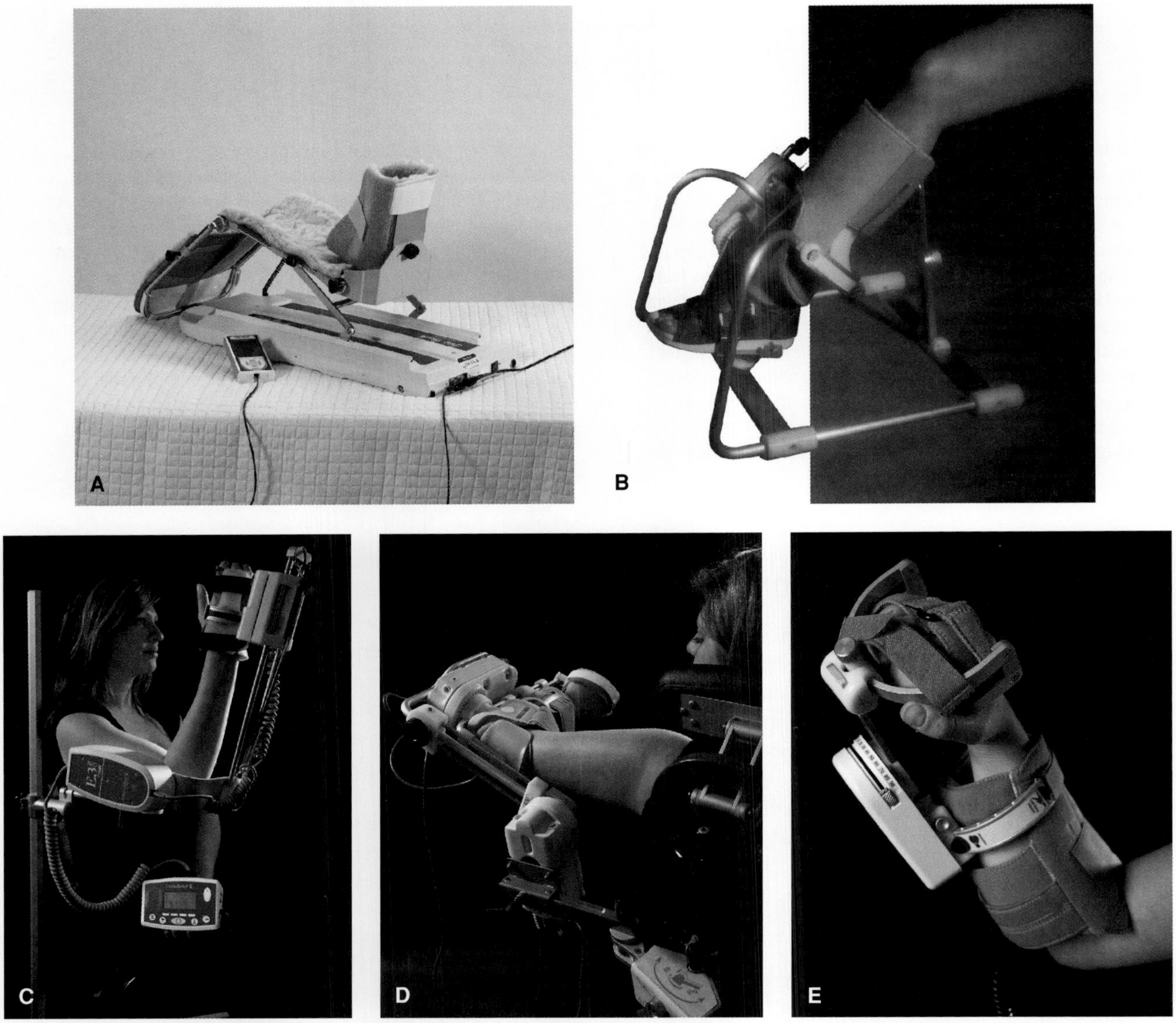

FIGURE 19-1 Typical continuous passive motion devices used for the knee (**A**), ankle (**B**), elbow (**C**), shoulder (**D**), and wrist (**E**). These devices are used with various bed- and chair-fitting accessories to accommodate different human segments and body positions. (Courtesy of Otto Bock HealthCare.)

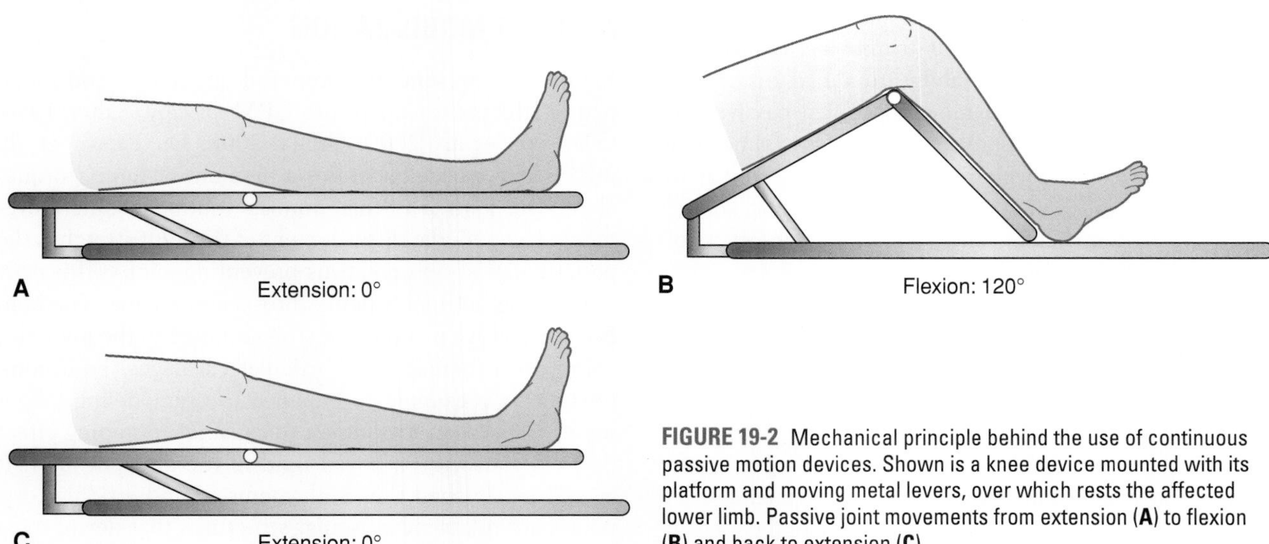

FIGURE 19-2 Mechanical principle behind the use of continuous passive motion devices. Shown is a knee device mounted with its platform and moving metal levers, over which rests the affected lower limb. Passive joint movements from extension (**A**) to flexion (**B**) and back to extension (**C**).

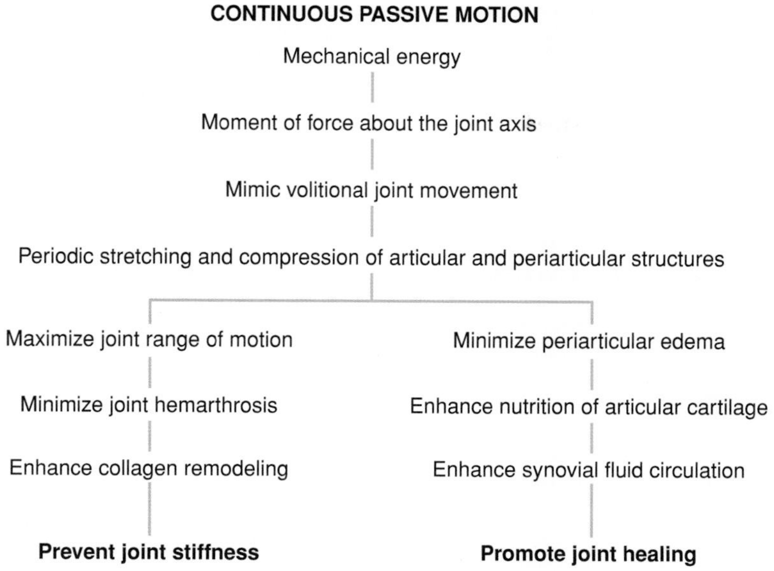

FIGURE 19-3 Proposed physiologic and therapeutic effects of continuous passive motion therapy.

of their nutrients from synovial fluid. Enhancing synovial fluid circulation is presumed to enhance joint nutrition, thus promoting joint healing. In addition to these primary specific mechanical effects, there is evidence from the literature that CPM therapy may also provide related clinical benefits such as (1) reducing the frequency and dosage of postoperative analgesics, (2) decreasing the length of hospitalization stay, and (3) decreasing the requirement for surgical manipulation.

B. RESEARCH-BASED INDICATIONS

The search for evidence behind the use of CPM therapy, displayed in the *Research-Based Indications* box, led to the collection of 70 English peer-reviewed human clinical studies. The methodology and criteria used to assess the strength of evidence and therapeutic effectiveness are described in Chapter 2. Of the 70 clinical trials, 68% (48) were conducted on the knee joint. As indicated, the strength of evidence is *moderate* for the knee, ankle, and shoulder joints. Therapeutic effectiveness is *conflicting* for the knee joint and minimally *substantiated* for both ankle and shoulder joints. There is dearth of clinical trials on the effect of CPM on the hip, elbow, wrist, and hand. Over all conditions, the strength of evidence behind the use of CPM is found to be *moderate* and its therapeutic effectiveness *conflicting*.

IV. DOSIMETRY

There is a consensus in the literature that CPM therapy should be initiated *as soon as possible* after surgery, usually in the recovery room or on the morning of the first day after surgery, for optimal results (Grella, 2008). Recall that the key therapeutic purposes of this mechanical agent are to prevent joint stiffness, minimize joint hemarthrosis and periarticular edema, promote early weight bearing, and enhance soft tissue healing. Listed and described in Table 19-1 are dosimetric parameters common to most CPM devices. ROM, speed of motion, and start/stop are the primary parameters (see later discussion). Secondary parameters, which modulate the time course of CPM, include warm-up, comfort zone, fast back, oscillation zone, progressive ROM, and pause. Safety parameters, such as the patient's handheld ON/OFF switch, reverse-on-load, and lockout, are also available. Many devices also include a compliance monitor for home therapy.

A. RANGE OF MOTION

The torque generated by the device passively moves the resting affected joint through a prescribed ROM, which is gradually increased over time until full ROM is achieved. For example, an initial ROM setting can be from 0 degrees extension to 90 degrees flexion, with increments of 5 degrees every 2 days, until the full 0- to 120-degree range is obtained. This range should be as large as possible and within the patient's tolerance for optimal results. When available on the device, set the desired torque, from low to high, according to the weight of the displaced body segments and the level of joint movement restriction. Program the device such as to increase, on a daily basis, the desired ROM until full ROM is achieved.

B. SPEED OF MOTION

This dosimetric parameter is defined as the number of degrees a joint is moved per minute (°/min) from the

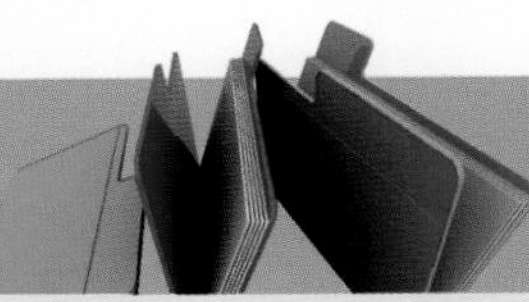

Research-Based Indications

CONTINUOUS PASSIVE MOTION

Health Condition	Benefit—Yes		Benefit—No	
	Rating	Reference	Rating	Reference
Knee	I	Gose, 1987	I	Bennett et al., 2005
	II	Lenssen et al., 2006	I	MacDonald et al., 2000
	II	Alfredson et al., 1999	I	Chiarello et al., 1997
	II	Colwell et al., 1992	I	McCarthy et al., 1993
	II	Friemert et al., 2005	II	Beaupre et al., 2001
	II	Johnson, 1990	II	Chen et al., 2012
	II	Johnson et al., 1992	II	Davies et al., 2003
	II	Lenssen et al., 2003	II	Denis et al., 2006
	II	London et al., 1999	II	Engstrom et al., 1995
	II	McInnes et al., 1992	II	Kumar et al., 1996
	II	Mullaji et al., 1989	II	Lau et al., 2001
	II	Ververeli et al., 1995	II	Leach et al., 2006
	II	Vince et al., 1987	II	Montgomery et al., 1996
	II	Walker et al., 1991	II	Nadler et al., 1993
	II	Wasilewski et al., 1990	II	Nielsen et al., 1988
	II	Witherow et al., 1993	II	Pope et al., 1997
	II	Maloney et al., 1990	II	Richmond et al., 1991
	II	Worland et al., 1998	II	Ritter et al., 1989
	II	Yashar et al., 1997	II	Rosen et al., 1992
	II	Harms et al., 1991	II	Bruun-Olsen et al., 2009
	II	Lenssen et al., 2008	II	Maniar et al., 2012
	II	Basso et al., 1987	II	Alkire et al., 2010
	II	Synder et al., 2004	II	Chen et al., 2000
	II	May et al., 1999	II	Erbold et al., 2012

Strength of evidence: Moderate
Therapeutic effectiveness: Conflicting

Health Condition	Benefit—Yes		Benefit—No	
	Rating	Reference	Rating	Reference
Ankle	II	McNair et al., 2001		
	II	Zeifang et al., 2005		
	II	Kasten et al., 2007		
	II	Farsetti et al., 2009		
	III	Grumbine et al., 1990		

Strength of evidence: Moderate
Therapeutic effectiveness: Substantiated

Health Condition	Benefit—Yes		Benefit—No	
Shoulder/Hand	II	Raab et al., 1996	II	Lastayo et al., 1998
	II	Lynch et al., 2005	II	Dundar et al., 2009
	II	Garofalo et al., 2010		
	II	Flowers et al., 1994	II	Ring et al., 1998
	III	Giudice, 1990	II	Schwartz et al., 2008
	III	Dirette et al., 1994	II	Trumble et al., 2010

Strength of evidence: Moderate
Therapeutic effectiveness: Conflicting

Fewer Than 5 Studies

Health Condition	Benefit—Yes		Benefit—No	
Elbow	II	Gates et al., 1992	II	Lindenhovius et al., 2009
	II	Aldridge et al., 2004		
Hip	II	Simkin et al., 1999		
	II	Wilk et al., 2004		
Wrist	III	Stevenson et al., 2005		

Strength of evidence: Pending
Therapeutic effectiveness: Pending

ALL CONDITIONS
Strength of evidence: Moderate
Therapeutic effectiveness: Conflicting

TABLE 19-1 DOSIMETRIC PARAMETERS* RELATED TO CONTINUOUS PASSIVE MOTION

Parameters	Description
ROM	Range from partial to full range of motion (ROM)
Speed of motion	Range from few to several degrees per minute (5 to180 degrees/min)
Start/Stop	Application duration set to minutes or hours
Warm-up	Increases the ROM from 50% of the programmed setting to the full setting over a certain number of cycles
Comfort zone	Reverses the direction and reduces the ROM by a few degrees, allowing the patient enough time to recover by not taking the joint into the painful ROM
Fast back	Increases the speed of motion in the nontherapeutic ROM (mid-range), leaving more time for the device to work, at the desired speed, in the therapeutic ROM (ends of range)
Oscillation zone	Reverses the direction of movement by a few degrees before returning to previous ROM; this reversal is repeated a few times (hence, the word *oscillation*), thus more time is spent in the therapeutic zone (ends of ROM).
Progressive ROM	Automatic increases (increments) of ROM, by a certain number of degrees per day, until final ROM is obtained
Pause	From 1 second to several minutes of hold motion at the end of ROM gains
ON/OFF switch	Manually controlled by patient for safety
Reverse-on-Load	Circuit will automatically reverse the direction of motion if the preset torque setting is exceeded
Lockout	Allows the device to be programmed and locked, preventing patient tampering during home therapy
Compliance monitor	Allows the practitioner to monitor patient's compliance with device during home therapy

*A handheld controller programs and controls all the above dosimetric parameters.

initial position to the target position and back to the initial position. For example, if the speed of motion is set at 60°/min, and ROM at 240°, this means that it will take 4 minutes to complete the full ROM cycle. As joint pain subsides, both ROM and speed of motion increase.

C. START/STOP

CPM devices may be applied continuously or intermittently for periods ranging from 1 hour to several hours per day. For example, if the application duration is set at 8 hours (480 min) per day and speed of motion is set at 60°/min, then the total number of joint motion cycles will be equivalent to 120. The application duration is usually several hours per day during the in-hospital period. These periods are shortened over the postoperative days, and the number of applications is usually increased. For example, the application duration for the first 4 postoperative days may have been, on average, 14 hours per day (a single application interrupted for a few minutes only for hygiene care and for a few hours for sleep). For the next 4 days, the application duration would be 4 hours, repeated three times a day.

V. APPLICATION, CONTRAINDICATIONS, AND RISKS

Prior to considering the application of CPM therapy, practitioners must first check for contraindications, consider the risks, and then go through key application steps and procedures designed to optimize treatment safety, efficacy, and effectiveness. It is important to always maintain a match between the device axis of rotation and that of the affected articular joint. Healing of surgical wounds may be affected by unduly pulling and tearing. To visualize and get more details on application, readers are invited to see selected **online videos**.

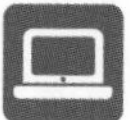

APPLICATION, CONTRAINDICATIONS, AND RISKS

Continuous Passive Motion

IMPORTANT: Although some have recommended that therapy be started the second day after surgery in order to minimize wound complications and blood loss (Maloney et al., 1990; Lotke et al., 1991, Pope et al., 1997), the general recommendation today is that therapy should begin as soon as possible after surgery (i.e., in the recovery room) for optimal results (Grella, 2008). Adequate prescription and monitoring during therapy should also minimize wound damage and blood loss.

NOTE: To describe the application protocol related to each device can be lengthy and repetitive. Presented next is a general protocol applicable to all continuous passive motion (CPM) devices. See **online videos**.

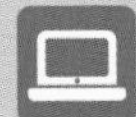

STEP	RATIONALE
1. Check for contraindications.	*Unstable fractures*—bone displacement and bone union delay during passive motion *Uncontrolled infection related to the affected joint*—wound complications and delayed healing *Muscle spasm and spasticity*—triggers unwanted muscle contraction during passive motion
2. Consider the risks.	*Post-surgical wound*—affects wound healing by unduly pulling or tearing the wound edges (Johnson, 1990; Maloney et al., 1990; Drez et al., 1991)
3. Position and instruct patient.	Ensure that the patient is comfortably positioned, and instruct to relax the treated limb segment.
4. Align joint in the device.	Align the joint axis with the device's axis of motion. Secure the limb segments about the treated joint with the device's fixation system. Plug line-powered CPM devices into ground-fault circuit interrupter (GFCI) receptacles to eliminate the risk of electrical macroshock (see Chapter 5 for details).
5. Set dosimetry.	Use Table 19-1 to set the parameters that will best meet the therapeutic goals.
6. Apply treatment.	Ensure adequate visual monitoring during treatment. Make sure that the patient holds the controller for optimal safety. Frequently check and adjust joint positioning in the CPM device. The rotational axis of the device should always match the functional axis of the joint to ensure optimal rotational movement. There may be a disparity between the true joint motion and the set CPM range of motion (Bible et al., 2009).
7. Conduct post-treatment inspection.	Inspect the surgical wounds on the joint, and question the patient on the level of sensation perceived during treatment. Document in the patient's file any unusual sensation felt by the patient during treatment.
8. Ensure post-treatment equipment maintenance.	Follow manufacturer recommendations. Immediately report all defects or malfunctions to technical maintenance staff.

CASE STUDIES

Presented are two case studies that summarize the concepts, principles, and applications of continuous passive motion (CPM) discussed in this chapter. Case Study 19-1 addresses the use of CPM for treatment following total knee arthroplasty affecting a male patient. Case Study 19-2 is concerned with the use of this agent for the treatment of frozen shoulder affecting a middle-aged woman. Each case is structured in line with the concepts of evidence-based practice (EBP), the International Classification of Functioning, Disability, and Health (ICF) disablement model, and SOAP (*s*ubjective, *o*bjective, *a*ssessment, *p*lan) note format (see Chapter 2 for details).

CASE STUDY 19-1: TOTAL KNEE ARTHROPLASTY

EVIDENCE-BASED CLINICAL DECISION MAKING PROTOCOL

1. Formulate the Case History

A 59-year-old male electrician, who has just undergone total right-knee arthroplastic surgery following severe osteoarthritis, is currently waking up in the hospital recovery room. You are asked to provide immediate post-surgical knee care until hospital discharge. There was no complication during surgery. The patient is medicated. The short-term therapeutic goals for CPM treatment of this patient are to decrease pain, prevent knee-joint stiffness, increase range of motion (ROM), and increase knee function. The longer-term goals are full weight bearing, normal walking over the next days, and return to work in the weeks to come.

2. Outline the Case Based on the ICF Framework

TOTAL KNEE ARTHROPLASTY		
BODY STRUCTURES AND FUNCTIONS	**ACTIVITIES**	**PARTICIPATION**
Knee prosthesis	Unable to mobilize knee	Inability to perform activities of daily living (ADLs)
Knee pain	Unable to bear weight	Inability to work full-time
Knee edema	Unable to walk	
Knee stiffness		

PERSONAL FACTORS	ENVIRONMENTAL FACTOR
Middle-aged man	Electrician
Healthy	

3. Outline Therapeutic Goals and Outcome Measurements

GOAL	OUTCOME MEASUREMENT
Decrease pain	Visual Analogue Scale (VAS)
Decrease stiffness	Goniometry
Decrease edema	Tape
Increase ability to do daily tasks	Western and Ontario Universities Osteoarthritis Index (WOMAC) questionnaire

4. Justify the Use of Continuous Passive Motion Based on the EBP Framework

PRACTITIONER'S EXPERIENCE	RESEARCH-BASED INDICATIONS	PATIENT'S EXPECTATION
Experienced in CPM	*Strength:* Moderate	Believes that CPM will be beneficial
Has used this agent in similar cases	*Effectiveness:* Conflicting	
Believes that CPM will be beneficial		

5. Outline Key Intervention Parameters

- **Treatment base:** Hospital
- **CPM device:** Knee
- **Patient position:** Lying supine in bed
- **First application:** In the recovery room
- **CPM method:** Move the knee joint from full extension (0 degrees) through increasing degrees of flexion.
- **Application protocol:** Follow the suggested application protocol in *Application, Contraindications, and Risks* box, and make the necessary adjustments for this case. See **online videos**.

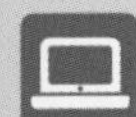

- **Day 1 (operative day):** ROM set at 0–60 degrees with speed of motion of 1°/s for 4 hours (120 cycles)
  Overnight: Device replaced with an extension knee splint
- **Day 2:** *Morning:* 0–65 degrees with speed of motion of 2°/s for 3 hours (166 cycles)
  Evening: 0–70 degrees with speed of motion of 2°/s for 3 hours (154 cycles)
  Overnight: Extension knee splint applied
- **Day 3:** *Morning:* 0–80 degrees with speed of motion of 3°/s for 3 hours (204 cycles)
  Afternoon: 0–85 degrees with speed of motion of 3°/s for 3 hours (190 cycles)
  Evening: 0–90 degrees with speed of motion of 3°/s for 3 hours (180 cycles)
  Overnight: Extension knee splint applied
- **Days 4–6 (discharge):** ROM increased 10 degrees a day and speed of motion increased 3 degrees a day for 3 hours until ceased on day 6
  Overnight: Extension knee splint applied
- **Concomitant therapy:** Postoperative nursing care
- *When indicated, the clinician also programs the CPM device for pause and reverse-on-load. For home therapy, the lockout and compliance monitor parameters are used.*

6. Report Pre- and Post-Intervention Outcomes

OUTCOME	PRE	POST
Pain (VAS score)	8/10	3/10
Knee flexion (ROM)	10 degrees	110 degrees
Knee edema	+3 cm	+1 cm
Knee function (WOMAC score)	200	100

7. Document Case Intervention Using the SOAP Note Format

S: Middle-aged male Pt presents with immediate R knee post-surgical condition following total knee arthroplasty.

O: *Intervention:* CPM to move knee joint from extension to flexion applied for 6 consecutive days; ROM and speed of motion increased daily; application duration of 3 hours repeated AM, afternoon, and evening; extension knee splint overnight. *Pre–post comparison:* Decreased pain: VAS 8/10 to 3/10; increased ROM: 10 degrees to 110 degrees flexion; decreased edema: +3 to +1 cm; increased knee function: WOMAC score 200 to 100.

A: Treatment very well tolerated. No adverse effect. Pt very pleased with therapeutic outcomes.

P: Further treatment required. Pt instructed to rent CPM device for home therapy until full knee extension is obtained. Pt also referred for full knee rehabilitation program following home therapy.

CASE STUDY 19-2: FROZEN SHOULDER

EVIDENCE-BASED CLINICAL DECISION MAKING PROTOCOL

1. Formulate the Case History

A retired 50-year-old woman presents with a left frozen shoulder (adhesive) after trauma that occurred 3 months ago. She did not see the need to consult, hoping that the condition would heal by itself without any complications. Physical examination reveals that the shoulder is in the stiff phase of the condition with marked flexion, abduction, internal/external rotation ROM limitations. She complains of pain particularly during shoulder movement. Left-handed, she is also very much concerned about her left shoulder lack of function. She prefers private clinic–based treatment. Her main goal is to regain full shoulder function in order to be able do all ADLs and play tennis occasionally.

2. Outline the Case Based on the ICF Framework

FROZEN SHOULDER		
BODY STRUCTURES AND FUNCTIONS	**ACTIVITIES**	**PARTICIPATION**
Shoulder pain	Difficulty to mobilize shoulder	Inability to perform ADLs
Shoulder stiffness	Severe ROM limitations	Inability to play tennis
PERSONAL FACTORS		**ENVIRONMENTAL FACTORS**
Middle-aged woman		Retired housewife
Healthy		Home living

3. Outline Therapeutic Goals and Outcome Measurements

GOAL	OUTCOME MEASUREMENT
Decrease pain	101-point Numerical Rating Scale (NRS-101)
Increase ROM	Goniometry
Increase shoulder function	Shoulder and Pain Disability Index (SPADI) questionnaire

4. Justify the Use of Continuous Passive Motion Based on the EBP Framework

PRACTITIONER'S EXPERIENCE	RESEARCH-BASED INDICATIONS	PATIENT'S EXPECTATION
Experienced in CPM	*Strength:* Moderate	Hopes that CPM will be beneficial
Has used this agent occasionally with similar cases	*Effectiveness:* Conflicting	
Believes that CPM will be beneficial		

5. Outline Key Intervention Parameters

- **Treatment base:** Private clinic
- **CPM device:** Shoulder mounted on a chair
- **Patient position:** Sitting
- **First application:** In the recovery room
- **CPM method:** Move the knee joint from full extension (0 degrees) through increasing degrees of flexion.
- **Application protocol:** Follow the suggested application protocol in *Application, Contraindications, and Risk* box, and make the necessary adjustments for this case. See **online videos**.

- **Treatment frequency:** Daily; 5 days a week
- **Week 1:** CPM device programmed to mobilize the left upper limb within the maximum tolerable ROM for *combined* abduction/adduction: internal/external rotation, vertical flexion/extension, horizontal abduction/adduction. Speed of motion is set at 4°/s. Application duration is 1 hour.
- **Weeks 2 to 4:** Progressive tolerable increases of ROM (+2 degrees) and speed of motion (+2°/s) based on previous measurements. Application duration remains at 1 hour.
- **Concomitant therapy:** Home stretching and pendulum exercises
- *When indicated, the clinician also programs the CPM device for pause and reverse-on-load.*

6. Report Pre- and Post-Intervention Outcomes

OUTCOME	PRE	POST
Pain (NRS-101 score)	55	15
Shoulder ROM	*Vertical flexion:* 80 degrees *Vertical extension:* 5 degrees *Abduction:* 65 degrees *Adduction:* Normal *Internal rotation:* 30 degrees *External rotation:* 5 degrees	150 degrees 15 degrees 90 degrees Normal 45 degrees 10 degrees
Shoulder function (SPADI score)	74%	35%

7. Document Case Intervention Using the SOAP Note Format

S: Retired middle-aged female Pt presents with left frozen shoulder following trauma.

O: *Intervention:* CPM to progressively move shoulder joint through combined flexion, extension, abduction, adduction, internal rotation and external rotation, daily, for 4 weeks. *Pre–post comparison:* Increased ROM: Flexion +70 degrees; extension +10 degrees; abduction +25 degrees; internal rotation +15 degrees; external rotation +5 degrees; improved SPADI score 74% to 35%.

A: Pt needed a few treatments to adjust to device. Well tolerated thereafter. No adverse effect.

P: Further home treatment required. Instructed to continue home shoulder program and to progressively engage in more ADLs, including playing tennis.

VI. THE BOTTOM LINE

- There is strong scientific evidence to show that CPM devices can effectively and safely mobilize human joints through full ROM and at various angular speeds.
- Motorized CPM devices generate mechanical energy, in the form of torque of moment of force, that move one or more joints through a preset ROM at a controlled speed for minimizing joint stiffness following trauma and surgery.
- The evidence suggests that CPM therapy tends to more beneficial in the initial phase of treatment—that is, in the first 4 postoperative weeks—because later on in the rehabilitation process there appears to be no difference between CPM therapy and manual joint mobilization.
- Although CPM devices are available for the treatment of several joints, the evidence presented in this chapter indicates that two thirds (68%) of clinical studies have focused on only one joint—the knee—following surgery.
- The overall body of evidence reported in this chapter shows the strength of evidence behind CPM to be *moderate* and its level of therapeutic effectiveness *conflicting*.
- The use of CPM devices as opposed to traditional manual early knee mobilization programs should be questioned.

VII. CRITICAL THINKING QUESTIONS

Clarification: What is meant by continuous passive motion (CPM) therapy?

Assumptions: You assume that motion is much better than rest or immobilization for the post-surgical treatment of joints. How do you justify making that assumption?

Reasons and evidence: Is there a difference between moving a joint using a CPM device and using your hand? If yes, what are the differences between these two therapeutic interventions?

Viewpoints or perspectives: How will you respond to a colleague who says that CPM therapy should not be used at home or after discharge from the hospital?

Implications and consequences: What are the implications and consequences if the patient involuntarily (e.g., a muscle spasm) or voluntarily offers resistance against the device during treatment?

About the question: What should the evidence-oriented clinician do in the face of strong conflicting evidence with regard to the use of a therapeutic agent for a given pathology? Why do you think I ask this question?

VIII. REFERENCES

Articles

Aldridge JM, Atkins TA, Gunneson EE, Urbaniak JR (2004) Anterior release of the elbow for extension loss. J Bone Joint Surg (A), 86; 1955–1960

Alfredson H, Lorentzon R (1999) Superior results with continuous passive motion compared to active motion after periosteal transplantation. A retrospective study of human patellar cartilage defect treatment. Knee Surg Sports Traumatol Arthrosc, 7: 232–238

Alkire MR, Swank ML (2010) Use of inpatient continuous passive motion versus no CPM in computer-assisted total knee arthroplasty. Orthop Nurs, 29: 36–40

Basso DM, Knapp L (1987) Comparison of two continuous passive motion protocols for patients with total knee implants. Phys Ther, 67: 360–363

Beaupre LA, Davies DM, Jones CA, Cinats JC (2001) Exercise combined with continuous passive motion or slider board therapy compared with exercise only: A randomized controlled trial of patients following total knee arthroplasty. Phys Ther 81: 1029–1037

Bennett LA, Brearley SC, Hart JA, Bailey MJ (2005) A comparison of two continuous passive motion protocols after total knee arthroplasty: A controlled and randomized study. J Arthroplasty, 20: 225–233

Bible JE, Simpson AK, Biswas D, Pelker RR, Grauer JN (2009) Actual knee motion during continuous passive motion protocols is less than expected. Clin Orthop Relat Res, 467: 2656–2661

Bruun-Olsen V, Heiberg KE, Mengshoel AM (2009) Continuous passive motion as an adjunct to active exercises in early rehabilitation following total knee arthroplasty: A randomized controlled trial. Disabil Rehabil, 31: 277–283

Chen B, Zimmerman JR, Soulen L, DeLisa JA (2000) Continuous passive motion after total knee arthroplasty: A prospective study. Am J Phys Med Rehab, 79: 421–426

Chen LH, Chen CH, Lin SY, Chien SH, Su JY, Huang CY, Wang HY, Chou CL, Tsai TY, Cheng YM, Huang HT (2012) Aggressive continuous passive motion exercise does not improve knee range of motion after total knee arthroplasty. J Clin Nurs, 22: 389–394

Chiarello CM, Gunderson L, O'Halloran T (1997) The effect of continuous passive motion duration and increment on range of motion in total knee arthroplasty patients. J Orthop Sports Phys Ther, 25: 119–127

Colwell CW, Morris BA (1992) The influence of continuous passive motion on the results of total knee arthroplasty. Clin Orthop Relat Res, 276: 225–228

Davies DM, Johnston DW, Beaupre LA, Lier DA (2003) Effect of adjunctive range-of-motion therapy after primary total knee arthroplasty on the use of health services after hospital discharge. Can J Surg, 46: 30–36

Denis M, Moffet H, Caron F, Ouellet D, Paquet J, Nolet L (2006) Effectiveness of continuous passive motion and conventional physical therapy after total knee arthroplasty: A randomized clinical trial. Phys Ther, 86: 174–185

Dirette D, Hinojosa J (1994) Effects of continuous passive motion on the edematous hands of two persons with flaccid hemiplegia. Am J Occup Ther, 48: 403–409

Drez D, Paine RM, Neuschwander DC, Young JC (1991) In vivo measurement of anterior tibial translation using continuous passive motion devices. Am J Sports Med, 19: 381–383

Dundar U, Toktas H, Cakir T, Evcik D, Kavuncu V (2009) Continuous passive motion provides good pain control in patients with adhesive capsulitis. Int J Rehabil Res, 32: 19–138

Engstrom B, Sperber A, Wredmark T (1995) Continuous passive motion in rehabilitation after anterior cruciate ligament reconstruction. Knee Surg Sports Traumatol Arthrosc, 3: 18–20

Erbold JA, Bonistall K, Blackburn M (2012) Effectiveness of continuous passive motion in an inpatient rehabilitation hospital after total knee replacement: A matched cohort study. Phys Med Rehabil, 4: 719–725

Farsetti P, Caterini R, Potenza V, De Luna V, De Maio F, Ippolito E (2009) Immediate continuous passive motion after internal fixation of an ankle fracture. J Orthop Traumatol, 10: 63–69

Flowers KP, Lastayo P (1994) Effect of total end range time on improving passive range of motion. J Hand Ther, 7: 150–157

Friemert B, Bach C, Schwarz W, Gerngross H, Schmidt R (2005) Benefits of active motion for joint position sense. Knee Surg Sports Traumatol Arthrosc, 14: 564–570

Garofalo R, Conti M, Notarnicola A, Maradei L, Giardella A, Castagna A (2010) Effects of one-month continuous passive motion after arthroscopic rotator cuff repair: Results at 1-year follow-up of a prospective randomized study. Musculoskelet Surg, 94: S79–S83

Gates HS, Sullivan FL, Urbaniak JR (1992) Anterior capsulotomy and continuous passive motion in the treatment of post traumatic flexion contracture of the elbow: A prospective study. J Bone Joint Surg (A), 74: 1229–1234

Giudice ML (1990) Effects of continuous passive motion and elevation on hand edema. Am J Occup Ther, 44: 914–921

Gose JC (1987) Continuous passive motion in the postoperative treatment of patients with total knee replacement. Phys Ther, 67: 39–42

Grumbine NA, Santoro JP, Chinn ES (1990) Continuous passive motion following partial ankle joint arthroplasty. J Foot Surg, 29: 557–566

Harms M, Engstrom B (1991) Continuous passive motion as an adjunct to treatment in the physical therapy management of the total knee arthroplasty patient. Physiotherapy, 77: 301–307

Johnson DP (1990) The effect of continuous passive motion on wound-healing mobility after knee arthroplasty. J Bone Joint Surg (A), 72: 421–426

Johnson DP, Eastwood DM (1992) Beneficial effects of continuous passive motion after total condylar knee arthroplasty. Ann R Coll Surg Engl, 74: 412–416

Kasten P, Geiger F, Zeifang F, Weiss S, Thomsen M (2007) Compliance with continuous passive movement is low after surgical treatment of idiopathic club foot in infants: A prospective, double-blinded clinical trial. J Bone Joint Surg (B), 89: 375–377

Kumar PJ, McPherson EJ, Dorr LD, Wan Z, Baldwin K (1996) Rehabilitation after total knee arthroplasty: A comparison of two rehabilitation techniques. Clin Orthop Relat Res, 331: 93–101

Lastayo PC, Wright T, Jaffe R, Hartzel J (1998) Continuous passive motion after repair of the rotator cuff. A prospective outcome study. J Bone Joint Surg (A), 80: 1002–1111

Lau SK, Chiu KY (2001) Use of continuous passive motion after total knee arthroplasty. J Arthroplasty, 16: 336–339

Leach W, Reid J, Murphy F (2006) Continuous passive motion following total knee replacement: A prospective randomized trial with follow-up to 1 year. Knee Surg Sports Traumatol Arthrosc, 14: 922–926

Lenssen AF, Crijns YH, Waltje EM, Roox GM, van Steyn MJ, Geesink RJ, van den Brandt PA, de Bie RA (2006) Effectiveness of prolonged use of continuous passive motion (CPM) as an adjunct to physiotherapy following total knee arthroplasty: Design of a randomized controlled trial. BMC Musculosket Disord, 23: 7–15

Lenssen AF, De Bie RA, Bulstra SK, Van Steyn MJ (2003) Continuous passive motion (CPM) in rehabilitation following total knee arthroplasty: A randomized controlled trial. Phys Ther Rev, 8: 123–129

Lenssen TA, van Steyn MJ, Crijns YH, Waltje EM, Roox GM, Geesink RJ, van den Brandt PA, De Bie RA (2008) Effectiveness of prolonged use of continuous passive motion (CPM), as an adjunct to physiotherapy, after total knee arthroplasty. BMC Musculoskelet Disord, 9: 60

Lindenhovius AL, van de Luijtgaarden K, Ring D, Jupiter J (2009) Open elbow contracture release: Postoperative management with and without continuous passive motion. JHS, 34A: 858–865

London NJ, Brown M, Newman RJ (1999) Continuous passive motion: Evaluation of a new portable low cost machine. Physiotherapy, 85: 610–612

Lotke PA, Faralli VJ, Orenstein EM, Ecker ML (1991) Blood loss after knee replacement. Effects of tourniquet release and continuous passive motion. J Bone Joint Surg (A), 73: 1037–1040

Lynch D, Ferraro M, Krol J, Trudell CM, Christos P, Volpe BT (2005) Continuous passive motion improves shoulder joint integrity following stroke. Clin Rehab, 19: 594–599

MacDonald SJ, Bourne RB, Rorabeck CH, McCalden RW, Kramer J, Vaz M (2000) Prospective randomized clinical trial of continuous passive motion after total knee arthroplasty. Clin Orthop Relat Res, 380: 30–35

Maloney WJ, Shurman DJ, Hangen D, Goodman SB, Edworthy S, Bloch DA (1990) The influence of continuous passive motion on outcome in total knee arthroplasty. Clin Orthop Relat Res, 256: 162–168

Maniar RN, Baviskar JV, Singhi T, Rathi SS (2012) To use or not to use continuous passive motion post-total knee arthroplasty presenting functional assessment results in early recovery. J Arthroplasty, 27: 193–200

May LA, Buss W, Zayac D, Whitridge MR (1999) Comparison of continuous passive motion machines and lower limb mobility boards in the rehabilitation of patients with total knee arthroplasty. Can J Rehab, 12: 257–263

McCarthy MR, Yates CK, Anderson MA, Yates-McCarthy JL (1993) The effect of immediate continuous passive motion on pain during the inflammatory phase of soft tissue healing following anterior cruciate ligament reconstruction. J Orthop Sports Phys Ther, 17: 96–101

McInnes J, Larson MG, Daltroy LH, Brown T, Fossel AH, Eaton HM, Shulman-Kirwan B, Steindorf S, Poss R, Liang MH (1992) A controlled evaluation of continuous passive motion in patients undergoing total knee arthroplasty. JAMA, 268: 1423–1428

McNair PJ, Dombroski EW, Hewson DJ, Stanley SN (2001) Stretching at the ankle joint: Viscoelastic responses to holds and continuous passive motion. Med Sci Sports Exerc, 33: 354–358

Montgomery F, Eliasson M (1996) Continuous passive motion compared to active physical therapy after knee arthroplasty: Similar hospitalization times in a randomized study of 68 patients. Acta Orthop Scand, 67: 7–9

Mullaji AB, Shahane MN (1989) Continuous passive motion for prevention and rehabilitation of knee stiffness: A clinical evaluation. J Postgrad Med, 35: 204–208

Nadler SF, Malanga GA, Zimmerman JR (1993) Continuous passive motion in the rehabilitation setting: A retrospective study. J Phys Med Rehab, 72: 162–165

Nielsen PT, Rechnagel K, Nielsen S (1988) No effects of continuous passive motion after arthroplasty of the knee. Acta Orthop Scand, 59: 580–581

Pope RO, Corcoran S, McCaul K, Howie DW (1997) Continuous passive motion after primary total knee arthroplasty. Does it offer any benefits? J Bone Joint Surg (B), 79: 914–917

Raab MG, Rzeszutko D, O'Conner W, Greatting MD (1996) Early results of continuous passive motion after rotator cuff repair. A prospective, randomized, blinded, controlled study. Am J Ortho, 25: 214–220

Richmond JC, Gladstone J, MacGillivray J (1991) Continuous passive motion after arthroscopically assisted anterior cruciate ligament reconstruction: Comparison of short- versus long-term use. Arthroscopy, 7: 39–44

Ring D, Simmons BP, Hayes M (1998) Continuous passive motion following metacarpophalangeal joint arthroplasty. J Hand Surg (A), 23: 505–511

Ritter MA, Gandolf VS, Holston KS (1989) Continuous passive motion versus physical therapy in total knee arthroplasty. Clin Ortho Relat Res, 244: 239–243

Rosen MA, Jackson DW, Atwell EA (1992) The efficacy of continuous passive motion in the rehabilitation of anterior cruciate ligament reconstructions. Am J Sports Med, 20: 122–127

Salter RB, Field P (1960) The effects of continuous compression on living articular cartilage. An experimental investigation. J Bone Joint Surg (A), 42: 31–49

Salter RB, Hamilton HW, Wedge JH, Tile M, Torode IP, O'Driscoll SW, Murnaghan JJ, Saringer JH (1984) Clinical application of basic research on continuous passive motion for disorders and injuries of synovial joints: A preliminary report of a feasibility study. J Orthop Res, 1: 325–342

Schwartz DA, Chafeltz R (2008) Continuous passive motion after tenolysis in hand therapy patients: A retrospective study. J Hand Surg, 21: 261–266

Simkin PA, de Lateur BJ, Alquist AD, Questad KA, Beardsley RM, Esselman PC (1999) Continuous passive motion for osteoarthritis of the hip: A pilot study. J Rheumatol, 26: 1987–1991

Stevenson JR, Blake JM, Douglas TF, Kercheval DM (2005) Does continuous passive motion during keyboarding affect hand blood flow and wrist function? A prospective case report. Work, 24: 145–155

Synder M, Kozlowski P, Drobniewski M, Grzegorzewski A, Glowacka A (2004) The use of continuous passive motion (CPM) in the rehabilitation of patients after total knee arthroplasty. Orthop Traumatol Rehabil, 6: 336–341

Trumble TE, Vedder NB, Seiler JG, Hnael DP, Diao E, Pettrone S (2010) Zone-II flexor tendon repair: A randomized prospective trial of active place-and-hold therapy compared with passive motion therapy. J Bone Joint Surg (A), 92: 1381–1389

Ververeli PA, Sutton DC, Hearn SL, Booth RE, Hozack WJ, Rothman RR (1995) Continuous passive motion after total knee arthroplasty: Analysis of costs and benefits. Clin Orthop Relat Res, 321: 208–245

Vince K, Kelly MA, Beck J, Insall JN (1987) Continuous passive motion after total knee arthroplasty. J Arthroplasty, 2: 281–284

Walker RH, Morris BA, Angulo DL, Schneider J, Colwell CW (1991) Postoperative use of continuous passive motion, transcutaneous electrical nerve stimulation, and continuous cooling pad following total knee arthroplasty. J Arthroplasty, 6: 151–156

Wasilewski SA, Woods LC, Torgerson WR, Healy WL (1990) Value of continuous passive motion in total knee arthroplasty. Orthopedics, 13: 291–295

Wilk M, Franczuk B (2004) Evaluating changes in the range of movement in the hip in patients with degenerative changes, before and after total hip replacement. Orthop Traumatol Rehabil, 6: 342–349

Witherow GE, Bollen SR, Pinczewski LA (1993) The use of continuous passive motion after arthroscopically assisted anterior cruciate ligament reconstruction: Help or hindrance? Knee Surg Sports Traumatol Arthrosc, 1: 68–70

Worland RL, Arredondo J, Angles F, Lopez-Jimenez FL, Jessup DE (1998) Home continuous passive motion machine versus professional physical therapy following total knee replacement. J Arthroplasty, 13: 784–788

Yashar AA, Venn-Watson E, Welsh T, Colwell CW, Lotke P (1997) Continuous passive motion with accelerated flexion after total knee arthroplasty. Clin Orthop Relat Res, 345: 38–43

Zeifang F, Carstens C, Schneider S, Thomsen M (2005) Continuous passive motion versus immobilisation in a cast after surgical treatment of idiopathic club foot in infants: A prospective, blinded, randomized, clinical study. J Bone Joint Surg (B), 87: 1663–1665

Review Articles

Du Plessis M, Eksteen E, Jenneker A, Kriel E, Mentoor C, Stucky T, van Staden D, Morris LD (2011) The effectiveness of continuous passive motion on range of motion, pain and muscle strength following rotator cuff repair: A systematic review. Clin Rehabil, 25: 291–302

Grella RJ (2008). Continuous passive motion following total knee arthroplasty: A useful adjunct to early mobilization. Phys Ther Rev, 13: 269–279

Lenssen AF, Koke AJ, DeBie RA, Geesink RG (2003) Continuous passive motion following primary total knee arthroplasty: Short-and long-term effects on range of motion. Phys Ther Rev, 8: 113–121

O'Driscoll SW, Giori NJ (2000) Continuous passive motion (CPM): Theory and principles of clinical application. J Rehab Res Dev, 37: 179–188

Salter RB (1982) Motion vs rest. Why immobilize joints? J Bone Joint Surg (B), 64: 251–254

Salter RB (1989) The biologic concept of continuous passive motion of synovial joints: The first 18 years of basic research. Clin Orthop, 242: 12–26

Salter RB (1994) The physiologic basis of continuous passive motion for articular healing and regeneration. Hand Clin, 10: 211–219

Salter RB (1996) History of rest and motion and the scientific basis for early passive motion. Hand Clin, 12: 1–11

Ultrasound

Chapter Outline

Learning Objectives

Remembering: Define and describe the biophysics of therapeutic ultrasound.

Understanding: Distinguish between conventional ultrasound (CUS), low-intensity pulsed ultrasound (LIPUS), and noncontact low-frequency ultrasound (NCLFUS).

Applying: Show the application steps for CUS, LIPUS, and NCLFUS.

Analyzing: Explain the proposed physiologic and therapeutic effects of CUS, LIPUS, and NCLFUS.

Evaluating: Formulate the dosimetric parameters associated with CUS, LIPUS, and NCLFUS.

Creating: Discuss the body of English-language, scientific evidence supporting the use of CUS, LIPUS, and NCLFUS therapy.

I. FOUNDATION

A. DEFINITION

Ultrasound, often designated by the acronym US, is sound traveling through a medium at frequencies above (hence, the prefix *ultra*) the upper-limit frequency of human audibility, which is measured to be approximately 20 kilohertz (kHz) (Leighton, 2007; O'Brien, 2007; Ter Haar, 2007). *Sound* is a form of mechanical acoustic energy, or pressure waves, that propagates through vibration in the air and in other media such as water and soft biologic tissues. Therapeutic ultrasound refers to the use of this mechanical acoustic energy for treating a variety of soft tissue pathologies, including bone fractures and dermal wounds. More specifically, its spectrum may be classified, as shown in Table 20-1, into three categories, namely conventional ultrasound (CUS), low-intensity pulsed ultrasound (LIPUS), and noncontact low-frequency ultrasound (NCLFUS). Therapeutic ultrasound is characterized based on the following parameters: frequency, intensity, delivery mode, application method, application technique, coupling agent, effect, and indication. Traditionally associated with the use of CUS is the practice of *sonophoresis,* also known as *phonophoresis,* which is defined as the application of acoustic energy (hence, the prefix *sono-* or *phono-*) for the transfer (*phoresis*) of drug ions through the skin for therapeutic purposes. In other words, sonophoresis is a form of drug iontophoresis (see Chapter 13) where mechanical energy is substituted for electrical energy. Coverage of sonophoresis is beyond the scope of this chapter because the human research-based literature is limited and dated, and results are conflicting (Griffin et al., 1967; Kleinkort et al., 1975; Wing, 1982; Halle et al., 1986; Pottenger et al., 1989; Stratford et al., 1989; Holdsworth et al., 1993; Saliba et al., 2007; Nagrale et al., 2009). To learn more about the broad use of sonophoresis in medicine, dentistry, and physical medicine, readers may consult the following recent review articles (Mitragotri et al., 2004; Mitragotri, 2005; Escobar-Chavez et al., 2009; Polat et al., 2010, 2011).

B. CONVENTIONAL ULTRASOUND

This first category, clinically introduced in the early 1950s, is called *conventional ultrasound* because it is the oldest and most conventional therapeutic type of ultrasound used today to treat soft tissues conditions (see Table 20-1). CUS is delivered at low and high frequencies and intensities using continuous or pulsed delivery modes. Its application technique is dynamic, and application is with contact or noncontact with the skin surface. Aquasonic gel and tap water are common coupling agents placed between the applicator faceplate and the skin surface to optimize acoustic energy transmission. CUS is used primarily for its thermomechanical effects on tendon, ligament, and muscle disorders (Robertson et al., 2001; Robertson, 2002; Robertson, 2008; Armijo-Olivo et al., 2013).

C. LOW-INTENSITY PULSED ULTRASOUND

Introduced in the 1980s, *low-intensity pulsed ultrasound* is characterized by ultrasonic energy delivered at medium frequency (1.5 megahertz [MHz]) and at much lower intensity (0.03 watts per square centimeter [W/cm^2]) than CUS (see Table 20-1). LIPUS is pulsed, and the stationary applicator makes contact with the skin surface overlying the bone fracture site. Ultrasonic gel is also required as coupling medium at the soundhead applicator–skin interface. LIPUS therapy is used for its mechanical effect on fresh and slow-to-heal bone fractures (Claes et al., 2007; Dijkman et al., 2009; Martinez et al., 2011).

D. NONCONTACT LOW-FREQUENCY ULTRASOUND

First introduced in the early 2000s, this most recent category is known as *noncontact low-frequency ultrasound.* It is characterized by ultrasonic energy delivered at a much lower frequency (40 kHz) with intensity in the lower range (0.5 W/cm^2). NCLFUS is pulsed, and its application technique is dynamic. It uses sterile saline water contained in a bottle as a coupling medium and

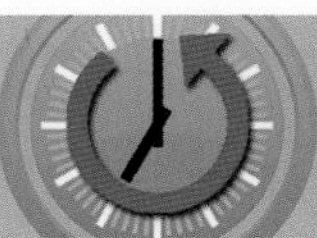

Historical Overview

The development of ultrasound as a means to treat human disorders dates back to the discovery, in the 1880s, of the *piezoelectric effect* by two French scientists, Pierre and Paul-Jacques Curie. This effect refers to the production of electrical energy, in certain nonconducting natural and synthetic crystals, by applying mechanical pressure on them (O'Brien, 2007). The word *piezo* is Greek for "pressure." In 1910, another French scientist, Paul Langevin, discovered the *reverse piezoelectric effect.* This effect is the production of mechanical energy in the crystals by applying electrical energy across them (O'Brien, 2007). Application of the reverse piezoelectric effect is the fundamental biophysical principle behind the manufacture of modern therapeutic, diagnostic, and industrial ultrasound devices.

TABLE 20-1 SPECTRUM OF THERAPEUTIC ULTRASOUND

Characteristics		CUS	LIPUS	NCLFUS
Frequency	Low (LF) Mid (MF) High (HF)	MF/HF 1–3 MHz	MF 1.5 MHz	LF 40 kHz
Intensity	Low (LI) High (HI)	LI/HI 0–3 W/cm^2	LI 0.03 W/cm^2	LI 0.5 W/cm^2
Delivery mode	Continuous (C) Pulsed (P)	C/P	P	P
Application technique	Stationary (S) Dynamic (D)	D	S	D
Application method	Contact (C) Noncontact (NC)	C/NC	C	NC
Coupling agent	Gel (G) Water (W)	G/W	G	W
Effect	Mechanical (M) Thermal (T)	M/T	M	M
Indication		Muscle, tendon, and ligament disorders	Bone fracture	Dermal wounds

CUS, conventional ultrasound; LIPUS, low-intensity pulsed ultrasound; NCLFUS, noncontact low-frequency ultrasound.

is applied in a dynamic noncontact fashion. This ultrasonic device creates ultrasonic waves that produce and propel a gentle mist of sterile saline water to the wound bed. This water mist facilitates the transfer of ultrasonic energy to the wound bed without direct contact. NCLFUS, also known under the commercial name *MIST Therapy System,* is used to promote dermal wound healing through its mechanical cleansing, debridement, and antibacterial effects.

E. ULTRASOUND DEVICES AND ACCESSORIES

1. Conventional Ultrasound

Figure 20-1 illustrates a typical line-powered CUS device made of an electrical generator to which is attached, via a cable, a handheld soundhead applicator that houses a piezoelectric transducer. Soundhead applicators come in different sizes to accommodate smaller to larger treatment surface areas. The delivery of ultrasound energy requires an ultrasonic coupling agent, such as a gel, gel pad, or tap water (noncontact), placed between the applicator and the skin overlying the treatment area. When there is risk of infection, sterile ultrasonic gel may be used. Gel temperature is kept constant by using a commercial ultrasound bottle warmer. Soundhead applicators, as well as reusable gel pads, should be cleaned with an antimicrobial solution after each application to minimize the risk of cross-infection (see Fig. 20-1).

2. Low-Intensity Pulsed Ultrasound

Figure 20-2 shows a battery-powered LIPUS device. Its applicator (transducer) may be applied in-cast, on-cast, or directly on the skin overlying a bone fracture site by using a specially designed retaining and fixating system placed over the fracture site. Ultrasonic gel is also required between the applicator and the skin overlying the fracture site.

3. Noncontact Low-Frequency Ultrasound

Figure 20-3 illustrates a line-powered NCLFUS device, which consists of an electrical generator to which is attached a handheld applicator that also houses a piezoelectric transducer. Attached to this applicator is a specially designed disposable applicator assembly system holding a sterile saline water bottle. Finger pressure on the applicator control button releases an ultrasonic flow of mist water through the transducer tip and over the wound bed primarily for the purpose of mechanical wound cleansing and debridement.

F. RATIONALE FOR USE

Ultrasound, a form of mechanical energy that can be transmitted in the human body as high-frequency acoustical pressure waves, has been widely used for therapeutic, diagnostic, and surgical purposes. This chapter focuses on the application of therapeutic ultrasound. The rationale

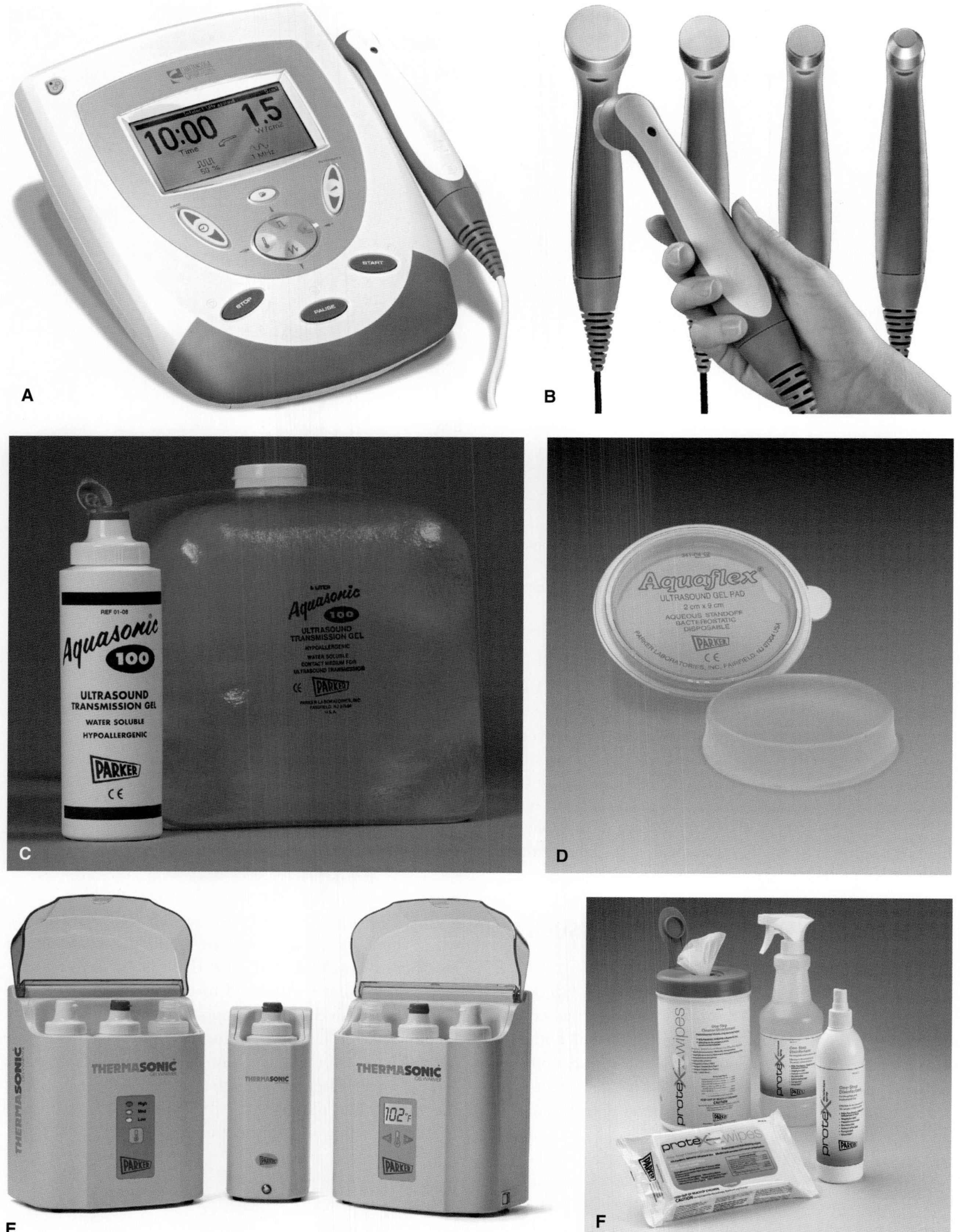

FIGURE 20-1 Typical conventional ultrasound device (**A**) with soundhead applicators of various sizes (**B**). Aquasonic gel (**C**), gel pad (**D**), gel bottle warmer (**E**), and soundhead cleaning solution (**F**). (A, B: Courtesy of DJO Global; C–F: Courtesy of Parker Laboratories Inc.)

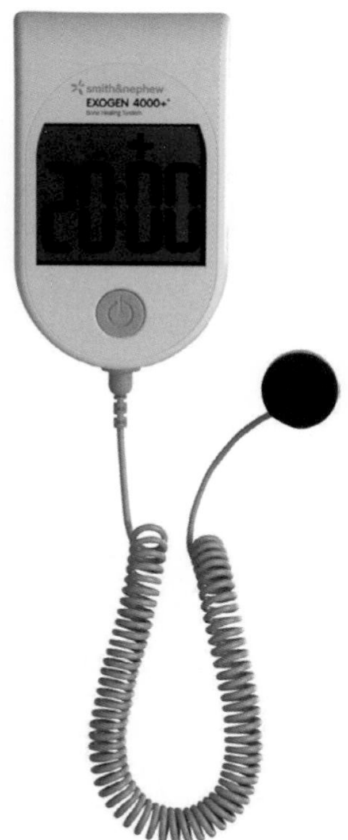

FIGURE 20-2 Low-intensity pulsed ultrasound device. (Courtesy of Smith & Nephew Inc.)

behind the use of CUS is to induce deep and localized thermal and mechanical effects in pathologic soft tissues, particularly in tissues rich in proteins, such as tendons, ligaments, and muscles, while inducing minimal effect on the overlying skin and subcutaneous tissues. The rationale for LIPUS therapy, on the other hand, is to promote and accelerate bone growth, through its mechanical effects, in cases of fresh and slow-to-heal bone fractures. Finally, the rationale for NCLFUS is to facilitate wound cleansing debridement through its noncontact mechanical effect, thus promoting dermal wound healing.

II. BIOPHYSICAL CHARACTERISTICS

A. ULTRASONIC WAVE FORMATION

Figure 20-4 schematizes the formation of an ultrasonic beam of energy generated by a therapeutic ultrasound device. The formation of sound, or mechanical waves, is based on the *reverse piezoelectric effect,* which states that when a high frequency, alternating electrical current (AC) is applied to the surface of a piezoelectric material, called a *transducer,* mechanical deformations of this transducer follow in the form of oscillations, or cycles of expansion and contraction. The soundhead applicator houses the transducer, which is made of a natural or synthetic piezoelectric material. The transducer converts the electrical energy applied against its surface into mechanical or acoustic energy. Attached to the transducer is the soundhead applicator metallic faceplate. The soundhead applicator transfers the acoustic energy from the transducer to the metallic faceplate interface and to soft tissues (see Fig. 20-4). The repeated high-frequency cycles of micro-expansion and micro-contraction of the transducer create an ultrasonic beam of energy described as acoustic, mechanical, or pressure waves having a sinusoidal shape and traveling in time in the medium. During the expansion phase of the transducer, high pressure develops in the soft tissues, bringing molecules closer together. During the contraction phase, however, low pressure develops, which sends molecules farther apart. Ultrasound waves are *longitudinal waves* because the motion of the

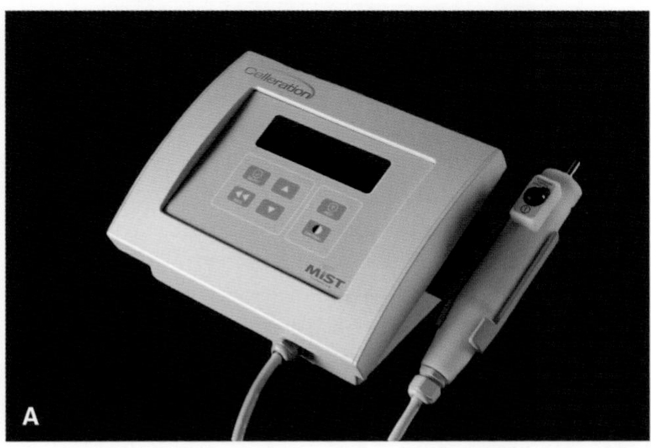

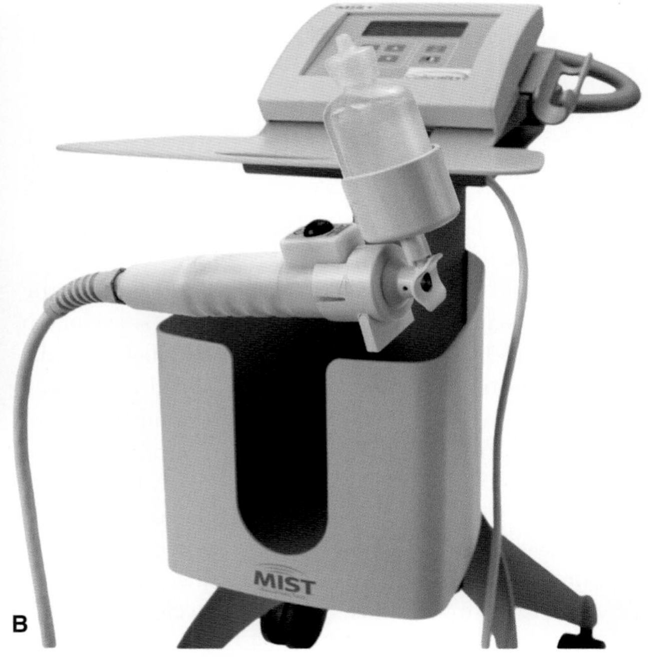

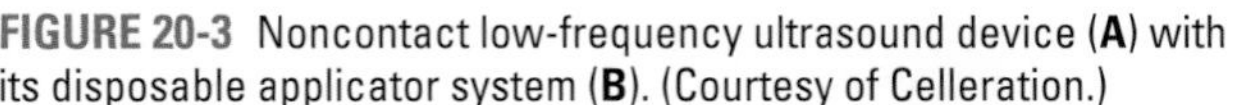

FIGURE 20-3 Noncontact low-frequency ultrasound device (**A**) with its disposable applicator system (**B**). (Courtesy of Celleration.)

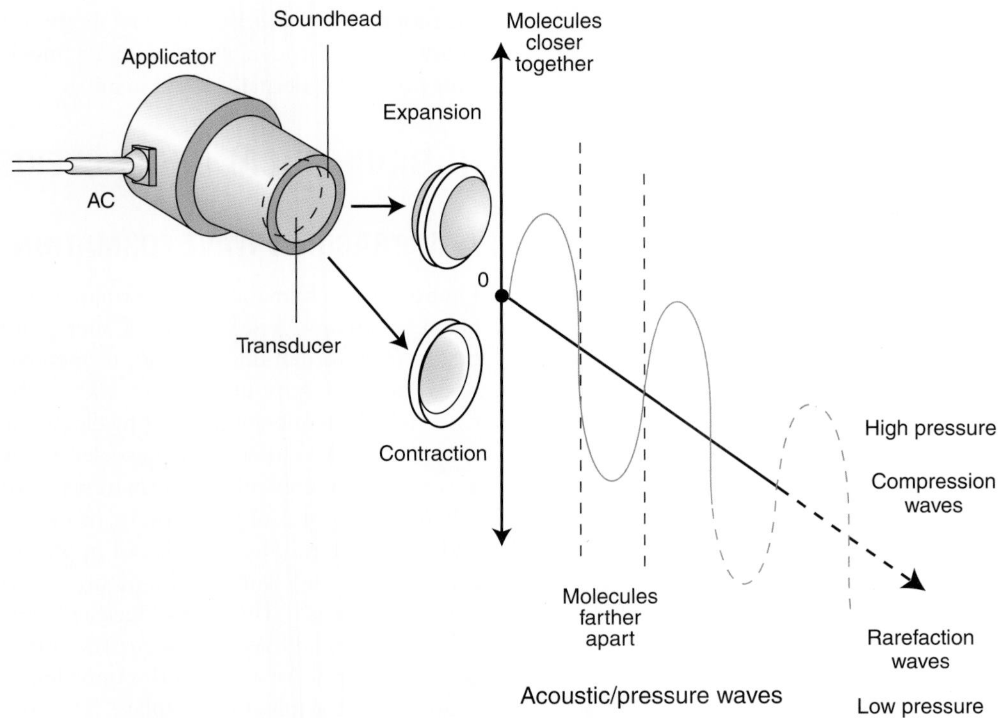

FIGURE 20-4 Production of an ultrasonic beam of energy. AC, alternating electrical current.

molecules in the medium is parallel to the direction of wave propagation (see Fig. 20-4).

B. ULTRASONIC BEAM PROJECTION

Figure 20-5 illustrates the spatial projection of the ultrasonic beam of energy emitted from a typical soundhead applicator. The beam region closest to the transducer faceplate is termed the *near field* or *Fresnel zone*. The region that immediately follows is called the *far field* or *Fraunhofer zone* (Frizzell et al., 1990). Biophysics has shown that the near field corresponds to the less divergent, or more focused, region of the beam emitted from the soundhead. The far field, in contrast, corresponds to the more divergent, or less focused, region of the beam. The length (L) of the near field, relative to the soundhead faceplate, corresponds to the boundary line separating these two fields or zones. This length (L) is directly related to the square radius (r^2) of the transducer's effective radiating area (ERA) and is inversely related to the ultrasonic beam's wavelength, where $L = r^2/\text{wavelength}$ (Ter Haar, 1996). Acoustic waves travel in aqueous media (e.g., gel, water, human tissues) at a speed or velocity (v) of approximately 1,500 meters per second (m/s). For example, the near-field length (L) of an ultrasonic beam emitted at 1 MHz, from a transducer ERA of 10 cm^2, equals 21.1 cm. This L value is calculated as follows. First, wavelength is proportional to the speed of transmission (v) and inversely related to frequency (f)—thus: Wavelength = v/f. In this example, wavelength equals 0.15 cm (0.15 cm = 1,500 m/s/1,000,000 cycles per

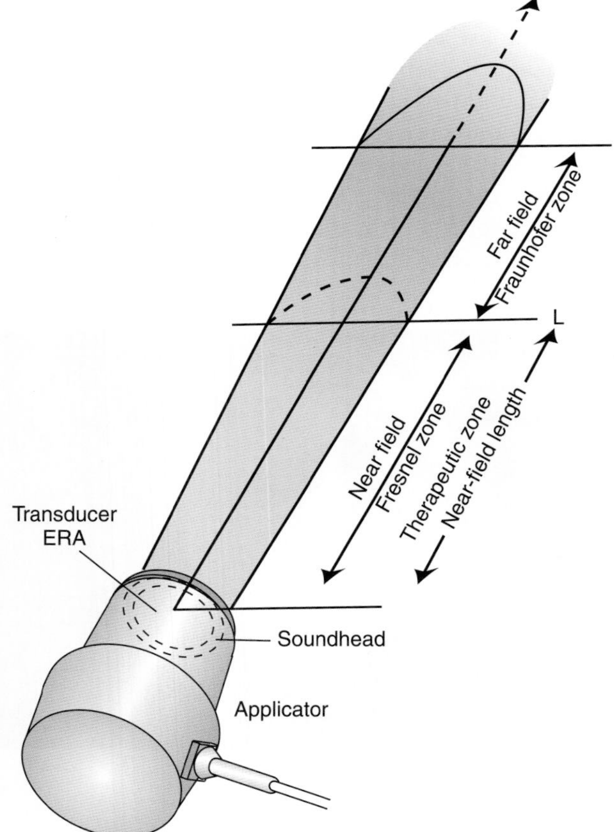

FIGURE 20-5 Spatial projection of an ultrasonic beam of energy showing the near-field (Fresnel) and far-field (Fraunhofer) zones. Note that the intensity of the ultrasonic beam is much more focused, or less divergent, in the near field than in the far field. ERA, effective radiating area; L, length.

second [cps]). Second, the radius (R) of a 10 cm^2 circular transducer (S) is 1.78 cm, where $S = \pi r^2$ (10 cm = 3.14 × 1.78^2 cm). Third, the near-field length (L) equals 21.1 cm, where $L = r^2$/wavelength (21.1 cm = 1.78^2 cm/0.15 cm). Practically speaking, the near field or Fresnel zone is the region of the ultrasonic beam where *therapeutic effects* occur in the tissues because the distances separating the piezoelectric transducer from the targeted tissues, in most clinical applications, are well within the length (L) of the near field (Ter Haar, 1996).

C. DELIVERY MODE

1. Continuous Versus Pulsed

Therapeutic CUS is delivered, as illustrated in Figure 20-6, using the continuous and pulsed modes. *Continuous mode* refers to the uninterrupted flow of acoustic energy during the entire treatment duration (see Fig. 20-6A). *Pulsed mode,* on the other hand, refers to periodic interruption of acoustic energy characterized by ON (flow) and OFF (no flow) periods (see Fig. 20-6B). Pulse frequency is the frequency with which ultrasonic pulses are delivered and is calculated as follows: f = 1/(ON + OFF). For example, a pulsed frequency (f) of 1,000 Hz will result from the combination of a pulse duration (ON time) of 0.2 milliseconds (ms) followed by an interpulse duration (OFF time) of 0.8 ms (1,000 Hz = 1/0.002 s + 0.008 s).

2. ON:OFF Ratio Versus Duty Cycle

The *ON:OFF ratio* expresses the relationship between the ON and OFF times. In the previous example, the ON:OFF ratio is 1:4 (0.002:0.008 = 1:4). This ratio means that the time during which ultrasound energy is delivered (ON) is four times shorter than the time value during which no ultrasound energy is delivered (OFF). *Duty cycle* (DC), on the other hand, refers to the duration, measured as a percentage (%), during which acoustic energy is delivered and is calculated using this formula: DC (%) = (ON/(ON + OFF)) × 100. Duty cycle related to the continuous mode is *always 100%* because there is no (zero) OFF time. In keeping with the example, the duty cycle related to the continuous mode equals 20%: 20% = (0.002 s/(0.002 s + 0.008 s)) × 100. This duty cycle means that ultrasonic energy is delivered for a period equivalent to 20% of the total treatment duration. In other words, if the total treatment duration is 6 minutes, acoustic energy would be delivered for a total of 1.2 minutes (1.2 min = 6 min × 20%), with delivery time being equivalent to one fifth (6 min/1.2 min), or 20%, of the total application duration. It follows from the earlier formula that the shorter the OFF time between given ultrasonic pulses (ON), the larger the duty cycle value and the larger the amount of acoustic energy delivered to the soft tissues. Duty cycle values are programmable and may range between 20% and 100% on most devices.

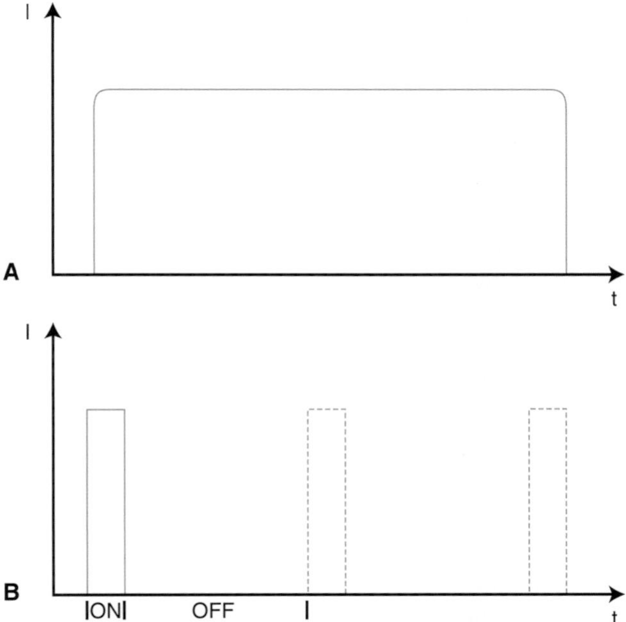

FIGURE 20-6 Ultrasound continuous (**A**) and pulsed (**B**) delivery modes.

D. TRANSDUCER EFFECTIVE RADIATING AREA

A soundhead applicator consists of a piezoelectric transducer covered by a steel plate; together they form a handheld soundhead applicator with a steel faceplate (see Fig. 20-1A,B). The term *effective radiating area,* measured in square centimeters (cm^2), is the area of the transducer from which ultrasound energy radiates. Transducer ERA is a key dosimetric parameter. Technically speaking, transducer ERA is always smaller (approximately 10%) that the soundhead applicator faceplate surface because the transducer is embedded in the applicator (see Figs. 20-4 and 20-5). Unfortunately, most manufacturers fail to make the distinction, when reporting technical specifications in their brochures, between transducer ERA and the applicator faceplate surface area. Most manufacturers report soundhead applicator using the term *size,* such as 1, 2, 5, and 10 cm^2. Not knowing what manufacturers refer to when reporting size (i.e., transducer ERA or soundhead applicator faceplate area), this chapter will assume, for the sake of simplifying dosimetry, that the soundhead applicator *size* is synonymous with transducer *ERA*.

E. ULTRASONIC INTENSITY

As ultrasound waves pass through soft tissues, they transport acoustic mechanical energy through them. *Energy* (E) is the ability to do work and is measured in joules (J). The rate of energy transport is known as power. *Power* (P) is the rate at which energy is transported and is measured in watts (W), where 1 watt equals 1 joule second (Js). Therapeutic ultrasound is produced in beams that are usually focused into small areas ranging from 1 to 10 cm^2. *Intensity* (I) is defined as the amount of acoustic power (P), measured in watts (W), per unit area of the transducer ERA, measured in square centimeters. It is expressed in watts per square centimeters based on this formula: $I = P/\text{ERA}$. For example, a power output (P) of 8 W applied through a transducer ERA of 5 cm^2 yields an intensity equal to 1.6 W/cm^2 (1.6 W/cm^2 = 8 W/5 cm^2). Because ultrasound energy is delivered using transducers with different ERAs (spatial domain), in both continuous and pulsed modes (temporal domain), the concept of intensity must be further defined in relation to these two domains.

1. Spatial Peak Intensity (I_{SP})

The term *spatial peak intensity* (I_{SP}) refers to the maximum, or peak, intensity delivered during the *continuous* delivery of ultrasound energy (see Fig. 20-6A). *Spatial peak intensity* (I_{SP}) is synonymous with *spatial average temporal peak intensity* (I_{SATP}).

2. Spatial Average Intensity (I_{SA})

Spatial average intensity (I_{SA}) refers to the mean, or average, intensity delivered during *pulsed* delivery of ultrasound energy (see Fig. 20-6B). Spatial average intensity (I_{SA}) is calculated by multiplying the spatial peak intensity (I_{SP}) of the device by its duty cycle (DC) using this formula: $I_{SA} = I_{SP} \times \text{DC}$. As discussed earlier, the duty cycle, expressed as a percentage (%), is derived from the ON and OFF times: DC (%) = (ON/(ON + OFF)) × 100. For example, the delivery of an I_{SP} equal to 1.6 W/cm^2, combined with a DC of 30%, yields an I_{SA} equal to 0.48 W/cm^2 (0.48 W/cm^2 = 1.6 W/cm^2 × 30%). The larger the duty cycle, the greater the spatial average intensity. *Spatial average intensity* (I_{SA}) is synonymous with *spatial average temporal average intensity* (I_{SATA}).

F. BEAM NONUNIFORMITY RATIO

Biophysics has shown that the ultrasonic beam delivered at the transducer faceplate is irregular, or *nonuniform,* meaning that the intensity is greater in the center (larger spikes) than at the edge (lower spikes) of the transducer (Dunn et al., 1990; Frizzell et al., 1990; Lehmann et al., 1990). The nonuniformity of an ultrasonic beam of energy is represented by its *beam nonuniformity ratio* (BNR) (Fig. 20-7). A transducer BNR is calculated as the ratio of its spatial peak intensity (I_{SP}) to its spatial average intensity (I_{SA}). In other words, it is the ratio between the peak intensity (highest spike at the center) and the average intensity of all other spikes (edges). For example, a BNR value of 5 (or 5:1) means that the spatial peak intensity generated by the device is five times larger than its spatial average intensity (5 = 5 W/cm^2 / 1 W/cm^2). BNR is determined by the intrinsic piezoelectric properties of the transducer. The better the piezoelectric quality of the transducer, the more uniform the beam intensity across its ERA, and the lower its BNR value. BNR values should range between 2 and 8.

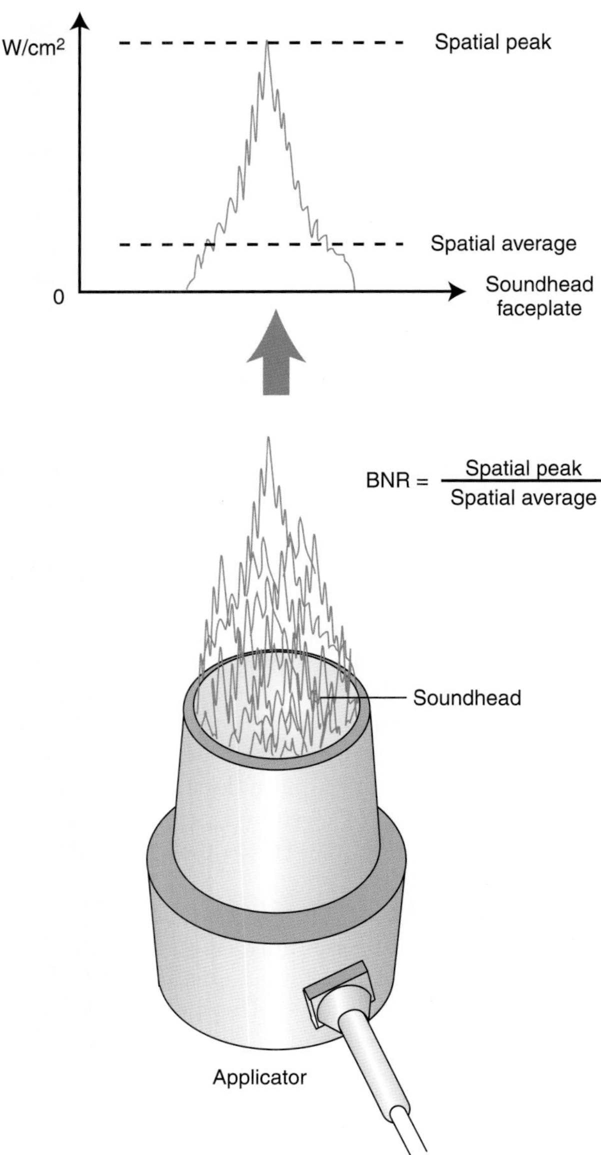

FIGURE 20-7 Ultrasonic beam nonuniformity ratio (BNR).

III. THERAPEUTIC EFFECTS AND INDICATIONS

Summarized in Figure 20-8, and discussed next, are the proposed physiologic and therapeutic effects associated with therapeutic ultrasound.

A. CONVENTIONAL ULTRASOUND

There is strong evidence in the literature to suggest that CUS can trigger significant thermomechanical effects on human soft tissues (see Lehmann et al., 1990; Alexander et al., 2010; Shanks et al., 2010; Tsai et al., 2011). Although the physiologic and therapeutic effects of CUS are traditionally separated into thermal and mechanical effects, there is evidence to suggest that both effects occur *concomitantly,* one dominating the other, depending on the dosimetry used (Erdogan et al., 2009).

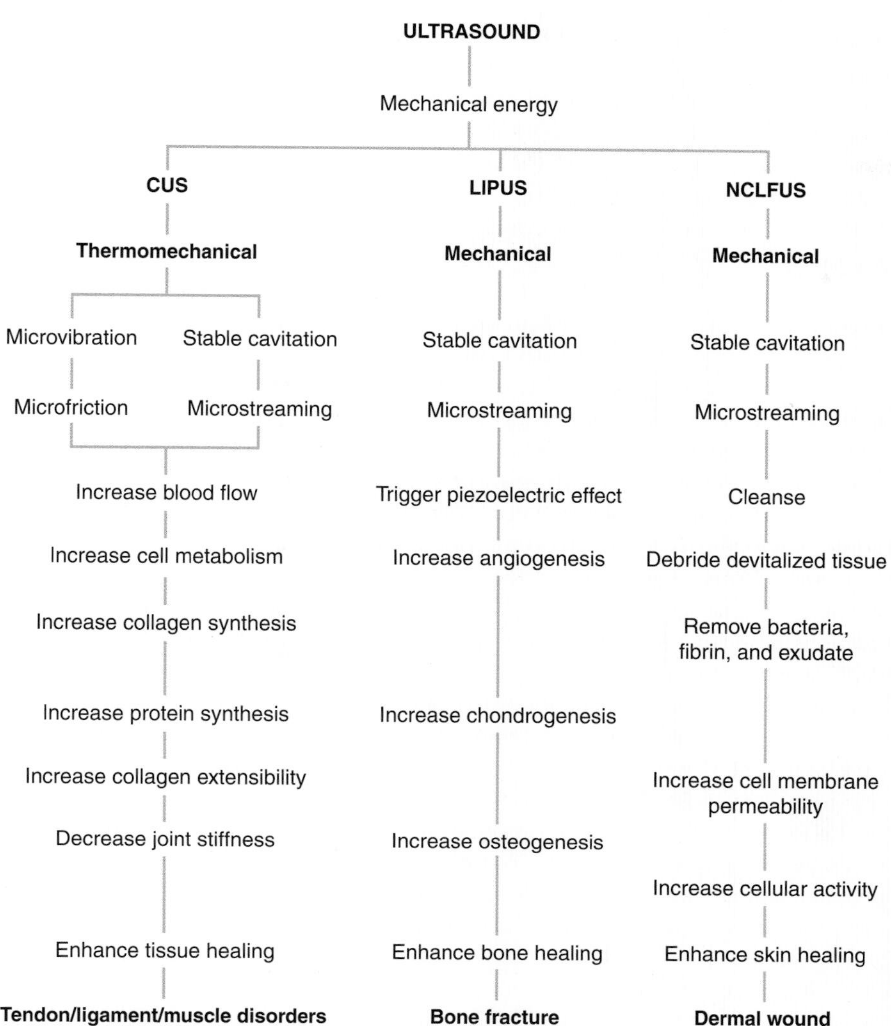

FIGURE 20-8 Proposed physiologic and therapeutic effects of ultrasound therapy. CUS, conventional ultrasound; LIPUS, low-intensity pulsed ultrasound; NCLFUS, noncontact low-frequency ultrasound.

1. Thermal Effect

When acoustic energy is absorbed as it penetrates soft tissues, molecules within the acoustic field are caused to vibrate under very high frequency cycles of compression waves (i.e., molecules moving closer together) and rarefaction waves (i.e., molecules moving farther apart). The higher the intensity of the ultrasonic beam and the more continuous the emission of acoustic waves, the more vigorous the molecular microvibration process. The more intense the molecular vibration, the more vigorous the microfriction between those millions of sonated molecules. The more vigorous the microfriction effect, the more intense the cellular kinetic energy, or frictional heat, generated in the tissue (Dyson, 1987, 1995).

2. Mechanical Effect

Concomitantly with the thermal effect induced in soft tissues is the mechanical effect triggered by the absorption of ultrasonic energy. Biophysics has shown that the delivery of ultrasonic energy to soft tissues triggers two interrelated mechanical effects—namely, stable cavitation and microstreaming (Kimmel, 2006; O'Brien, 2007). The word *cavitation* is derived from the Latin word *cavus,* meaning "hollow" and refers to the formation, in fluids or solids, of empty spaces or cavities resulting from the formation of microbubbles. Ultrasonic cavitation, triggered by the absorption of sound energy, begins when minute gas pockets that infiltrate most biologic fluids, termed *nuclei,* develop into microscopic bubbles, thus causing cavities in these fluids and the surrounding soft tissues. Under the sustained influence of acoustic radiation, these microscopic bubbles expand and contract (pulsate or oscillate) at the same carrier frequency at which the acoustic waves are produced. Depending on the frequency and intensity level of acoustic energy, two types of cavitation can occur in soft tissues: stable and unstable. *Stable cavitation* occurs when the bubbles begin to pulsate—that is, compress during the high-pressure waves and expand during the low-pressure waves. This phenomenon triggers *molecular movement* as molecules move closer together during the compression phase and farther apart during the rarefaction phase of the acoustic waves. This movement in the fluid is called *microstreaming,* which is defined as localized high-velocity streams of fluids created by ultrasonic energy in a liquid (Erdogan et al., 2009). Microstreaming causes movement and transfer of intracellular and extracellular ions affecting cellular membrane permeability. *Unstable cavitation,* on the other hand, occurs when the bubbles, subjected to strong cycles of compression and expansion, *collapse* or *implode,* releasing very high temperature and pressure changes in their vicinity in the fluid. Biophysics has shown that therapeutic ultrasound devices do not have the intensity and frequency outputs necessary to produce unstable cavitation. The occurrence of unstable cavitation during CUS therapy, therefore, poses no therapeutic concern.

3. Targeted Tissues

For thermomechanical effects to occur, ultrasonic energy must be absorbed by soft tissues. *Attenuation* reflects on the weakening of sound energy as it propagates through a medium such as soft tissues. It results from the combined effect of absorption and scattering. *Absorption* is the conversion of ultrasound energy to other forms of energy, such as thermal and mechanical energy. *Scattering* is the reflection of sound waves in directions other than its original direction of propagation. Biophysicists express the extent of ultrasound attenuation by using attenuation coefficients. An *attenuation coefficient* is a measure that characterizes how easily a material or tissue can be penetrated by a beam of ultrasound energy. In other words, attenuation coefficient is a measure of the capacity of a material or tissues to absorb ultrasonic energy. The attenuation coefficient is the sum of the individual coefficients for absorption and scatter. In soft tissues, the absorption coefficient accounts for 60% to 90% of the attenuation, and scatter accounts for the remainder (Hendee et al., 2002). Consequently, the terms *attenuation coefficient* and *absorption coefficient* are generally used interchangeably in the literature. Practically speaking, the larger the attenuation coefficient of a tissue, the greater is its capacity to absorb ultrasonic energy. Biophysicists have measured the attenuation coefficients of several soft tissues when exposed to ultrasound energy delivered at 1 MHz (Frizzell et al., 1990, p. 393). The results show that soft tissue attenuation or absorption coefficients tend to *increase* with protein content and *decrease* with water content. Clinically speaking, this means that protein-rich deeper tissues, such as bones (collagen), tendons (collagen), ligaments (elastin), and muscles (actin/myosin) can absorb greater amounts of ultrasonic energy than in those more superficial tissues, such as skin and fat, both of which contain less protein and more water. Together, the thermomechanical effects of CUS are presumed to increase blood flow, cell metabolism, collagen synthesis, protein synthesis, and collagen extensibility, thus decreasing joint stiffness while enhancing connective (tendon and ligament) and muscular tissue healing (see Fig. 20-8).

B. LOW-INTENSITY PULSED ULTRASOUND

Contrary to the application of CUS, the delivery of LIPUS energy to soft tissues causes *only mechanical effects* (see Fig. 20-8). There is minimal to no thermal (athermal) effect because the pulsed ultrasonic beam of energy is delivered at a very low intensity (30 mW/cm^2). In other words, minimal microvibration or microfriction effects occur, leading to very low levels of molecular kinetic energy that are unable to heat up soft tissues. There is strong evidence to show that the main, and only, target tissue for LIPUS therapy is bone (Malizos et al., 2006; Griffin et al., 2008; Busse et al., 2009; Erdogan et al., 2009; Mundi et al., 2009; Watanabe et al., 2010; Kasturi et al., 2011; Bashardoust et al., 2012; Riboh et al., 2012). Why is it so? First, bone, among all human soft tissues, has the highest ultrasound absorption coefficient, which is approximately three times higher than those coefficients measured for tendons, ligaments, and muscles (Frizzell et al., 1990). This means that the application of low-level ultrasonic energy is capable of triggering physiologic effects in bone without causing any thermomechanical effect on the soft tissues surrounding it. Second, ultrasound application generates the piezoelectric effect in bone. The piezoelectric effect is the property of some materials, such as bone, to convert mechanical energy to electrical current. In the 1950s, Fukada et al. (1957) first discovered and described the piezoelectric property of bone, and Corradi et al. (1953) made the first observation that ultrasound stimulates fracture healing in humans. In 1983, Xavier (1983) and Duarte (1983), using *animal models,* demonstrated the effectiveness of LIPUS for bone fractures. In the same year, Xavier and Duarte (1983) showed the benefit of using LIPUS for the treatment of human bone fractures. As shown in Figure 20-8, the application of LIPUS mechanically stresses the bone, thus triggering the piezoelectric effect—that is, the production of electrical potential across the bone. This effect, in turn, induces and increases bone reparative processes such as angiogenesis, chondrogenesis, and osteogenesis, which together enhance fracture healing (Ying et al., 2012).

C. NONCONTACT LOW-FREQUENCY ULTRASOUND

In contemporary wound care, a plethora of topical treatments is available that are aimed at accelerating the healing of chronic wounds (Sussman et al., 2012). Among them, cleansing and debriding procedures are critical to optimal dermal wound healing. NCLFUS, commercially known as the *MIST Therapy System,* is a mechanical agent that uses low-frequency ultrasonic energy to atomize saline water and deliver it as mist to the wound (Driver et al., 2011; Voigt et al., 2011; Escandon et al., 2012). The water mist generated has a relatively uniform droplet size that acts a *conduit* for transmitting ultrasound energy to the treatment site. The use of NCLFUS for treating open wounds first originated in the early 2000s from the studies of Ennis and colleagues on humans (2005, 2006). As illustrated in Figure 20-8, the application of NCLFUS triggers mechanical effect only—that is, stable cavitation and microstreaming. Ultrasound energy is used to mechanically cleanse and debride devitalized tissues covering the wound. In doing so, NCLFUS mechanically removes bacteria, fibrin, and exudates, and increases cell membrane permeability, thus increasing cellular activity leading to enhanced wound healing.

D. RESEARCH-BASED INDICATIONS

The search for evidence behind the use of CUS, LIPUS, and NCLFUS, displayed in the *Evidence-Based Indications* box, led to a collection of 150 English peer-reviewed human clinical studies. The methodologies and criteria used to assess the strength of evidence and therapeutic effectiveness are described in Chapter 2. Of the 150 studies, 102 studies are associated with the study of CUS, 34 studies with LIPUS, and 13 studies with NCLFUS. For CUS therapy, the results reveal 60 studies showing benefit and 42 showing no benefit. Considering all conditions treated with CUS, results indicate that the strength of evidence is *moderate* and therapeutic effectiveness *conflicting*. For both LIPUS and NCLFUS therapies, the strength of evidence is *moderate* and therapeutic effectiveness *substantiated*.

IV. DOSIMETRY

A. CONVENTIONAL ULTRASOUND

Table 20-2 lists the main dosimetric parameters considerations from which clinicians must choose to prescribe and apply CUS therapy. Let us discuss and exemplify each of them.

TABLE 20-2 DOSIMETRIC PARAMETERS FOR CONVENTIONAL ULTRASOUND THERAPY

Parameters	Basis for Selection
Frequency	• *Criteria:* Depth of lesion • *Deeper lesion:* 1 MHz • *More superficial lesion:* 3 MHz
Delivery mode	• *Criteria:* Thermal effect required • *More thermal effect:* Continuous mode • *More mechanical effect:* Pulsed mode
Transducer ERA	• *Criteria:* Treatment surface area • *Optimal applicator size to treatment surface area ratio:* 1:3
Application method and coupling medium	• *Criteria:* Geometry and sensitivity of body surface area overlying the lesion • *Contact with gel:* Over flat and insensitive surface • *Contact via gel pad:* Over moderately irregular and hyposensitive surface • *Noncontact via tap water:* Over severely irregular and hypersensitive surface
Application technique	• *Criteria:* Avoid hot spots • Dynamic only
Dosage	• *Criteria:* Desired thermomechanical effects • Dosage depends on intensity, application duration, transducer ERA, and treatment surface area • See Table 20-3 for details.

ERA, effective radiating area.

1. Frequency

Frequency is selected based on the depth of the lesion in relation to the skin surface overlying it. Ultrasonic energy emitted at 1 MHz penetrates soft tissues deeper because of its longer wavelength (see Ultrasonic Beam Projection section for details). In other words, the therapeutic zone (near-field length or Fresnel zone) is longer at 1 MHz than at 3 MHz because of its inverse relationship with wavelength.

2. Delivery Mode

Delivery mode is selected based on the amount of thermal effect needed for treatment. The more continuous the flow of ultrasonic energy delivered to the tissues, the greater the acoustic intensity delivered, and the larger the thermal effect. Pulsating the acoustic beam of energy, by manipulating its duty cycle, can either minimize or maximize the thermal or mechanical effect. For example, larger duty cycles will maximize thermal effect and minimize mechanical effect. Smaller duty cycles, on the other hand, will induce opposite effects.

3. Transducer Effective Radiating Area

Therapeutic soundhead applicators used to deliver CUS are available in various sizes (see Fig. 20-1C). To avoid confusion, we will assume that the term *size,* used in most corporate brochures, is synonymous with transducer *ERA*. The selection of applicator size is based on the treatment surface area under consideration. The optimal recommended ratio between transducer size and treatment surface area is 1:3. Practically speaking, this means that to treat a surface area of 15 cm^2, a transducer size of 5 cm^2 or larger should be used. Using a smaller applicator size implies longer treatment duration in order to deliver the same acoustic energy in each square centimeter of tissue as well as less thermal effect due to the recooling of previously sonated tissues during application.

4. Application Method and Coupling Medium

Both the selection of application methods and coupling media are guided by the geometry and sensitivity level of the treatment area. The contact method is recommended over relatively flat surface areas that can

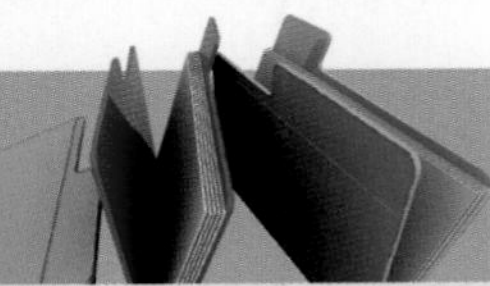

Research-Based Indications

ULTRASOUND

Health Condition	Benefit—Yes Rating	Benefit—Yes Reference	Benefit—No Rating	Benefit—No Reference
CONVENTIONAL ULTRASOUND				
Shoulder disorders	I	Ebenbichler et al., 1999	I	Van der Heijden et al., 1999
	I	Munting, 1978	I	Downing et al., 1986
	II	Ebenbichler et al., 1997	I	Ainsworth et al., 2007
	II	Aldes et al., 1954a	I	Perron et al., 1997
	II	Aldes et al., 1954b	I	Inaba et al., 1972
	II	Cline, 1963	I	Kurtais Gursel et al., 2004
	II	Roden, 1952	II	Nykänen, 1995
	II	Grynbaum, 1954	II	Hamer et al., 1976
	II	Flax, 1964		
	II	Herrera-Lasso et al., 1993		
	II	Shehab et al., 2000		
	II	Shomoto et al., 2002		
	II	Echternach, 1965		
	III	Bundt, 1958		
	III	Bearzy, 1953		
	III	Gorkiewicz, 1984		
Strength of evidence: Moderate **Therapeutic effectiveness:** Substantiated				
Dermal wounds	I	McDiarmid et al., 1985	I	Ericksson et al., 1991
	I	Callam et al., 1987	I	Ter Riet et al., 1996
	I	Dyson et al., 1976	II	Lundeberg et al., 1990
	I	Roche et al., 1984	II	Watson et al., 2011a
	II	Nussbaum et al., 1994	II	Watson et al., 2011b
	II	Paul et al., 1960		
	II	Ferguson, 1981		
	II	Franek et al., 2004		
	II	Taradaj et al., 2008		
	II	Bierman, 1954		
Strength of evidence: Moderate **Therapeutic effectiveness:** Substantiated				
Arthritic disorders	I	Huang et al., 2005a	I	Falconer et al., 1992
	II	Kazanoglu et al., 2003	I	Mueller et al., 1954
	II	De Preux, 1952	II	Aldes et al., 1952
	II	Svarcova et al., 1988	II	Ulus et al., 2012
	II	Swartz, 1953		
	II	Lehmann et al., 1954		
	II	Huang et al., 2005b		
	II	Ozgonenel et al., 2009		
Strength of evidence: Moderate **Therapeutic effectiveness:** Substantiated				
Mixed soft tissue disorders	II	Patrick, 1978	I	Roman, 1960
	II	Middlemast et al., 1978		
	II	Soren, 1965		
	II	Klaiman et al., 1998		
Strength of evidence: Moderate **Therapeutic effectiveness:** Substantiated				
Epicondylitis	I	Binder et al., 1985	I	Haker et al., 1991
	II	Aldes, 1956	II	Lundeberg et al., 1988
	II	Davidson et al., 2001		
Strength of evidence: Moderate **Therapeutic effectiveness:** Substantiated				
Perineal lesions	I	McLaren, 1984	I	Everett et al., 1992
	III	Fieldhouse, 1979	I	Creates, 1987
			I	Grant et al., 1989
Strength of evidence: Strong **Therapeutic effectiveness:** Unsupported				
Post-exercise muscle soreness			I	Hasson et al., 1990
			I	Craig et al., 1999
			I	Stay et al., 1998
			I	Plaskett et al., 1999
			I	Brock Symons et al., 2004
Strength of evidence: Strong **Therapeutic effectiveness:** Unsupported				

Health Condition	Benefit—Yes Rating	Benefit—Yes Reference	Benefit—No Rating	Benefit—No Reference
Ankle sprain	II	Makuloluwe et al., 1977	I	Williamson et al., 1986
			I	Nyanzi et al., 1999
			I	Zammit et al., 2005
			I	Oakland et al., 1993

Strength of evidence: Strong
Therapeutic effectiveness: Unsupported

Fewer Than 5 Studies

Health Condition	Benefit—Yes Rating	Benefit—Yes Reference	Benefit—No Rating	Benefit—No Reference
Back pain	I	Nwuga, 1983		
	I	Ansari et al., 2006b		
	II	Ebadi et al., 2012		
	II	Aldes et al., 1958		
Carpal tunnel syndrome	I	Ebenbichler et al., 1998	I	Oztas et al., 1998
	II	Bakhtiary et al., 2004	I	Yildiz et al., 2011
Postherpetic neuralgia	II	Garrett et al., 1982		
	II	Payne, 1984		
	II	Jones, 1984		
Myofascial pain	II	Talaat et al. 1995	I	Gam et al., 1998
	II	Esenyel et al., 2000		
Tendinopathy	II	Lanfear et al., 1972	I	Warden et al., 2008
	II	Chester et al., 2008	II	Stasinopoulos et al., 2004
Plantar warts	I	Cherup et al., 1963		
	II	Vaughn, 1973		
	II	Kent, 1959		
Dupuytren's contracture	III	Markham et al., 1980		
Hip contracture	II	Lehmann et al., 1961		
Phantom pain	II	Tepperberg et al., 1953		
Reflex sympathetic dystrophy	III	Portwood et al., 1987		
Neuroma	II	Uygur et al., 1995		
Meniscus tear	III	Muche, 2003		
Sinusitis	II	Ansari et al., 2007		
Plantar fasciitis	II	Clarke et al., 1976		
Tibial periostitis	II	Smith et al., 1986		
Heel pain	I	Crawford et al., 1996		
Dental pain			I	Hashish et al., 1986
			I	Hashish et al., 1988
Spasticity			II	Sahin et al., 2011
			III	Ansari et al., 2006a
Fibrotic muscles			I	Klemp et al., 1982
Breast engorgement			I	McLachlan et al., 1991

Strength of evidence: Pending
Therapeutic effectiveness: Pending

ALL CONDITIONS
Strength of evidence: Moderate
Therapeutic effectiveness: Substantiated

LOW-INTENSITY PULSED ULTRASOUND (LIPUS)

Health Condition	Benefit—Yes Rating	Benefit—Yes Reference	Benefit—No Rating	Benefit—No Reference
Bone fracture	I	Heckman et al., 1994	I	Emami et al., 1999a
	I	Dudda et al., 2011	I	Emami et al., 1999b
	I	Kristiansen et al., 1997	I	Lubbert et al., 2008
	I	Leung et al., 2004	I	Rue et al., 2004
	I	Ricardo, 2006	I	Handolin et al., 2005a
	II	Xavier et al., 1983	I	Handolin et al., 2005b
	II	El-Mowafi et al., 2005	I	Handolin et al., 2005c
	II	Tsumaki et al., 2004	II	Mayr et al., 2000
	II	Rutten et al., 2007		
	II	Rutten et al., 2008		
	II	Pigozzi et al., 2004		
	II	Roussignol et al., 2012		
	II	Corradi et al., 1953		
	II	Cook et al., 1997		
	II	Gebauer et al., 2005a		
	II	Jingushi et al., 2007		
	II	Gebauer et al., 2005b		
	II	Nolte et al., 2001		
	II	Lerner et al., 2004		
	III	Stein et al., 2005		
	III	Gold et al., 2005		
	III	Hemery et al., 2011		
	III	Giannini et al., 2004		

Strength of evidence: Moderate
Therapeutic effectiveness: Substantiated

Fewer Than 5 Studies

Health Condition	Benefit—Yes Rating	Benefit—Yes Reference	Benefit—No Rating	Benefit—No Reference
Congenital pseudoarthrosis	III	Okada et al., 2003		
Calcaneal osteoporosis			II	Warden et al., 2001

Health Condition	Benefit—Yes Rating	Benefit—Yes Reference	Benefit—No Rating	Benefit—No Reference
Chronic epicondylitis			I	D'Vaz et al., 2006
Strength of evidence: Pending **Therapeutic effectiveness:** Pending				
ALL CONDITIONS **Strength of evidence:** Moderate **Therapeutic effectiveness:** Substantiated				
NONCONTACT LOW-FREQUENCY ULTRASOUND (NCLFUS)				
Dermal wounds	I	Ennis et al., 2005		
	II	Kavros et al., 2007a		
	II	Kavros et al., 2007b		
	II	Kavros et al., 2008		
	II	Ennis et al., 2006		
	II	Escandon et al., 2012		
	II	Peschen et al., 1997		
	II	Weichenthal et al., 1997		
	II	Bell et al., 2008		
	II	Cole et al., 2009		
	II	Haan et al., 2009		
	III	Waldrop et al., 2008		
	III	Gehling et al., 2007		
Strength of evidence: Moderate **Therapeutic effectiveness:** Substantiated				

tolerate the pressure exerted by the soundhead applicator during treatment. Apply *medium pressure* over the skin, considering that too much pressure will wash away the coupling medium, thus decreasing the transfer of energy; too little pressure will cause improper coupling. When dealing with irregular body surfaces, both the contact with gel pad and noncontact with tap water methods can be used. Noncontact with tap water is the method of choice with very irregular and hypersensitive treatment surface areas.

5. Application Technique

The application technique is dynamic only because maintaining the soundhead stationary over the treated area will induce hot spots causing pain and potentially tissue burn, especially when the level of intensity used is elevated, which often is the case with the use of CUS therapy. Hot spots are caused by stationary or standing waves, which are formed when two waves of equal frequency that are traveling in opposite directions collide. Practically speaking, standing waves are high-energy waves concentrated in a small area that can be avoided by the continuous displacement of the soundhead applicator over the treated surface area.

6. Dosage

Dosage is based on the desired thermomechanical effects required for treatment. It is by far the most challenging, and sometime the most confusing, parameter to determine. For the very large majority of clinicians and authors of textbooks on electrophysical agents, *dosage* is simply express using two parameters: *intensity* and duration of *application*. For example, to document dosage as "*2 W/cm² for 8 minutes*" in patient files or research manuscripts is incomplete and misleading. Why is this so? Such a dosage expression is *no longer acceptable,* as discussed later, because it does not reflect the dose of ultrasonic energy delivered to the sonated tissues. To calculate the ultrasonic dose, one must take into consideration two other dosimetric parameters—namely, the *transducer ERA* and the *treatment surface area* (S). The product of intensity (I), measured in watts per square centimeter (W/cm²), and application duration (T), measured in seconds (s), corresponds to the energy density per treatment (E_D), measured in joules per square centimeter (J/cm²). It is calculated using the formula $E_D = I \times T$, where watts times seconds (W × s) equals joules. In the previous example, to report dosage as "2 W/cm² for 8 minutes" is to report that the energy density per treatment is equal to 980 J/cm². As demonstrated next, to report energy density per treatment is not to report the dose per treatment.

a. Dosage Calculation

Table 20-3 presents dosimetric examples related to continuous and pulsed applications of CUS therapy. These examples are designed to clarify the concept of dosage, which rests on the definition of dose. *Dose per treatment* is defined as the amount of ultrasonic energy delivered per square centimeter of tissue at the applicator–skin interface. To facilitate calculation, readers are invited to use the **Online Dosage Calculator: Ultrasound**.

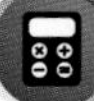

i. Continuous Mode

Spatial peak intensity (I_{SP}) is calculated by dividing the device's power (P), measured in watts (W), by the transducer faceplate effective radiating area (ERA), measured in square centimeters (cm²). It is expressed in units of watts per square centimeter (W/cm²) based on this formula: $I_{SP} = P/\text{ERA}$. In both examples shown in Table 20-3, I_{SP} equals 2 W/cm² (2 W/cm² = 10 W/5 cm²). Energy density is the product of intensity (W/cm²) and application duration measured in seconds ($E_D = I_{SP} \times T$).

TABLE 20-3 DOSAGE EXAMPLES FOR CONTINUOUS ULTRASOUND THERAPY

Parameters	Delivery Mode			
	Continuous*		Pulsed**	
Power (P)	10 W	10 W	10 W	10 W
Transducer effective radiating area (ERA)	5 cm^2	5 cm^2	5 cm^2	5 cm^2
Treatment surface area (S)	10 cm^2	15 cm^2	10 cm^2	15 cm^2
Spatial peak intensity (I_{SP})	2 W/cm^2	2 W/cm^2	2 W/cm^2	2 W/cm^2
Application duration (T)	480 s	480 s	480 s	480 s
Duty cycle (DC)	100%***	100%***	20%	20%
Energy density (E_D)	960 J/cm^2	960 J/cm^2	192 J/cm^2	192 J/cm^2
Spatial average intensity (I_{SA})	NA	NA	0.4 W/cm^2	0.4 W/cm^2
Total energy (E_T)	4,800 J	4,800 J	960 J	960 J
Dose per treatment (D_T)	**480 J/cm^2**	**320 J/cm^2**	**96 J/cm^2**	**64 J/cm^2**

* Continuous: $I_{SP} = P/ERA$; $E_D = I_{SP} \times T$; $E_T = I_{SP} \times ERA \times T$; $D_T = E_T/S$
** Pulsed: $I_{SA} = I_{SP} \times DC$; $E_D = I_{SA} \times T$; $E_T = I_{SA} \times ERA \times T$; $D_T = E_T/S$
*** DC: Always equal to 100% because there is no OFF time.

Use Online Dosage Calculator: Ultrasound

In both examples, application durations are identical at 8 minutes or 480 s. Energy density is equal to 960 J/cm^2 in both examples (960 J/cm^2 = 2 W/cm^2 × 480 s). Total energy (E_T), measured in Joules (J), is the product of three parameters: intensity (I_{SP}), transducer ERA, and application duration (T). It is calculated as follows: $E_T = I_{SP} \times ERA \times T$ (J = ((W/cm^2/cm^2) × T); J = W.s). In other words, this parameter refers to the total amount of ultrasonic energy delivered under the transducer ERA during the entire application duration. In both examples, E_T equals 4,800 J (4,800 J = 2 W/cm^2 × 5 cm^2 × 480 s). As mentioned earlier, the dose per treatment (D_T) refers to the amount of ultrasonic energy delivered per square centimeter of tissue at the applicator–skin interface. The dose per treatment takes into account the total energy (E_T) delivered and the treatment surface area (S) measured in square centimeters (cm^2). It is expressed in joules per square centimeters (J/cm^2) based on the following formula: $D_T = E_T/S$. In the first and second examples, doses per treatment equal 480 J/cm^2 (4,800 J/10 cm^2) and 320 J/cm^2 (4,800 J/15 cm^2), respectively. The dose per treatment is *smaller* in the second example because the same total energy is spread, or distributed, over a larger treatment (from 10 to 15 cm^2) area, within the same application duration (8 min), thus leaving less energy per square centimeter of tissue at the applicator–skin interface (see Table 20-3). Stated differently, dose per treatment (D_T) is said to be directly proportional to intensity, transducer ERA, and application duration, and inversely proportional to treatment surface area ($D_T = (I_{SP} \times \text{ERA} \times T)/S$).

ii. Pulsed Mode

When the flow of energy is interrupted or pulsed, the spatial average intensity needs to be calculated and taken into consideration. Spatial average intensity (I_{SA}) is calculated, as shown in Table 20-3, by multiplying the spatial peak intensity (I_{SP}) of the device by its duty cycle (DC), using this formula: $I_{SA} = I_{SP} \times$ DC. Recall that the duty cycle, expressed as a percentage (%), is derived from the selected ON and OFF times: DC = (ON/(ON + OFF)) × 100. In both examples, DC values are set at 20%, which yield spatial average intensities (I_{SA}) equal to 0.4 W/cm^2 (0.4 W/cm^2 = 2 W/cm^2 × 20%). Energy densities (E_D), measured at 192 J/cm^2, are identical in both examples (192 J/cm^2 = 0.4 W/cm^2 × 480 s). Keeping the application duration times (T) identical at 480 seconds or 8 minutes, total energy (E_T), in both examples, equals 960 J. The resulting dose per treatment (D_T) is, however, smaller than in the second example (64 J/cm^2) when compared to the first example (96 J/cm^2), because the treatment surface area (S) in the second example is larger (15 cm^2 vs. 10 cm^2).

b. Summing Up on the Concept of Dosage

Dosage is defined as the amount of ultrasonic energy delivered per square centimeter of tissue at the applicator–skin interface. To express dosage as the product of intensity and application duration i.e., W/cm^2, which is unfortunately routinely done in clinical settings, is incomplete and misleading because it reflects the *energy density* ($E_D = I \times T$), not the *dose*, delivered to soft tissues. To determine the dose per treatment (D_T), practitioners must take into consideration the transducer ERA (used to calculate total energy) and the treatment surface area (S), because the larger the treatment surface area for a given total energy, the smaller the dose per treatment. There is evidence to suggest that better treatment effectiveness using CUS is achieved when larger doses per treatment are delivered to soft tissues (Alexander et al., 2010).

7. Importance of Periodic Device Maintenance and Calibration

There is strong consensus in the literature to support the view that CUS devices are highly susceptible to *decalibration* after use. The extent of decalibration can have negative impacts on dosimetry and clinical effectiveness (Stewart et al., 1974; Allen et al., 1978; Stewart et al., 1980; Snow, 1982; Hekkenberg et al., 1986; Rivest et al., 1987; Chartered Society of Physiotherapy, 1990; Pye et al., 1994; Pye, 1996; Kimura et al., 1998; Artho et al., 2002; Johns et al., 2007; Straub et al., 2008). This situation may explain why different clinical outcomes are observed with seemingly identical devices and dosimetry (Holcomb et al., 2003; Merrick et al., 2003). As a result, it is strongly recommended that all CUS devices be inspected and calibrated several times a year and weekly if used frequently.

8. Need for Ultrasonic Coupling Media

For ultrasound energy to be effective, it must be properly transmitted to the soft tissues. The opposition to the transmission or flow of sound through a medium is called *acoustic impedance.* The specific acoustic impedance of a medium is defined as its density times its sound propagation velocity, and is measured in unit of newton second per cubic meter (N-s/m^3). For example, because of its low density and propagation velocity, *air* has a very low acoustic impedance (413 N-s/m^3) in comparison to *water* (1,440,000 N-s/m^3) and *steel* (45,000,000 N-s/m^3). *For maximal (100%) transmission of ultrasonic energy from one medium to the next, the acoustic impedance of the two media needs to be the same.* The greater the difference in acoustic impedance at the interface between the two media, the greater the amount of energy that is reflected back. The greater the reflection, the smaller the amount of ultrasound energy transmitted at the interface. Practically speaking, to penetrate soft tissues, the ultrasound beam has to overcome the *soundhead steel faceplate–air interface.* Biophysics has established that approximately 99.99% of ultrasound energy is reflected by air, meaning no transmission, because the very large difference (approximately 100,000 fold) between the acoustic impedance of steel and that of air (45,000,000 N-s/cm^3/413 N-s/cm^3). To optimize ultrasonic energy transmission, a suitable coupling medium is therefore required, to replace air at the soundhead faceplate–skin interface. Tap water is an ideal coupling medium because its acoustic impedance (1,440,000 N-s/m^3) closely matches that of soft tissues (1,350,000 N-s/m^3). Commercial aquasonic gels are also excellent coupling media, with transmissivity percentages ranging from 95% to 100% (Klucinec, 1997; Klucinec et al., 2000; Oshikoya et al., 2000; Myrer et al., 2001; Merrick et al., 2002; Casarotto et al., 2004; Gulick et al., 2005; Poltawski et al., 2007).

B. LOW-INTENSITY PULSED ULTRASOUND

The dosimetry related to LIPUS therapy, contrary to that of CUS discussed previously, is much simpler because there is only one dosimetric protocol used for treatment (Table 20-4). All of the dosimetric parameters relate to this research-based dosimetric protocol. Clinicians need only to turn the device on, and the desired dosage is ready to be delivered at the bone fracture site. This standardized dosage is based on data gathered from both animal research and human clinical trials. LIPUS is routinely applied at very low intensity (0.03 W/cm^2), for 20 minutes (1,200 s), using a 4 cm^2 transducer ERA. The ultrasonic beam is pulsed with a 20% duty cycle (ON:OFF ratio 1:4). ON time (i.e., pulse duration) is fixed at 200 μs, and pulse frequency is preset at 1,000 Hz. The application is stationary with the transducer ERA covering the fracture site area (S), which is 4 cm^2 because it is equivalent to transducer ERA. The *dose per treatment* (D_T), in this case, equals 36 J/cm^2: 36 J/cm^2 = (0.03 W/cm^2 × 4 cm^2 × 1,200 s)/4 cm^2. LIPUS may be applied directly on the skin overlying the bone fracture site, or in-cast or on-cast situations using a specially designed retaining and fixating system. The application method is stationary because the ultrasonic intensity level is very low (0.03 or 30 mW/cm^2), thus posing minimal to no risk for the occurrence of hot spots. The application duration is fixed at 20 minutes per treatment, and treatments are applied daily until satisfactory bone healing is achieved. The device will automatically shut itself off with an audible beep when the 20 minutes is complete.

C. NONCONTACT LOW-FREQUENCY ULTRASOUND

The dosimetry and application of NCLFUS, shown in Table 20-5, is standardized based on research data from human clinical trials. NCLFUS delivers continuous low-frequency (40 kHz) and low-intensity (0.5 W/cm^2) ultrasound energy to the wound bed via a fine mist of sterile water that acts as a conduit for transmitting the energy from the transducer faceplate to the treatment site. The applicator tip makes no contact with the wound bed and is held perpendicular to the wound surface, with its tip approximately 0.5 to 1.5 cm (0.2 to 0.6 in) away from the wound. The application technique is dynamic, with the applicator moved vertically and horizontally across the wound using multiple passes. Application duration is variable and is directly related to wound size. The larger the wound size, the longer the application duration (Bell et al., 2008; Driver et al., 2011; Voigt et al.,

TABLE 20-4 STANDARDIZED DOSIMETRIC PARAMETERS AND PROTOCOL FOR LOW-INTENSITY PULSED ULTRASOUND THERAPY

Parameters	LIPUS
Frequency (Hz)	1.5 MHz
Delivery mode	Pulsed: *Pulse frequency:* 1,000 Hz *Pulse duration:* 200 μs *Duty cycle:* 20% *ON:OFF ratio:* 1:4
Intensity (I)	Spatial average intensity (I_{SA}) = 0.03 W/cm^2
Transducer ERA	4 cm^2
Treatment surface area (S)	4 cm^2
Application method and coupling medium	Contact with aquasonic gel On the skin surface overlying the bone fracture site In-cast or on-cast application
Application technique	*Stationary:* Transducer placed immediately over the bone fracture line
Application duration (T)	1,200 s (20 min)
Treatment frequency	Daily
Dose per treatment (D_T)	**36 J/cm^2**

LIPUS, low-intensity pulsed ultrasound; ERA, effective radiating area.

2011; Escandon et al., 2012). Upon entering the wound size (cm^2) on the unit console, the corresponding application time will appear. For example, duration from 3 to 20 minutes may be necessary to treat a wound size ranging from 10 to 30 cm. Treatment frequency is every second day. It is impossible to calculate the exact dose per treatment because the applicator to wound distance will fluctuate throughout the application duration, inducing water mist ERA variation, and because clinicians may spend more time debriding a certain area of wound over other areas, causing variable energy absorption per square centimeter of tissue.

TABLE 20-5 STANDARDIZED DOSIMETRIC PARAMETERS AND PROTOCOL FOR NONCONTACT LOW-FREQUENCY ULTRASOUND THERAPY

Parameters	NCLFUS
Frequency (Hz)	40 kHz
Delivery mode	Continuous
Intensity (I)	Spatial peak intensity (I_{SP}) = 0.5 W/cm^2
Application method	Noncontact
Application technique	Dynamic
Applicator to wound distance	0.5 to 1.5 cm
Application duration (T)	3 to 20 minutes, depending on wound size
Treatment frequency	Every second day

NCLFUS, noncontact low-frequency ultrasound.

V. APPLICATION, CONTRAINDICATIONS, AND RISKS

Prior to considering the application of therapeutic ultrasound, practitioners must first consider the contraindications and risks associated with it and then turn their attention to those key application steps and procedures designed to optimize treatment safety, efficacy, and effectiveness. To further facilitate and visualize the application of therapeutic ultrasound, readers are invited to view related **online videos**.

APPLICATION, CONTRAINDICATIONS, AND RISKS

Ultrasound

IMPORTANT: Conduct a thermal skin discrimination test prior to first application. Cleanse the soundhead faceplate with cleansing solution *after* each use to prevent spreading of nocosomial infection (Schabrun et al., 2006). Illustrated, as examples, are the applications of conventional ultrasound (Fig. 20-9) and noncontact low-frequency ultrasound (Fig. 20-10).

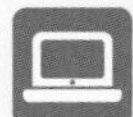

See **online videos.**

CONVENTIONAL ULTRASOUND (CUS)

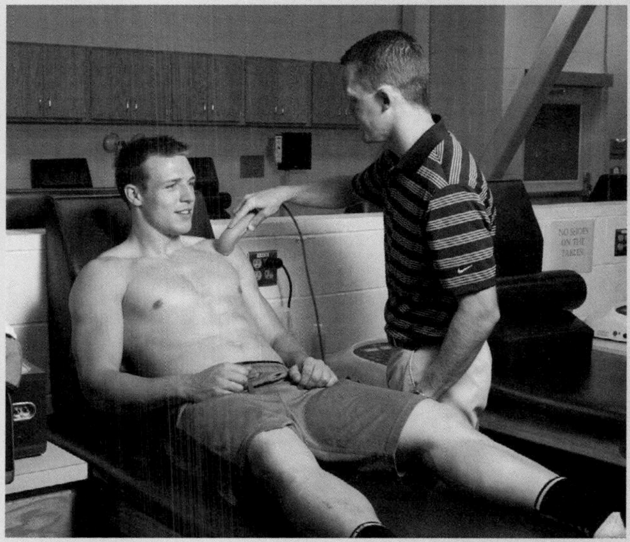

STEP	RATIONALE
1. Check for contraindications.	*Over malignant area*—increases tumor growth
	Over hemorrhagic area—increases hemorrhagic response
	Over ischemic area—increases ischemia resulting from the vascular system's inability to meet the increased metabolic demand induced by the induced-heat response
	Over area of thrombosis—thrombus detachment leading to embolism
	Over infected lesion—spread of infection
	Over gonads—infertility
	Over the eye—cavitation of humor fluid leading to damage to the retina
	Over the pelvic abdominal and lumbar areas of women who are pregnant—disruption of fetal development
	Over the pelvic and lumbar areas of women who are menstruating—increases menstrual flow
	Over the spinal cord after laminectomy—cavitation of cerebrospinal fluid leading to damage to the spinal cord
	Over plastic and cemented implants—heating can cause damage to plastic, cement, and surrounding soft tissues. CUS can be safely used over or around metallic implants (Gersten, 1958; Lehmann et al., 1958, 1959, 1961; Skoubo-Kristensen et al., 1982).
	Near or over all electronic implants—electronic malfunction
2. Consider the risks.	*Over epiphyseal plate*—may alter normal bone growth (Nussbaum et al., 2006)
	With patients who have received radiotherapy—wait at least 6 months after the last radiotherapy treatment before using CUS over cancerous areas
3. Position and instruct patient.	Ensure comfortable body positioning, and inform the patient that a sensation of heat may be present during treatment.

FIGURE 20-9 Application of conventional ultrasound over the shoulder area. (Reprinted with permission from Knight KL, Draper DO. Therapeutic Modalities: The Art and Science. 2nd ed. Philadelphia: Lippincott Williams & Wilkins, 2013.)

STEP	RATIONALE
4. Prepare treated area.	Cleanse the skin overlying the targeted area with rubbing alcohol. Shave or clip excess hair over treatment area because air bubbles tend to cling to them, thus reducing ultrasound transmission.
5. Select application method.	Choose between *contact* and *noncontact* methods. Noncontact is recommended when the treated surface area is too irregular or too painful for contact by the applicator.
6. Select coupling medium.	• *For contact method:* Use commercial ultrasonic gel for optimal ultrasonic transmissivity (Poltawski et al., 2006). Avoid gel and degassed water in latex gloves or condoms (Klucinec, 1997). Use thinner gel pads to optimize transmissivity (Draper et al., 2010). Apply a thin layer of ultrasonic gel at the applicator/pad–skin interface. Keep ultrasonic coupling media at room temperature for optimal thermal effect (Oshikoya et al., 2000). • *For noncontact method:* Immerse both body segment and applicator in a plastic bath or tub filled with tap or degassed water. Keep the soundhead faceplate at a distance of 2–3 cm for the skin overlying affected tissue, because the farther away it is, the less the temperature elevation in the tissues (Robertson et al., 1996). To compensate for thermal energy loss to water, increase dosage with distance (Draper et al., 1993b; Robertson et al., 1996). Air bubbles will accumulate on both the applicator faceplate and irradiated skin surface during treatment. Wipe off the bubbles periodically, using a stick or with a brush of one's finger, to ensure maximum transmission at all times during the application.
7. Prepare device.	Keep ultrasound devices at least 5 m (15 ft) away from functioning shortwave diathermy devices to prevent electromagnetic interference. Plug line-powered devices into ground-fault circuit interrupter (GFCI) receptacles to eliminate the risk of electrical macroshock (see Chapter 5). Make sure that the ultrasound device is properly calibrated and that its beam nonuniformity ratio (BNR) value is between 2 and 8.
8. Estimate lesion depth and surface area.	Estimate the depth of the lesion (in centimeters) from the skin surface as well as its surface area (in square centimeters). Information about tissue depth will guide the selection of frequency. Estimation of the lesion surface area will guide the selection of transducer effective radiating area (ERA).
9. Select frequency.	Choose between 1 and 3 MHz. The deeper the lesion, the shorter the frequency.
10. Select applicator size (ERA).	Applicators in different sizes or ERAs are available (see Fig. 20-1B). Transducer ERA (applicator size) is directly related to the treatment surface area under consideration. Keep a ratio of less than 3 between these two surface areas, such that the treated surface area (S) is no more than 3 times greater than the transducer ERA (Chan et al., 1998). For example, the maximum surface area that can be treated with a transducer of 5-cm^2 ERA is 15 cm^2.
11. Select delivery mode.	Choose between the *continuous* and *pulsed* modes. Theoretically, the continuous mode will always deliver more ultrasonic energy to the tissues per unit of time, and consequently more thermal effects, than the pulsed mode.
12. Select application technique.	Use the dynamic technique because the stationary technique is likely to cause hot spots. Slowly move the applicator at low speed (2–7 cm/s), and with a light pressure, over the treatment area (Weaver et al., 2006). These movements should not be too fast, because the faster the movements, the less the absorption of ultrasonic energy into the soft tissues per unit of time. Do a series of up-and-down, side-to-side, and overlapping circular movements while attempting to cover the entire treatment surface area evenly. Keep the applicator faceplate perpendicular to the treatment surface to minimize reflection.
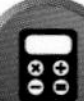 **13. Set dosimetry.**	Use Table 20-2 as a guideline. See Table 20-3 for dosimetric calculation. Use the **Online Dosage Calculator: Ultrasound**.
14. Apply treatment.	Apply the soundhead faceplate over the treatment surface, and turn the device ON.

STEP	RATIONALE
15. Conduct post-treatment procedures.	Wipe off excess ultrasonic gel or water. Inspect the exposed skin area, and record any adverse reaction.
16. Ensure post-treatment equipment maintenance.	Clean and disinfect the applicator faceplate to ensure optimal hygiene and prevent cross-contamination between patients (Schabrun et al., 2006). Follow manufacturer recommendations. Immediately report all defects or malfunctions to technical maintenance staff.

LOW-INTENSITY PULSED ULTRASOUND (LIPUS)

STEP	RATIONALE
1. Check for contraindications.	*Near or over all electronic implants*—electronic interference
2. Position and instruct patient.	Ensure comfortable body positioning, and inform the patient that no sensation should be felt during treatment.
3. Prepare treated area.	Cleanse the skin surface overlying the targeted fracture site area with rubbing alcohol and dry. Clip or shave excessive hair if necessary.
4. Locate the fracture site.	Put an X mark on the skin overlying the bone fracture site with a dermal pen.
5. Position the retaining and alignment fixture (RAF).	The RAF is composed of an adjustable strap and a cap (see online video). Positioned the strap with the cap placed directly over the fracture as marked on the skin. Apply a layer of ultrasonic gel onto the transducer faceplate, place the transducer into the RAF, and snap the cap to close.
6. Set dosimetry.	All dosimetric parameters are preset. See Table 20-4.
7. Apply treatment.	The device is powered by a nonrechargeable lithium battery that can be changed after a lifetime of more than 150 treatment periods of 20 minutes each. It will deliver low-intensity pulsed ultrasound energy, run for 20 minutes, and then turn itself off.
8. Conduct post-treatment procedure.	Remove the RAF. Inspect the skin, and record any adverse reactions. Open cap. Remove transducer from RAF, and wipe off gel from the transducer using a soft cloth. Wipe off any gel remaining on skin with a soft cloth.
9. Ensure post-treatment equipment maintenance.	Follow manufacturer recommendations. Immediately report all defects or malfunctions to technical maintenance staff.

NONCONTACT LOW-FREQUENCY ULTRASOUND (NCLFUS)

STEP	RATIONALE
1. Check for contraindications.	*Near or over all electronic implants*—electronic interference
2. Consider the risks.	Treatment of open wounds always presents a risk of cross-contamination. The wearing of goggles, mask, gown, and gloves is highly recommended.

STEP	RATIONALE
3. Position and instruct patient.	Ensure comfortable body positioning, and inform the patient about the feeling of a fine water mist over the wound area during treatment.
4. Prepare wound treatment area.	Expose the wound and then measure its size (in square centimeters) using a ruler or a planimeter.
5. Prepare the device.	Keep the device at least 5 m (15 ft) away from functioning shortwave diathermy devices to prevent electromagnetic interference. Plug line-powered devices into GFCI receptacles to eliminate the risk of electrical macroshock (see Chapter 5). The device is composed of a generator and handheld transducer, to which is attached a single-use disposable applicator (see Fig. 20-3B and online videos). Press the applicator onto the transducer tip in one continuous motion. Place the refillable saline bottle upright into the applicator. Turn the generator ON.
6. Set dosimetry.	All dosimetric parameters are *preset* with the exception of wound size (see Table 20-5). Enter wound size (in square centimeters) into the console. The corresponding application time will automatically appear. Larger wound beds will require longer-duration applications. When treating wounds with sizes greater than 30 cm^2 on the same patient, it will be necessary to refill the saline bottle, using sterile saline water, during treatment.
7. Apply treatment.	Position and maintain the applicator perpendicular to the wound with the leading edge of the applicator approximately 0.5 to 1.5 cm (0.2 to 0.6 in) from the wound surface (Fig. 20-10). Depress and release the control button to initiate the saline flow. Move the applicator over the wound surface using slow vertical and horizontal multiple strokes or passes. The applicator tip must not touch the wound.
8. Conduct post-treatment procedure.	Inspect the wound, and record any adverse reactions. Remove the applicator from the transducer. Discard the applicator and saline bottle. Clean and disinfect the applicator, cable, and device to ensure optimal hygiene and prevent cross-contamination between patients.
9. Ensure post-treatment equipment maintenance.	Follow manufacturer recommendations. Immediately report defects or malfunctions to technical maintenance staff.

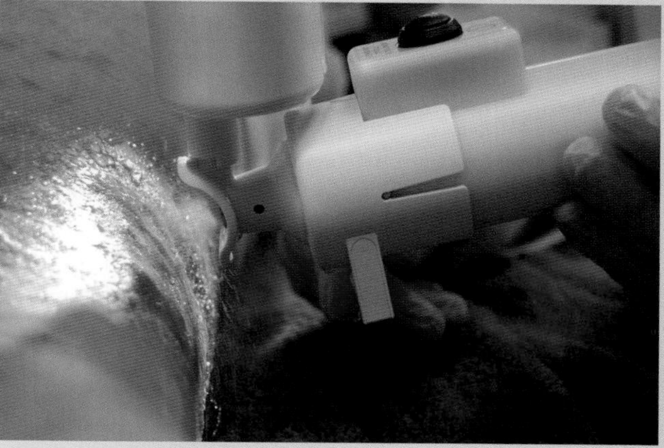

FIGURE 20-10 Application of noncontact low-frequency ultrasound to an open wound. Ultrasonic effervescence is visible in the form of a bubbling or frothing action at the wound surface. (Courtesy of Celleration.)

CASE STUDIES

Three case studies summarize the concepts, principles, and applications of therapeutic ultrasound discussed in this chapter. Case Study 20-1 addresses the use of conventional ultrasound (CUS) for a shoulder tendinosis affecting a middle-aged man. Case Study 20-2 is concerned with the use of low-intensity pulsed ultrasound (LIPUS) for the treatment of a slow-to-heal humeral bone fracture affecting a woman. Case Study 20-3 addresses the use of noncontact low-frequency ultrasound (NCLFUS) for an open infected wound affecting a man who is diabetic. Each case is structured in line with the concepts of evidence-based practice (EBP), the International Classification of Functioning, Disability, and Health (ICF) disablement model, and SOAP (*s*ubjective, *o*bjective, *a*ssessment, *p*lan) note format (see Chapter 2 for details).

CASE STUDY 20-1: CONVENTIONAL ULTRASOUND FOR SHOULDER TENDINOSIS

EVIDENCE-BASED CLINICAL DECISION MAKING PROTOCOL

1. Formulate the Case History

A 44-year-old right-handed commercial painter, diagnosed with a rotator cuff tendonitis to his right shoulder 4 months ago, is referred for conservative treatment before considering surgery. The shoulder condition has evolved from a state of tendinitis to tendinosis. Radiologic imaging reveals no calcification. This patient has a surgical history that reveals a metallic implant associated with a past injury to his right acromioclavicular joint. His main complaint is pain during movement and at palpation and restricted right shoulder function. Goniometric evaluation reveals deficits in range of motion (ROM) of 20 degrees in abduction and 30 degrees in elevation. The affected tendons are estimated to be at a depth of approximately 3 cm from the overlying skin surface. Treatment surface area is estimated at 10 cm^2. Past treatments included oral and injected analgesic and anti-inflammatory drugs. This therapeutic approach gave less than satisfactory results. The patient continues taking analgesic drugs to control his chronic shoulder pain. He works 3 days a week, and with his right arm, doing only those painting tasks that are below shoulder height. His goal is to resume full-time work with no functional limitation as soon as possible and without having to undergo surgical treatment.

2. Outline the Case Based on the ICF Framework

SHOULDER TENDINOSIS		
BODY STRUCTURES AND FUNCTIONS	**ACTIVITIES**	**PARTICIPATION**
Pain	Difficulty with painting tasks	Unable to work full-time
Decrease ROM	Difficulty with some shoulder activities of daily living (ADLs)	

PERSONAL FACTORS	ENVIRONMENTAL FACTOR
Healthy man	Home construction
Outdoor character	

3. Outline Therapeutic Goals and Outcome Measurements

GOAL	OUTCOME MEASUREMENT
Decrease pain	Visual Analogue scale (VAS)
Increase shoulder ROM	Goniometry
Avoid surgery and accelerate return to full-time work	Constant Shoulder Score (CSS)

4. Justify the Use of Conventional Ultrasound Based on the EBP Framework

PRACTITIONER'S EXPERIENCE	RESEARCH-BASED INDICATIONS	PATIENT'S EXPECTATION
Experienced in CUS	*Strength:* Moderate	Has no opinion on CUS treatment
Has used CUS in previous cases	*Effectiveness:* Conflicting	Hopes to avoid surgery
Is unsure about treatment effectiveness		Wants to return to full-time work

5. Outline Key Intervention Parameters

- **Treatment base:** Private clinic
- **Ultrasound device:** Cabinet-type CUS. The thermomechanical effects are expected to enhance the proliferative and maturation phase of tendon healing, thus facilitating normal function.
- **Contraindication:** None, because metallic implants are present in the right shoulder area, *not* metallic implants.
- **Application protocol:** Follow the suggested application protocol for CUS in *Application, Contraindications, and Risks* box, and make the necessary adjustments for this case. See **online videos.**
- **Dosimetry*:** See Table 20-2, Table 20-3, and following information.
- **Frequency:** 1 MHz
- **Delivery mode:** Pulsed
- **Duty cycle:** 50%
- **Patient's positioning:** Lying supine
- **Applicator type:** Handheld
- **Treatment surface area:** 10 cm^2
- **Transducer effective radiating area (ERA):** 5 cm^2
- **Application method:** Contact
- **Coupling medium:** Aquasonic gel
- **Application technique:** Dynamic
- **Spatial average intensity (I_{SA}):** 0.5 W/cm^2
- **Application duration:** 420 s (7 min)
- **Energy density (E_D):** 210 J/cm^2
- **Total energy (E_T):** 1,050 J
- **Dose per treatment (D_T):** 105 J/cm^2
- **Treatment frequency:** 3 times per week
- **Intervention period:** 4 weeks
- **Concomitant therapies:** Regimen of shoulder flexibility and strengthening exercises. Home-based program focused on maintaining shoulder movements.
- **Use the Online Dosage Calculator: Ultrasound.**

6. Report Pre- and Post-Intervention Outcomes

OUTCOME	PRE	POST
Pain (VAS score)	4/10	2/10
Shoulder ROM	*Abduction:* 20% restriction *Elevation:* 30% restriction	5% restriction 5% restriction
CSS	45%	70%
Work status	Part-time	Full-time

7. Document Case Intervention Using the SOAP Note Format

S: Middle-aged male Pt presents with a moderate case of rotator cuff tendinosis to right shoulder.

O: *Intervention:* CUS at 1 MHz; Pulsed; DC 50%; applicator ERA 5 cm^2; contact application with aquasonic gel; I_{SA} 0.5 W/cm^2; application duration 7 min; E_D 210 J/cm^2; E_T 1,050 J; dose per treatment (D_T) 105 J/cm^2. *Pre–post comparison:* Pain decrease (VAS 4/10 to 2/10); ROM increase: abduction from 20% to 5% restriction; elevation from 30% to 5% restriction; improved shoulder function: CSS score from 45% to 70%; improved work status: part-time to full-time.

A: No adverse effect.

P: No further treatment required. Pt instructed to minimize the use of his right upper limb for painting tasks above shoulder height. High risk of aggravation of his shoulder condition because of the nature of his employment (repeated use of his right upper limb for painting commercial buildings). This patient will need to strengthen his right shoulder and make judicious use (using the left upper limb more often) of his right shoulder at work. Otherwise, the need for additional CUS treatments is very likely over the months or years to come. Surgery as a last resort cannot be ruled out if further conservative treatments fail, and if the patient is then willing to accept it.

CASE STUDY 20-2: LOW-INTENSITY PULSED ULTRASOUND FOR NONUNION HUMERAL FRACTURE

EVIDENCE-BASED CLINICAL DECISION MAKING PROTOCOL

1. Formulate the Case History

An active 57-year-old woman broke her left humerus about 11 months ago in a bad fall while skiing. Despite traditional orthopedic management and regular follow-up for her condition (surgery involving metallic rod, plates, and screws followed by cast immobilization), she is diagnosed today with nonunion of her fracture. Her main complaint is residual pain, combined with the limited use of her upper right arm in the course of her daily activities. She is eager to resume her daily activities, including skiing. Her goal is to achieve complete union or resolution of the fracture without further surgery. To accelerate bone healing and the complete resolution of this fracture, the orthopedic surgeon refers this patient for LIPUS therapy. The purpose is to initiate treatment at the hospital and then to instruct and train her for home therapy for the remaining weeks of treatment. The patient is asked to come to the hospital for periodic radiographs to monitor the resolution of her bone fracture.

2. Outline the Case Based on the ICF Framework

NONUNION HUMERAL FRACTURE		
BODY STRUCTURES AND FUNCTIONS	**ACTIVITIES**	**PARTICIPATION**
Pain	Limited ability to do ADLs	Unable to resume skiing
Bone nonunion at fracture site		

PERSONAL FACTORS	ENVIRONMENTAL FACTORS
Healthy woman	Housewife
Athletic character	Recreational sports
Retired	Fitness and leisure

3. Outline Therapeutic Goals and Outcome Measurements

GOAL	OUTCOME MEASUREMENT
Decrease pain	101-point Numerical Rating Scale (NRS-101)
Achieve complete bone calcification and union	Serial radiography
Upper arm function	Patient-Specific Functional Scale (PSFS)

4. Justify the Use of Low-Intensity Pulsed Ultrasound Based on the EBP Framework

PRACTITIONER'S EXPERIENCE	RESEARCH-BASED INDICATIONS	PATIENT'S EXPECTATION
Minimal experience in LIPUS	*Strength:* Moderate	Hopeful that the treatment will work
Has occasionally used LIPUS in previous cases	*Effectiveness:* Substantiated	Wants to recover full upper limb function
Is convinced that LIPUS will be beneficial		

5. Outline Key Intervention Parameters

- **Treatment base:** Hospital first and home thereafter
- **Ultrasound device:** Battery-operated LIPUS device. LIPUS is expected to promote osteogenesis, thus building the necessary callus for complete union of bone.
- **Contraindication:** There is no known contraindication to the use of LIPUS therapy.
- **Patient's positioning:** Sitting with upper arm resting on table
- **Application protocol:** Follow the suggested application protocol for LIPUS therapy in *Application, Contraindications, and Risks* box, and make the necessary adjustments for this case. See **online videos**.

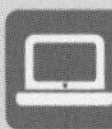

- **Dosimetry:** See Table 20-4 and following information.
- **Frequency:** 1.5 MHz
- **Delivery mode:** Pulsed
- **Duty cycle:** 20%
- **Treatment surface area:** Longitudinal fracture zone; estimated at 5 cm^2
- **Transducer ERA:** 5 cm^2
- **Application method:** Contact
- **Applicator fixation:** The transducer is kept in place with a plastic retaining and alignment fixture strapped in position over the marking on the skin that identifies the nonunion fracture site.
- **Fracture site identification:** Marked on the skin using a dermatologic pen

- **Coupling medium:** Aquasonic gel
- **Application technique:** Stationary—applicator applied directly over the bone fracture site
- **Spatial average intensity (I_{SA}):** 0.03 W/cm^2
- **Application duration:** 20 minutes (1,200 s)
- **Treatment frequency:** Daily
- **Intervention period:** Until satisfactory bone union
- **Concomitant therapy:** Home-based program focused on maintaining shoulder movements

6. Report Pre- and Post-Intervention Outcomes

OUTCOME	PRE	POST
Pain (NRS-101 score)	45	10
Bone healing		Consolidation
Upper arm function (PSFS score)	60%	90%

7. Document Case Intervention Using the SOAP Note Format

S: Female Pt presents with a case of nonunion humeral bone fracture following a skiing accident.

O: *Intervention:* LIPUS 1.5 MHz; Pulsed; DC 20%; applicator ERA 5 cm^2; contact application with aquasonic gel; application duration 20 min; I_{SA} 0.03 W/cm^2; E_D 36 J/cm^2; E_T 180 J; dose per treatment (D_T) 36 J/cm^2.

Pre–post comparison: Pain decrease: NRS-101 from 45 to 10; complete bone healing and consolidation; improved upper function: PSFS score from 60% to 90%.

A: No adverse effect. Pt overwhelmed with the result.

P: No further treatment required.

CASE STUDY 20-3: NONCONTACT LOW-FREQUENCY ULTRASOUND FOR RECALCITRANT DIABETIC ANKLE ULCER

EVIDENCE-BASED CLINICAL DECISION MAKING PROTOCOL

1. Formulate the Case History

A 54-year-old man with diabetes, diagnosed 5 months ago with a right ankle ischemic ulcer, is referred for treatment. The wound does not respond to treatment with multi-layered compression bandages. Physical examination reveals the presence of yellow slough, fibrin, tissue exudates, and bacteria in the wound bed. The wound has been recalcitrant to standard care (manual debridement and dressing), which has delayed healing. The therapeutic goal is for wound cleansing and debridement leading to wound healing. The ulcer is located below the medial malleolus. The wound size is irregular, with a surface area corresponding to 15 cm^2. The patient has difficulty wearing shoes and walking, both of which have a negative impact on his ADLs and work (no car; must use public transportation to commute to work). Pain is always present and is aggravated by ankle joint movement. The patient is anxious. He desperately wants to keep his ability to walk so that he is able to commute to work.

2. Outline the Case Based on the ICF Framework

RECALCITRANT DIABETIC ANKLE ULCER		
BODY STRUCTURES AND FUNCTIONS	**ACTIVITIES**	**PARTICIPATION**
Pain	Difficulty walking	Difficulty commuting (walking) to work
Open infected wound	Difficulty with ADLs	

PERSONAL FACTORS	ENVIRONMENTAL FACTOR
Middle-aged man	Home and leisure
Worker	
College educated	

3. Outline Therapeutic Goals and Outcome Measurements

GOAL	OUTCOME MEASUREMENT
Decrease pain	Visual Analogue Scale (VAS)
Eliminate wound infection	Serial bacterial counts
Increase wound healing	Serial digital photographs (wound surface area)
Improve walking	Patient-Specific Functional Scale (PSFS)

4. Justify the Use of Noncontact Low-Frequency Ultrasound Based on the EBP Framework

PRACTITIONER'S EXPERIENCE	EVIDENCE-BASED INDICATIONS	PATIENT'S EXPECTATION
Experienced in NCLFUS	*Strength:* Moderate	No opinion on treatment
Has used NCLFUS in previous cases	*Effectiveness:* Substantiated	Just wants to resume normal walking
Believes that NCLFUS can be beneficial		

5. Outline Key Intervention Parameters

- **Treatment base:** Hospital
- **Ultrasound device:** Line-powered NCLFUS system. NCLFUS is expected to cleanse and disinfect the wound through effective debridement and thus facilitate and accelerate wound healing.
- **Contraindication:** None
- **Application protocol:** Follow the suggested application protocol for NCLFUS therapy in *Application, Contraindications, and Risks* box, and make the necessary adjustments for this case. See **online videos**.

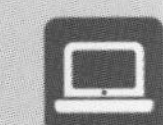

- **Dosimetry:** See Table 20-5 and following information.
- **Frequency:** 40 kHz
- **Delivery mode:** Continuous
- **Patient's positioning:** Lying on bed with leg extended
- **Transducer ERA:** 1 cm^2
- **Treatment surface area:** 15 cm^2
- **Application method:** Noncontact
- **Application technique:** Dynamic—slow, even, repeated vertical and horizontal passes over wound bed
- **Applicator to wound distance:** 1 cm
- **Coupling medium:** Sterile water in a bottle
- **Spatial peak intensity (I_{SP}):** 0.5 W/cm^2
- **Application duration:** 4 minutes
- **Treatment frequency:** Every second day
- **Intervention period:** Until wound closure
- **Concomitant therapy:** Home-based wound care

6. Report Pre- and Post-Intervention Outcomes

OUTCOME	PRE	POST
Pain (VAS score)	6/10	0/10
Bacterial count	Present	Eliminated
Wound healing	*Open wound surface area:* 15 cm^2	Wound closed
Walking status	Limited	Normal

7. Document Case Intervention Using the SOAP Note Format

S: Male Pt presents with diabetic recalcitrant leg ulcer.

O: *Intervention:* NCLFUS; 40 kHz; continuous; applicator ERA 1 cm^2; noncontact—mist of sterile water; dynamic application; applicator to wound distance 1 cm; application duration 4 min; I_{SP} 0.5 W/cm^2. *Pre–post comparison:* Pain decrease: VAS 6/10 to 0/10; wound infection eliminated; complete wound closure; normal walking.

A: No adverse effect. Pt extremely pleased with the result.

P: No further treatment required. To prevent recurrence, the patient needs to control his diabetic condition and wear adequate shoes.

VI. THE BOTTOM LINE

- There is strong scientific evidence to show that ultrasound energy, delivered at frequencies ranging from 40 kHz to 3 MHz and at intensities up to 3 W/cm^2, can induce significant therapeutic thermal and mechanical effects on human soft tissues.
- Ultrasound energy is the production of mechanical acoustic waves resulting from the reversed piezoelectric property of natural or synthetic materials called *transducers.*
- The thermal effects of ultrasonic acoustic waves are caused by molecular microfriction.
- The mechanical effects of ultrasonic waves are caused by stable cavitation and microstreaming.
- The delivery of ultrasonic energy to soft tissues requires the use of a coupling medium.
- Dosage, or dose per treatment, is defined as the amount of ultrasonic energy delivered per square centimeter of tissues at the applicator–skin interface and is measured in joules per square centimeter (J/cm^2).
- To express dosage as the product of intensity and application duration—for example, "1.5W/cm^2 for 6 minutes"—is incomplete and misleading, and therefore no longer acceptable, because it reflects the *energy density, not the dose per treatment,* delivered to soft tissues.
- To determine the dose per treatment, practitioners must take into consideration four parameters: intensity, application duration, transducer ERA, and treatment surface area.
- Therapeutic ultrasound is delivered in three forms: CUS, LIPUS, and NCLFUS.
- Ultrasound energy is absorbed primarily by high protein–low water content soft tissues such as bones, tendons, ligaments, and muscles.
- CUS is used primarily for the treatment of pathologies affecting connective (tendons and ligaments) and muscular tissues.
- LIPUS is dedicated to the treatment of delayed-union and nonunion bone fractures.
- NCLFUS is used to cleanse and debride open wounds.
- The evidence behind the use of CUS is *conflicting,* whereas that related to both LIPUS and NCLFUS is *substantiated.*

VII. CRITICAL THINKING QUESTIONS

Clarification: What is meant by CUS, LIPUS, and NCLFUS therapy?

Assumptions: You assume that the thermomechanical effects of CUS are frequency and intensity dependent. How do you justify making this assumption?

Reasons and evidence: What leads you to believe that the reverse piezoelectric phenomenon is responsible for the production of acoustic waves?

Viewpoints or perspectives: How will you respond to a colleague who says that the use of LIPUS therapy is similar to using CUS therapy in its pulsed mode and at low intensity?

Implications and consequences: What are the implications and consequences of using CUS for its thermal effect on a patient wearing an implanted Medtronic neurostimulation system?

About the question: What is the difference between intensity and dose per treatment? Why do you think I ask this question?

VIII. REFERENCES

Articles

Ainsworth R, Dziedzic K, Hiller L, Daniels J, Bruton A, Broadfield J (2007) A prospective double blind placebo-controlled randomized trial of US in the physiotherapy treatment of shoulder pain. Rheumatology, 48: 815–820

Aldes JH (1956) Ultrasonic radiation in the treatment of epicondylitis. Gen Pract, 13: 89–96

Aldes JH, Grabin S (1958) Ultrasound in the treatment of intervertebral disc syndrome. Am J Phys Med, 37: 199–202

Aldes JH, Jadeson WJ (1952) Ultrasonic therapy in the treatment of hypertrophic arthritis in elderly patients. Ann West Med Surg, 6: 545–550

Aldes JH, Jadeson WJ, Grabinsky S (1954a) A new approach to the treatment of subdeltoid bursitis. Am J Phys Med, 33: 79–88

Aldes JH, Klaras T (1954b) Use of ultrasonic radiation in the treatment of subdeltoid bursitis with and without calcareous deposits. West J Surg Obstet Gynecol, 62: 369–376

Allen KG, Battye CK (1978) Performance of ultrasonic therapy instruments. Physiotherapy, 64: 174–179

Ansari NN, Adelmanesh F, Nafhdi S, Tabtabaei A (2006a) The effect of physiotherapeutic ultrasound on muscle spasticity in patients with hemiplegia: A pilot study. Electromyogr Clin Neurophysiol, 46: 247–252

Ansari NN, Ebadi S, Talebian S, Naghdi S, Mazaheri H, Olyaei G, Jalaie S (2006b) A randomized single blind placebo controlled clinical trial on the effect of continuous ultrasound on low back pain. Electromyogr Clin Neurophysiol, 46: 329–336

Ansari NN, Haghdi S, Farhadi M, Jalaie S (2007) A preliminary study into the effect of low-intensity pulsed ultrasound on chronic maxillary and frontal sinusitis. Physiother Theory Pract, 23: 211–218

Artho PA, Thyme JG, Warring BP, Willis CD, Brismee JM, Latman NS (2002) A calibration study of therapeutic ultrasound units. Phys Ther, 82: 257–263

Bakhtiary AH, Rashid-Pour A (2004) Ultrasound and laser therapy in the treatment of carpal tunnel syndrome. Aust J Physiother, 50: 147–151

Bearzy HJ (1953) Clinical applications of ultrasonic energy in treatment of acute and chronic subacromial bursitis. Arch Phys Med Rehabil, 34: 228–231

Bell Al, Cavorsi J (2008) Noncontact ultrasound therapy for adjunctive treatment of nonhealing wounds: Retrospective analysis. Phys Ther, 88: 1517–1524

Bierman W (1954) Ultrasound in the treatment of scars. Arch Phys Med Rehabil, 35: 209–214

Binder A, Hodge G, Greenwood AM, Hazelman BL, Page TD (1985) Is therapeutic ultrasound effective in treating soft tissue lesions? Br Med J, 290: 512–514

Brock Symons T, Clasey JL, Gater DR, Yates JW (2004) Effects of deep heat as a preventive mechanism on delayed onset muscle soreness. J Strength Cond Res, 18: 155–161

Bundt FB (1958) Ultrasound therapy in supraspinatus bursitis. Phys Ther Rev, 38: 826–827

Callam MJ, Harper DR, Dale JJ, Ruckley CV, Prescott RJ (1987) A controlled trial of weekly ultrasound therapy in chronic leg ulceration. Lancet, 2: 204–206

Casarotto RA, Adamowski JC, Fallopa F, Bacanelli F (2004) Coupling agents in therapeutic ultrasound: Acoustic and thermal behavior. Arch Phys Med Rehabil, 85: 162–165

Chan AK, Myer JW, Measom GJ, Draper DO (1998) Temperature changes in human patellar tendon in response to therapeutic ultrasound. J Athl Train, 33: 130–135

Chartered Society of Physiotherapy (1990) Guidelines for the safe use of ultrasound physiotherapy equipment. Physiotherapy, 76: 683–684

Cherup N, Urben J, Bender LF (1963) Treatment of plantar warts with ultrasound. Arch Phys Med Rehabil, 44: 602–604

Chester R, Costa Ml, Shepstone L, Cooper A, Donell ST (2008) Eccentric calf muscle training compared with therapeutic ultrasound for chronic Achilles tendon pain—a pilot study. Man Ther, 13: 484–491

Clarke GR, Stenner L (1976) Use of therapeutic ultrasound. Physiotherapy, 62: 185–190

Cline PD (1963) Radiographic follow-up of ultrasound therapy in calcific bursitis. Phys Ther, 43: 16–18

Cole PS, Quinsberg J, Melin MM (2009) Adjuvant use of acoustic pressure wound therapy for treatment of chronic wounds: A retrospective analysis. J Wound Ostomy Continence Nurs, 36: 171–177

Cook SD, Ryaby JP, McCabe J, Frey JJ, Heckman JD, Kristiansen TK (1997) Acceleration of tibial and distal radius fracture healing in patients who smoke. Clin Orthop, 337: 198–207

Corradi C, Cozzolino A (1953) Ultrasound and bone callus formation during function. Arch Orthop, 66: 77–98

Craig JA, Bradley J, Walsh DM, Baxter GD, Allen JM (1999) Delayed onset muscle soreness: Lack of effect of therapeutic ultrasound. Arch Phys Med Rehabil, 80: 318–323

Crawford F, Snaith M (1996) How effective is therapeutic ultrasound in the treatment of heel pain? Ann Rheumatol Dis, 55: 265–267

Creates V (1987) Study of ultrasound treatment to the painful perineum after childbirth. Physiotherapy, 73: 162–165

Davidson JH, Vandervoort A, Lessard L, Miller L (2001) The effect of acupuncture versus ultrasound on pain level, grip strength and disability in individuals with lateral epicondylitis: A pilot study. Physiother Can, 53: 195–202

De Preux T (1952) Ultrasonic wave therapy in osteoarthritis of the hip joint. Br J Phys Med, 15: 14–19

Downing DS, Weinstein A (1986) Ultrasound therapy of subacromial bursitis: A double blind trial. Phys Ther, 66: 194–199

Draper DO, Edvalson CG, Knight KL, Eggett D, Shurtz J (2010) Temperature increases in the human Achilles tendon during ultrasound treatments with commercial ultrasound gel and full-thickness and half-thickness gel pads. J Athl Train, 45: 333–337

Draper DO, Sunderland S, Kirkendall DT, Ricard MD (1993b) A comparison of temperature rise in human calf muscles following applications of underwater and topical gel ultrasound. J Orthop Sports Phys Ther, 17: 247–251

Duarte LR (1983) The stimulation of bone growth by ultrasound. Orthop Trauma Surg, 101: 153–159 (Animal study)

Dudda M, Hauser J, Muhr G, Esenswein SA (2011) Low-intensity pulsed ultrasound as a useful adjuvant during distraction osteogenesis: A prospective, randomized controlled trial. J Trauma, 71: 1276–1380

D'Vaz AP, Ostor AJ, Speed CA, Jenner JR, Bradley M, Prevost AT, Hazleman BL (2006) Pulsed low-intensity ultrasound therapy for chronic lateral epicondylitis: A randomized controlled trial. Rheumatology (Oxford), 45: 566–570

Dyson M, Franks C, Suckling J (1976) Stimulation of healing of varicose ulcers by ultrasound. Ultrasonics, 14: 232–236

Ebadi S, Nakhostin AN, Naghdi S, Jalaei S, Sadat M, Bagheri H, Vantulder MW, Hwnaxhke N, Fallah E (2012) The effect of continuous ultrasound on chronic non-specific low back pain: A single blind placebo-controlled randomized trial. BMC Musculoskelet Disord, 13: 59

Ebenbichler GR, Erdogmus CB, Resh KL, Funovics MA, Kainberger F, Barisani G, Aringer M, Nicolakis P, Wiesinger GF, Baghestanian M, Preisinger E, Fialka-Moser V (1999) Ultrasound therapy for calcific tendonitis of the shoulder. N Engl J Med, 340: 1533–1538

Ebenbichler GR, Resch, KL, Graninger WB (1997) Resolution of calcium deposits after ultrasound of the shoulder. J Rheumatol, 24: 235–236

Ebenbichler GR, Resch, KL, Nicolakis P, Wiesinger GF, Uhl F, Ghanem AH, Filaka, V (1998) Ultrasound treatment for treating the carpal tunnel syndrome: Randomized sham controlled trial. Br Med J, 316: 731–735

Echternach JL (1965) Ultrasound: An adjunct treatment for shoulder disabilities. Phys Ther, 45: 865–869

El-Mowafi H, Mohsen M (2005) The effect of low-intensity pulsed ultrasound on callus maturation in tibial distraction osteogenesis. Int Orthop, 29: 121–124

Emami A, Larsson A, Petren-Mallmin M (1999b) Serum bone markers after intramedullary fixed tibial fractures. Clin Orthop Relat Res, 368: 220–229

Emami A, Petren-Mallmin M, Larsson S (1999a) No effect of low-intensity ultrasound on healing time of intramedullary fixed tibial fractures. J Orthop Trauma, 13: 252–257

Ennis WJ, Foremann P, Mozen N, Massey J, Conner-Kerr T, Meneses P (2005) Ultrasound therapy for recalcitrant diabetic foot ulcers: Results of a randomized, double-blind, controlled, multicenter study. Ostomy Wound Manage, 51: 24–59

Ennis WJ, Valdes W, Gainer M, Meneses P (2006) Evaluation of clinical effectiveness of MIST ultrasound therapy for the healing of chronic wounds. Adv Skin Wound Care, 19: 437–446

Ericksson SV, Lundeberg T, Malm M (1991) A placebo-controlled trial of ultrasound therapy in chronic leg ulceration. Scand J Rehab Med, 23: 211–213

Escandon J, Vivas AC, Perez R, Kirsner R, Davis S (2012) A prospective pilot study of ultrasound therapy effectiveness in refractory venous leg ulcers. Int Wound J, 9: 570–578

Esenyel M, Caglar N, Aldemir T (2000) Treatment of myofascial pain. Am J Phys Med Rehabil, 79: 48–52

Everett T, McIntosh J, Grant A (1992) Ultrasound therapy for persistent post-natal perineal pain and dyspareunia: A randomized placebo-controlled trial. Physiotherapy, 78: 263–267

Falconer J, Hayes KW, Chang RW (1992) Effect of ultrasound on mobility in osteoarthritis of the knee. A randomized clinical trial. Arthritis Care Res, 5: 29–35

Ferguson HN (1981) Ultrasound in the treatment of surgical wounds. Physiotherapy, 67: 43

Fieldhouse C (1979) Ultrasound for relief of painful episiotomy scars. Physiotherapy, 65: 217

Flax HJ (1964) Ultrasound treatment of peritendonitis calcerea of the shoulder. Am J Phys Med, 43: 117–124

Franek A, Chmielewska D, Brzezinska-Wcislo L, Siezak A, Blaszczak E (2004) Application of various power densities of ultrasound in the treatment of leg ulcers. J Dermatol Treat, 15: 379–386

Fukada E, Yasuda I (1957). On the piezoelectric effect of bone. J Physiol Soc Jpn, 12: 1158–1162

Gam AM, Warming S, Larsen LH, Jensen B, Hoydolsmo O, Alloni, Anderson B, Gotzchen E, Petersen M, Mathiesen B (1998) Treatment of myofascial trigger-points with ultrasound combined with massage and exercise: A randomized controlled trial. Pain, 77: 73–79

Garrett AS, Garrett M (1982) Ultrasound therapy for herpes zoster pain. J R Coll Gen Pract, 32: 709–711

Gebauer D, Correl J (2005a) Pulsed low-intensity ultrasound: A new salvage procedure for delayed unions and nonunions after leg lengthening in children. J Pediatr Orthop, 25: 750–754

Gebauer D, Mayr E, Orthner E, Ryaby JP (2005b) Low-intensity pulsed ultrasound: Effects on nonunions. Ultrasound Med Biol, 31: 1391–1402

Gehling ML, Samies JH (2007) The effect of noncontact, low-intensity, low frequency therapeutic ultrasound on lower-extremity chronic wound pain: A retrospective chart review. Ostomy Wound Manage, 53: 44–50

Gersten JW (1958) Effects of metallic objects on temperature rises produced in tissue by ultrasound. Am J Phys Med, 37: 75–82 (Animal study)

Giannini S, Giombini A, Moneta MR, Massazza G, Pigozzi F (2004) Low-intensity pulsed ultrasound in the treatment of traumatic hand fracture in an elite athlete. Am J Phys Med Rehabil, 83: 921–925

Gold SM, Wasserman R (2005) Preliminary results of tibial bone transports with pulsed low intensity ultrasound (Exogen). J Orthop Traum, 19: 10–16

Gorkiewicz R (1984) Ultrasound for subacromial bursitis. Phys Ther, 64: 46–47

Grant A, Sleep J, McIntosh J, Ashurst H (1989) Ultrasound and pulsed electromagnetic energy treatment for perineal trauma: A randomized placebo-controlled trial. Br J Obstet Gynaecol, 96: 434–439

Griffin JE, Echternach JL, Price RE, Touchtone JC (1967) Patients treated with ultrasonic driven hydrocortisone and with ultrasound alone. Phys Ther, 47: 594–601

Grynbaum BB (1954) An evaluation of the clinical use of ultrasonics. Am J Phys Med, 33: 75–78

Gulick DT, Ingram N, Krammes T, Wilds C (2005) Comparison of tissue heating using 3 MHz ultrasound with T-Prep versus Aquasonic gel. Phys Ther Sports, 6: 131–136

Haan J, Lucich S (2009) A retrospective analysis of acoustic pressure wound therapy: Effects on the healing progression of chronic wounds. J Am Coll Cert Wound Spec, 1: 28–34

Haker E, Lundeberg T (1991) Pulsed ultrasound treatment in lateral epicondylalgia. Scand J Rehab Med, 23: 115–118

Halle JS, Franklin RJ, Kralfa BL (1986) Comparison of four treatment approaches for lateral epicondilytis of the elbow. J Orhtop Sports Phys Ther, 8: 62–68

Hamer J, Kirk JA (1976) Physiotherapy of the frozen shoulder: A comparative trial of ice and ultrasonic therapy. N Z Med J, 83: 191–192

Handolin L, Kiljunen V, Arnala I, Kiuru MJ, Pajarinen J, Pertio EK, Rokkanen P (2005a) Effect of ultrasound therapy on bone healing of lateral malleolar fractures of the ankle joint fixed with bioarsorbable screws. J Orthop Sci, 10: 391–395

Handolin L, Kiljunen V, Arnala I, Kiuru MJ, Pajarinen J, Pertio EK, Rokkanen P (2005b) No long-term effects of ultrasound therapy in bioabsorbable screw-fixed lateral malleolar fracture. Scand J Surg, 94: 239–242

Handolin L, Kiljunen V, Arnala I, Kiuru MJ, Pajarinen J, Pertio EK, Rokkanen P (2005c) The effect of low intensity ultrasound and bioabsorbable self-reinforced poly-L-lactide screw fixation on bone in lateral malleolar fractures. Arch Orthop Trauma Surg, 125: 317–321

Hashish I, Hai H, Harvey W (1988) Reproduction of postoperative pain and swelling by ultrasound treatment: A placebo effect. Pain, 33: 303–311

Hashish I, Harvey W, Harris M (1986) Anti-inflammatory effects of ultrasound therapy: Evidence for a major placebo effect. Br J Rheumatol, 25: 77–81

Hasson S, Mundorf R, Barnes W, Williams J, Fijii M (1990) Effect of pulsed ultrasound versus placebo on muscle soreness perception and muscular performance. Scand J Rehab Med, 22: 199–205

Heckman JD, Ryabi JP, Mccabe J, Frey JJ, Kilcoyne RF (1994) Acceleration of tibial fracture-healing by noninvasive, low-intensity pulsed ultrasound. J Bone Joint Surg (A), 76: 26–34

Hekkenberg RT, Oosterbaan WA, van Beekum WT (1986) Evaluation of ultrasound therapy devices. Physiotherapy, 72: 390–395

Hemery X, Ohl X, Saddiki R, Barresi L, Dehoux E (2011) Low-intensity pulsed ultrasound for non-union treatment: A 14-case series evaluation. Orthop Traumatol Surg Res, 97: 51–57

Herrera-Lasso I, Mobarak L, Fernandez-Dominguez L, Cardiel MH, Alargon-Segovia D (1993) Comparative effectiveness of packages of treatment including ultrasound or transcutaneous electrical nerve stimulation in painful shoulder syndrome. Physiotherapy, 79: 251–253

Holcomb WR, Joyce CJ (2003) A comparison of temperature increases produced by 2 commonly used ultrasound units. J Athl Train, 38: 24–27

Holdsworth LK, Anderson DM (1993) Effectiveness of ultrasound used with a hydrocortisone coupling medium or epicondylitis clasp to treat lateral epicondylitis: Pilot study. Physiotherapy, 79: 19–25

Huang MH, Lin YS, Lee CL, Yang RC (2005a) Use of ultrasound to increase effectiveness of isokinetic exercise for knee osteoarthritis. Arch Phys Med Rehabil, 86: 1545–1551

Huang MH, Yang RC, Lee CL, Chen TW, Wang MC, Huang MH (2005b) Preliminary results of integrated therapy for patients with knee osteoarthritis. Arthritis Rheum, 53: 812–820

Inaba MK, Piorkowski M (1972) Ultrasound in treatment of painful shoulders in patients with hemiplegia. Phys Ther, 52: 737–741

Jingushi S, Mizuno K, Matsushita T, Itoman M (2007) Low-intensity pulsed ultrasound treatment for postoperative delayed union or nonunion of long bone fracture. J Orthop Sci, 12: 35–41

Johns LD, Straub SJ, Howard SM (2007) Analysis of effective radiation area, power, intensity, and field characteristics of ultrasound transducers. Arch Phys Med Rehabil, 88: 124–129

Jones RJ (1984) Ultrasonic therapy: Report on a series of twelve patients. Physiotherapy, 70: 94–96

Kavros CJ, Liedl DA, Boon AJ, Miller JL, Hobbs JA, Andrews KL (2008) Expedited wound healing with noncontact, low-frequency ultrasound therapy in chronic wounds: A retrospective analysis. Adv Skin Wound Care, 21: 415–423

Kavros CJ, Miller JL, Hanna SW (2007a) Treatment of ischemic wound with noncontact, low-frequency ultrasound: The Mayo Clinic experience, 2004–2006. Adv Skin Wound Care, 20: 221–226

Kavros SJ, Schenck EC (2007b) Use of noncontact low-frequency ultrasound in the treatment of chronic foot and leg ulcerations: A 51-patient analysis. J Am Podiatr Med Assoc, 97: 95–101

Kazanoglu E, Basaran S, Guzel R, Guler-Uysal F (2003) Short term efficacy of ibuprofen phonophoresis versus continuous ultrasound therapy in knee osteoarthritis. Swiss Med Wkly, 133: 333–338

Kent H (1959) Plantar wart treatment with ultrasound. Arch Phys Med Rehabil, 40: 15–18

Kimura IF, Gulick DT, Shelly J, Ziskin MC (1998) Effects of two ultrasound devices and angles of application on the temperature of tissue phantom. J Orthop Sports Phys Ther, 27: 27–31

Klaiman MD, Shrader JA, Danoff JV, Hicks JE, Pesce WJ, Ferland J (1998) Phonophoresis versus ultrasound in the treatment of common musculoskeletal conditions. Med Sci Sports Exerc, 30: 1349–1355

Kleinkort JA, Wood JA (1975) Phonophoresis with 1 percent versus 10 percent hydrocortisone. Phys Ther, 55: 1320–1324

Klemp P, Staberg B, Korsgård J, Nielsen HV, Crone P (1982) Reduced blood flow in fibromyotic muscles during ultrasound therapy. Scand J Rehab Med, 15: 21–23

Klucinec B (1997) The effectiveness of the Aquaflex gel pad in the transmission of acoustic energy. J Athl Train, 31: 313–317

Klucinec B, Scheidler M, Denegar C, Dohmholdt E, Burgess S (2000) Transmissivity of coupling agents used to deliver ultrasound through indirect methods. J Orthop Sports Phys Ther, 30: 263–269

Kristiansen TK, Ryaby JP, McCabe J, Frey JJ, Roe LR (1997) Accelerated healing of distal radial fractures with the use of specific, low-intensity ultrasound. J Bone Joint Surg (A), 79: 961–973

Kurtais Gursel Y, Ulus Y, Bilgic A (2004) Adding ultrasound in the management of soft-tissue disorders of the shoulder: A randomized placebo-controlled trial. Phys Ther, 84: 336–343

Lanfear RT, Clarke WB (1972) The treatment of tenosynovitis in industry. Physiotherapy, 58: 128–129

Lehmann JF, Brunner GD, Martinis AJ, McMillan JA (1959) Ultrasonic effects as demonstrated in live pigs with surgical metallic implants. Arch Phys Med Rehabil, 40: 483–488 (Animal study)

Lehmann JF, Brunner GD, McMillan JA (1958) Influence of surgical metal implants on temperature distribution in thigh specimen exposed to ultrasound. Arch Phys Med Rehabil, 39: 692–695 (Animal study)

Lehmann JF, Erickson DJ, Martin GM, Krusen FH (1954) Comparison of ultrasonic and microwave diathermy in the physical treatment of periarthritis of the shoulder. Arch Phys Med Rehabil, 35: 627–634

Lehmann JF, Fordyce WE, Rathbun LA, Larson, RE, Wood DH (1961) Clinical evaluation of a new approach in the treatment of contracture associated with hip fracture after internal fixation. Arch Phys Med Rehabil, 42: 95–100

Lerner A, Stein H, Soudry M (2004) Compound high-energy limb fractures with delayed union: Our experience with adjuvant ultrasound stimulation (Exogen). Ultrasonics, 42: 915–917

Leung KS, Lee WS, Tsui HF, Liu PP, Cheung WH (2004) Complex tibial fracture outcome following treatment with low-intensity pulsed ultrasound. Ultrasound Med Biol, 30: 389–395

Lubbert PH, van der Rijt RH, Hoornjte LE, van de Werken C (2008) Low-intensity pulsed ultrasound (LIPUS) in fresh clavicle fractures: A multi-centre double blind randomised trial. Injury, 39: 1444–1452

Lundeberg T, Abrahamsson P, Haker E (1988) A comparative study of continuous ultrasound, placebo ultrasound and rest in epicondylalgia. Scand J Rehab Med, 20: 99–101

Lundeberg T, Nordström F, Brodda-Jensen G, Ericksson SV, Kjartansson J, Samuelson VE (1990) Pulsed ultrasound does not improve healing of venous ulcers. Scand J Rehab Med, 22: 195–197

Makuloluwe RTB, Mouzas GL (1977) Ultrasound in the treatment of sprained ankles. Practitioner, 218: 586–588

Markham DE, Wood MR (1980) Ultrasound for Dupuytren's contracture. Physiotherapy, 66: 55–58

Mayr E, Frankel V, Ruter A (2000) Ultrasound—an alternative healing method for nonunions? Arch Orthop Trauma Surg, 120: 1–8

McDiarmid T, Burns PN, Lewith GT, Machin D (1985) Ultrasound and the treatment of pressure sores. Physiotherapy, 71: 66–70

McLachlan Z, Milne EJ, Lumley J, Walker BL (1991) Ultrasound treatment for breast engorgement: A randomized double blind trial. Aust J Physiother, 37: 23–28

McLaren J (1984) Randomized controlled trial of ultrasound therapy for the damaged perineum. Clin Phys Physiol Meas, 5: 40–46

Merrick MA, Bernard KD, Devor ST, Williams JM (2003) Identical 3-MHz ultrasound treatments with different devices produce different intramuscular temperatures. J Orthop Sports Phys Ther, 33: 379–385

Merrick MA, Mihalyov MR, Roethemeier JL, Cordova ML, Ingesoll CD (2002) A comparison of intramuscular temperatures during ultrasound treatments with coupling gel or gel pads. J Orthop Sports Phys Ther, 32: 216–220

Middlemast S, Chatterjee DS (1978) Comparison of ultrasound and thermography for soft-tissue injuries. Physiotherapy, 64: 331–332

Muche JA (2003) Efficacy of therapeutic ultrasound treatment of a meniscus tear in a severely disabled patient: A case report. Arch Phys Med Rehabil, 84: 1558–1559

Mueller EE, Mead S, Schulz BF, Vaden MR (1954) A placebo-controlled study of ultrasound treatment for periarthritis. Am J Phys Med, 33: 31–35

Munting E (1978) Ultrasonic therapy for painful shoulders. Physiotherapy, 64: 180–181

Myrer JW, Measom GJ, Fellingham GW (2001) Intramuscular temperature rises with topical analgesics used as coupling agents during therapeutic ultrasound. J Athl Train 36: 20–26

Nagrale AV, Herd CR, Ganvir S, Ramteke G (2009) Cyriax physiotherapy versus phonophoresis with supervised exercise in subjects with lateral epicondylalgia: A randomized clinical trial. J Man Manip Ther, 17: 171–178

Nolte PA, Van der Krans A, Patka P, Janssen IM, Ryaby JP, Albers GH (2001) Low-intensity pulsed ultrasound in the treatment of nonunions. J Trauma, 51: 693–702

Nussbaum EL, Blemann I, Mustard B (1994) Comparison of ultrasound/ultraviolet-C and laser treatment of pressure ulcers in patients with spinal cord injury. Phys Ther, 74: 812–823

Nwuga VC (1983) Ultrasound in treatment of back pain resulting from prolapsed intervertebral disc. Arch Phys Med Rehabil, 64: 88–89

Nyanzi CS, Landgride J, Heyworth JR, Mani R (1999) Randomized controlled study of ultrasound therapy in the management of acute lateral ligament sprains of the ankle joint. Clin Rehab, 13: 16–22

Nykänen M (1995) Pulsed ultrasound treatment of the painful shoulder: A randomized, double-blind, placebo-controlled study. Scand J Rehab Med, 27: 105–108

Oakland C, Rapier C (1993) Comparison of the efficacy of the topical NSAID felbinac and ultrasound in the treatment of acute ankle injury. Br J Clin Res, 4: 89–96

Okada K, Miyakoshi N, Yalahashi S, Ishigaki S, Nishida J, Itoi E (2003) Congenital pseudoarthrosis of the tibia treated with low-intensity pulsed ultrasound stimulation (LIPUS). Ultrasound Med Biol, 29: 1061–1064

Oshikoya CA, Shultz SJ, Mistry D, Perrin DH, Arnold BL, Gansneder BM (2000) Effect of coupling medium temperature on the rate of intramuscular temperature rise using continuous ultrasound. J Athl Train, 35: 417–421

Ozgonenel L, Aytekin E, Durmu OL, Lu G (2009) A double-blind trial of clinical effects of therapeutic ultrasound in knee osteoarthritis. Ultrasound Med Biol, 35: 44–49

Oztas O, Turan B, Bora I, Karakaya MK (1998) Ultrasound therapy effect in carpal tunnel syndrome. Arch Phys Med Rehabil, 79: 1540–1544

Patrick MK (1978) Applications of therapeutic pulsed ultrasound. Physiotherapy, 64: 103–104

Paul BJ, Lafratta CW, Dawson AR, Baab E, Bullock F (1960) Use of ultrasound in the treatment of pressure sores in patients with spinal cord injury. Arch Phys Med Rehab, 41: 438–440

Payne C (1984) Ultrasound for post-herpetic neuralgia: A study to investigate the results of treatment. Physiotherapy, 70: 96–97

Perron M, Malouin F (1997) Acetic acid iontophoresis and ultrasound for the treatment of calcifying tendinitis of the shoulder: A randomized controlled trial. Arch Phys Med Rehabil, 78: 379–384

Peschen M, Weichenthal M, Schopf E, Vanscheidt W (1997) Low-frequency ultrasound treatment of chronic venous leg ulcers in an outpatient therapy. Acta Derm Venereol, 77: 311–314

Pigozzi F, Moneta MR, Giombini A, Giannini S, Di Cesare A, Fagnani F (2004) Low-intensity pulsed ultrasound in the conservative treatment of pseudoarthrosis. J Sports Med Phys Fitness, 44: 173–178

Plaskett C, Tiidus P, Livingston L (1999) Ultrasound treatment does not affect postexercise muscle strength recovery or soreness. J Sport Rehabil, 8: 1–9

Poltawski L, Watson T (2007) Relative transmissivity of ultrasound coupling agents commonly used by therapists in the UK. Ultrasound Med Biol, 33, 120–128

Portwood MM, Lieberman JS, Taylor RG (1987) Ultrasound treatment of reflex sympathetic dystrophy. Arch Phys Med Rehabil, 68: 116–118

Pottenger FJ, Karalfa BL, (1989) Utilization of hydrocortisone phonophoresis in United States Army physical therapy clinics. Mil Med, 154: 355–358

Pye S (1996) Ultrasound therapy equipment—does it perform? Physiotherapy, 82: 39–44

Pye SD, Milford C (1994) The performance of ultrasound physiotherapy machines in Lothian Region, Scotland, 1992. Ultrasound Med Biol, 20: 347–359

Riboh JC, Leversedge FJ (2012) The use of low-intensity pulsed ultrasound bone stimulators for fractures of the hand and upper extremity. J Hand Surg (A), 37: 1456–1461

Ricardo M (2006) The effect of ultrasound on the healing of muscle-pediculated bone graft in scaphoid non-union. Int Orthop, 30: 123–127

Rivest M, Quirion-DeGirardi C, Seaborne D, Lambert J (1987) Evaluation of therapeutic ultrasound devices: Performance stability over 44 weeks of clinical use. Physiother Can, 39: 77–86

Robertson VJ, Ward AR (1996) Limited interchangeability of methods of applying 1 MHz ultrasound. Arch Phys Med Rehabil, 77: 379–383

Roche C, West J (1984) A controlled trial investigating the effect of ultrasound on venous ulcers referred from general practitioners. Physiotherapy, 70: 475–477

Roden D (1952) Ultrasonic waves in the treatment of chronic adhesive subacromial bursitis. J Irish Med Assoc, 30: 85–88

Roman MP (1960) A clinical evaluation of ultrasound by use of a placebo technique. Phys Ther Rev, 40: 649–652

Roussignol X, Currey C, Dupard F, Dujardin F (2012) Indications and results for the Exogen ultrasound system in the management of non-union: A 59-case pilot study. Orthop Traumatol Surg Res, 98: 206–213

Rue JP, Armstrong DW, Frassica FJ, Deafenbaugh M, Wilckens JH (2004) The effect of pulsed ultrasound in the treatment of tibial stress fractures. Orthopedics, 27: 1192–1195

Rutten S, Nolte PA, Guit GL, Bouman DE, Albers GH (2007) Use of low-intensity pulsed ultrasound for posttraumatic nonunions of the tibia: A review of patients treated in the Netherlands. J Trauma, 62: 902–908

Rutten S, Nolte PA, Korstjens CM (2008) Low intensity pulsed ultrasound increases bone volume, osteoid thickness and mineral apposition rate in the area of fracture healing in patients with a delayed union of the osteotomized fibula. Bone, 43: 348–354

Sahin N, Ugurlu H, Karahan AY (2011) Efficacy of therapeutic ultrasound in the treatment of spasticity: A randomized controlled study. NeuroRehabilitation, 29: 61–66

Saliba S, Mistry DJ, Perrin DH, Gieck J, Weltman A (2007) Phonophoresis and the absorption of dexamethasone in the presence of an occlusive dressing. J Athl Train, 42: 349–354

Schabrun S, Chipchase L, Rikard H (2006) Are therapeutic ultrasound units a potential vector for nocosomial infection? Physiother Res Int, 11: 61–71

Shehab D, Adham N (2000) Comparative effectiveness of ultrasound and transcutaneous electrical stimulation in treatment of periarticular shoulder pain. Physiother Can, 52: 208–210

Shomoto K, Katsuhiko T, Morishita S (2002) Effects of ultrasound therapy on calcified tendinitis of the shoulder. J Jap Phys Ther Assoc, 5: 7–11

Skoubo-Kristensen E, Sommer J (1982) Ultrasound influence on external fixation with a rigid plate in dogs. Arch Phys Med Rehabil, 63: 371–373 (Animal study)

Smith W, Winn F, Parette R (1986) Comparative study versus four modalities in shinsplint treatments. J Orthop Sports Phys Ther, 8: 77–82

Snow CJ (1982) Ultrasound therapy units in Manitoba and Northwestern Ontario: Performance evaluation. Physiother Can, 34: 185–189

Soren A (1965) Evaluation of ultrasound treatment in musculoskeletal disorders. Physiotherapy, 51: 214–217

Stasinopoulos D, Stasinopoulos I (2004) Comparison of effects of exercise programme, pulsed ultrasound and transverse friction in the treatment of chronic patellar tendinopathy. Clin Rehabil, 18: 347–352

Stay JC, Ricard MD, Draper DO, Schulties SS, Durrant E (1998) Pulsed ultrasound fails to diminish delayed-onset muscle soreness symptoms. J Athl Train, 33: 341–346

Stein H, Lerner A (2005) How does pulsed low-intensity ultrasound enhance fracture healing? Orthopedics, 28: 1161–1163

Stewart HF, Abzug JL, Harris GR (1980) Considerations in ultrasound therapy and equipment performance. Phys Ther, 60: 424–428

Stewart HF, Harris GR, Herman BA, et al. (1974) Survey of use and performance of ultrasonic therapy equipment in Pinellas County, Florida. Phys Ther, 54: 707–714

Stratford PW, Levy DR, Gauldie S, Miseferi D, Levy K (1989). The evaluation of phonophoresis and friction massage as treatments for extensor carpi radialis tendinitis: A randomized controlled trial. Physiother Can, 41: 93–99

Straub SJ, Johns LD, Howard SM (2008) Variability in effective radiating area at 1 MHz affects ultrasound treatment intensity. Phys Ther, 88: 50–57

Svarcova J, Trnavsky K, Zvarova J (1988) The influence of ultrasound, galvanic currents and shortwave diathermy on pain intensity with osteoarthritis. Scand J Rheumatol (Suppl), 67: 83–85

Swartz FZ (1953) Ultrasonics in osteoarthritis. J Med Assoc Al, 22: 182–185

Talaat AM, El-Dibany MM, El-Garf A (1995) Physical therapy in the management of myofascial pain dysfunction syndrome. Ann Otol Rhinol Laryngol, 95: 225–228

Taradaj J, Franek A, Brzezinska-Wcislo L, Cierpka L, Dolibog P, Chmielewska D, Blaszczak E, Kusz D (2008) The use of therapeutic ultrasound in venous leg ulcers: A randomized, controlled trial. Phlebology, 23: 178–183

Tepperberg I, Marjey E (1953) Ultrasound therapy of painful postoperative neurofibromas. Am J Phys Med, 32: 27–30

Ter Riet G, Kessels AG, Knipschild P (1996) A randomized clinical trial of ultrasound in the treatment of pressure ulcers. Phys Ther, 76: 1301–1312

Tsumaki N, Kakiuchi M, Sasaki J (2004) Low-intensity pulsed ultrasound accelerates maturation of callus in patients treated with opening-wedge high tibial osteotomy by hemicallotasis. J Bone Joint Surg, 86: 2399–2405

Ulus Y, Tander B, Akyol Y, Durmus D, Buyukakincak O, Gul U, Canturk F, Bilgici A, Kuru O (2012) Therapeutic ultrasound versus sham ultrasound for the management of patients with knee osteoarthritis: A randomized double-blind controlled clinical trial. In J Rheum Dis, 15: 197–206

Uygur F, Sener G (1995) Application of ultrasound in neuromas: Experience with seven below-knee strumps. Physiotherapy, 81: 758–762

Van der Heijden GJ, Leffers P, Wolters PH, Verheijden JJ, van Mameren H, Hoiber JP, Bouter LM, Knipscheild, PG (1999) No effect of bipolar interferential electrotherapy and pulsed ultrasound for soft tissue shoulder disorders: A randomized controlled trial. Ann Rheum Dis, 58: 530–540

Vaughn DT (1973) Direct method versus underwater method in the treatment of plantar warts with ultrasound. Phys Ther, 53: 396–397

Waldrop K, Serfass A (2008) Clinical effectiveness of noncontact, low-frequency, nonthermal ultrasound in burn care. Ostomy Wound Manage, 54: 66–69

Warden SJ, Bennel KL, Matthews DJ, Brown DJ, McMeeken JM, Wark JD (2001) Efficacy of low-intensity pulsed ultrasound in the prevention of osteoporosis following spinal cord injury. Bone, 29: 431–436

Warden SJ, Metcalf BR, Kiss ZS, Cook JL, Purdam CR, Bennell KL, Crossley KM (2008) Low-intensity pulsed ultrasound for chronic patellar tendinopathy: A randomized, double blind, placebo-controlled trial. Rheumatol, 47: 467–471

Watson JM, Kangombe AR, Soares MO, Chuang LH, Wortht G, Bland JM, Iglesias C, Cullum N, Torgerson D, Nelson EA (2011a) Use of weekly, low dose, high frequency ultrasound for hard to heal venous leg ulcers: The VenUS III randomised controlled trial. BMJ, 342: d1092

Watson JM, Kangombe AR, Soares MO, Chuang LH, Wortht G, Bland JM, Iglesias C, Cullum N, Torgerson D, Nelson EA (2011b) VenUS III: A randomized controlled trial of therapeutic ultrasound in the management of venous leg ulcers. Health Technol Assess, 15: 1–192

Weaver SL, Demchak TJ, Stone MB, Brucker JB, Burr PO (2006) Effect of transducer velocity on intramuscular temperature during a 1-MHz ultrasound treatment. J Orthop Sports Phys Ther, 36: 320–325

Weichenthal M, Morh P, Stegmann W, Breitbart EW (1997) Low-frequency ultrasound treatment of chronic venous ulcers. Wound Repair Regen, 5: 18–22

Williamson JB, George TK, Simpson DC, Hannah B, Bardbury E (1986) Ultrasound in the treatment of ankle sprains. Injury, 17: 176–178

Wing M (1982) Phonophoresis with hydrocortisone in the treatment of temporomandibular joint dysfunction. Phy Ther, 62: 32–33

Xavier CA (1983) Stimulation of bone repair by ultrasound. Brasil Orthop, 18: 73–80 (Animal study)

Xavier CA, Duarte LR (1983) Ultrasonic stimulation on bone callus: Clinical application. Rev Brazil Orthop, 18: 73–80

Yildiz N, Atalay NS, Gungen GO, Sanal E, Akkaya N, Topuz O (2011) Comparison of ultrasound and ketoprofen phonophoresis in the treatment of carpal tunnel syndrome. J Back Musculoskelet Rehabil, 24: 39–47

Zammit E, Herrington L (2005) Ultrasound therapy in the management of acute lateral ligament sprains of the ankle joint. Phys Ther Sports, 6: 116–121

Review Articles

Conventional Ultrasound

Alexander LA, Gilman DR, Brown DR, Brown JL, Houghton PE (2010) Exposure to low amounts of ultrasound energy does not improve tissue shoulder pathology: A systematic review. Phys Ther, 90: 14–25

Armijo-Olivo S, Fuentes J, Muir I, Gross DP (2013) Usage patterns and beliefs about therapeutic ultrasound by Canadian physical therapists: An exploratory population-based cross-sectional survey. Physioth Can, 65: 289–299

Dyson M (1987) Mechanisms involved in the therapeutic ultrasound. Physiotherapy, 73: 116–120

Kimmel E (2006) Cavitation bioeffects. Crit Rev Biomed Eng, 34: 105–161

Leighton TG (2007) What is ultrasound? Prog Biophys Mol Biol, 93: 1–83

O'Brien WD (2007) Ultrasound-biophysics mechanisms. Prog Biophys Mol Biol, 93: 212–255

Robertson VJ (2002) Dosage and treatment response in randomized clinical trials of therapeutic ultrasound. Phys Ther Sports, 3: 124–133

Robertson VJ (2008) Electrophysical agents and research: From instinct to evidence. Phys Ther Rev, 13: 377–385

Robertson VJ, Baker KG (2001) A review of therapeutic ultrasound: Effective studies. Phys Ther, 81: 1339–1350

Shanks P, Curran M, Fletcher P, Thompson R (2010) The effectiveness of therapeutic ultrasound for musculoskeletal conditions of the lower limb: A literature review. Foot (Edinb), 20: 133–139

Ter Haar G (2007) Therapeutic applications of ultrasound. Prog Biophys Mol Biol, 93: 111–129

Tsai WC, Tang SF, Liang FC (2011) Effect of therapeutic ultrasound on tendons. Am J Phys Med Rehabil, 90: 1068–1073

Low-Intensity Pulsed Ultrasound

Bashardoust Tajali S, Houghton P, McDermid JC, Grewal R (2012) Effects of low-intensity pulsed ultrasound therapy on fracture healing: A systematic review and meta-analysis. Am J Phys Med Rehabil, 91: 349–367

Busse JW, Kaur J, Mollon B, Bhandari M, Tornetta P, Schunemann HJ, Guyatt GH (2009) Low intensity pulsed ultrasonography for fractures: Systematic review of randomized controlled trials. BMJ, 338: b351

Claes L, Willie B (2007) The enhancement of bone regeneration by ultrasound. Prog Biophys Mol Biol, 93: 384–398

Dijkman BG, Sprague S, Bhandari M (2009) Low-intensity ultrasound: Nonunions. Indian J Orthop, 43: 141–148

Erdogan O, Esen E (2009) Biological aspects and clinical importance of ultrasound therapy in bone healing. J Ultrasound Med, 28: 765–776

Griffin XL, Costello I, Costa M (2008) The role of low intensity pulsed ultrasound therapy in the management of acute fracture: A systematic review. J Trauma, 65: 1446–1452

Kasturi G, Adler RA (2011) Mechanical means to improve bone strength: Ultrasound and vibration. Curr Rheumatol, 13: 251–256

Malizos KN, Hantes ME, Protopappas V, Papachristos A (2006) Low-intensity pulsed ultrasound for bone healing: An overview. Injury, 37: S56–S62

Martinez de Albornoz P, Khanna A, Longo UG, Forriol F, Maffulli N (2011) The evidence of low-intensity pulsed ultrasound for in vitro, animal and human fracture healing. Br Med Bull, 100: 39–57

Mundi R, Petis S, Kaloty R, Shetty V, Bhandari M (2009) Low-intensity pulsed ultrasound: Fracture healing. Indian J Orthop, 43: 132–140

Watanabe Y, Matsushita T, Bhandari M, Zdero R, Schemitsch EH (2010) Ultrasound for fracture healing: Current evidence. J Orthop Trauma, 24, Suppl 1: S56–S61

Ying ZM, Lin T, Yan SG (2012) Low-intensity pulsed ultrasound therapy: A potential strategy to stimulate tendon-bone junction healing. Biomed Biotechnol, 13: 955–963

Noncontact Low-Frequency Ultrasound

Driver VR, Yao M, Miller CJ (2011) Noncontact low-frequency ultrasound therapy in the treatment of chronic wounds: A meta-analysis. Wounds Repair Regen, 19: 475–480

Voigt J. Wendelken M, Driver V, Alvarez OM (2011) Low-frequency ultrasound (20–40 kHz) as an adjunctive therapy for chronic wound healing: A systematic review of the literature and meta-analysis of eight randomized controlled trials. Int J Low Extrem Wounds, 10: 190–199

Sonophoresis

Escobar-Chavez JJ, Bonilla-Martinez D, Villegas-Gonzales MA, Rodriguez-Cruz IM, Dominguez-Delgado CL (2009) The use of sonophoresis in the administration of drugs throughout the skin. J Pharm Pharm Sci, 12: 88–115

Mitragotri S (2005) Healing sound: The use of ultrasound in drug delivery and other therapeutic applications. Nat Rev Drug Discov, 4: 255–260

Mitragotri S, Kost J (2004) Low-frequency sonophoresis: A review. Adv Drug Deliv Rev, 27: 589–601

Polat BE, Blankschtein D, Langer R (2010) Low-frequency sonophoresis: Application to the transdermal delivery of macromolecules and hydrophilic drugs. Expert Opin Drug Deliv, 7: 1415–1432

Polat BE, Hart D, Langer R, Blankschtein D (2011) Ultrasound-mediated transdermal drug delivery: Mechanism, scope and emerging trends. J Control Rel, 152: 330–348

Chapters of Textbooks

Dunn F, Frizzell LA (1990) Bioeffects of ultrasound. In: Therapeutic Heat and Cold, 4th ed. Lehmann JF (Ed). Williams & Wilkins, Baltimore, pp 398–416

Dyson M (1995) Role of ultrasound in wound healing. In: Wound Healing: Alternatives in Managements, 2nd ed. McCulloch JM, Kloth LC, Feedar JA (Eds). FA Davis, Philadelphia, pp 318–345

Frizzell LA, Dunn F (1990) Biophysics of ultrasound. In: Therapeutic Heat and Cold, 4th ed. Lehmann JF (Ed). Williams & Wilkins, Baltimore, pp 362–397

Lehmann JF, De Lateur BJ (1990) Therapeutic heat. In: Therapeutic Heat and Cold, 4th ed. Lehmann JF (Ed). Williams & Wilkins, Baltimore, pp 504–581

Nussbaum EL, Berhens BJ (2006) Therapeutic ultrasound. In: Physical Agents: Theory and Practice, 2nd ed. In: Behrens BJ, Michlovitz SL (Eds). FA Davis, Philadelphia, pp 56–79

Ter Haar G (1996) Electrophysical principles. In: Clayton's Electrotherapy, 10th ed. Kitchen S, Bazin S (Eds). WB Saunders, London, pp 3–30

Textbooks

Hendee WR, Ritenour ER (2002) Medical Imaging Physics, 4th ed. Wiley-Liss, London

Sussman C, Bates-Jensen B (2012) Wound Care. A Collaborative Practice Manual for Health Professionals, 4th Ed. Lippincott Williams & Wilkins, Baltimore

Internet Resource

http://thePoint.lww.com: Online Dosage Calculator: Ultrasound

Chapter 21

Extracorporeal Shockwave Therapy

Chapter Outline

Learning Objectives

Remembering: List and describe the four types of generators used to produce therapeutic shock waves.
Understanding: Compare focused versus radial extracorporeal shockwave therapy (ESWT).
Applying: Demonstrate how to apply focused and radial ESWT.
Analyzing: Explain the physiologic and therapeutic effects of ESWT.
Evaluating: Argue the rationale for using ESWT for the management of chronic soft-tissue disorders.
Creating: Formulate the strength of evidence behind the use of therapeutic ESWT, and write a recommendation on its overall effectiveness.

I. FOUNDATION

A. DEFINITION

Extracorporeal shock wave therapy, commonly designated under the acronym ESWT, is the application of pressure mechanical waves outside of the body (*extracorporeal*) that violently impact (*shock*) biologic tissues for therapeutic purposes (Rompe, 2002; Maier et al., 2005; Gerdesmeyer et al., 2007a, b; Gleitz, 2011). A *shock wave* is defined as a low- to large-amplitude wave formed by the sudden mechanical compression of the medium through which the wave moves. Based on their propagation pattern, shock waves are divided

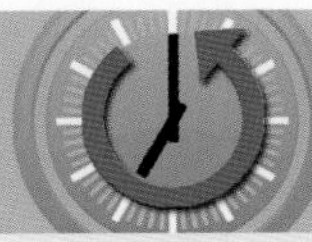

Historical Overview

Shock waves accompany our daily life and can, sometimes, create catastrophic effects. For example, earthquakes create gigantic shock waves that are broadcasted over very long distances, causing massive land damages. The first time that the effect of shock waves was observed in humans was during the Second World War (1939–1945), when observation was made that swimming castaways suffered lethal lung damage when water bombs were detonated in a wide radius. What caught attention was that shock waves were able to travel though body connective, muscular, and bone tissues without causing major damage to them (Haake et al., 2007). The first idea to use extracorporeal shock waves for therapeutic purpose (ESWT) came in the early 1970s with the introduction of a technique called *lithotripsy,* which is to disintegrate (*tripsy*) kidney stones (*litho*). The late 1980s saw the introduction of other ESWT devices used in the treatment for a variety of chronic and recalcitrant tendinopathies affecting the shoulder, elbow, and knee and for plantar fasciopathies. In 2006, ESWT was approved by the U.S. Food and Drug Administration (FDA) for the treatment of plantar fasciitis. The use of ESWT is seen, today, as an alternative treatment to surgery for the management of chronic and recalcitrant tendinopathies and fasciopathies that have failed conservative treatments.

into two categories: focused and unfocused. *Unfocused* shock waves are referred to in the literature as *radial* shock waves. These waves are produced pneumatically using compressed air to accelerate a projectile onto a solid applicator that is in contact with the skin surface overlying the affected tissue. *Focused* shock waves, on the other hand, are produced using electrohydraulic, electromagnetic, and piezoelectric systems. The repetitive delivery of shock waves causes mechanical energy that is absorbed by soft tissues and leads to physiologic and therapeutic effects.

B. EXTRACORPOREAL SHOCKWAVE DEVICES

Typical ESWT devices include those that deliver high-energy focused ESWT (f-ESWT), those that deliver low-energy radial ESWT (r-ESWT), and dual or combined-type units. The f-ESWT device is mounted with an integrated image guiding system that can be adjusted along its axis to allow precise localization for therapy. The multi-joint articulated arm allows individual adjustment for all treatment positions with the patient lying or sitting. Various applicators can be mounted at the extremity of the articulated arm for specific treatments. The r-ESWT device is made of a pneumatic system to which a handheld pistol-like applicator is attached with a cable. No image guiding system is required because of the radial or divergent projection of the waves. Dual or combined-type units, mounted with an image guiding system, allow the delivery of both f-ESWT and r-ESWT (for example, see www.storzmedical.ch).

C. APPLICATOR TYPE AND COUPLING MEDIA

Various applicators are used to deliver f- and r-ESWT. A coupling medium is required for mechanical energy created by the shock waves to be transmitted and absorbed by soft tissues. Adjustable dome membranes that are filled with either gas, water, or gel are used as coupling media with focused-type applicators. For radial-type applicators, standard aquasonic gel is used.

D. RATIONALE FOR USE

The rationale behind the development and use of ESWT lies with the need to provide a safer, noninvasive alternative to surgery for chronic and recalcitrant tendinopathies and delayed/nonunion fractures by stimulating the healing process of tendons and bones. To stimulate soft-tissue healing using shock waves (*orthotripsy*) contrasts with the original and classic use of ESWT in urology, which is to disintegrate (*lithotripsy*) kidney and ureteral stones.

II. BIOPHYSICAL CHARACTERISTICS

Table 21-1 lists key biophysical parameters useful to distinguish between focused and radial shock waves in ESWT. Let us consider each of them.

A. GENERATOR

Four types of generators, schematized in Figure 21-1, are used to produce extracorporeal shock waves: electrohydraulic, electromagnetic, piezoelectric, and ballistic (for details, see Ogden et al., 2001b; Maier et al., 2005; Gerdesmeyer et al., 2007a, b). The first three generators rest on the conversion of electrical energy to mechanical energy and generate focused shock waves (f-ESWT). The fourth generator, called *ballistic,* rests on the pneumatic principle and generates radial shock waves (see Table 21-1). The basic concept behind these sources is similar and rests on the principle that the acoustic impedances within human tissues are very similar to those of water.

1. Electrohydraulic

The *electrohydraulic* generator rests on the application of a high voltage across a spark plug, which discharges rapidly

TABLE 21-1 COMPARISON BETWEEN FOCUSED AND RADIAL EXTRACORPOREAL SHOCKWAVE THERAPY

Parameters	f-ESWT	r-ESWT
Generator	Electrohydraulic Electromagnetic Piezoelectric	Ballistic
Propagation	Focused (convergent)	Radial (divergent)
Penetration depth	Deep at focal point >5 cm	Superficial on skin surface <5 cm
Localization method	Image guided	Clinical focusing/palpation
Compressive pressure* (P+)	Up to 120 MPa Up to 1,200 bar	Up to 0.5 MPa Up to 5 bar
Tensile pressure (P–)	~1/10 of P+	~1/10 of P+
Rise time (RT)	<0.1 μs	<10 μs
Pulse duration (PD)	<0.5 μs	<500 μs
Energy flux density (EFD)	Up to 2.0 mJ/mm^2	Up to 0.5 mJ/mm^2
Coupling medium	Fluid (water or gas)-filled balloon	Thin layer of aquasonic gel
Applicator	Bulkier and more difficult to manipulate	Smaller and easier to manipulate
Local analgesia	Often required to prevent pain during treatment	Not required
Indication	For smaller, more focused, and deeper area	For larger, less focused, and more superficial area

f-ESWT, focused extracorporeal shockwave therapy; r-ESWT, radial extracorporeal shockwave therapy.
*1 MPa = 10 bar.

within a water-filled ellipsoid reflector (see Fig. 21-1A). The resultant spark heats and vaporizes the surrounding water, thus generating a gas bubble. This bubble expands and contracts, creating a shock wave. Shock waves are reflected by the surface of the ellipsoid reflector, which leads to the production of focused shock waves (Ogden et al., 2001b).

2. Electromagnetic

This generator uses a coil acting on a metal membrane contained in a fluid (see Fig. 21-1B). Coil discharges create strong electromagnetic fields in the opposite membrane and cause shock waves in the surrounding water medium. These shock waves are then focused on the target tissue using an acoustic lens.

3. Piezoelectric

High voltage applied to a spherical piezoelectric crystal causes it to expand and collapse, thus generating shock waves in the surrounding water medium. These shock waves are then focused on the tissue by means of the crystal's spherical shape (see Fig. 21-1C).

4. Ballistic

This generator consists of compressed air rapidly accelerating a projectile, which hits the impact surface of the applicator and causes a shock wave (see Fig. 21-1D). This wave immediately propagates in the tissues in a radial (like radii of a circle) fashion, resulting in unfocused shock waves.

B. PROPAGATION

As illustrated in Figure 21-1, electrohydraulic, electromagnetic, and piezoelectric generators deliver shock waves to soft tissues that propagate in a focused-like fashion—that is, over a small and precise location. Pneumatic generators, on the other hand, deliver shock waves in an unfocused or radial-like fashion to the tissues (Maier et al., 2005).

C. PENETRATION DEPTH

The convergent nature of focused shock waves allows them to penetrate deep into the tissues. In contrast, the

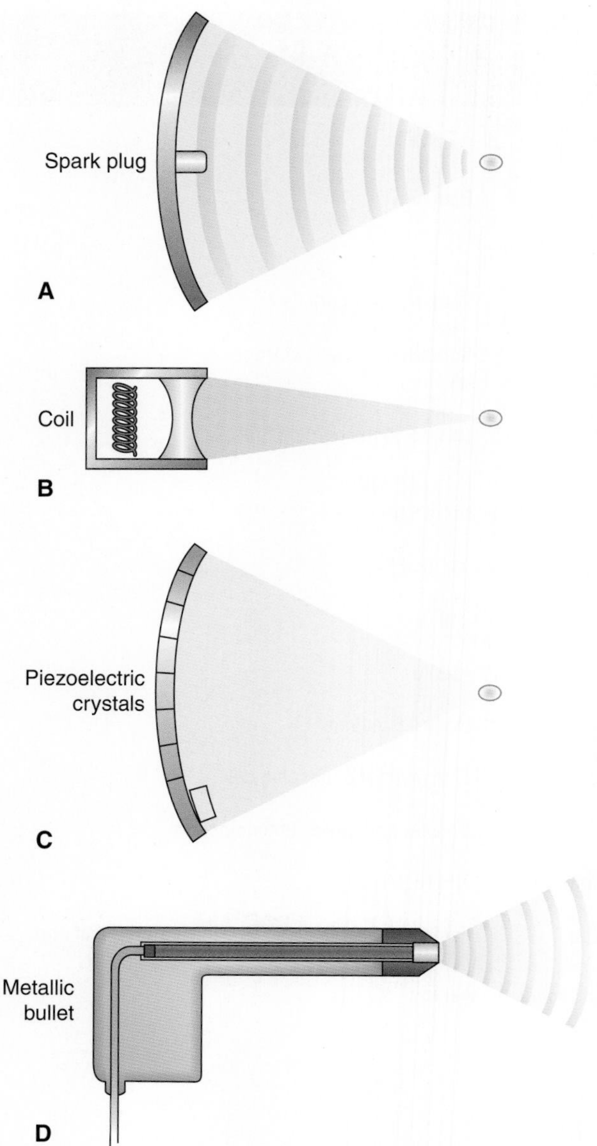

FIGURE 21-1 Simplified schematic drawings of electrohydraulic (**A**), electromagnetic (**B**), piezoelectric (**C**), and ballistic (**D**) extracorporeal shockwave generators.

divergent nature of radial these waves limits them to a more superficial penetration depth (Table 21-1).

D. LOCALIZATION METHOD

f-ESWT is delivered to smaller and deeper target tissue areas with great precision using either in-line or off-line image guiding systems such as ultrasound, fluoroscopy, or x-rays. r-ESWT, on the other hand, is directed to larger and more superficial target tissues using a method called *clinical focusing* or *palpation*. This method relies on the manual localization of the painful area to which the impact surface of the handheld pistol-like applicator is applied (Table 21-1).

E. WAVEFORM AND PARAMETER

1. Waveform

Figure 21-2 presents typical waveforms associated with focused and radial ESWT. Both waveforms are characterized by a *compressive* phase followed by a *tensile* phase. Radial shock waves, when compared to focused shock waves, present much lower compressive and tensile pressures and much longer time courses.

2. Compressive Versus Tensile Pressure

Positive peak pressure (P_p+) is defined as the difference between maximum positive peak pressure of the shock wave and ambient pressure (baseline). P+ represents the pressure exerted during the positive compressive phase of the shock wave. *Negative peak pressure* (P–), on the other hand, relates to the maximum negative peak pressure exerted during the tensile phase of the shock wave. Pressure is commonly measured and expressed in units of megapascal (Mpa) or bar, where 10 bar is equivalent to 1 MPa. Tensile pressure amplitudes are equivalent to approximately 10% (1/10) of P+. Focused shock waves can reach compressive pressure (P+) amplitudes as high as 120 MPa (1,200 bar), with amplitudes being approximately 120 times larger than those achieved by radial shock waves (see Table 21-1).

3. Rise Time and Pulse Duration

The waveform associated with the compressive or positive phase of a shock wave is characterized by its

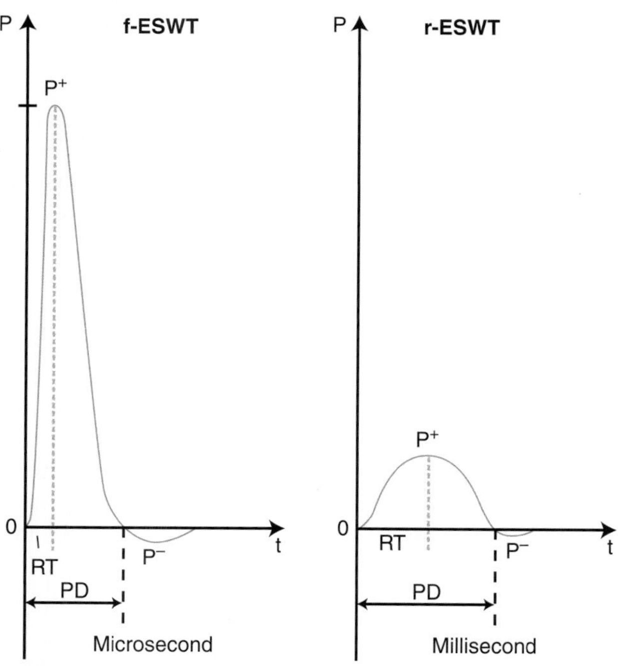

FIGURE 21-2 Graphic representation of a focused versus radial standard shock wave. f-ESWT, focuses extracorporeal shockwave therapy; r-ESWT, radial extracorporeal shockwave therapy; P+, positive compressive phase; RT, rise time; PD, pulse duration; P–, negative tensile phase.

rise time (RT) and pulse duration (PD). *Rise time* is defined as the time interval during which P+ rises from baseline to peak value. *Pulse duration* is defined as the interval between the beginning and ending of the compressive phase. As shown in Figure 21-2, focused-type shock waves display much faster pressure rise times and pulse durations (microsecond range) than those related to radial shock waves (millisecond range).

4. Energy and Energy Flux Density

The mechanical or acoustic *energy* (E) contained in a shock wave is expressed in millijoules (mJ). It is calculated by taking the time integral over the pressure/time curve or function (see Fig. 21-2). As is the case with ultrasound therapy (Chapter 20), the therapeutic effects of shock waves are affected by whether the shockwave energy is distributed over a large treatment area or concentrated on a narrow treatment area. The concentration of shockwave energy per area is thus an important dosimetric parameter. A measure of shockwave energy concentration or density is obtained by calculating the *energy flux density* (EFD), which is defined as the amount of mechanical acoustic energy per unit area (A) per shock (Cleveland et al., 2007; Foldager et al., 2012). EFD is calculated as follows: $EDF = E/A$. EFD is measured in millijoules per square millimeter (mJ/mm^2). The EFD level may be classified as low, medium, or high (Haake et al., 2007). Focused shock waves have much larger EFDs than radial shock waves because they contain much more energy (larger pressure/time curve; see Fig. 21-2) distributed over a much smaller area (focused). Because radial shock waves (r-ESWT) have significantly lower pressures and longer pulse durations than focused shock waves, calculation of EFDs may not be suitable to accurately represent such waves. An alternative and perhaps more accurate representation is to simply report the pressure level, in bar, used to drive and accelerate the projectile (Gleitz, 2011). Practically speaking, this means that practitioners, using certain types of r-ESWT devices, may have to select pressure rather than EFD from the console (see the Dosimetry section).

5. Coupling Medium

To deliver shockwave acoustic energy to soft tissues, as with ultrasonic acoustic energy (Chapter 20), requires the use of a coupling medium to optimize energy transmission to soft tissues. An acoustic fluid-filled adapter is used at the applicator–skin interface to deliver f-ESWT. To deliver R-ESWT, a thin layer of acoustic gel is applied over the applicator contact surface (Table 21-1).

6. Applicator

ESWT is delivered using various applicators, also referred to as headpieces or handpieces. Generally speaking, applicators used to deliver r-ESWT are smaller and easier to manipulate than those used for f-EWST.

7. Local Analgesia

The application of high-energy f-ESWT over a very small target tissue area can be particularly painful. To minimize pain during therapy, local analgesia, often in the form of lidocaine cream, is applied over the skin surface overlying the target area prior to treatment. There is evidence to show that local analgesia may reduce therapeutic effectiveness (Rompe et al., 2005; Klonschinski et al., 2011). This means that local analgesia should be avoided to optimize treatment effectiveness.

8. Indication

The use of focused over radial ESWT is based on the depth and size of the targeted soft-tissue lesion. The divergent propagation of r-ESWT is best suited for larger, more superficial soft-tissues lesions (Table 21-1).

III. THERAPEUTIC EFFECTS AND INDICATIONS

A. MICROTRAUMA

Figure 21-3 summarizes the proposed physiologic and therapeutic effects associated with ESWT. Both focused and radial shock waves produce the same effects (Zelle et al., 2010; van der Worp et al., 2012; Al-Abbad et al., 2013). It is postulated that delivery of mechanical or acoustic energy contained in shock waves causes microtrauma, which creates fresh micro-injuries within the

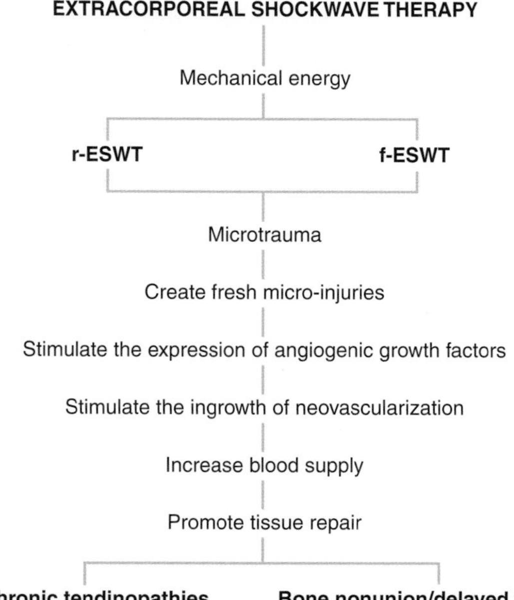

FIGURE 21-3 Proposed physiologic and therapeutic effects of extracorporeal shockwave therapy. r-ESWT, radial extracorporeal shockwave therapy; f-ESWT, focused extracorporeal shockwave therapy.

targeted soft tissue. These micro-injuries are presumed to stimulate the expression of angiogenic growth factors and the ingrowth of neovascularization (Gerdesmeyer et al., 2007a, b). Together, these biologic effects are presumed to increase the blood supply, which promotes soft-tissue repair in cases of chronic tendinopathies and delayed fractures of bone.

B. RESEARCH-BASED INDICATIONS

The search for evidence behind the use of ESWT, as displayed in the *Research-Based Indications* box, led to the collection of 113 English peer-reviewed human clinical studies. The methodologies and criteria used to assess the strength of evidence and therapeutic effectiveness are described in Chapter 2. As indicated, the strength of evidence is ranked as *moderate* for shoulder, elbow, Achilles, and patellar tendinopathies, as well as for shoulder calcific tendinitis, plantar fasciopathy, chronic heel pain, nonunion and delayed-union bone fracture, and osteonecrosis. Analysis is pending for all other remaining conditions because fewer than five studies could be collected. Over all conditions, the strength of evidence behind ESWT is determined to be *moderate* and its therapeutic effectiveness *substantiated*.

IV. DOSIMETRY

Table 21-2 lists key dosimetric parameters from which clinicians must choose when prescribing and applying ESWT. These parameters are *arbitrarily* chosen because there is no evidence, as yet, to show that a particular dose may be better than another. Let us discuss and exemplify each of them. First, the *number of shocks per treatment* is determined. This number may range between 1,000 and 4,000 shocks. Second, *shock frequency*, expressed in shocks per second (Hz), is selected. This frequency may range between 50 and 250 shocks per minute. Third, EFD, previously calculated by the manufacturer, is selected from the console. EDF is classified as low, medium, or high. Fourth, the number of treatments is determined; the number may vary between 1 and 4 treatments separated over days or weeks. From these selected parameters, the corresponding dose per treatment (D) and total energy dose (TED) may be calculated. Dose per treatment (D), measured in mJ/mm^2, corresponds to the product of EDF times the number of shocks per treatment (D = EFD × Number of shocks per treatment). Total energy dose is the total amount of mechanical energy delivered to the target soft tissue (TED = D × Number of treatments). For example, as shown in Table 21-2, the delivery of 1,800 focused shock waves per treatment using an EDF set at 0.38 mJ/mm^2 corresponds to a dose per treatment of 684 mJ/mm^2. Considering that two treatments are being delivered, the total energy dose received by the patient would be 1.368 J/mm^2. To facilitate dosimetry, use the **Online Dosage Calculator: Extracorporeal Shockwave Therapy**. Note that it may not be possible to select EFD values on some ballistic r-ESWT devices, thus making the calculation and recording of D and TED impossible. In such a case, select pressure and express dosage as follows: for example, 4 bar/3,000 shocks/6 Hz.

TABLE 21-2 DOSIMETRIC EXAMPLES OF EXTRACORPOREAL SHOCKWAVE THERAPY

Parameters	f-ESWT	r-ESWT
Number of shocks per treatment	1,800	2,000
Shock frequency	3 Hz	5 Hz
Energy flux density (EFD)	0.38 mJ/mm^2	0.18 mJ/mm^2
Dose per treatment (D)*	684 = 0.38 mJ/mm^2 × 1,800 684 mJ/mm^2	540 = 0.18 mJ/mm^2 × 2,000 360 mJ/mm^2
Pressure**	NA	4 bar
Number of treatments	2	3
Total energy dose (TED)***	1.368 J/mm^2	1.080 J/mm^2

f-ESWT, focused extracorporeal shockwave therapy; r-ESWT, radial extracorporeal shockwave therapy.
*D = EFD × Number of shocks per treatment.
**EFD is not always an available parameter to select on r-ESWT devices. Instead, practitioners have to select pressure (see the Dosimetry section for details).
***TED = D × Number of treatments.

Use the Online Dosage Calculator: Extracorporeal Shockwave Therapy.

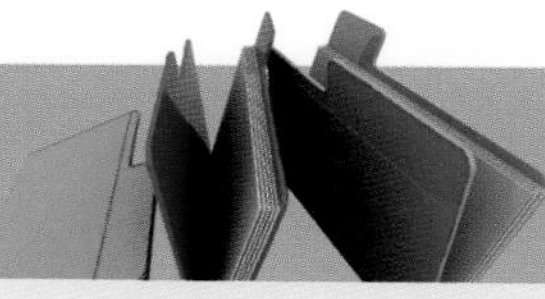

Research-Based Indications

EXTRACORPOREAL SHOCKWAVE THERAPY

Health Condition	Benefit—Yes Rating	Benefit—Yes Reference	Benefit—No Rating	Benefit—No Reference
Shoulder tendinopathy	I	Loew et al., 1999	I	Speed et al., 2002b
	I	Wang et al., 2003	I	Schmitt et al., 2001
	II	Haake et al., 2002b	II	Melegati et al., 2000
	II	Krasny et al., 2005	II	Schofer et al., 2009
	II	Pan et al., 2003	II	Engebretsen et al., 2011
	II	Sabeti-Aschraf et al., 2005		
	II	Albert et al., 2007		
	II	Loew et al., 1995		
	II	Wang et al., 2001b		
	II	Rompe et al., 2001c		
	II	Rompe et al., 1995		
	II	Moretti et al., 2005a		
	II	Pigozzi et al., 2000		
	II	Daecke et al., 2002		
Strength of evidence: Moderate **Therapeutic effectiveness:** Substantiated				
Shoulder calcific tendinitis	I	Consentino et al., 2003		
	I	Gerdesmyer et al., 2003		
	II	Mangone et al., 2010		
	II	Perlick et al., 2003		
	II	Hearnden et al., 2009		
	II	Hsu et al., 2008		
	II	Cacchio et al., 2006		
	II	Peters et al., 2004		
	II	Rompe et al., 1998		
	II	Avancini-Dobrovic et al., 2011		
	III	Spindler et al., 1998		
Strength of evidence: Moderate **Therapeutic effectiveness:** Substantiated				

Health Condition	Benefit—Yes Rating	Benefit—Yes Reference	Benefit—No Rating	Benefit—No Reference
Plantar fasciopathy	I	Malay et al., 2006	I	Buchbinder et al., 2002
	I	Kudo et al., 2006	I	Haake et al., 2003
	I	Theodore et al., 2004	I	Speed et al., 2003
	I	Rompe et al., 2003	I	Marks et al., 2008
	I	Ogden et al., 2001a	II	Rompe et al., 2010b
	I	Ogden et al., 2004		
	I	Ibrahim et al., 2010		
	II	Dorotka et al., 2006		
	II	Chuckpaiwong et al., 2009		
	II	Wang et al., 2002b		
	II	Porter et al., 2005		
	II	Hammer et al., 2002		
	II	Hammer et al., 2003		
	II	Hammer et al., 2005		
	II	Rompe et al., 2002		
	II	Rompe et al., 2005		
	II	Furia, 2005b		
	II	Hyer et al., 2005		
Strength of evidence: Moderate **Therapeutic effectiveness:** Substantiated				
Elbow tendinopathy	I	Rompe et al., 2004	I	Melikyan et al., 2003
	I	Pettrone et al., 2005	I	Speed et al., 2002a
	II	Chung et al., 2005	I	Haake et al., 2002c
	II	Melegati et al., 2004	I	Chung et al., 2004
	II	Rompe, 1996a	II	Lebrun, 2005
	II	Spacca et al., 2005	III	Krischek et al., 1999
	II	Crowther et al., 2002		
	II	Ko et al., 2001		

Health Condition	Benefit—Yes Rating	Benefit—Yes Reference	Benefit—No Rating	Benefit—No Reference
	II	Rompe et al., 1996b		
	II	Furia, 2005a		
	II	Radwan et al., 2008		
	II	Rompe et al., 2001a		
	II	Wang et al., 2002a		
	II	Ilieva et al., 2012		
Strength of evidence: Moderate **Therapeutic effectiveness:** Substantiated				
Achilles tendinopathy	I	Rompe et al., 2007c	I	
	II	Rompe et al., 2008		
	II	Fridman et al., 2008		
	II	Furia, 2006		
	II	Rompe et al., 2009a		
		Rasmussen et al., 2008		
	II	Vulpiani et al., 2007a		
Strength of evidence: Moderate **Therapeutic effectiveness:** Substantiated				
Patellar tendinopathy	II	Zwerver et al., 2010	I	Zwerver et al., 2011
	II	Wang et al., 2007		
	II	Vulpiani et al., 2007b		
	II	Taunton et al., 2003		
	II	Peers et al., 2003		
Strength of evidence: Moderate **Therapeutic effectiveness:** Substantiated				
Chronic heel pain	I	Rompe et al., 1996c		
	II	Chow et al., 2007		
	II	Yalcin et al., 2012		
	II	Moretti et al., 2005b		
	II	Chen et al., 2001		
	II	Hammer et al., 2000		
	II	Cosentino et al., 2001		
Strength of evidence: Moderate **Therapeutic effectiveness:** Substantiated				

Health Condition	Benefit—Yes Rating	Benefit—Yes Reference	Benefit—No Rating	Benefit—No Reference
Nonunion and delayed-union bone fracture	II	Wang et al., 2001a		
	II	Schaden et al., 2001		
	II	Vogel et al., 1997		
	II	Cacchio et al., 2009		
	II	Rompe et al., 2001b		
	II	Elster et al., 2010		
	II	Xu et al., 2009		
		Valchanou et al., 1991		
	III	Schleberger et al., 1992		
Strength of evidence: Moderate **Therapeutic effectiveness:** Substantiated				
Osteonecrosis	I	Wang et al., 2008a		
	II	Wang et al., 2008b		
	II	Wang et al., 2005		
	II	Ludwig et al., 2001		
	III	Lin et al., 2006		
Strength of evidence: Moderate **Therapeutic effectiveness:** Substantiated				
Fewer Than 5 Studies				
Hamstring tendinopathy	II	Cacchio et al., 2011		
Medial tibial stress syndrome	II	Rompe et al., 2010a		
Trochanteric pain syndrome	II	Furia et al., 2009		
	II	Rompe et al., 2009b		
Chronic diabetic foot ulcer	II	Wang et al., 2009		
Bicipital tenosynovitis	I	Liu et al., 2012		
Spasticity	I	Vidal et al., 2011		
Strength of evidence: Pending **Therapeutic effectiveness:** Pending				

ALL CONDITIONS
Strength of evidence: Moderate
Therapeutic effectiveness: Substantiated

V. APPLICATION, CONTRAINDICATIONS, AND RISKS

Prior to considering the application of ESWT, practitioners must first consider the contraindications and risks associated with it and then turn their attention to those key application steps and procedures designed to optimize treatment safety, efficacy, and effectiveness. To further facilitate and visualize the application of therapeutic ESWT, readers are invited to view related **online videos**.

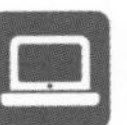

APPLICATION, CONTRAINDICATIONS, AND RISKS

Extracorporeal Shock Wave Therapy

IMPORTANT: Prior to treatment, inform patients that clinical benefits are not immediate and make take several days, and perhaps weeks, before manifesting themselves. In addition, inform patients that immediately after treatment, their conditions may worsen for a few hours or days and then get much better.

See **online videos** for more details.

FOCUSED EXTRACORPOREAL SHOCKWAVE THERAPY

STEP	RATIONALE
1. Check for contraindications.	*Over gas-filled tissues such as lung and intestine*—severe tissue damage *Over uterus*—disrupts fetal development *Over electronic implant*—electronic interference *Blood coagulation therapy*—severe bleeding *Over acute injury*—increases inflammatory process *Over large vessel and nerve*—damage to sensitive tissue *Over epiphyseal plates*—alters normal bone growth
2. Consider the risks.	*Pain, swelling, ecchymosis, and bruising*—repetitive pressure impacts cause local tissue microvascular damages that may trigger one or many of these risks
3. Position and instruct patient.	Ensure comfortable body positioning. Instruct to minimize movement of the treated body segment during therapy. Inform the patient that he or she may feel light to uncomfortable pain and vibration during treatment.
4. Prepare treatment area.	Expose bare skin.
5. Select device type and delivery mode.	Choose between electrohydraulic-, electromagnetic-, and piezoelectric-type f-ESWT devices. f-ESWT is used when the objective is to deliver focused high energy level (higher than 0.29 mJ/mm^2) shock waves to smaller and deeper (depth greater than 5 cm) soft-tissue areas. Note that all three types produce similar shock waves.
6. Select application mode.	• *Image guiding:* Application of f-ESWT may require the use of an in- or off-line image guiding system, mounted on the applicator head, to direct the small focused shockwave beam area over the targeted tissue area. • *Local analgesia:* Because the delivery of high-energy shock waves may be too painful for the patient to bear during therapy, the use of local or intravenous analgesia may be required.

STEP	RATIONALE
7. Select applicator.	There are several applicators with different shapes and attached coupling media to choose from. Select the one that best matches the geometry of the treated area.
8. Prepare f-ESWT device.	Connect the applicator to the extremity of the device's adjustable mechanical arm. Power on the device.
9. Apply coupling medium and position the applicator.	Apply aquasonic gel between the applicator surface and the skin surface to maximize the acoustic transmission. Place the applicator in a way to match the focused shockwave beam with the tissue target area using the imaging system.
10. Set dosimetry.	Use Table 21-2 as a guideline. Because the shockwave beam is focused and delivered at higher energy level, general sedation or localized analgesia may be required depending on the patient's tolerance to pain. Use **Online Dosage Calculator: Extracorporeal Shock Wave Therapy.**
11. Apply treatment.	Ensure adequate monitoring. If the patient moves during f-ESWT, refocusing of the applicator on the targeted treatment area is needed.
12. Conduct post-treatment inspection.	Remove the applicator. Inspect the treated skin area for any side effects, such as skin reddening, light bruising or swelling. Reassure the patient that these are normal side effects that will disappear within a few hours or days.
13. Ensure post-treatment equipment maintenance.	Follow manufacturer recommendations. Immediately report defects or malfunctions to technical maintenance staff.

See **online video** for more details.

RADIAL EXTRACORPOREAL SHOCKWAVE THERAPY

STEP	RATIONALE
1–4.	Repeat steps 1–4 in the f-ESWT section.
5. Select device type and delivery mode.	Select radial mode. All r-ESWT devices are ballistic-type devices. r-ESWT is used when the objective is to deliver divergent (radial) low to medium energy level (less than 0.29 mJ/mm^2) shock waves to larger and more superficial (less than 5 cm for the skin surface) soft-tissue areas.
6. Select application mode.	r-ESWT requires no image guiding system because the shockwave beam of energy propagates from the skin surface down in a radial fashion to cover the targeted tissue area. Instead clinical focusing—that is, the patient's own localization of the painful area to which is applied the impact surface of the handheld pistol-like applicator—is used. Because radial shock waves are delivered at lower energy levels, they are much less painful to bear during therapy, thus requiring no sedation or local analgesia.
7. Select applicator.	All applicators have a pistol-like shape (handpiece). Select the one that best matches the geometry of the treated area.
8. Prepare r-ESWT device.	Connect the handheld applicator, via its cable, to the device. Power the device ON.
9. Apply coupling medium and position the applicator.	Localize the treatment area (most painful area) by palpation based on the patient's feedback (clinical focusing). Mark the skin over the treatment area. Apply aquasonic gel over the area to be treated. Manually apply and hold the applicator surface against the skin overlying the painful area.

STEP	RATIONALE
10. Set dosimetry.	Use Table 21-2 as a guideline. No sedation or local analgesia is required because the shockwave beam propagates in a divergent or radial fashion at lower energy levels. Use **Online Dosage Calculator: Extracorporeal Shock Wave Therapy.**
11. Apply treatment.	Ensure adequate monitoring.
12. Conduct post-treatment inspection.	Remove the applicator. Inspect the treated skin area for any side effects, such as skin reddening, light bruising, or swelling. Reassure the patient that these are normal side effects that will disappear within a few hours or days.
13. Ensure post-treatment equipment maintenance.	Follow manufacturer recommendations. Immediately report defects or malfunctions to technical maintenance staff.

CASE STUDIES

Presented are two case studies summarizing the concepts, principles, and applications of extracorporeal shockwave therapy (ESWT) discussed in this chapter. Case Study 21-1 addresses the use of focused ESWT (f-ESWT) for the management of chronic calcific shoulder tendinitis affecting a middle-aged man. Case Study 21-2 is concerned with the application of radial ESWT (r-ESWT) for chronic plantar fasciitis affecting an elite male marathoner. Each case is structured in line with the concepts of evidence-based practice (EBP), the International Classification of Functioning, Disability, and Health (ICF) disablement model, and SOAP (subjective, *o*bjective, *a*ssessment, *p*lan) note format (see Chapter 2 for details).

CASE STUDY 21-1: CHRONIC CALCIFIC SHOULDER TENDINOSIS

EVIDENCE-BASED CLINICAL DECISION MAKING PROTOCOL

1. Formulate the Case History

A 53-year-old man presents with a chronic recalcitrant calcific right shoulder tendinosis. Recent x-ray examination shows a type II Bosworth calcific deposit located in the supraspinatus muscle. Pain first appeared 9 months ago and has gradually increased since then. It is present at rest, during sleep, and at work. His condition has failed all conventional treatments thus far, including analgesic and anti-inflammatory drugs, rest, and two joint infiltrations. Before considering surgery, his physician refers him for ESWT. The patient is apprehensive about this treatment. He asks for pain sedation during treatment. The patient is right-handed and works as a carpenter. He wants to avoid surgery. He can only work part-time because of his condition.

2. Outline the Case Based on the ICF Framework

CHRONIC CALCIFIC SHOULDER TENDINOSIS		
BODY STRUCTURES AND FUNCTIONS	**ACTIVITIES**	**PARTICIPATION**
Pain	Difficulty with arm movement	Unable to work full-time
Calcium deposit	Difficulty with activities of daily living (ADLs)	

PERSONAL FACTORS	ENVIRONMENTAL FACTORS
Middle-aged man	Home construction
Manual worker	Works with tools
College educated	

3. Outline Therapeutic Goals and Outcome Measurements

GOAL	OUTCOME MEASUREMENT
Decrease pain	Visual Analogue scale (VAS)
Eliminate calcium deposit	X-ray
Improve ability with ADLs and resume full-time work	Constant Murley Scale (CMS)

4. Justify the Use of Extracorporeal Shockwave Therapy Based on the EBP Framework

PRACTITIONER'S EXPERIENCE	RESEARCH-BASED EVIDENCE	PATIENT'S EXPECTATION
Experienced in f-ESWT	*Strength:* Moderate	No opinion on ESWT
Has used f-ESWT in previous cases	*Effectiveness:* Substantiated	Wants to return to full-time work
Believes that f-ESWT can be beneficial		Wants to avoid surgery

5. Outline Key Intervention Parameters

- **Treatment base:** Private clinic
- **ESWT device:** Focused (f-ESWT)—electrohydraulic generator
- **Application protocol:** Follow the suggested application protocol for f-ESWT therapy in *Application, Contraindications, and Risks* box, and make the necessary adjustments for this case. See **online videos**.

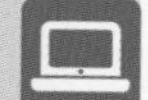

- **Patient's positioning:** Seated with the shoulder abducted at 45 degrees, elbow flexed at 90 degrees, and forearm resting on a flat surface
- **Localization method:** Fluoroscopy to localize calcium deposit
- **Analgesia:** Local—analgesic cream
- **Applicator type:** Cylindrical handpiece
- **Applicator alignment:** In the direction of the calcium deposit
- **Coupling medium:** Aquasonic gel
- **Dosimetry:** See Table 21-2 and below.
- **Number of shocks:** 1,500 per treatment session
- **Shock frequency:** 150/minute
- **Energy flux density (EFD):** 0.32 mJ/mm^2 per treatment
- **Number of treatment sessions:** 2 at 14-day interval
- **Intervention period:** 2 weeks
- **Dose per treatment (D):** 480 mJ/mm^2 per treatment
- **Treatment duration (T):** 10 minutes
- **Total energy dose (TED):** 960 mJ/mm^2 or 0.96 J/mm^2
- **Concomitant therapy:** None
- Use the **Online Dosage Calculator: Extracorporeal Shockwave Therapy**.

6. Report Pre- and Post-Intervention Outcomes

OUTCOME	PRE	POST
VAS score	7/10	1/10
CMS score	65	90
Calcium deposit size	1.2 cm^2	0.2 cm^2
Work status	Part-time	Full-time

7. Document Case Intervention Using the SOAP Note Format

S: Male Pt presents with chronic case of R calcific shoulder tendinosis.

O: *Intervention:* f-ESWT; localization using fluoroscopy; local analgesia; 1,500 shock waves; 150 shock waves/min; EDF: 0.32 mJ/mm^2; dose per treatment: 480 mJ/mm^2; total of 2 treatments; TED: 0.96 J/mm^2. *Pre–post comparison:* Pain decrease VAS 7/10 to 1/10; significant decrease calcium deposit 1.2–0.2 cm^2; CMS score increase from 65 to 90; resume full-time work.

A: Treatment well tolerated. Sign of hematoma, reddening, and swelling after each treatment all spontaneously disappeared within 36 hours. Pt extremely satisfied with the results.

P: No further treatment required. Patient discharged.

CASE STUDY 21-2: CHRONIC PLANTAR FASCIITIS

EVIDENCE-BASED CLINICAL DECISION MAKING PROTOCOL

1. Formulate the Case History

A 25-year-old elite male marathoner presents with a chronic right plantar fasciitis now lasting for approximately 10 months. Despite numerous conservative treatments, including insoles and numerous shoe changes, the condition is still present. Pain increases with millage. This runner is getting more and frustrated as he prepares to compete in the next world championship. Surfing the Internet, he discovers that ESWT might be beneficial. After discussing this treatment approach with the medical and training staff, he agrees to it. He refuses to undergo surgery.

2. Outline the Case Based on the IFC Framework

CHRONIC PLANTAR FASCIITIS		
BODY STRUCTURES AND FUNCTIONS	**ACTIVITIES**	**PARTICIPATION**
Pain at rest	Difficulty to run	Unable to engage in full training
Morning pain (first steps)		

PERSONAL FACTORS	ENVIRONMENTAL FACTORS
Young man	Running
Elite athlete	Performance and competition

3. Outline Therapeutic Goals and Outcome Measurements

GOAL	OUTCOME MEASUREMENT
Decrease pain	101-point Numerical Rating Scale (NRS-100)
Performance	Training log

4. Justify the Use of Extracorporeal Shockwave Therapy Based on the EBP Framework

PRACTITIONER'S EXPERIENCE	RESEARCH-BASED EVIDENCE	PATIENT'S EXPECTATION
Experienced in ESWT	*Strength:* Moderate *Effectiveness:* Substantiated	Believes that ESWT will be beneficial
Has used ESWT in similar cases		
Believes that ESWT will be beneficial		

5. Outline Key Intervention Parameters

- **Treatment base:** Sports clinic
- **ESWT device:** Radial (r-ESWT)—ballistic generator
- **Application protocol:** Follow the suggested application protocol for r-ESWT therapy in *Application, Contraindications, and Risks* box, and make the necessary adjustments for this case. See **online video**.
- **Patient's positioning:** Lying prone with feet hanging free on the edge of table
- **Localization method:** Palpation—feedback from patient
- **Analgesia:** None
- **Applicator type:** Handheld pistol like
- **Applicator alignment:** Over most tender area of fascia
- **Coupling medium:** Aquasonic gel
- **Dosimetry:** See Table 21-2 and below.
- **Number of shocks:** 2,000 per treatment
- **Shock frequency:** 200/minute
- **Energy flux density (EFD):** 0.12 mJ/mm^2 per treatment
- **Number of treatment sessions:** 3 at 1-week intervals
- **Intervention period:** 3 weeks
- **Dose per treatment (D):** 240 mJ/mm^2 per treatment
- **Treatment duration (T):** 10 minutes
- **Total energy dose (TED):** 720 mJ/mm^2 or 0.72 J/mm^2
- **Concomitant therapy:** None
- Use the **Online Dosage Calculator: Extracorporeal Shockwave Therapy**.

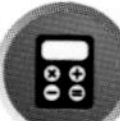

6. Report Pre- and Post-Intervention Outcomes

OUTCOME	PRE	POST
Pain (NRS-101)	85/100	20/100
Running performance		Distance—increase by 25% Able to run 42 km (26 miles)

7. Document Case Intervention Using the SOAP Note Format

S: Elite male runner presents with R chronic plantar fasciitis causing difficulty with training and performance.

O: *Intervention:* r-ESWT; localization by palpation; 2,000 shock waves; 200 shock waves/min; EDF: 0.12 mJ/mm^2; dose per treatment: 240 mJ/mm^2; total of 3 treatments at 1-week intervals; TED: 0.72 J/mm^2. *Pre–post comparison:* Pain decrease in NRS-101 score from 85 to 20; increase performance level by 25% leading to full marathon distance.

A: Treatment shows important benefit. No adverse effect. Treatment well tolerated. Patient extremely satisfied. More than happy to avoid surgery.

P: No more treatment required. Pt discharged.

VI. THE BOTTOM LINE

- ESWT is the external application of shock waves to soft tissues for the purpose of promoting tissue repair and healing.
- Shock waves are high-amplitude sound waves that propagate in tissue with a sudden rise from ambient pressure to maximum compressive pressure (P+) followed by a lower tensile pressure (P–).
- A shock wave is a pressure or acoustic wave characterized by high pressure (P) and short rise time (RT) and pulse duration (PD).
- There are two types of shock waves: focused (f-ESWT) and radial (r-ESWT).
- Focused shock waves are created using three types of generators: electrohydraulic, electromagnetic, and piezoelectric. All three have in common that the waves are generated in water (inside the applicator) because the acoustic impedance of water and biologic tissues are comparable.
- Radial shock waves are created using a ballistic generator—that is, using compressed air to drive and accelerate a projectile.
- The proposed biologic and therapeutic effects of ESWT are to create fresh micro-injuries to stimulate revascularization, thus promoting soft-tissue repair.
- Localization of the treatment site or target tissue is determined by means of palpation (r-ESWT) or by using computerized imaging techniques (f-ESWT).
- The use of local analgesia over the treated area during therapy should be avoided because there is evidence to show that it may decrease treatment effectiveness.
- Main complications associated with ESWT are local reddening, ecchymosis, and mild hematoma that spontaneously recover.
- ESWT appears as a viable and useful alternative therapy to surgery for the management of chronic soft-tissue conditions.
- r-ESWT is a better choice than f-ESWT because it is more affordable and easier to administer.

- The research-based evidence presented in this chapter supports the use of ESWT for chronic soft-tissue conditions, particularly for tendinopathies and delayed bone union.
- When used to treat tendinopathy, it is best to apply ESWT in the latter stages of healing.
- ESWT is a noninvasive therapeutic intervention that has the potential of replacing surgery for the management of many chronic soft tissue disorders.

VII. CRITICAL THINKING QUESTIONS

Clarification: What is meant by extracorporeal shockwave therapy (ESWT)?

Assumptions: Many of your colleagues assume that there is no difference between a focused versus a radial shock wave. How can you approve or disprove this assumption?

Reasons and evidence: Your colleague argues that using ESWT to treat chronic soft-tissue disorders makes no sense because of the higher risk of causing pain, ecchymosis, or hematoma following treatment. How can you rebut this argument?

Viewpoints or perspectives: How will you respond to a colleague who says that there is no similarity between ESWT and surgery for the management of chronic soft-tissue disorders?

Implications and consequences: What are the implications and consequences of not quantifying dosimetry—that is, to know the amount of mechanical energy delivered to the target tissue?

About the question: What are the main differences between focused and radial ESWT? Why do you think I ask this question?

VIII. REFERENCES

Articles

Albert JD, Meadeb J, Guggenbuhl P, Marin F, Benkalfate T, Thomazeau H (2007) High-energy extracorporeal shock-wave therapy for calcifying tendinitis of the rotator cuff: A randomized trial. J Bone Joint Surg (B), 89: 335–341

Avancini-Dobrovic V, Frlan-Vrgoc L, Stamenkovic D, Pavlovic I, Vrbanic TS (2011) Radial extracorporeal shock wave therapy in the treatment of shoulder calcific tendinitis. Coll Antropol, 35: 221–225

Buchbinder R, Ptasznik R, Gordon J, Buchanan J, Prabaharan V, Forbes A (2002) Ultrasound-guided extracorporeal shock wave therapy for plantar fasciitis: A randomized controlled trial. JAMA, 288: 1364–1372

Cacchio A, Giordano L, Colafarina O, Rompe JD, Travernese E, Lopolo F, Flamini S, Spacca G, Santili V (2009) Extracorporeal shock-wave therapy compared with surgery for hypertrophic long-bone nonunions. J Bone Joint Surg (A), 91: 2589–2597

Cacchio A, Paoloni M, Barile A, Don R, de Paulis F, Cjalvisi V (2006) Effectiveness of radial shock-wave therapy for calcific tendinitis of the shoulder: Single-blind, randomized clinical trial. Phys Ther, 86: 672–682

Cacchio A, Rompe JD, Furia JP, Susi P, Santilli V, De Paulis F (2011) Shockwave for the treatment of chronic proximal hamstring tendinopathy in professional athletes. Am J Sports Med, 39: 146–153

Chen HS, Chen LM, Huang TW (2001) Treatment of painful heel syndrome with shock waves. Clin Orthop Rel Res, 387: 41–46

Chow IH, Cheing GL (2007) Comparison of different energy densities of extracorporeal shock wave therapy (ESWT) for the management of chronic heel pain. Clin Rehabil, 21: 131–141

Chuckpaiwong B, Berkson EM, Theodore GH (2009) Extracorporeal shock wave for chronic proximal plantar fasciitis: 225 patients with results and outcome predictors. J Foot Ankle Surg, 28: 148–155

Chung B, Wiley JP (2004) Effectiveness of extracorporeal shock wave therapy in the treatment of previously untreated lateral epicondylitis: A randomized controlled trial. Am J Sports Med, 32: 1660–1667

Chung B, Wiley JP, Rose MS (2005) Long-term effectiveness of extracorporeal shockwave therapy in the treatment of previously untreated lateral epicondylitis. Clin J Sports Med, 15: 305–312

Cleveland RO, Chitnis PV, McClure SR (2007) Acoustic field of ballistic shock wave therapy device. Ultrasound Mol Biol, 33: 1327–1335

Cosentino R, De Stefano R, Selvi E, Frati E, Manca S, Frediani B, Marcolongo R (2003) Extracorporeal shock wave therapy for chronic calcific tendinitis of the shoulder: Single blind study. Ann Rheum Dis, 62: 248–250

Cosentino R, Falsetti P, Manca S (2001) Efficacy of extracorporeal shock wave treatment in calcaneal enthesophytosis. Ann Rheum Dis, 60: 1064–1067

Crowther MA, Bannister GC, Huma H, Rooker GP (2002) A prospective randomized study to compare extracorporeal shock wave therapy and injection of steroid for the treatment of tennis elbow. J Bone Joint Surg (B), 84: 678–679

Daecke W, Kusnierczak D, Loew M (2002) Long-term effects of extracorporeal shock wave therapy in chronic calcific tendinitis of the shoulder. J Shoulder Elbow Surg, 11: 476–480

Dorotka R, Sabeti M, Jimenez-Boj E, Goll A, Schubert S, Trieb K (2006) Location modalities for focused extracorporeal shock wave application in the treatment of chronic plantar fasciitis. Foot Ankle Int, 27: 943–947

Elster EA, Stojadinovic A, Forsberg J, Shawen S, Andersen RC, Schaden W (2010) Extracorporeal shock wave therapy for nonunion of the tibia. J Orthop Trauma, 24: 133–141

Engebretsen K, Grotel M, Bautz-Holter E, Ekeberg OM, Juel NG, Brox JI (2011) Supervised exercises compared with extracorporeal shock-wave therapy for subacromial shoulder pain: 1-year results of a single-blind randomized controlled trial. Phys Ther, 91: 37–47

Fridman R, Cain J, Weil L, Well L (2008) Extracorporeal shockwave therapy for the treatment of Achilles tendinopathies: A prospective study. J Am Podiatr Med Assoc, 98: 466–468

Furia JP (2005a) Safety and efficacy of extracorporeal shock wave therapy for chronic lateral epicondylitis. Am J Orthop, 34: 13–19

Furia JP (2005b) The safety and efficacy of high energy extracorporeal shock wave therapy in active, moderately active, and sedentary patients with chronic plantar fasciitis. Orthopedics, 28: 685–692

Furia JP (2006) High energy extracorporeal shock wave therapy as treatment for insertional Achilles tendinopathy. Am J Sports Med, 34: 733–740

Furia JP, Rompe JD, Maffulli N (2009) Low-energy extracorporeal shock wave therapy as a treatment for greater trochanteric pain syndrome. Am J Sports Med, 37: 1806–1813

Gerdesmeyer L, Wagenpfeil S, Haake M, Maier M, Loew M, Wortler K, Lampe R, Seil R, Handle G, Gassel S, Rompe JD (2003) Extracorporeal shock wave therapy for the treatment of chronic calcifying tendonitis of the rotator cuff: A randomized controlled trial. JAMA, 290: 2573–2580

Haake M, Buch M, Schoellner, Goebel F, Vogel M, Mueller I, Hausdorf J, Zamzow I, Schade-Brittinger C, Mueller HH (2003) Extracorporeal shock wave therapy for plantar fasciitis: A randomized controlled multicenter trial. BMJ, 327: 75–80

Haake M, Deike B, Thon A, Schmitt J (2002b) Exact focusing of extracorporeal shock wave therapy for calcifying tendinopathy. Clin Orthop, 397: 323–331

Haake M, Konig IR, Decker T, Riedel C, Buch M, Muller HH (2002c) Extracorporeal shock wave therapy in the treatment of lateral epicondylitis: A randomized multicenter trial. J Bone Joint Surg (A), 84: 1982–1991

Hammer D, Adam F, Kreutz A, Kohn D, Seil R (2003) Extracorporeal shock wave therapy (ESWT) in patients with chronic proximal plantar fasciitis: A 2-year follow-up. Foot Ankle Int, 24: 823–828

Hammer D, Adam F, Kreutz A, Rupp S, Kohn D, Seil R (2005) Ultrasonic evaluation at 6-month follow-up of plantar fasciitis after extracorporeal shock wave therapy. Arch Orthop Trauma Surg, 125: 6–9

Hammer D, Rupp S, Kreutz A, Pape D, Kohn D, Seil R (2002) Extracorporeal shock wave therapy (ESWT) in patients with chronic proximal plantar fasciitis. Foot Ankle Int, 23: 309–313

Hammer DS, Rupp S, Ensslin S, Kohn D, Seil R (2000) Extracorporeal shock wave therapy in patients with tennis elbow and painful heel. Arch Orthop Trauma Surg, 120: 304–307

Hearnden A, Desai A, Karmegan A, Flannery M (2009) Extracorporeal shock wave therapy in chronic calcific tendinitis of the shoulder—is it effective? Acta Orthop Belg, 75: 25–31

Hsu CJ, Wang DY, Tseng KF, Fong YC, Hsu HC, Jim YF (2008) Extracorporeal shock wave therapy for calcifying tendinitis of the shoulder. J Shoulder Elbow Surg, 17: 55–59

Hyer CF, Vancourt B, Block A (2005) Evaluation of ultrasound-guided extracorporeal shock wave therapy (ESWT) in the treatment of chronic plantar fasciitis. J Foot Ankle Surg, 44: 137–143

Ibrahim MI, Donatelli RA, Schmitz C, Hellman MA, Buxbaum F (2010) Chronic plantar fasciitis treated with two sessions of radial extracorporeal shock wave therapy. Foot Ankle Int, 31: 391–397

Ilieva EM, Minchev RM, Petrova NS (2012) Radial shock wave therapy in patients with lateral epicondylitis. Folia Med, 54: 35–41

Klonschinski T, Ament SJ, Schlereth T, Rompe JD, Birklein F (2011) Application of local anesthesia inhibits effects of low-energy extracorporeal shock wave treatment (ESWT) on nociceptors. Pain Med, 12: 1532–1537

Ko JY, Chen HS, Chen LM (2001) Treatment of lateral epicondylitis of the elbow with shock waves. Clin Orthop Rel Res, 387: 60–67

Krasny C, Enenkel M, Aigner N, Wlk M, Landsiedl F (2005) Ultrasound-guided needling combined with shock wave therapy for the treatment of calcifying tendonitis of the shoulder. J Bone Joint Surg (B), 87: 501–507

Krischek O, Hopf C, Nafe B, Rompe JD (1999) Shock wave therapy for tennis and golfer's elbow: 1 year follow-up. Arch Orthop Trauma Surg, 119: 62–66

Kudo P, Dainty K, Clarfield M, Coughlin L, Lavoie P, Lebrun C (2006) Randomized, placebo-controlled, double-blind clinical trial evaluating the treatment of plantar fasciitis with an extracorporeal shock wave therapy (ESWT) device: A North American confirmatory study. J Orthop Res, 25: 115–123

Lebrun CM (2005) Low-dose extracorporeal shock wave therapy for previously untreated lateral epicondylitis. Clin J Sports Med, 15: 401–402

Lin PC, Wang CJ, Yang KD, Wang FS, Ko JY, Huang CC (2006) Extracorporeal shockwave treatment of osteonecrosis of the femoral head in systemic lupus erythematosis. J Arthroplasty, 21: 911–915

Liu S, Zhai L, Shi, Z, Jing R, Zhao B, Xing G (2012) Radial extracorporeal pressure pulse therapy for the primary long bicipital tenosynovitis: A prospective randomized controlled study. Ultrasound Med Biol, 38: 727–735

Loew M, Daecke W, Kusnierczak D, Rahmanzadeh M, Ewerbeck V (1999) Shock wave therapy is effective for chronic calcifying tendinitis of the shoulder. J Bone Joint Surg (B), 81: 863–867

Loew M, Jurgowski W, Mau HC (1995) Treatment of calcifying tendinitis of rotator cuff by extracorporeal shock waves: A preliminary report. J Shoulder Elbow Surg, 4: 101–106

Ludwig J, Lauber S, Lauber HJ, Dreisilker U, Raedel R, Hotzinger H (2001) High-energy shock wave treatment of femoral head necrosis in adults. Clin Orthop Relat Res, 387: 119–126

Malay DS, Pressman MM, Assili A (2006) Extracorporeal shockwave therapy versus placebo for the treatment of chronic proximal plantar fasciitis: Results of a randomized, placebo-controlled, double-blinded, multicenter intervention trial. J Foot Ankle Surg, 45: 196–201

Mangone G, Vella A, Postiglione M, Viliani T, Pasquetti P (2010) Radial extracorporeal shock-wave therapy in rotator cuff calcific tendinosis. Clin Cases Min Bone Metabol, 7: 91–96

Marks W, Jackiewicz A, Witkowski Z, Kot J, Deja W, Lasek J (2008) Extracorporeal shock-wave therapy with a new-generation pneumatic device in the treatment of heel pain. A double blind randomized controlled trial. Acta Orthop Belg, 74: 98–101

Melegati G, Tornese D, Bandi M (2000) Effectiveness of extracorporeal shock wave therapy associated with kinesitherapy in the treatment of subacromial impingement: A randomized, controlled study. J Sports Traumatol Rel Res, 22: 58–64

Melegati G, Tornese D, Bandi M, Rubini M (2004) Comparison of two ultrasonographic localization techniques for the treatment of lateral epicondylitis with extracorporeal shock wave therapy: A randomized study. Clin Rehabil, 18: 366–370

Melikyan EY, Shahin E, Miles J (2003) Extracorporeal shock wave treatment for tennis elbow. A randomized double-blind study. J Bone Joint Surg (B), 85: 852–855

Moretti B, Garofalo R, Genco S, Patella V, Moushsine E (2005a) Medium-energy shock wave therapy in the treatment of rotator cuff calcifying tendonitis. Knee Surg Sports Traumatol Arthrosc, 13: 405–410

Moretti B, Garofalo R, Patella V, Sisti GL, Corrado M, Mouhsine E (2005b) Extracorporeal shock wave therapy in runners with a symptomatic heel spur. Knee Surg Sports Traumatol Arthrosc, 14: 1–4

Ogden JA, Alvarez R, Levitt R, Cross GL, Marlow M (2001a) Shock wave therapy for chronic proximal plantar fasciitis. Clin Orthop Rel Res, 387: 47–59

Ogden JA, Alvarez R, Levitt R, Johnson JE, Marlow ME (2004) Electrohydraulic high-energy shock-wave treatment for chronic plantar fasciitis. J Bone Joint Surg (A), 86: 2216–2228

Ogden JA, Toth-Kischkat A, Schultheiss R (2001b) Principles of shock wave therapy. Clin Orthop Rel Res, 387: 8–17

Pan PJ, Chou CL, Chiou HJ, Ma HL, Lee HC, Chan RC (2003) Extracorporeal shock wave therapy for chronic calcific tendinitis of the shoulders: A functional and sonographic study. Arch Phys Med Rehabil, 84: 988–993

Peers KH, Lysens R, Brys P, Bellemans J (2003) Cross-sectional outcome analysis of athletes with chronic patellar tendinopathy treated surgically and by extracorporeal shock wave therapy. Clin J Sport Med, 13: 79–83

Perlick L, Luring C, Bathis H, Perlick C, Kraft C, Diedrich O (2003) Efficacy of extracorporeal shock wave treatment for calcific tendinitis of the shoulder: Experimental and clinical results. J Orthop Sci, 8: 777–783

Peters J, Luboldt W, Schwarz W, Jacob V, Herzog C, Vogl TJ (2004) Extracorporeal shock wave therapy in calcific tendinitis of the shoulder. Skeletal Radiol, 33: 712–718

Pettrone FA, McCall BR (2005) Extracorporeal shock wave therapy without local anesthesia for chronic lateral epicondylitis. J Bone Joint Surg (A), 87: 1297–1304

Pigozzi F, Giombini A, Parisi A, Casciello G, Di Salvo V, Santori N, Mariani PP (2000) The application of shock waves therapy in the treatment of resistant chronic painful shoulder. A clinical experience. J Sports Med Phys Fit, 40: 356–361

Porter MD, Shadbolt B (2005) Intralesional corticosteroid injection versus extracorporeal shock wave therapy for plantar fasciopathy. Clin J Sport Med, 15: 119–124

Radwan YA, Elsobi G, Badawy W, Reda A, Khalid S (2008) Resistant tennis elbow: Shock-wave therapy versus percutaneous tenotomy. Int Orthop, 32: 671–677

Rasmussen S, Christensen M, Mathieson I, Simonsen O (2008) Shock-wave therapy for chronic Achilles tendinopathy: A double-blind, randomized clinical trial of efficacy. Acta Orthop, 79: 249–256

Rompe JD, Burger R, Hopf C, Eysel P (1998) Shoulder function after extracorporeal shock wave therapy for calcific tendonitis. J Shoulder Elbow Surg, 7: 505–509

Rompe JD, Cacchio A, Furia JP, Maffulli N (2010a) Low-energy extracorporeal shock wave therapy as a treatment for medial tibial stress syndrome. Am J Sports Med, 38: 125–132

Rompe JD, Cacchio A, Weil L, Furia JP, Haist J, Reiners V, Schnitz C, Maffulli N (2010b) Plantar fascia-specific stretching versus shock-wave therapy as initial treatment of plantar fasciopathy. J Bone Joint Surg (A), 92: 2514–2522

Rompe JD, Decking J, Schoellner C, Nafe B (2003) Shock waves application for chronic plantar fasciitis in running athletes. A prospective, randomized, placebo-controlled trial. Am J Sports Med, 31: 268–275

Rompe JD, Decking J, Schoellner C, Theis C (2004) Repetitive low-energy shock wave treatment for chronic lateral epicondylitis in tennis players. Am J Sports Med, 32: 734–743

Rompe JD, Furia J, Maffulli N (2008) Eccentric loading compared with shock wave treatment for chronic insertional Achilles tendinopathy. J Bone Joint Surg (A), 90: 52–61

Rompe JD, Furia JP, Maffulli N (2009a) Eccentric loading versus eccentric loading plus shockwave treatment for midportion Achilles tendinopathy: A randomized controlled trial. Am J Sports Med, 37: 463–470

Rompe JD, Hopf C, Kullmer K, Heine J, Burger R (1996a) Analgesic effect of extracorporeal shock wave therapy on chronic tennis elbow. J Bone Joint Surg (B), 78: 233–237

Rompe JD, Hopf C, Kullmer K, Heine J, Burger R, Nafe B (1996b) Low-energy extracorporeal shock wave therapy for persistent tennis elbow. Int Orthop, 20: 23–27

Rompe JD, Hopf C, Nafe B, Burger R (1996c) Low-energy extracorporeal shock wave therapy for painful heel: A prospective controlled single-blind study. Arch Orthop Trauma Surg, 115: 75–79

Rompe JD, Meurer A, Nafe B, Hofmann A, Gerdesmeyer L (2005) Repetitive low-energy shock wave application without local anesthesia is more efficient than repetitive low-energy shock wave application with local anesthesia in the treatment of chronic plantar fasciitis. J Orthop Res, 23: 931–941

Rompe JD, Nafe B, Furia J, Maffulli N (2007) Eccentric loading, shockwave treatment or a wait-and-see policy for tendinopathy of the main body of the tendo Achilles: A randomized controlled trial. Am J Sports Med, 35: 374–383

Rompe JD, Riedel C, Betz U, Fink C (2001a) Chronic lateral epicondylitis of the elbow: A prospective study of low-energy shock wave therapy and low-energy shock wave therapy plus manual therapy of the cervical spine. Arch Phys Med Rehabil, 82: 578–582

Rompe JD, Rosendahl T, Schollner C, Theis C (2001b) High-energy extracorporeal shock wave treatment of nonunions. Clin Orthop Rel Res, 387: 102–111

Rompe JD, Rumler F, Hopf C, Nafe B, Heine J (1995) Extracorporeal shock wave therapy for calcifying tendonitis of the shoulder. Clin Orthop Rel Res, 321: 196–201

Rompe J, Schoellner C, Nafe B (2002) Evaluation of low-energy extracorporeal shock wave application for treatment of chronic plantar fasciitis. J Bone Joint Surg (A), 84: 335–341

Rompe JD, Segal NA, Cacchio A, Furia JP, Morral A, Maffulli N (2009b) Home training, local corticosteroid injection, or radial shock wave therapy for greater trochanter pain syndrome. Am J Sports Med, 37: 1981–1990

Rompe JD, Zoellner J, Nafe B (2001c) Shock wave therapy versus conventional surgery in the treatment of calcifying tendinitis of the shoulder. Clin Orthop Rel Res, 387: 72–82

Sabeti-Aschraf M, Dorotka R, Goll A, Trieb K (2005) Extracorporeal shock wave therapy in the treatment of calcific tendonitis of the rotator cuff. Am J Sports Med, 33: 1365–1368

Schaden W, Fischer A, Sailler A (2001) Extracorporeal shock wave therapy of nonunion or delayed osseous union. Clin Orthop Rel Res, 387: 90–94

Schleberger R, Senge TH (1992) Noninvasive treatment of long-bone pseudoarthrosis by shock wave (ESWT). Arch Orthop Trauma Surg, 111: 224–227

Schofer MD, Hinrichs F, Peterlein CD, Arendt M, Schmitt J (2009) High- versus low-energy extracorporeal shock wave therapy of rotator cuff tendinopathy: A prospective, randomised, controlled study. Acta Orthop Belg, 75: 452–458

Schmitt J, Haake M, Tosch A, Hildebrand R, Deike B, Griss P (2001) Low-energy extracorporeal shock-wave treatment (ESWT) for tendinitis of the supraspinatus. A prospective, randomised study. J Bone Joint Surg (B), 83: 873–876

Spacca G, Necozione S, Cacchio A (2005) Radial shock wave therapy for lateral epicondylitis: A prospective randomised controlled single-blind study. Eura Medicophys, 41: 17–25

Speed CA, Nichols D, Richards C, Humphreys H, Wies JT, Burnet S, Hazleman BL (2002a) Extracorporeal shock wave therapy for lateral epicondylitis—a double blind randomized controlled trial. J Orthop Res, 20: 895–898

Speed CA, Nichols D, Wies J, Humphreys H, Richards C, Burnet S, Hazleman BL (2003) Extracorporeal shock wave therapy for plantar fasciitis: A double-blind randomized controlled trial. J Orthop Res, 21: 937–940

Speed CA, Richards C, Nichols D, Burnet S, Wies JT, Humphreys H, Hazleman BL (2002b) Extracorporeal shock wave therapy for tendonitis of the rotator cuff: A double-blind, randomized, controlled trial. J Bone Joint Surg (B), 84: 509–512

Spindler A, Berman A, Lucero E, Braier M (1998) Extracorporeal shock wave treatment for chronic calcific tendinitis of the shoulder. J Rheumatol, 25: 1161–1163

Taunton KM, Taunton JE, Khan KM (2003) Treatment of patellar tendinopathy with extracorporeal shock wave therapy. BCMJ, 45: 500–507

Theodore GH, Buch M, Amendola A, Bachmann C, Fleming LL, Zingas C (2004) Extracorporeal shock wave therapy for the treatment of plantar fasciitis. Foot Ankle Int, 25: 290–297

Valchanou VD, Michailov P (1991) High energy shock waves in the treatment of delayed and nonunion of fractures. Int Orthop, 15: 181–184

Vidal X, Norral A, Costa L, Tur M (2011) Radial extracorporeal shock wave therapy (rESWT) in the treatment of spasticity in cerebral palsy: A randomized, placebo-controlled clinical trial. NeuroRehabilitation, 29: 413–419

Vogel J, Hopf C, Eysel P (1997) Application of extracorporeal shock waves in the treatment of pseudoarthrosis of lower extremity. Preliminary results. Arch Orthop Trauma Surg, 116: 480–483

Vulpiani MC, Trischitta D, Trovato P, Vetrano M, Ferretti A (2007a) Extracorporeal shockwave therapy (ECSWT) in Achilles tendinopathy. A long-term follow-up observational study. J Sports Med Phys Fit, 49: 171–176

Vulpiani MC, Vetrano M, Savoia W (2007b) Jumper's knee treatment with extracorporeal shock wave therapy: A long-term follow-up observational study. J Sports Med Phys Fit, 47: 323–328

Wang CJ, Chen HS (2002a) Shock wave therapy for patients with lateral epicondylitis of the elbow: A one-to two-year follow-up study. Am J Sports Med, 30: 422–425

Wang CJ, Chen HS, Chen, CE, Yang KD (2001a) Treatment of nonunions of long bone fractures with shock waves. Clin Ortho Rel Res, 387: 95–101

Wang CJ, Chen HS, Huang TW (2002b) Shock wave therapy for patients with plantar fasciitis: A one-year follow-up study. Foot Ankle Int, 23: 204–207

Wang CJ, Ko JY, Chan YS, Weng LH, Hsu SL (2007). Extracorporeal shock-wave for chronic patellar tendinopathy. Am J Sports Med, 35: 972–978

Wang CJ, Ko JY, Chen HS (2001b) Treatment of calcifying tendinitis of the shoulder with shock wave therapy. Clin Orthop, 387: 83–89

Wang CJ, Kuo YR, Wu RW, Liu RT, Hsu CS, Wang FS, Yang KD (2009) Extracorporeal shockwave treatment for chronic diabetic foot ulcers. J Surg Res, 152: 96–103

Wang CJ, Wang FS, Huang CC, Yang KD, Weng LH, Huang HY (2005) Treatment of osteonecrosis of the femoral head: Comparison of extracorporeal shock waves with core decompression and bone-grafting. J Bone Joint Surg (A), 87: 2380–2387

Wang CJ, Wang FS, Ko JY, Huang HY, Chen CJ, Sun YC (2008a) Extracorporeal shockwave therapy shows regeneration in hip necrosis. Rheumatology, 47:542–546

Wang CJ, Wang FS, Yang KD, Huang CC, Lee MS, Chan YS (2008b) Treatment of osteonecrosis of the hip: Comparison of extracorporeal shockwave with shockwave and alendronate. Arch Orthop Trauma Surg, 128: 901–908

Wang CJ, Yang KD, Wang FS, Chen HH, Wang JW (2003) Shock wave therapy for calcific tendinitis of the shoulder: A prospective clinical study with two-year follow-up. Am J Sports Med, 31: 425–430

Xu ZH, Jiang Q, Chen DY (2009) Extracorporeal shock wave treatment in nonunions of long bone fractures. Int Orthop, 33: 789–793

Yalcin E, Akca AK, Selcuk B, Kurtaran A, Akyuz M (2012) Effects of extracorporeal shock wave therapy on symptomatic heel spurs: A correlation between clinical outcome and radiographic changes. Rheumatol Int, 32: 343–347

Zwerver J, Dekker F, Pepping GL (2010) Patient guided Piezo-electric Extracorporeal Shockwave Therapy as treatment for chronic severe tendinopathy: A pilot study. J Back Musculoskelet Rehabil, 23: 111–115

Zwerver J, Hartgens F, Verhagen E, van der Worp H, van den Akker-Scheek I, Diercks RL (2011) No effect of extracorporeal shockwave therapy on patellar tendinopathy in jumping athletes during the competitive season: A randomized clinical trial. Am J Sports Med, 39: 1191–1199

Review Articles

Al-Abbad H, Simon JV (2013) The effectiveness of extracorporeal shock wave therapy on chronic Achilles tendinopathy: A systematic review. Foot Ankle Int, 34: 33–41

Foldager CB, Kearney C, Spactor M (2012) Clinical application of extracorporeal shock wave therapy in orthopedics: Focused versus unfocused shock waves. Ultrasound Med Biol, 38: 1673–1680

Van der Worp H, van der Akker-Scheek, van Schie H, Zwerver J (2012) ESWT for tendinopathy: Technology and clinical implications. Knee Surg Sports Traumatol Arthrosc, 21: 1451–1458

Zelle BA, Gollwitzer H, Zlowodski M, Buhren V (2010) Extracorporeal shock wave therapy: Current evidence. J Orthop Trauma, 24: S66–S70

Chapters of Textbooks

Gerdesmeyer L, Henne M, Gobel M, Diehl P (2007a) Physical principles and generation of shockwaves. In: Extracorporeal Shockwave Therapy. Clinical Results, Technologies, Basics. Gerdermeyer L, Weil LS (Eds). Data Trace Publishing, Towson, 11–20

Haake M, Gerdesmeyer L (2007) History of extracorporeal shockwave therapy. In: Extracorporeal Shockwave Therapy. Clinical Results, Technologies, Basics. Gerdermeyer L, Weil LS (Eds). Data Trace Publishing, Towson, 1–9

Maier M, Tischer T, Gerdesmeyer L (2005) Physical-technical principles of ESWT. In: Therapeutic Energy Applications in Urology. Chaussy C, Haupt G, Jocham D, Kohrmann KU, Wilbert D (Eds). Thieme, Stuttgart, 144–153

Novak P (2011) Physical basics. In: Shock Wave Therapy in Practice: Myofascial Syndromes & Trigger Points. Gleitz M (Ed). Level 10, Heilbroon, 17–33

Textbooks

Gerdesmeyer L, Weil LS (2007b) Extracorporeal Shockwave Therapy: Clinical Results, Technologies, Basics. Data Trace Publishing, Towson

Gleitz M (2011) Shock Wave Therapy in Practice: Myofascial Syndromes & Trigger Points. Gleitz M (Ed). Level 10, Heilbroon

Rompe JD (2002) Shock Wave Applications in Musculoskeletal Disorders. Thieme, Stuttgart

Internet Resources

www.ismst.com: International Society for Medical Shockwave Treatment (ISMST)

http://thePoint.lww.com: Online Dosage Calculator: Extracorporeal Shockwave Therapy

Suggested Review Articles

Alves EM, Angrisani AT, Santiago MB (2009) The use of extracorporeal shock waves in the treatment of osteonecrosis of the femoral head: A systematic review. Clin Rheumatol, 28: 1247–1251

Chang KV, Chen AY, Chen WS, Tu YK, Chien KL (2012) Comparative effectiveness of focused shock wave therapy of different intensity levels and radial shock wave therapy for treating plantar fasciitis: A systematic review and network meta-analysis. Arch Phys Med Rehabil, 93: 1259–1268

Huisstede BM, Gebremariam L, van der Sande R, Hay EM, Koes BW (2011) Evidence for effectiveness of Extracorporal Shock-Wave Therapy (ESWT) to treat calcific and non-calcific rotator cuff tendinosis—a systematic review. Man Ther, 16: 419–433

Lee SY, Chen B, Grimmer-Somers K (2011) The midterm effectiveness of extracorporeal shockwave therapy in the management of chronic calcific shoulder tendinitis. J Shoulder Elbow Surg, 20: 845–854

Lin TC, Lin CY, Chou CL, Chiu CM (2012) Achilles tendon tear following shock wave therapy for calcific tendinopathy of the Achilles tendon: A case report. Phys Ther Sport, 13: 189–192

Mouzopoulos G, Stamatakos M, Mouzopoulos D, Tzurbakis M (2007) Extracorporeal shock wave treatment for calcific tendinitis: A systematic review. Skelet Radiol, 36: 803–811

Schmitt C, Depace R, (2009) Pain relief by extracorporeal shockwave therapy: An update on the current understanding. Urol Res, 37: 231–234

Seco J, Kovacs FM, Urrutia G (2011) The efficacy, safety, effectiveness, and cost-effective of ultrasound and shock wave therapies for low back pain: A systematic review. Spine J, 11: 966–977

Van Leeuwen MT, Zwerver J, van den Akker-scheek I (2009) Extracorporeal shockwave therapy for patellar tendinopathy: A review of the literature. Br J Sports Med, 43: 163–168

Wang CJ (2012) Extracorporeal shockwave therapy in musculoskeletal disorders. J Orthop Surg Res, 7: 11

INDEX

Note: Page number followed by f, t and b indicate figure, table and box respectively.